Estimated Safe and Adequate Daily Dietary Intakes of Additional Selected Vitamins and Minerals*

	Vitamins			Trace Elements†						Electrolytes		
Age (years)	Vitamin K (μg)	Biotin (μg)	Panto-thenic Acid (mg)	Copper (mg)	Man-ganese (mg)	Fluoride (mg)	Chro-mium (mg)	Sele-nium (mg)	Molyb-denum (mg)	Sodium (mg)	Potas-sium (mg)	Chloride (mg)
INFANTS												
0-0.5	12	35	2	0.5-0.7	0.5-0.7	0.1-0.5	0.01-0.04	0.01-0.04	0.03-0.06	115-350	350-925	275-700
0.5-1	10-20	50	3	0.7-1.0	0.7-1.0	0.2-1.0	0.02-0.06	0.02-0.06	0.04-0.08	250-750	425-1275	400-1200
CHILDREN AND ADOLESCENTS												
1-3	15-30	65	3	1.0-1.5	1.0-1.5	0.5-1.5	0.02-0.08	0.02-0.08	0.05-0.1	325-975	550-1650	500-1500
4-6	20-40	85	3-4	1.5-2.0	1.5-2.0	1.0-2.5	0.03-0.12	0.03-0.12	0.06-0.15	450-1350	775-2325	700-2100
7-10	30-60	120	4-5	2.0-2.5	2.0-3.0	1.5-2.5	0.05-0.2	0.05-0.2	0.1-0.3	600-1800	1000-3000	925-2775
11+	50-100	100-200	4-7	2.0-3.0	2.5-5.0	1.5-2.5	0.05-0.2	0.05-0.2	0.15-0.5	900-2700	1525-4575	1400-4200
ADULTS	70-140	100-200	4-7	2.0-3.0	2.5-5.0	1.5-4.0	0.05-0.2	0.05-0.2	0.15-0.5	1100-3300	1875-5625	1700-5100

From Recommended Dietary Allowances, Revised 1979. Food and Nutrition Board National Academy of Sciences–National Research Council, Washington, D.C.

*Because there is less information on which to base allowances, these figures are not given in the main table of the RDA and are provided here in the form of ranges of recommended intakes.

†Since the toxic levels for many trace elements may be only several times usual intakes, the upper levels for the trace elements given in this table should not be habitually exceeded.

Nutrition Throughout the Life Cycle

Nutrition Throughout The Life Cycle

Edited by

Sue Rodwell Williams, Ph.D., M.P.H., R.D.

President, SRW Productions, Inc., and Director, The Berkeley Nutrition Group, Berkeley, California; Metabolic Nutritionist, Kaiser-Permanente Northern California Regional Newborn Screening and Metabolic Program, Kaiser-Permanente Medical Center, Oakland; Field Faculty, M.P.H.-Dietetic Internship Program and Coordinated Undergraduate Program in Dietetics, University of California, Berkeley, California

Bonnie S. Worthington-Roberts, Ph.D., R.D.

Professor and Director, Nutritional Sciences, Chief Nutritionist, Child Development and Mental Retardation Center, Clinical Training Unit, University of Washington, Seattle, Washington

Co-Authors

Eleanor D. Schlenker, Ph.D., R.D.

Associate Professor and Chair, Nutritional Sciences, University of Vermont, Burlington, Vermont

Peggy Pipes, M.S., R.D.

Assistant Chief, Nutrition Section, Child Development and Mental Retardation Center, Clinical Training Unit, University of Washington, Seattle, Washington

Jane M. Rees, M.S., R.D.

Director, Adolescent Nutrition Services and Education, Child Development and Mental Retardation Center, University of Washington, Seattle, Washington

L. Kathleen Mahan, M.S., R.D.

Consulting Nutritionist, Private Practice, Seattle, Washington

With 133 Illustrations

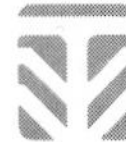

TIMES MIRROR/MOSBY COLLEGE PUBLISHING

St. Louis • Toronto • Santa Clara 1988

Publisher: Nancy K. Roberson
Editor: Ann Trump
Editorial Assistant: Susan Clancy
Project Manager: Teri Merchant
Production Editor: Robert A. Kelly
Editing and Production: EDP, Inc.
Design: Rey Umali

A Division of the C. V. Mosby Company
11830 Westline Industrial Drive
St. Louis, MO 63146

Printed in the United States of America

Library of Congress Cataloging-in-Publication Data

Williams, Sue Rodwell.

Nutrition throughout the life cycle.

Includes bibliographies and index.

1. Nutrition. I. Worthington-Roberts, Bonnie S., 1943- II. Pipes, Peggy L. III. Title.
[DNLM: 1. Nutrition. W727n]
TX354.N87 1988 613.2 87-18106
ISBN 0-8016-5639-7
TS/VH/VH 9 8 7 6 5 4 3 2 1 1/C/034

To Nancy K. Roberson
editor, publisher, friend—
whose ideas and support started this project on its way

Preface

This new book, *Nutrition Throughout the Life Cycle,* is true to its title. Here the six authors of the highly successful Mosby Life Cycle Series books bring together in one comprehensive book our unique backgrounds and working knowledge of each stage of human development. In this project we provide for students, teachers, and practitioners a unified view of the life cycle as one whole, supported in each stage by the nutrition essential for this development.

This underlying developmental concept of human life—the unifying thread throughout the life cycle—has become increasingly significant in today's modern world as our life span has lengthened but for many persons has not improved in quality. We recognize anew that the quality of this lengthened life, genetically programmed from conception but dependent on a nourishing environment for fulfillment of this genetic potential, builds at each stage upon a complex of all past and present life experiences.

We also recognize that our environment is rapidly changing and affecting individual lives in many ways, ways that are not always kind. In the midst of these changes, we are made increasingly aware that nutritional needs—so fundamental to human growth and development—do not exist in a vacuum. At each life stage they are always interwoven with many other personal, socioeconomic, and cultural factors that make up the whole of life and influence positive growth and development and health in both subtle and obvious ways.

This new book reflects these far-reaching changes. Its guiding principle continues to be the commitment, along with that of our publisher, to the integrity of each of our previous individual books. Our expanded goal here is to produce a new book for today's needs, with new design and format and sound content to meet the expectations and changing needs of students, faculty, and practitioners in nutrition and health promotion—for all ages.

Objectives of the Book

This text is designed primarily for students in upper division courses in life cycle nutrition and for health professionals working in both individual and community health programs. It approaches nutrition from a developmental, person-centered view of individual integrity. It seeks to build nutritional needs as growth proceeds on the basis of both physical growth and psychosocial development. Its focus throughout is on positive health for which nutrition provides a fundamental foundation.

Major Characteristics of This New Book

In a very real sense, then, this first edition is a new book for our times and needs. To accommodate the demands of our rapidly developing science and society, yet retain a clearly understood writing style, we have rewritten all age-group background material from our individual life cycle books in the new format here, written important new chapters, and made major changes throughout to increase the usefulness of this new comprehensive text.

1. **Coordinated Life Cycle Chapters.** Chapters 4 through 10 present a coordinated and comprehensive view of the entire life cycle. Each author presents material on human growth and development needs at each age: pregnancy and lactation, infancy, childhood, adolescence, adults and the aging process, and special needs of elderly persons in our aging population.
2. **Special Chapters.** These special chapters underscore our book's comprehensive approach. They provide new understanding of the changing body at each stage in the human life cycle, ways of determining nutritional status and needs along the way, the special needs of persons carrying increased risk at different ages and stressful life situations, and new approaches to nutrition education for health promotion.
3. **Book Format and Design.** The chapter format enhances the appeal of this book and encourages its use. Clear chapter concepts and overview, illustrations, tables, charts, and topic headings and subheadings make the text easier and more interesting to read.
4. **Learning Aids.** A number of educational aids have been developed to assist both student and instructor in the teaching-learning process. These aids are described later in this preface in detail.
5. **Illustrations.** We have selected many illustrations, including artwork, graphs, charts, and photographs, to help both students and practitioners better understand the concepts and health care practices we are presenting.
6. **Enhanced Readability and Student Interest.** We have written our text in a style that helps "unfold" the material. We want to make developmental nutrition *come alive* in real situations. We want to create new interest and help students understand basic concepts better by expanded explanations to "flesh out" the human development and needs at each life stage discussed.

Special Features of This New Text

Throughout all its chapters, this text is distinctive in its breadth of topics discussed, its comprehensive research base, and its many practical and helpful applications to meet individual and group situations. Its major references bring current scientific knowledge to a variety of modern situations and problems. Students can then further apply this up-to-date comprehensive knowledge to needs they discover for themselves. We have tried to provide a basis for students to weigh pros and cons and understand why the scientific method in thinking through a problem is important, because often there are no "cookbook" answers to complex life problems, and basic principles must be the guiding light. Such principles and concepts are highlighted here in many ways to help students see just how nutrition "works" in the lives of people at all ages.

THE CORE LIFE CYCLE CHAPTERS: THE DEVELOPMENTAL CONCEPT

Chapters 4 through 10 provide the strong core of this text. As a whole unit, they show clearly the overall developmental concept of life itself—constant dynamic change and balance. To the discussion of each life stage, the authors bring their unique knowledge and experience, their caring and sensitivity to meet human needs. In-depth reviews of early fetal growth and development during pregnancy and breast-feeding of the newborn infant probe fundamental relationships of nutrition to maternal health and the outcome of pregnancy, and to the following process of lactation. A clear foundation is laid for the varying nutritional needs of rapid infant growth and the slowed erratic growth of young children, revealing the lifetime importance of these early family and cultural food experiences and learned behaviors. An especially sensitive discussion of the volatile nature of rapid adolescent growth and sexual maturation displays the increased nutritional and personal needs of these teenagers "coming of age" in an increasingly complex modern society. For young and middle adults, the important theme of health promotion through the building of healthy life-styles provides the basis for helping adults reduce their risks of health problems: those that affect food intake and use and thus nutritional status and those leading to chronic disease.

THE SUPPORT CHAPTERS: THE COMMON HUMAN THREADS

A second group of chapters strengthens the basic emphasis of this new text. Following a brief introductory chapter that sets needed direction for the reader, four significant chapters, two preceding and two following the core life cycle chapters, provide essential foundation and follow-up for dealing with individual and community nutritional needs. They weave their common human threads throughout life and determine much of our individual nutritional status and its measure.

1. **Body Composition and Nutrition Assessment.** These chapters meet current needs for a sound working knowledge of important aspects of nutritional status and needs of persons throughout the life cycle. Based on the concepts of body balance and compartments, Chapter 2 lays the necessary foundation for understanding the variable nature of individual body composition, methods of its measure, and how it changes throughout the human life cycle pattern of growth, maintenance, and decline. Based on changing concepts of health and health care that express increasing concern for human values, Chapter 3 outlines goals and methods for assessing nutritional status of both communities and individuals and for determining needs as a basis for planning wise nutritional care.

2. **High-Risk Populations.** Chapter 11 addresses the multiple interrelated factors, both physiologic and psychosocial, that create nutrition and health problems in high-risk populations. This chapter is unique, however, in the underlying foundation it lays on the basic effect of *stress,* which in our increasingly complex society is becoming a

pervading high-risk factor in modern disease. Today's health care professionals are giving increased attention to this ever-present factor, whatever their discipline, as a necessary approach for realistic and effective health care. Particularly vulnerable age groups in the life cycle are identified, along with the stress effects of trauma and disease, the changing nature of work in our changing economy, our changing environment, and especially the devastating stress of poverty. All of these stress-related problems have nutrition and health components. To help reduce high levels of stress and provide better nutritional care for these persons, some suggestions for stress management are provided.

3. **Nutrition Education.** Chapter 12 relates nutrition knowledge, motivation, and food behavior to the learning process, food guides, and nutrition education. It provides guidance for developing and evaluating nutrition education programs based on sound communications theory and suggests principles for selecting appropriate materials and resources. A number of current strategies in nutrition education are described, as well as ways that realistic nutrition education may be involved in food assistance programs such as school lunch, WIC, and meals for the aged.

Learning Aids Throughout the Text

As indicated, this book is especially significant in its use of many learning aids throughout the text.

1. **Chapter Openers.** To immediately draw students into the topic for study, each chapter opens with a concise list of the basic concepts involved and a brief chapter overview leading into the topic to "set the stage."

2. **Chapter Headings.** Throughout each chapter, the major headings and subheadings in special type indicate the organization of the chapter material. This makes for easy reading and understanding of the key ideas. Main concepts and terms are also emphasized with bold type and italics.

3. **Boxes.** At different places in the text special related material is placed in boxes to provide further explanation or application.

4. **Definitions of Terms.** Key terms important to the student's understanding and application of the material in nutritional care are presented in two ways. First, they are identified in the body of the text, often with interesting derivation and description of the words. Second, they are listed in a summary glossary at the back of the book for quick reference.

5. **Illustrations.** Careful selection of illustrations throughout the text creates interest and helps the student better understand important concepts and illustrations.

6. **Chapter Summaries.** Brief paragraphs review chapter highlights and help students see the "big picture." Then they can return to any part of the material for repeated study and clarification of details as needed.

7. **Review Questions.** To help the student understand and think through key parts of the chapter or to apply these concepts to health care problems, questions are given after each chapter for review and analysis of the material presented.

8. **Case Studies.** At the end of appropriate chapters, case studies have been highlighted separately to focus the student's attention on related health needs or problems. Each case is accompanied by questions for case analysis. Students can use these examples for similar situations in their individual or community learning experiences.

9. **Cited References.** Background references throughout the text provide resources for students who may want to dig further into a particular topic of interest.

10. **Further Annotated Readings.** To encourage further reading of useful materials for expanding knowledge of key concepts or applying the material in practical ways for nutritional care and education, a brief list of annotated resources is provided at the end of each chapter.

11. **Appendices.** A number of appendices are provided for reference tools. These include weight-height tables for children and adults, growth charts, assessment references, and food guides. Since this text is for use by upper division students, who already have basic food value tables in introductory texts, these references are not repeated here.

Acknowledgments

A realistic and useful college textbook is never the work of one person or even a team of authors as in this case. It develops into the planned product through the committed hands and hearts of a number of persons. It would be impossible to name all the individuals involved here, but several groups deserve special recognition.

First, we are indebted to the Times Mirror/Mosby College Publishing Company and the many persons there, new and old friends, who have had a part in this project. Especially do we thank our publisher and editorial staff, including Nancy Roberson, Ann Trump, Susan Clancy, Bob Kelly, and our outside project editor, Brad Fisher. All of these skilled persons have helped shape the manuscript and support our efforts and goals.

Second, we are grateful to the reviewers who gave their valuable time and skills to help us strengthen the final manuscript:

Joanne Lupton
Texas A&M University

Kathleen Stitt
University of Alabama, Tuscaloosa

Karen Graves
University of North Carolina, Greensboro

Bernice Kopel
Oklahoma State University

Margaret McCarthy
Eastern Kentucky University

Third, as the overall coordinating editor on this writing team, responsible for producing the full manuscript through its several production stages, Sue Rodwell Williams is grateful to her own production staff, especially to her expert systems analyst, Jim Williams, who has developed and set up her expanded computer system, a true joy to work with. And to Tony Rinella, friend and computer expert, who has responded with grace to her calls for help at all sorts of odd hours, she gives special thanks for being there when she needed him.

Fourth, to our many students and interns, colleagues, clients, and patients over the years who have enriched our professional and personal lives, we give our thanks. Each one has taught us something about human experience, and we are grateful for these opportunities for personal growth. Especially do the authors of Chapter 8 wish to thank their colleagues Leona Eggert, Margaret McIntyre, Robin Rosebrough, Mary Storey, and Lanita Wright who wrote original chapters in their background book *Nutrition in Adolescence,* from which portions of Chapter 8 here were taken.

And finally, but most of all, we want to thank our families—our "home teams." These beautiful people never cease to provide loving support for all our work, and to each one we are eternally grateful.

Sue Rodwell Williams
Bonnie S. Worthington-Roberts

Contents

3 Nutrition Assessment 39

Sue Rodwell Williams

4 Maternal Nutrition and the Course and Outcome of Pregnancy 69

Bonnie S. Worthington-Roberts

Nutrition Throughout the Life Cycle

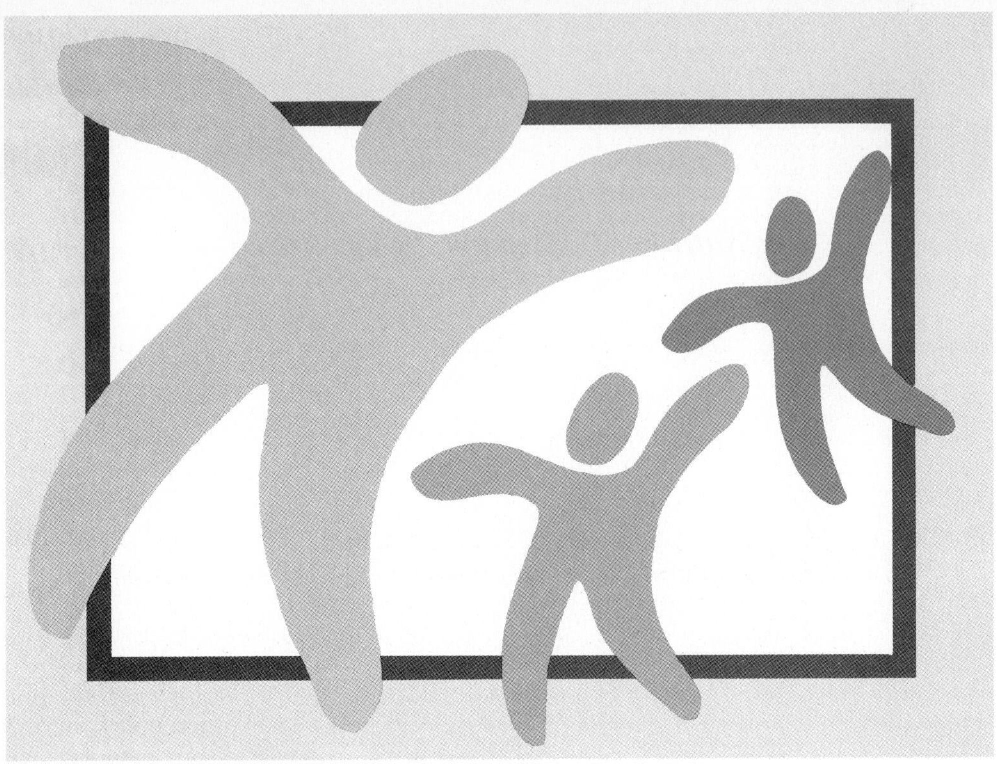

Basic Concepts

1. Each stage of the life cycle is associated with a distinct set of nutritional priorities.
2. All persons throughout life need the same nutrients but in varying amounts.
3. Health maintenance and disease prevention are the underlying goals throughout the life cycle.
4. In some cases, especially in the later years, disease management may impact significantly on dietary planning.

Chapter One

Introduction

Bonnie S. Worthington-Roberts

Growth and development, and the maintenance of health, require attention to diet and nutrition throughout the life cycle. Each stage of life presents a unique set of challenges, including those related to nutritional priorities and diet planning. Although needs may vary with increasing age, at all times the major goal is the same: selecting a variety of foods to include all necessary nutrients while avoiding excessive intake of kilocalories and in some cases other food constituents such as saturated fat and sodium.

Life Cycle Nutritional Needs

From the moment of conception, the human organism depends on nutrition for growth, development, and long-term survival. Prior to birth, the fetus must draw from maternal nutrient supplies and this process may continue after birth if the mother chooses to breast-feed her baby. Ultimately, an outside food supply provides the ongoing nutritional support for life. This nutritional support may come from both animal and plant food sources. An unlimited number of food combinations are known to satisfy nutrient needs. Consequently, peoples of the world consuming vastly different foods and food mixtures demonstrate satisfactory growth and health.

STAGES OF THE LIFE CYCLE

Fetal and Maternal Needs

The mammalian fetus is completely dependent on nutritional support from the mother. The quantitative requirements are very small in the beginning but increase gradually until birth. During this time it is absolutely essential that a correct equilibrium be maintained among the various nutrients circulating in the maternal blood. This required biochemical milieu depends entirely on the mother's diet, her nutritional stores, and her metabolic indiosyncrasies. The adverse effects of nutritional-biochemical imbalance during gestation have been examined most frequently in animal models. Fortuitous observations of human experience, however, have contributed to our slowly growing knowledge base in this field. In general, the repercussions of abnormal nutrition depend on the stage at which a given nutrient factor acts, the nature of the nutrient considered, the intensity of the disequilibrium, and the species or strain of the animal studied. The types of repercussion are very different. They include death, tissue alterations, delayed growth, alterations of cellular differentiation, and malformations. Improvement in pregnancy outcome depends in part on motivating the pregnant woman to establish satisfactory diet and supplementation practices.[1]

Lactation

Establishment of lactation and continued production of sufficient high-quality milk also demands that the mother consume an adequate diet. While lactation is a high-priority physiologic process maintained even in the face of serious nutritional deprivation, without continuing nutritional support the quantity of milk production is generally hampered and milk quality eventually deteriorates. In either case, the nutritional well-being of the mother will be compromised as will eventually her health and preparedness for "mothering."[1,2]

Infancy

The first year after birth is a time in the life cycle when many changes occur in relation to food and nutrient intake. A number of factors influence these dramatic changes: (1) a rapid then gradually declining rate of physical growth, (2) maturation of oral structures and functions, (3) development of fine and gross motor skills, and (4) establishment of relationships with parents and family. As a result of these tremendous changes, infants prepared at birth to suck liquids from a nipple are at one year of age making attempts to feed themselves table foods with culturally defined utensils. The need for nutrients and energy depends on the infant's requirement for physical growth, maintenance, and energy expenditure. The foods offered to infants reflect culturally accepted practices. Infants' acceptance of food is influenced by neuromotor maturation and by their interactions with their parents. Well-nourished children at any month during infancy will consume a variety of food combinations.[3]

Preschool Years

During the preschool years, the decreased rates of growth bring decreased appetites. Children learn to understand language and to talk and ask for food. Development of gross motor skills permits them to learn to feed themselves and to prepare simple foods such as cereal and milk and sandwiches. They learn about food and the way it feels, tastes, and smells. Preschool children learn to eat a wider variety of textures and kinds of food, give up the bottle, and drink from a cup. They demand independence and refuse help in many tasks, such as self-feeding, in which they are not yet skillful. As they grow older, they become less interested in food and more interested in their environment. They test and learn the limits of acceptable behavior.[3]

School-Age Children

Between preschool and adolescence, children continue to grow slowly and demonstrate maturation of fine and gross motor skills. Individual personality develops and degree of independence increases. All of these changes influence the amounts of food consumed, the manner in which it is eaten, and the acceptability of specific foods. Food habits, likes and dislikes are established, some of which are transient, but many of which form the base for a lifetime of food experiences. Environmental influences and parental behaviors reinforce or extinguish food-related behaviors. Parents need to provide appropriate foods and supportive guidance so that appropriate food patterns develop. The nutrition knowledge of the parents and other care providers positively influences children's requests for and acceptance of various foods. School feeding programs provide an opportunity for nutrition education.[3]

Adolescence

The adolescent period is a unique stage in the process of growth and development. It is characterized by a wide variability in norms of growth, increasingly independent behavior, and the testing of adult roles. This critical period of human development occurs at physiologic, psychologic, and social levels. These tumultuous changes do not occur simultaneously but at varying rates. Although adolescence may be defined as the teenage years between twelve and twenty, physical maturation and changes in nutrient requirements actually begin at younger years and sometimes extend into the third decade.[3,4]

Teenagers assume greater responsibility for decision-making in their own lives. In contrast to younger children, adolescents themselves most often determine their food intake. Their food choices reflect various factors including family eating patterns, peer influence, media, appetite, and food availability. Some of these factors can be positive for nutritional quality and others may leave a lot to be desired. Body image plays a very important role in the eating behaviors of adolescents. Eating disorders account for a large number of nutritional concerns during adolescence.[3,4]

Adulthood

The adult years span a number of decades during which nutritional needs change very little, but family circumstances and lifestyle often undergo substantial change. Marital status, living environment, job setting and responsibilities, income, and a variety of other factors significantly impact upon specific food choices and long-term dietary patterns. Ideally, a major focus during these years is health promotion and disease prevention. This goal entails, among other things, establishing nutritional practices that will maximize health and minimize risk for developing preventable chronic diseases. Appropriate practices vary somewhat among individuals owing in large part to differences in genetic bases. Of primary concern, however, is maintaining desirable body fatness by eating moderate amounts of a wide variety of wholesome foods.[5-7]

Older Adults

Persons who are 65 years old and over comprise the fastest growing segment of the population in most developed countries. Of these older individuals, 95% live within the community, many of them on incomes barely sufficient for survival. Financial limitations adversely affect food purchasing power. But an assortment of other factors also contribute to the increased prevalence of malnutrition in this age group. Important contributors to the problem include loneliness, depression, oral discomfort, and chronic diseases, all of which add to poor appetite. Physical and mental handicaps may limit the ability to shop for food or to prepare it. Use of an assortment of drugs, both prescription and over-the-counter, may further interfere with the maintenance of satisfactory nutritional status. The aging process itself may reduce nutrient absorption, increase urinary loss, and interfere with normal pathways of nutrient utilization.[8]

Health Maintenance and Disease Prevention

THE ROLE OF NUTRITION: A CHANGED FOCUS

During the past ten years, understanding has improved about the role of nutrition in health promotion and disease prevention. Relationships between specific nutrient deficiencies and inferior health status have long been recognized. But in recent years, diet has been associated with a number of chronic diseases, such as cardiovascular disease, cancer, and diabetes. The focus of concern about human nutrition has moved from the issues of nutritional deficiencies toward increased emphasis on chronic disease prevention and health maintenance in all phases of the life cycle.

NATIONAL HEALTH OBJECTIVES

As a result of this increased concern and changed focus, nutrition has been included as a separate priority area in the Surgeon General's 1990 Health Objectives for the Nation. These objectives, defined in the 1980 Public Health Service report *Promoting Health/Preventing Disease: Objectives for the Nation,*[9] reflect a major initiative of the U.S. Department of Health and Human Services. Fifteen priority areas are defined and one of these is nutrition (see box). The target date for achieving these objectives is 1990. Some progress has been made to date in achieving the nutrition objectives. (See Table 11–6.) The amount of progress reflects both the degree to which national nutrition concern has begun to affect actual behavior and the relative immaturity of the nutrition field. Unfortunately, a number of the objectives are not measurable. Equally unfortunate is the obvious persistence of overweight in the American population and the supporting epidemiologic evidence suggesting increased risk of chronic disease linked to this condition. On the other hand, heartening data are available on the level of public awareness about the danger of being overweight and the basic requirements of decreased dietary kilocalories and increased physical exercise necessary to control weight.[10,11]

Diet Therapy as a Component of Disease Management

While the maintenance of health and prevention of disease is a priority focus throughout the life cycle, circumstances arise in every stage of life when dietary inter-

THE PUBLIC HEALTH SERVICE NATIONAL NUTRITION OBJECTIVES FOR 1990

1. By 1990, the proportion of pregnant women with iron deficiency anemia should be reduced to 3.5%.
2. By 1990, growth retardation of infants and children caused by inadequate diets should have been eliminated in the United States as a public health problem.
3. By 1990, the prevalence of significant overweight among the U.S. adult population should be decreased to 10% of men and 17% of women, without nutritional impairment.
4. By 1990, 50% of the overweight population should have adopted weight loss regimens, combining appropriate balance of diet and physical activity.
5. By 1990, the mean serum cholesterol level in the adult population 18 to 74 years of age should be at or below 200 mg/dl.
6. By 1990, the mean serum cholesterol level in children aged one to 14 should be at or below 150 mg/dl.
7. By 1990, the average daily sodium ingestion for adults should be reduced to at least the 3 to 6 g range.
8. By 1990, the proportion of women who breastfeed their babies should be increased to 75% at hospital discharge and to 35% at 6 months of age.
9. By 1990, the proportion of the population which is able to correctly associate the principal dietary factors known or strongly suspected to be related to disease should exceed 75% for each of the following diseases: heart disease, high blood pressure, dental caries, and cancer.
10. By 1990, 70% of adults should be able to identify the major foods which are: low in fat content, low in sodium content, high in calories, high in sugars, good sources of fiber.
11. By 1990, 90% of adults should understand that to lose weight people must either consume foods that contain fewer calories or increase physical activity, or both.
12. By 1990, the labels of all packaged foods should contain useful calories and nutrient information to enable consumers to select diets that promote and protect good health. Similar information should be displayed where nonpackaged foods are obtained or purchased.
13. By 1990, sodium levels in processed food should be reduced by 20% from present levels.
14. By 1990, the proportion of employee and school cafeteria managers who are aware of and actively promoting USDA/DHHS dietary guidelines should be greater than 50%.
15. By 1990, all states should include nutrition education as part of required comprehensive school health education at the elementary and secondary levels.
16. By 1990, virtually all routine health contacts with health professionals should include some element of nutrition education and nutrition counseling.
17. Before 1990, a comprehensive national nutrition status monitoring system should have the capability for detecting nutritional problems in special population groups, as well as for obtaining baseline data for decisions on national nutrition policies.

ventions are required to treat disease, trauma, or other undesirable situations. The basic principles governing diet therapy are simple: meet nutritional needs while modifying the diet to satisfy the health problem under treatment. Some changes in diet may be easily implemented, but others require much special planning and in some cases major changes from established food habits. The degree to which an individual—with the help of family, friends, health-care providers, and others—is able to follow short-term or permanent changes in diet varies in each case. The needed diet changes may impact significantly on quality of life and in some cases even on chances of survival. While the focus of this book is health maintenance and disease prevention, some discussion of necessity will include selected problems that require diet and nutrition intervention.

Summary

Growth, development, reproduction, and the maintenance of health require that the human organism satisfy basic biologic needs. Nutrition is a basic need that can be met minimally to prevent death or optimally to help achieve maximal genetic potential. The goal of this book is to approach the issue of optimal nutrition from the developmental framework of specific stages of the life cycle. Attention to normal needs and feeding practices will predominate but management strategies for selected special problems will be addressed. For more detailed coverage of special problems requiring diet therapy, the reader is referred to other available sources of information.[12-17]

Review Questions

1. Define key nutritional concerns at each stage of the life cycle.
2. Discuss the 1990 Nutrition Objectives for the United States and indicate progress made toward achieving these objectives as of 1986.

REFERENCES

1. Worthington-Roberts, B., Vermeersch, J., and Williams, S.R.: Nutrition in pregnancy and lactation, ed. 3, St. Louis, 1985, Times Mirror/Mosby College Publishing.
2. Lawrence, R.A.: Breast-feeding: a guide for the medical profession, ed. 2, St. Louis, 1985, Times Mirror/Mosby College Publishing.
3. Pipes, P.: Nutrition in infancy and childhood, ed. 3, St. Louis, 1985, Times Mirror/Mosby College Publishing.
4. Mahan, L.K., and Rees, J.M.: Nutrition in adolescence, St. Louis, 1984, Times Mirror/Mosby College Publishing.
5. Pennington, J.A.T.: Dietary patterns and practices, Clin. Nutr. **5**(1):17, January-February 1986.
6. Crosetti, A.F., and Guthrie, H.A.: Alternate eating patterns and the role of age, sex, selection, and snacking in nutritional quality, Clin. Nutr. **5**(1):34, January-February 1986.
7. Lecos, C.: America's changing diet, FDA Consumer, October 1985, p. 4.
8. Schlenker, E.D.: Nutrition in aging, St. Louis, 1984, Times Mirror/Mosby College Publishing.

9. United States Department of Health and Human Services, Public Health Service: Promoting health/preventing disease: Objectives for the nation, Washington, D.C., 1980, U.S. Government Printing Office.
10. Thornberry, O.T., Wilson, R.W., and Golden, P.M.: Health promotion data for the 1990 objectives, Estimates from National Health Interview Survey of Health Promotion and Disease Prevention: United States, 1985, Advance Data No. 126, September 19, 1986.
11. Kaufman, M., and others: Progress toward meeting the 1990 nutrition objectives for the nation: nutrition services and data collection in state/territorial agencies, Am. J. Public Health 77(3):299, March 1987.
12. Kerner, J.A.: Manual of pediatric parenteral nutrition, New York, 1983, John Wiley & Sons, Inc.
13. Suskin, R.M.: Textbook of pediatric nutrition, New York, 1981, Raven Press.
14. American Academy of Pediatrics: Pediatric nutrition handbook, Elk Grove Village, Ill., 1985, American Academy of Pediatrics.
15. American Dietetic Association: Handbook of clinical dietetics, New Haven, 1981, Yale University Press.
16. Dietetic Staffs of the Mayo Clinic, Mayo Clinic diet manual: a handbook of dietary practices, ed. 5, Philadelphia, 1981, W.B. Saunders Co.
17. Williams, S.R.: Nutrition and diet therapy, ed. 5, St. Louis, 1985, Times Mirror/Mosby College Publishing.

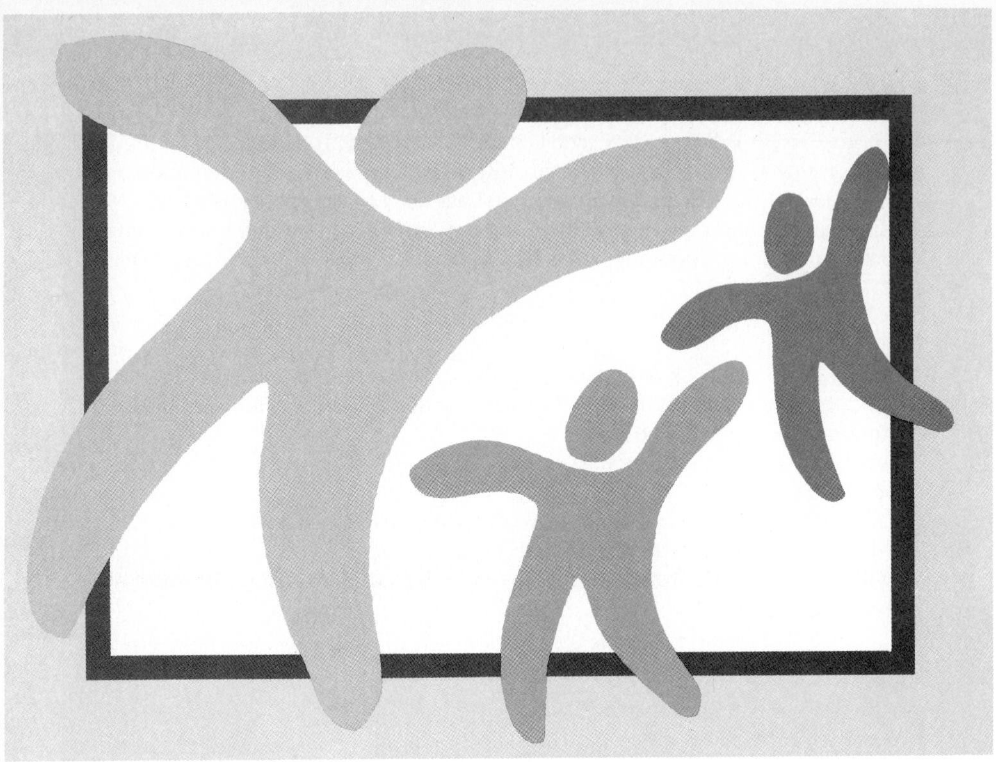

Basic Concepts

1. Perpetual change and balance among the basic components of the body and its environment according to need maintain human life.
2. Within the limits of genetic potential, body composition varies widely among healthy individuals.
3. Body compartments are designations of collective amounts of basic body materials and functional aspects of body composition.
4. Body composition changes throughout the normal human life cycle to maintain homeostasis and health, but this dynamic balance may be influenced in abnormal ways by disease.

Chapter Two

Body Composition

Sue Rodwell Williams

Throughout the life cycle the physical composition of the human body is changing. From conception and birth, through childhood growth and adult aging, to old age decline and death, the human body and its basic components change and adapt in a remarkable fashion to meet physiologic needs. Given the genetic imprint of its heritage and the physical and psychosocial nature of its environment, the human body, in the most literal sense, is the product of its nutrition throughout life. Through profound and fascinating transformations, food makes possible the living body and all its functions, and the varying mass of tissue it produces and maintains.

Is there an "ideal" or "standard" body composition? Hardly, that is, except in the laboratory for purposes of study. In reality we shall see that this is a hazardous assumption, for within the limits of genetic potential, individuals differ widely. There is a great variability among healthy persons in both body composition and body response to internal and external environmental influences and to disease. Thus an analysis of body composition provides an important basis for determining the nutritional status of individuals of all ages, as well as the many influencing factors that shape it.

In this chapter we will look at body composition in terms of its components and their balance within the body. We shall see how this balance changes throughout life, both in normal growth and aging and in disease. Then in following chapters we will apply this background to nutrition assessment and ways of meeting nutritional needs through all of life's stages.

The Concept of Body Balance

Basic to an understanding of body composition throughout life's changes is the concept of body balance. The human body is a dynamic organism. It maintains a balancing interchange with its external environment, as well as a life-sustaining balance among its parts within its internal environment. Consider first, then, the nature of this human body balance and the factors that work together to maintain it.

FACTORS INFLUENCING BODY BALANCE

External Intake-Output Balance

The intake of needed nutrients and the output of these nutrients and their metabolites according to need determine the overall body supply of vital substances essential for maintaining body mass and metabolism. Various body systems govern the many processes that control essential intake-output balances. For example, the gastrointestinal system takes in necessary water and food, processes them for body use, and together with the renal system expels the unneeded remainder in normal output. Similarly, the respiratory system takes in vital oxygen from the air and exchanges it for the metabolic product carbon dioxide, which it then expels in exhalation.

Internal Dynamic Equilibrium

In balance with its external environment, the body maintains an exquisite state of dynamic equilibrium—*homeostasis*—within its internal milieu. In the ebb and flow of this warm, watery environment, through its myriad of biochemical processes, the body produces a life-sustaining "steady state." Numerous biochemical agents such as enzymes and hormones, as well as physical forces such as the hydrostatic-osmotic pressure balances of capillary dynamics controlling fluid shifts, govern this state of physiologic homeostasis. Since the body is an open system, interfacing constantly with its external environment, these adaptive homeostatic mechanisms enable it to adjust to varying external events and situations.

Personal Characteristics

Individual characteristics such as genetic heritage, sex, and age also influence body balance. For example, a genetic lack of sufficient specific enzyme to metabolize a given nutrient causes an imbalance of that nutrient and its metabolites in the body. In the genetic disease *phenylketonuria (PKU),* a lack of phenylalanine hydroxylase to metabolize the essential amino acid phenylalanine causes elevated levels of that amino acid, a deficiency of its normal metabolic product tyrosine, and an accumulation of abnormal metabolites instead. In aging persons, calcium imbalance contributes to *osteoporosis* due to the abnormal loss of mineral mass from the bone compartment. Iron imbalance during the reproductive years may cause *anemia* in iron-deficient women.

Disease

Illness generally curtails appetite, reduces food intake and its use by the body, and produces both energy and nutrient imbalances. Hypermetabolic disease such as cancer demands vigorous nutritional support to offset imbalances due to increased need in the face of diminished intake. The chronic disease diabetes mellitus creates a glucose imbalance with elevated blood sugar.

Psychosocial Influences

Work and family stress, social and cultural attitudes and practices, or economic pressures can cause body imbalances. For example, social attitudes that value thinness in women, reinforced in the media, contribute to the development of a distorted body image in adolescent girls and young women, sometimes leading to severe eating disorders such as anorexia nervosa and bulimia.

ENERGY BALANCE: BODY WEIGHT

The body's weight reflects the overall balance between energy intake as fuel in foods—kilocalories—and energy expenditure in metabolic requirements and physical activity. This balance is fairly equal in the steady state. It becomes positive during weight gain and negative during weight loss. Of particular significance is the relative body leanness and fatness.

Positive and Negative Energy Balance

When energy intake exceeds energy expenditure, weight gain occurs and relative obesity, or more correctly overfatness, may result. When energy intake is less than energy expenditure, weight loss occurs and relative underweight or underfatness may result.

Leanness and Fatness

If energy expenditure is increased by physical activity, even though gross body weight may remain the same or even increase somewhat, the body fatness in relation to leanness decreases. Many trained athletes, for example, are often "overweight" by standard height-weight tables but seldom overfat. The gross body weight, to the extent that it represents the size of the body cell mass, or more specifically lean body mass, has metabolic significance through its influence on the basal metabolic rate (BMR) and the energy cost of physical activity. Ultimately, however, its major importance lies in its association with body fatness. The amount of body fat reflects the body's energy balance.

ENERGY EXPENDITURE: COSTS AND REQUIREMENTS

Balanced against energy intake, mainly in the form of carbohydrates and fats, is the large metabolic energy cost of maintaining the body plus the lesser but variable energy cost of physical activity. The internal balance between tissue buildup and breakdown is part of this overall body energy balance, which influences relative body composition.

Types of Metabolic Reactions

The two types of metabolic activity, *anabolism* and *catabolism,* are continually going on in energy balance. Each requires energy.

1. **Anabolism** synthesizes more complex substances. Energy is required to drive this synthesis. The more complex the substance formed, the greater is its potential or bound energy.
2. **Catabolism** breaks down body tissue compounds to simpler substances. It releases free energy, but there must also be some free energy available to initiate the breakdown.

Body Energy Stores

When food is not available, as in fasting or starvation, the body must draw on its own tissue reserves for needed energy: (1) **glycogen** in liver and muscle provides only a 12- to 48-hour energy supply, which is quickly depleted; (2) **adipose** tissue can store virtually unlimited amounts of fat, but the supply of stored fat varies from person to person and in a given person at different times; and (3) **muscle mass** provides limited energy, and is not a major body fuel form.

Basal Metabolic Needs

Basal metabolism is the sum of all internal activities that maintain the body at rest. The basal metabolic rate (BMR) is a measure of the energy required by these activities of resting tissue. The major predictor of BMR is the lean body mass component of the individual body composition (see box opposite).

Measuring BMR

The common indirect method of measuring BMR in health care today is through laboratory tests of thyroid function. Since the thyroid hormone regulates BMR, thyroid function tests used in clinical practice can serve as indirect measures. These tests include measures of serum protein bound iodine (PBI), radioactive iodine uptake, and serum thyroxine levels. In the PBI test, the amount of iodine bound to circulating blood protein relates to the level of thyroid hormone produced. In the iodine uptake test, the amount of orally administered radioactive "tagged" iodine taken up by the thyroid gland also measures the activity of the thyroid hormone. In the serum thyroxine tests most commonly used, the free thyroxine index (FTI) is based on the product of T_3 (triiodothyronine) and T_4 (thyroxine) levels. These two compounds are produced in the final two stages of thyroid hormone (thyroxine) synthesis in the thyroid gland. This product ($T_3 \times T_4$) reflects the relative functioning of the thyroid gland and the amount of circulating hormone activity influencing the BMR.

Factors Influencing BMR

In addition to the main effect of lean body mass as indicated above, several other factors influence BMR. These factors relate to life cycle stages, disease, and the environment:

1. **Pregnancy**. The BMR rises during pregnancy, which is a period of rapid tissue growth. The metabolic rate increases as a result of increases in muscle mass of the uterus, size of mammary glands, fetal mass and placenta, and maternal cardiac work and respiratory rate. This totals a 20% to 25% increase over the non-pregnant state.
2. **Childhood growth.** Metabolic work requirements increase during the anabolic periods of growth at different ages, influenced by the growth hormone (GH). GH stimulates cell metabolism and raises BMR 15% to 20%. Thus the BMR slowly rises during the first 5 years of life, levels off, rises again just before and during puberty, and then declines into old age. If BMR is expressed in terms of body surface area (kcal per square meter per hour) as the child grows larger, it would be a declining figure, leveling off in adulthood and declining further in later years.

THE DIFFERENCE BETWEEN SAM AND JOE

Sam and Joe are both healthy, 35-year-old accountants who are 175 cm (5 ft, 10 in) tall, weigh 74.2 kg (165 lb), and jog 3.2 km (2 miles) a day. They need the same number of kilocalories to get through the day, right? Not necessarily.

Tradition dictates that energy requirements are based on basal needs plus physical activity. Since basal requirements are said to depend on the three factors of sex, age, and body composition, then Sam and Joe should have the same basal needs.

However, current researchers have taken a second look at an old study that concluded that these three factors could predict basal energy needs and found that only one—*body composition*—really makes a difference. After analyzing data about the original 223 subjects, the current investigators found *lean body mass (LBM)* to be the *only* predictor of BMR:

$$\text{BMR (kcal/day)} = 500 + 22 \text{ (LBM in kg)}$$

Sam and Joe may weigh the same, but if Sam's weight is made up of more fatty tissue than Joe's, his requirements may be lower. But suppose Sam and Joe have the same amount of LBM, which you may suspect because of their similar activity levels. Would their energy levels be the same? The answer again is not necessarily. The assumptions that energy needs for physical activity are the same among individuals or stay the same within the same individual over time have both been questioned.

As far back as 1947, a study showed that workers performing similar tasks had a wider range of energy intake (kilocalories) than energy output, which means that some persons burn their kilocalories more efficiently than others. The same study, whose results have been repeated over the years by other researchers, also showed that individuals varied widely in the amount of energy spent doing the same work over a week's time, *even when changes in weight were accounted for,* which means that the individual might be more energy-efficient at certain times than at others. One study suggests that the differences might be due to the body's attempt to regulate the amount of energy stored in the body.

Joe always seems to eat more than Sam. Sam wonders about this difference when they seem so much alike in their size and activity, but he does not know about the internal metabolism of his energy-efficient friend. Old and new energy balance studies are helping provide some of the answers.

References

Cunningham, J.J.: A reanalysis of the factors influencing basal metabolic rate in normal adults, Am. J. Clin. Nutr. 33(11):2372, 1980.

Cunningham, J.J.: An individualization of dietary requirements for energy in adults, J. Am. Diet. Assoc. 80:335, April 1982.

Sukhatme, P.V., and Margen, S.: Autoregulatory homeostatic nature of energy balance, Am. J. Clin. Nutr. 35(2):335, 1982.

3. **Fever and disease.** Fever increases BMR about 7% for each .83 degree Centigrade (1 degree Fahrenheit) rise. Also, diseases involving increased cell activity such as cancer, certain anemias, cardiac failure, hypertension, and respiratory problems such as emphysema usually increase BMR. In the abnormal states of starvation and malnutrition, the BMR is lowered.
4. **Cold climate.** BMR rises in response to lower temperatures as a compensatory mechanism to maintain body temperature, unless, of course, sufficient additional clothing is worn.

Food Intake Effect

Food ingestion separately stimulates metabolic work requiring energy to meet the multiple activities of digestion, absorption, and transport of nutrients. This overall stimulating effect of food is called *dietary thermogenesis,* or food's *specific dynamic action (SDA).* About 10% of the body's total energy need is attributed to activities related to metabolizing food.

Physical Activity Needs

Exercise involved in work and recreation or physical training accounts for wide individual variations in energy intake needs. Mental work as such or heightened emotional states alone do not increase metabolic activity, but they may bring added energy needs because they involve increased muscle tension, restlessness, or agitated movements.

Total Energy Requirements

The energy demands of BMR, especially during growth periods, those of food intake and use, and the variable requirements of physical activity make up an individual's total energy requirement. To maintain daily energy balance, the total energy requirement of an individual is the number of kilocalories necessary to replace daily metabolic loss plus loss from exercise and other physical activities.

WATER BALANCE: BODY HYDRATION

Earth is a watery planet. Human lives, and those of all other life forms sharing this planet, are sustained by an ever-moving cycle of water. It is the one nutrient most vital to human existence. Human beings can survive far longer without food than without water. Only the need for air is more pressing. Meeting the need for a continuous supply of life-giving water and maintaining the body's water composition are major nutritional and physiologic tasks, as well as environmental concerns. Finely balanced homeostatic mechanisms protect the essential supply and distribution of this vital body water.

Overall Water Balance: Intake and Output

The average adult processes from 2.5 to 3.0 L of water a day in a constant turnover balanced between intake and output. Normally water enters and leaves the body by various routes, controlled by two basic mechanisms:

1. **Thirst and drinking.** These mechanisms are complex interactions involving con-

trol centers located in the brain's hypothalamus and related hormonal regulation of intake. Thirst is a distinct physical sensation and a conscious demand for water caused by: (1) extracellular dehydration; (2) low cardiac output or hemorrhage; (3) intracellular dehydration; and (4) dryness of the mouth. In elderly persons the sensation of thirst may be decreased, requiring close attention to detect and correct such problems early and prevent fluid-balance disorders.[1]

2. **Hormonal controls.** Two hormones regulate renal water excretion to maintain body water balance. These are *vasopressin,* the antidiuretic hormone (ADH) from the pituitary gland, and *aldosterone,* the sodium- and water-conserving hormone from the adrenal glands.

Sources of Water Intake

Body water intake comes from three sources: (1) preformed water alone or in other beverages provides the main source, about 1200 to 1500 ml of liquid daily; (2) preformed water in foods provides a variable source, about 700 to 1000 ml daily; and (3) water of oxidation from the metabolizing of food, about 200 to 300 ml daily. This makes a total daily intake of about 2100 to 2800 ml.

Routes of Water Output

Water leaves the body by four routes: (1) **Kidneys.** Normal adult kidneys excrete about 1 to 2 L of urine daily, depending upon the amount they are "obligated" to excrete to expel the body's load of metabolic end products, and the variable amount according to body need and the renal tubular reabsorption rate. (2) **Skin.** About 350 ml of water is lost daily through the skin by diffusion (called *insensible water loss* because it is automatic), another 100 ml in normal perspiration, and additional amounts in heavier sweating, about 250 ml according to heat and exercise. Drinking to replace these heavier losses is stimulated when the body water volume decreases by 0.5% to 1.0%, but there is a delay in the body rehydration effect.[2] (3) **Lungs.** About 350 ml of water is lost daily through normal respiration vapor, varying with the climate—least in hot, humid weather and greatest in very cold temperature. (4) **Feces.** A small amount of water, about 150 to 200 ml, is usually lost daily through intestinal elimination, with larger losses in abnormal conditions such as diarrhea.

On the average, daily water output from the adult body, in balance with water intake, totals about 2600 ml, as summarized in Table 2-1.

Body Water Distribution

A woman's body is about 50% to 55% water. A man's body is about 55% to 60% water. The higher water content in most men results from their greater muscle mass. Striated muscle contains more water than any body tissue other than blood. The remaining 40% of a man's weight is about 18% protein and related substances, 15% fat, and 7% minerals. A woman's remaining body composition is about the same, except for a somewhat smaller muscle mass and larger fat deposit. The body's water performs three essential life functions: (1) it helps give structure and form to the body through the turgor it provides to tissue; (2) it creates the water environment necessary for cell metabolism; and (3) it provides the means for maintaining a stable body temperature.

TABLE 2-1 Approximate Daily Adult Intake and Output of Water

	Intake (replacement) ml/Day		Output (loss) Obligatory (insensible) ml/Day	Additional (according to need) ml/Day
Preformed		Lungs	350	
Liquids	1200-1500	Skin		
In foods	700-1000	Diffusion	350	
Metabolism	200- 300	Sweat	100	±250
(oxidation		Kidneys	900	±500
of food)		Feces	150	
	2100-2800	TOTAL	1850	750
TOTAL (approx. 2600 ml/day)			(aprox. 2600 ml/day)	

The total body water is interbalanced between its two compartments: (1) **extracellular fluid (ECF)**, all water outside of cells; and (2) **intracellular fluid (ICF)**, all water inside of cells (Fig. 2-1). Their respective content of electrolytes and protein maintains water balance between these two compartments.

Electrolyte Control of Body Hydration

Ionized sodium (Na+) is the chief cation of ECF. Ionized potassium (K+) is the chief cation of ICF. These two major electrolytes, with others present in smaller

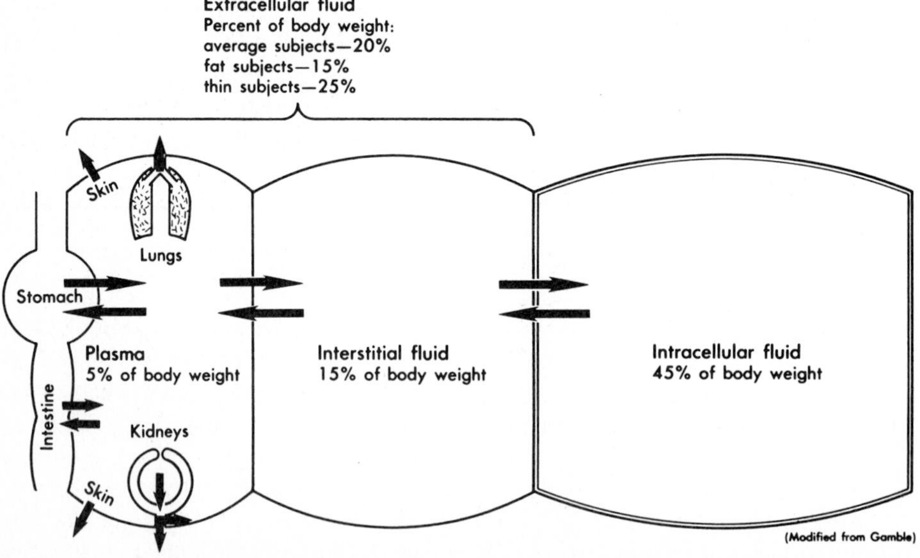

FIG. 2-1 Body fluid compartments. Note the relative total quantities of water in the intracellular compartment and in the extracellular compartment.

amounts, control the amount of water to be retained in a given compartment. The usual reason for shifts of water from one compartment to another is a change in the ECF concentration of these electrolytes. The terms *hypertonic dehydration* and *hypotonic dehydration* refer to the electrolyte concentration of the water outside the cell, which in turn causes a shift of water into or out of the cell.

Protein Control of Body Hydration

Protein influences the internal shifting of body water in three areas: (1) **Plasma protein**, mainly albumin, controls water exchange across capillary membranes. (2) **Cell protein**, along with cell $K+$, controls water exchange across cell membranes. (3) **Lymph protein** drains excess water from tissue spaces.

Gastrointestinal Water Balance

Interfacing with the blood circulation is the "gastrointestinal circulation" of water and secretions. Plasma water, containing ions in patterns that vary according to numerous factors, is converted by the appropriate secretions of the gastrointestinal tract into digestive secretions. These secretions, produced daily, function throughout the alimentary system in the processes of digestion and absorption. They circulate constantly between the plasma and secreting cells. Finally, in the distal portion of the intestine, most of the water and electrolytes are reabsorbed into the plasma to circulate again. In an average-size adult, the total amount of body water involved in this important "gastrointestinal circulation" has been variously estimated at 7500 to 10,000 ml daily. Because of the large amounts of water and electrolytes involved, it is not surprising that loss of gastrointestinal secretions in persistent vomiting or diarrhea is the most common cause of clinical water and electrolyte problems. The general distribution of the total volume in the various secretions is given in Table 2-2.

Renal Water Circulation

The major responsibility for maintaining water and electrolyte balance in the body belongs to the kidneys. Through their functional units, the *nephrons,* the kidneys protect vital body water. The nephron is an exquisite example of a highly complex, minute tissue unit, adapted in fine structural detail to its vital function of maintaining an internal fluid environment compatible with life (Fig. 2-2). Important body fluids

TABLE 2-2 Approximate Total Volume of Digestive Secretions Produced in 24 Hours by Adult of Average Size

Secretion	Amount
Saliva	1500 ml
Gastric	2500
Bile	500
Pancreatic	700
Intestinal	3000
TOTAL	8200 ml

From Gamble, J.L.: Chemical anatomy, physiology and pathology of extracellular fluid, ed. 6, Cambridge, Mass., 1954, Harvard University Press.

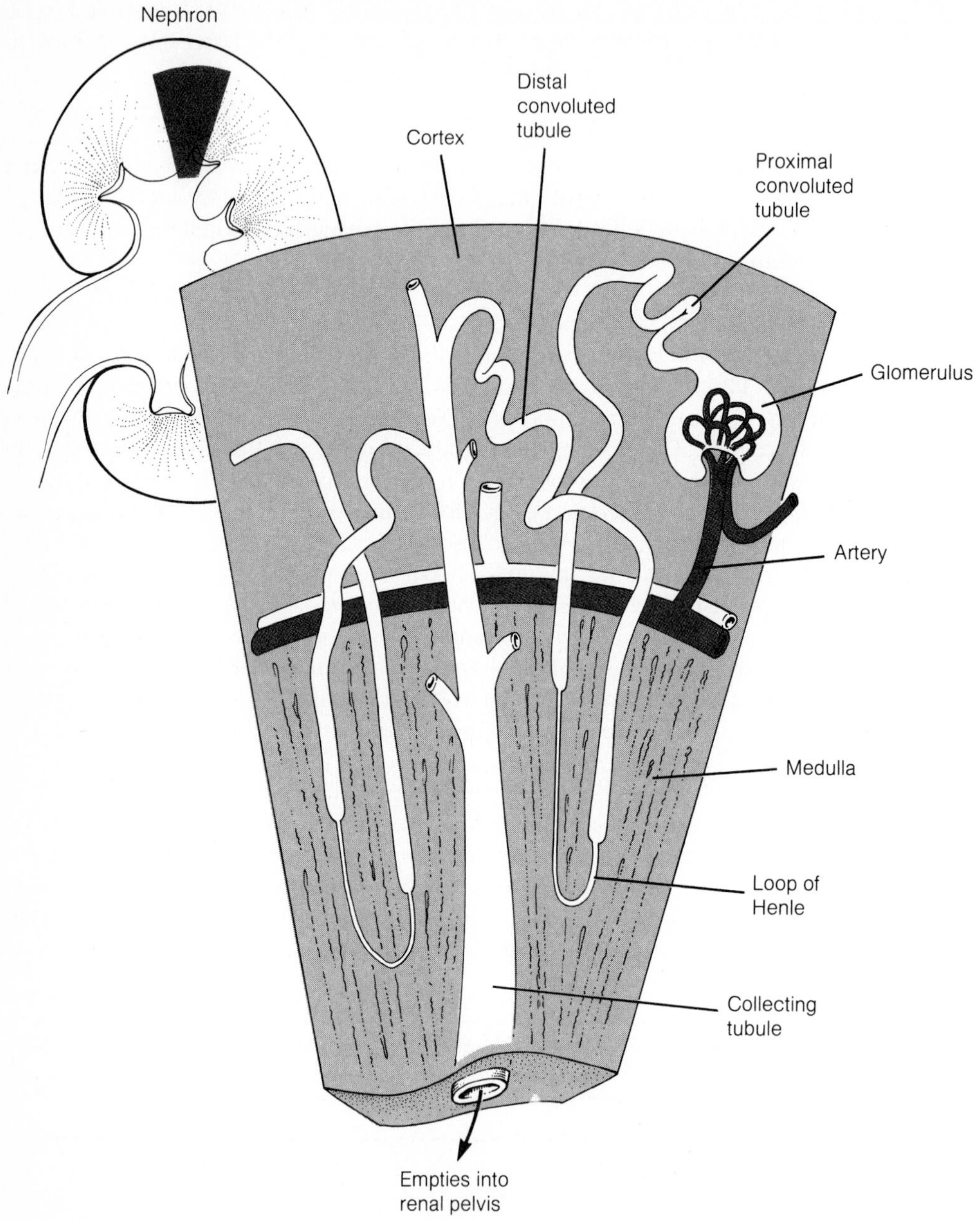

FIG. 2-2 The nephron-functional unit of the kidney.

flow through the successive sections of some one million nephrons in each kidney. Two hormones, vasopressin and aldosterone (p. 15), control the reabsorption of water and electrolytes according to need. Together they protect the integrity of the blood volume and maintain adequate blood circulation despite real or threatened deprivation of water or sodium.

NUTRIENT BALANCE: BODY NUTRITIONAL STATUS

Balances among the various nutrients, as well as intake-output balance for individual nutrients, determine the nutritional status. In turn, the body composition reflects the nature of this individual nutritional status, in both body structure and function. For example, just as energy balance largely depends on fuel intake of adequate carbohydrate and fat, so protein balance depends on an adequate intake of food protein to build and maintain the body's tissue protein mass.

Protein Balance

The primary function of dietary protein is to supply amino acids in the amount and kind necessary for growth and maintenance of body tissue protein. Thus protein intake must balance with protein consumption by the lean body mass, the internal tissue protein turnover and metabolic amino acid pool, as well as with overall nitrogen balance.

1. **Protein turnover.** The use of radioactive isotopes has clearly demonstrated that the body's protein tissues are continually being broken down into amino acids and then resynthesized into new tissue proteins.[3] When "labeled" amino acids are fed, they are rapidly incorporated into various body tissue proteins. The rate of this turnover varies in different tissues. It is highest in intestinal mucosa, liver, pancreas, kidney, and plasma. It is lower in muscle, brain, and skin tissue. It is much slower in structural tissues such as bone.
2. **Protein compartment balance.** Body protein exists in a balance between two compartments, the tissue protein compartment and the plasma protein compartment. These internal stores are further balanced with dietary protein intake. Protein from one compartment may be drawn to supply a need in the other. But even when the intake of protein and other nutrients is adequate, the tissue proteins are still continually being broken down and reformed. The body's state of stability, then, results from this dynamic balance between the rates of protein breakdown and synthesis. In periods of growth, the synthesis (anabolic) rate is higher so that new tissue will form. Conversely, in conditions of hunger and disease, and more gradually in the aging process, the breakdown (catabolic) rate exceeds that of synthesis, and the body slowly deteriorates.
3. **Metabolic amino acid pool.** The biologic term *pool* is useful to describe the body's internal collective supply of amino acids scattered in various parts of the body tissues and organs. This metabolic pool of amino acids provides a reserve of available amino acids for tissue synthesis. Amino acids from tissue breakdown and from dietary protein digestion and absorption make up the metabolic pool. A balance of amino acids that satisfies the body's needs is maintained. Shifts and balances between these two sources ensure the constant availability of a balanced mixture of

amino acids. From this amino acid reserve pool, specific amino acids can be supplied as needed for specific protein synthesis. This important overall balance is illustrated in Fig. 2-3.

4. **Nitrogen balance.** A measure of protein balance is provided by the body's overall nitrogen balance, although nitrogen is also found in body compounds other than amino acids. Total nitrogen balance is the net result of all nitrogen gains and losses in all protein compartments of the body, though it gives no picture of the shifts in distribution of nitrogen. Nevertheless, in most cases the total nitrogen balance is a useful measure of nitrogen equilibrium and hence general nutritional status (p. 60).

Mineral Balance

To protect the mineral component of its composition, mainly the skeletal mass, the body maintains an intake-output balance as well as an internal mineral balance. For example, intake of the major mineral calcium balances with the bone compartment calcium, which in turn balances with the ionized plasma calcium. Similar balances exist with other minerals, and with vitamins, to ensure the body's overall sound nutritional status and healthy body composition.

Body Composition Components

BODY COMPARTMENTS BASED ON METABOLIC ACTIVITY

Basic Concepts of Compartments and Balance

Using the two basic concepts of body compartments and balance for a foundation, we may seek an appropriate means of identifying and describing the gross compo-

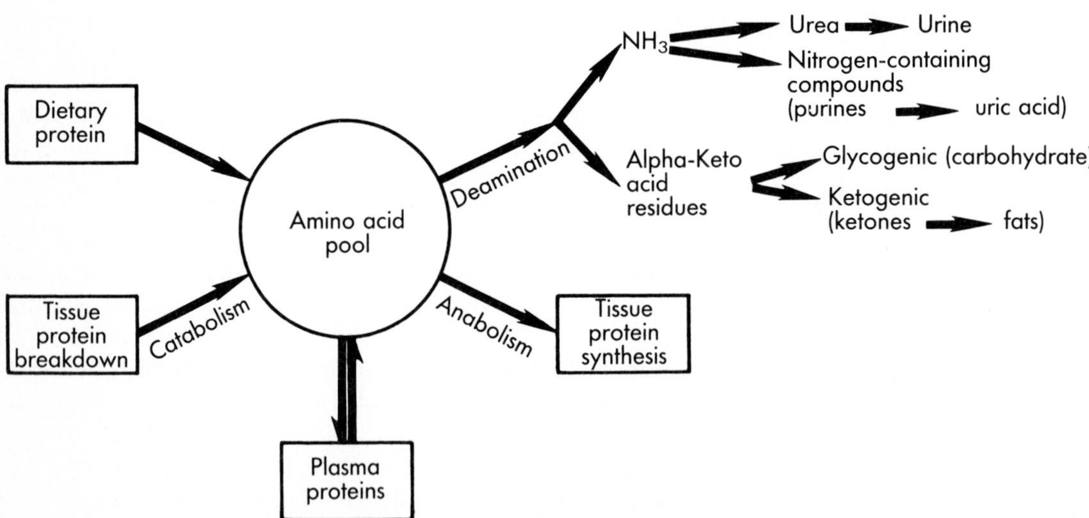

FIG. 2-3 Balance between protein compartments and amino acid pool.

nents of body composition, especially in relation to our basic interest here in body changes and nutrition needs through the life cycle. The concept of balance provides us with a dynamic view of the body, ever changing and adjusting to its external and internal environments. The concept of compartments gives us a comprehensive view, not of static mechanical parts, but of a dynamic, interrelated whole. The nutritional needs of individuals throughout growth and development can be understood through the application of these two basic concepts.

Traditional Approaches

A number of approaches have been used to classify the basic components of body composition. Holliday[4] used the traditional divisions of body systems to develop a model based on functional aspects of body composition in four categories: (1) organ systems such as liver, heart, etc.; (2) locomotion—the muscle mass; (3) energy storage—adipose tissue; and (4) extracellular fluid and supporting structures such as bone. In this model the first two categories, organ systems and muscle mass, account for the bulk of the body protein. However, traditional approaches based on kinds of body parts such as cartilaginous skeleton, bony skeleton, and voluntary muscle, or on body systems, such as skeletal system, nervous system, and muscular system, fail to satisfy on two counts: (1) measurement of relative components in the living body, and (2) body nutritional status and relative sensitivity to nutritional effects.[5]

Other Influencing Factors

Other factors influencing the relative composition of body components must also be taken into consideration. These factors include varying tissue densities, body temperature, state of body hydration, and weight status in terms of obesity or underweight.

Metabolic Activity

Since our interest here is in nutrition, particularly nutritional status as a means of determining nutritional needs throughout life, we will use the criterion of metabolic activity to define the gross components of body composition. On this basis many researchers commonly distinguish four main components in two divisions: (1) those parts that are most active in energy metabolism, and (2) those parts that are relatively inactive. The parts that are relatively inactive in energy metabolism are the **body fat,** the **extracellular water**, and the **mineral mass** of the bones and smaller structural parts. The remaining body compartment most active in energy metabolism is the **lean body mass.** This component has also been variously termed the body protein compartment, the active tissue mass, the body cell mass, or the cell residue.

LEAN BODY MASS COMPARTMENT

The body's lean cell mass is the primary determinant of its energy requirements. Thus the overall body composition in terms of this major body compartment largely determines the body's nutrient needs. Its relative size and metabolic activity, as well as its relation to weight changes, are important considerations.

Compartment Size and Metabolic Activity

In various individuals the lean body mass, as a collective compartment of the body's active fat-free mass of cells, will account for anything from 30% to 65% of the total body weight. However, in any person it accounts for almost all of the energy consumption. As a percentage of body weight, for example, the values for this lean cell mass will range from low levels in very fat, sedentary persons who are also edematous, to higher levels in very muscular persons who are also dehydrated.

Relation to Weight Changes

When persons gain or lose weight due to diet changes, it is not merely a reflection of changes in the body fat mass but also in the lean body mass. Numerous studies have shown that the density of the tissue added or lost is never that of pure fat.[5] The density of the nonfat lean part also changes with nutritional status. Added exercise enhances its relative size.

BODY FAT COMPARTMENT

Compartment Size

The gross amount of the body fat component can vary widely according to individual degrees of obesity. In general, the fat compartment reflects the number and size of fat cells—*adipocytes*—making up the adipose tissue. However, adipose tissue is not pure fat. It also contains parts of other compartments such as blood vessels, connective tissue, cell membranes, and water. The body fat compartment has been variously estimated in healthy persons in relation to a standard "reference body" and from body water measurements to range in an adult man, for example, from about 14% to 28% of the total body weight. The woman's "reference body" would have a somewhat larger fat compartment, about 15% to 29% of total body weight. These percentages vary with factors such as age, climate, exercise, and fitness. About half of the total body fat is in the subcutaneous fat layers, which serve the important task of helping to maintain body temperature.

Relation to Health

Extremes in size of the body fat compartment can affect individual health status. For example, some athletes, especially compulsive runners, may strive for a very low level of body fat, even in some cases to an unhealthy deficit. Conversely, at the other extreme, massively obese sedentary persons carry increased health risks from an excessively large body fat mass. However, common beliefs that even moderate overweight brings poorer health and a shorter life span are unfounded. Population studies show that it is the extremes of both underweight and obesity that increase health risks. In a recent study of elderly persons, Mattila[6] found that higher mortality rates occurred with underweight and obese persons, concluding that moderate amounts of overweight may actually be a health protection.

BODY WATER COMPARTMENT

Total Body Water

The total body water content varies widely with relative body composition in terms of leanness and fatness, since lean muscle tissue contains more water than any body tissue other than blood. It also varies with age, being relatively higher in infants, and with hydration status, being lower in conditions causing dehydration and higher in conditions causing edema or ascities. In pregnancy the total maternal body water increases normally to support the increased metabolic work, and sometimes abnormally when complications of pregnancy-induced hypertension occur. As indicated the total body water is divided into two sub-compartments—the collective water inside the cells and the remaining collective water outside of cells. The water inside of cells is part of the active cell mass or lean body mass. So it is the remaining collective water outside of cells, the extracellular fluid (ECF), that makes up this designated water compartment of gross body composition.

ECF Compartment

Since the size of the ECF compartment varies with individual fatness or leanness, it is higher in thin persons and lower in fat persons. In average weight adults, the collective water outside cells makes up about 20% of the total body weight. In fat persons, it accounts for about 15% of the total weight; in thin persons, about 25%. The ECF consists of four parts: (1) *blood plasma,* which accounts for approximately 25% of the ECF and 5% of body weight; (2) *interstitial fluid,* the water surrounding the cells; (3) *secretory fluid,* the circulating water in transit; and (4) *dense tissue fluid,* the water in dense connective tissue, cartilage, and bone (see Fig. 2-1).

BODY MINERAL COMPARTMENT

The body's major mineral content by far is found in its large skeletal mass, with much smaller amounts in teeth, nails, and hair. Of all the minerals in the human body, calcium is present in far greater amounts than any other, comprising about 2% of the total body weight.

Skeletal Mass

The human skeleton is a relatively large structure, comprising in the living body about one-sixth of the total body mass. Most of the body calcium—about 99%—is in the skeleton, accounting for most of the body mineral compartment. Other minerals occur in varying lesser amounts in the body mineral compartment.

Mineral Ash

Only a small part of the skeletal mass, however, is comprised of bone mineral matter. The other components of bone—water, protein, and fat—are accounted for in their respective body composition compartments. In its dried defatted state, the skeleton represents only about 6% of the gross body weight. Bone mineral mass as estimated from bone ash values is about 5% of total body weight.

Methods of Measuring Body Composition

A number of methods have been developed by researchers to study the composition of the human body. The initial direct method of postmortem examination has provided important data but has obvious limitations. Current indirect research methods continue to provide more important information. All of these methods have their limitations, but a growing body of knowledge about the human body has developed through contributions of each approach. Here we will briefly describe two of these methods that have emerged from research for use in general practice along with the basic tools of anthropometrics.

DIRECT AND INDIRECT METHODS

Direct Method

Direct analyses of human body composition are done by postmortem examination of the main components of whole bodies.[5] However, many technical and legal problems greatly limit available data from these direct sources. Nonetheless, the value of these data lies in: (1) validation of current indirect methods of measuring body composition; and (2) demonstration of the wide range of human variability in body composition. This latter fact is sometimes forgotten in the frequent assumptions of body composition constancy, which though reasonable on the average do not hold in individual cases. Grande and Keys[5] have studied several reports of gross body composition from direct chemical analyses of adult male bodies, with results expressed as percentage of total body weight: Water 63%, protein or lean body mass 16%, fat 15%, and mineral ash 6%.

Indirect Methods

A number of indirect methods for measuring the various compartments of the living body have been developed for use in research, field situations, and clinical work. These methods are based on such physiologic and biochemical principles as tissue density, water dilution and displacement, radioactive body emissions, light absorption and reflection, ultrasonics, electrical conductivity and resistance, radiation absorption, and related estimates from body size and anatomic features. All of these methods have limitations that must be considered in applying results. Most of them require sophisticated equipment and hence are used mainly in research centers and in population studies. Nonetheless, they have helped to develop and validate procedures and standards for simpler methods such as anthropometrics. Two of these research methods, infrared interactance and absorptiometry, are briefly described here because they have emerged from the laboratory in redesigned smaller form and are appearing in health-care offices and clinics for use in current practice. Response to their use with clients and patients is mixed. They need evaluation.

INFRARED INTERACTANCE

Principles

The infrared interactance (IRI) method of analyzing body composition was developed by a team of scientists at the Agricultural Research Service of the U.S. Department of Agriculture. It is based on principles of light absorption and reflection by materials of differing densities. It uses near-infrared rays in the light spectrum and measures radiation response.

Method

A single-beam rapid scanning instrument directs the infrared-area rays of the light spectrum. A fiber-optic probe or "wand" conducts the light scan to selected body sites and collects the interactive radiation, which is then measured by spectrophotometry.[7] The body sites used are the five common ones used in surface skinfold measures: triceps, biceps, subscapular, suprailiac, and thigh. Of these sites, the biceps measure alone seems to give a good estimate of body fat.[8] Derived values for body density and body fat are calculated. Currently the ARS team is developing a simple portable instrument, a small-scale model of their computerized spectrophotometer, which may prove to be a useful tool for office and clinic practice.

PHOTON ABSORPTIOMETRY

Principles

In a similar method, but using a different form of radiation, absorptiometry is based on principles of varying radiation absorption rates by body tissues of differing densities. For example, the mineral mass of harder bone tissue would have a different radiation absorption rate from that of the lean-fat content of soft tissue.

Method

Controlled low-dose radiation scans (1-2 mrem) of the body are done and a special instrument measures the degree of absorption by body tissues. Mazess and associates[9] have developed methods of using dual-photon external radiation beams of the rare element gadolinium (^{153}Gd) in low doses (1-2 mrem) for absorption scans to measure skeletal mineral mass, as well as total body composition of lean and fat compartments.

Current Use in Osteoporosis

Because of its sensitive measure of bone mass, dual-photon absorptiometry (DPA) is currently considered by some observers to be the best detection technique for osteoporosis, a condition of increased bone mass loss.[10] Influenced by increasing media attention to this "in" disorder, some 500 or more osteoporosis screening clinics using this method have opened recently across the country. These clinics use two tests: (1) single-photon absorptiometry (SPA), which measures the density of bones in the forearm; and (2) dual-photon absorptiometry (DPA), which measures density of the vertebrae. However, other observers, researchers and consumers alike, question such indiscriminate marketing to the public, which at best seems premature with claims that are unjustified by current research.[11] Cummings and Black,[12] in a recent review of the medical literature, indicate that DPA is not a sure risk assessment of vertebral fracture associated with osteoporosis, and should be reserved for use with diagnosed high-risk women as a clinical monitoring tool, which, along with other tools, can be used to determine medical treatment. They warn that no test can accurately predict who will suffer a hip fracture in old age, since researchers themselves do not know what degree of bone loss can serve as a marker. Further, SPA used alone, as it is in many of the screening centers, has no real value, since osteoporosis of the hip and spine, the most common fracture sites, has little or no relation to bone loss in the forearm.

ANTHROPOMETRICS

Principles

Anthropometric measures of body size and contours, together with caliper-measured skinfold thicknesses at selected sites, provide useful tools in general practice for estimating relative body composition. The thickness of the subcutaneous fat layer is related to total body fat, regardless of the individual body frame or type. Thus skinfold measures, taken with accurate technique, are simple yet valid indicators for estimating body fat content. Together with outer circumference measures at special sites such as the upper arm (triceps), they also help to estimate skeletal muscle mass from calculated inner midarm muscle circumference values. Anthropometric measures vary with age, sex, body build, and physical activity. They may be distorted by illness. These factors must be considered in interpreting values obtained in practice. However, studies comparing anthropometrics with some of the more sophisticated research methods have shown remarkably close correlations.[7,9]

Methods

Detailed procedures for various anthropometric measures of body composition are described in the following chapter on nutrition assessment.

Body Composition Changes During the Life Cycle

THE CONCEPT OF HUMAN GROWTH

Normal human growth and development is not only a period of highly visible changes in exterior body size. It is also a cycle of important changes in the interior body composition. The word "cycle" is significant here. It indicates a set, progressive course relating the twin concepts of human *growth* and *development* to the concepts of *velocity* and *acceleration.* In the changing physical human body, the term "growth" refers to an increase in cell number and size. The associated term "development" refers to an increased functional ability of these cells or groups of cells (tissues and organs). At different times in the cycle of human growth and its associated body development, the "velocity" of that growth, that is, the general rate of movement along its set direction or course, will vary. At times it will be rapid and at other times it will be slower. Then at certain set points in the cycle, the growth will speed up or "accelerate." For example, this growth acceleration is particularly evident at the beginning of puberty when hormones flood the body and speed up its metabolic machinery for rapid movement or "velocity" of growth during this adolescent period. Then at the end of puberty, the growth rate decelerates and maintains a slower and gradually declining velocity through adulthood.

This pattern of growth during the life cycle is described below, but each person's movement along this cycle is individual. Within healthy ranges, each person moves along at his or her own speed. Also, throughout this fundamental life process, the relative composition of the body and its parts will be influenced by weight gain or loss and degrees of physical training, as well as by diseases that may occur. The normal human growth pattern, genetically set and nurtured by nutritional and psychosocial support, follows distinct phases from its beginning in fetal life to its decline in old age.

NORMAL LIFE CYCLE GROWTH PATTERN

Fetal Life

The most rapid growth and development of the human body occurs during the short 9 months of embryonic-fetal life. From the early 8 weeks of embryonic growth and differentiation of major organs and tissues, through the intensive fetal growth of the remaining months to term, the newborn has reached an average birth weight of about 3.2 kg (7 lb).

Infancy

During the first year of life the infant's rapid growth continues, with the rate tapering off somewhat in the latter half of the year. At age 6 months an infant will probably weigh twice what it weighed at birth and at one year may weigh three times its birth weight.

Latent Period of Childhood

During the years between infancy and adolescence, the rate of growth slows and becomes erratic. At some periods there are plateaus; at others small spurts of growth occur. The overall erratic rate affects appetite accordingly.

Adolescence

The second rapid rate of growth occurs during adolescence, when the body undergoes the enormous physical changes of puberty. Hormonal influences bring multiple body changes, including the growth and development of long bones, sex characteristics, and fat and muscle mass.

Adulthood

In the final phase of the normal life cycle, growth in body size levels off in the adult plateau, with continued cell growth and reproduction maintaining the body. Then there is a gradual decline in old age.

MATERNAL-FETAL GROWTH AND DEVELOPMENT

Highly important maternal-fetal body changes occur during pregnancy. You will find details of this unique maternal-fetal-placental relationship that nurtures the beginnings of human growth and development in Chapter 4. All of these vital changes support the pregnancy and bring it to a healthy and successful outcome.

Maternal Body Composition Changes

Sufficient increases in body size and composition are essential to support the demands of pregnancy. These changes in the major components of body composition reflect the maternal body's normal physiologic adaptation. In a biologic sense, the maternal organism, fetus, and placenta all interact to create a new balanced whole, not existing before, and produce a total effect greater than and different from the mere sum of their parts. This is a prime example of biologic *synergism,* all for the purpose of sustaining and nurturing the pregnancy and its offspring. All major maternal body components are affected:

1. **Body weight.** About 900 to 1800 g (2 to 4 lb) is an average gain during the first trimester. Thereafter, about 450 g (1 lb) a week during the remainder of the pregnancy is usual, although an individual woman may gain more or less depending on her pre-conception weight and nutrition status. The nutritional quality of the gain is the important factor in nourishing the pregnancy with positive energy and protein balances to fulfill the increased metabolic and tissue growth needs.
2. **Body water.** Of the total tissue gained in an average pregnancy, the largest component—62%—is water. Water is also the most variable component of tissue gained, accounting for a range of from 8 kg (18 lb) to as much as 11 kg (24 lb). Of the 8 kg of water usually gained, about 5.5 kg (12 lb) is associated with the fetal tissues and other maternal tissues gained during pregnancy. The remaining 2.5 kg (6 lb) of water accumulates in the maternal interstitial tissue spaces. The connective tissue becomes more *hygroscopic,* that is, has a greater affinity for water, due to estrogen-induced changes in the ground substance.[13] The connective tissue thus becomes softer and more easily distended to facilitate delivery through the cervix and vaginal canal. Also the increased total body water is necessary to handle the increased metabolic work and circulation of the many resulting metabolites essential for fetal growth.
3. **Body protein mass.** Nitrogen-balance studies give some indication of the large amounts of nitrogen used by the mother and child during pregnancy. The increased maternal body protein mass is made up of: (1) the enlargement of the uterus, mammary glands, and placenta; (2) the increased plasma protein required by the increased circulating blood volume to maintain normal serum albumin levels for shifting water and nutrients to and from the tissue fluids bathing the cells; and (3) storage reserves for labor, delivery, and lactation.
4. **Body fat.** Fat accounts for 31% of the total body tissue gained in an average pregnancy. These additional maternal stores provide energy support to fetal growth during the latter part of pregnancy and to lactation. These maternal stores are variable, about 1800-3600 g (4-8 lb).
5. **Body mineral mass.** The maternal bone-mineral mass remains relatively unchanged during the pregnancy. The major mineral storage is the rapid mineralization of the fetal skeletal tissue.

Fetal Body Composition Changes

During the gestation period the fetus grows rapidly, especially during the latter phase when the major growth in body size occurs.[14] The increase in size of body composition compartments during the latter weeks of growth is indicated in Table 2-3.

1. **Body water.** During the final week of gestation, the fetal body water increases about 9 ml a day. This rate gives an indication of the rapid increase in total body water during the final body growth period.
2. **Lean body mass.** The protein stores increase rapidly in proportion to the increase in body size. By week 40 of gestation, the near-term fetus is increasing in body protein mass by 2.5 g a day.
3. **Body fat.** The body fat compartment also increases in proportion as the body grows larger. At near term, the average fetus is gaining body fat at a rate of 5 g a day.
4. **Skeletal bone mass.** Two-thirds of the full-term infant's total body mineral content is deposited during the last 2 months of fetal life. This reflects a faster rate of skeletal mineralization shortly before birth than during the first 6 months of infancy.

Comparison of Premature and Full-Term Infants

Since much of the fetal growth occurs in the final weeks of gestation, the premature infant lacks this important completion of body composition components before birth. Thus the premature infant's body composition differs from that of full-term infants in significant ways: (1) they have more water and less protein and minerals per kg body weight; (2) there is little subcutaneous fat; and (3) bones are poorly calcified.

INFANT BODY COMPOSITION CHANGES

Infant growth is very rapid during the first 4-6 months, following a brief adjustment to life outside the uterus. Then the rate slows somewhat over the second half of the infant's first year. Increases and adjustments in body composition relate to this rapid growth pattern.[15]

Body Water

During the first 4 months, the average infant increases body weight by about 3.5 kg (7.7 lb), of which 45.3% is water. By the end of the first year, another 3.5 kg is added, of which 56.6% is water. The infant's total body water makes up a greater proportion of total body weight than does the adult's; infants need more water relative to size than do adults to manage renal excretion. Also, a greater proportion of the infant's total body water is outside of cells (ECF) and therefore more vulnerable to loss.

TABLE 2-3 Near-term Fetal Growth in Weight and Body Composition Gains

Fetal Age (weeks)	Body Composition (g)			Weight (g)
	Water	LBM*	Fat	
36–37	35.7	4.83	5.6	35.7
37–38	21.4	4.34	5.6	31.4
38–39	15.4	3.44	5.4	24.3
39–40	9.6	2.50	5.0	17.1

Adapted from Rosso, P.: Nutritional needs of the human fetus, Clinical Nutrition, 2(5):4, September-October, 1983.
*Lean body mass

Body Fat

Of the average infant's weight gain of 3.5 kg during the first 4 months, 41.6% is fat. This rapid increase in body fat during the first half year demands a high caloric intake per kg body weight. During the remaining months of the first year, another 3.5 kg increase in weight occurs, about 19% of which is fat. This overall increase in body fat supplies fuel, support and protection for vital organs, and control of body temperature by the subcutaneous fat layer.

Body Protein Mass

The protein component of the 3.5 kg gain during the first 4 months of life is 11.4% protein tissue. By the end of the first year, another 3.5 kg is gained, 21% of which is protein tissue.

Body Mineral Mass

Of the first 4 months weight gain of 3.5 kg, the remaining 1.7% is composed of other material, mainly body mineral mass. Of the second 3.5 kg weight increase during the remainder of the first year, 3.3% is mineral mass.

A summary of these body composition increases during the infant year is given in Table 2-4.

CHILDHOOD BODY COMPOSITION

Toddler (1-3 Years)

Following the first year of rapid growth, the rate of childhood growth slows. Although the rate of gain is less, the pattern of growth produces significant gradual overall changes in body form and composition. The legs become longer, and the child begins losing baby fat. There is less total body water and more water inside the cells. The young child begins to look and feel less like a baby and more like a child. There are fewer energy demands because of the slackened growth. However, important muscle development is taking place. Muscle mass development accounts for about one-half of the total weight gain during this period. As the child begins to walk and stand erect, more muscle is needed to strengthen the body. There is special need, for example, for the big muscles of the back, buttocks, and thighs. The overall rate of skeletal growth slows, but there is more deposit of mineral to build bone density rather than lengthening the bones.

TABLE 2-4 Infant and Early Childhood Growth in Weight and Body Composition

Age (months)	Body Composition of Gain (%)				Weight Gain (kg)
	Water	LBM*	Fat	Other†	
0-4	45.3	11.4	41.6	1.7	3.5
4-12	56.6	21.0	19.1	3.3	3.5
12-24	69.4	20.3	6.8	3.5	2.5
24-36	68.5	20.9	3.4	7.2	2.0

Adapted from Paige, D.M.: Infant growth and nutrition, Clinical Nutrition, 2(5):15, September-October 1983.
*Lean body mass
†Mainly mineral mass

Preschooler (3-6 Years)

Slow, erratic growth continues through these preschool years of young childhood. Protein needs continue to be relatively high as lean body mass develops. The continuing development of skeletal muscles brings increases in intracellular water, since skeletal muscle cells have a high water content. As age advances the proportion of extracellular water decreases. The proportion of body fat, though variable, remains fairly constant with small periodic increases. A similar pattern of slow development is seen in the mineral mass component.

School-Aged Child (6-12 Years)

The school-age period has been called the latent time of growth. It is like a film in slow motion, the lull before the storm, awaiting the burst of adolescence. The gradually developing pattern of body composition continues. As the rate of growth slows, body changes occur in similar fashion. However, beneath the surface resources are being stored for the rapid adolescent growth ahead. By now the body type has been established, and growth rates vary widely. Girls usually outdistance boys by the latter part of the period.

ADOLESCENT BODY COMPOSITION CHANGES

General Pattern of Development

With the onset of puberty, under the stimulus of growth and sex hormones, the growth rate accelerates markedly and proceeds at a greater velocity during this final period of childhood growth and development. Maturation during this time varies so widely that chronological age is a less useful reference point. *Physiologic age* becomes more important in dealing with individual boys and girls. It accounts for wide variability in metabolic rates and body composition changes. Dramatic body changes result from hormones regulating the development of sex characteristics. The rate of these changes also varies widely and is particularly distinct in growth pattern differences that emerge between the sexes.

Height and Weight

During this period of rapid growth, in each facet of body change we see two basic characteristics very clearly: (1) magnitude and (2) variability. They are large changes and they vary widely. In height, adolescents achieve 15% to 25% of their adult stature over a 3 to 4 year time span.[16] In boys the "peak height velocity"—the year in which the greatest increase in height occurs—is reached at about age 14. In girls it occurs earlier at about age 12. We see similar patterns in weight changes. In boys from age 10 to 17, the average weight increase is 32 kg (70 lb), accounting for 51% of the adult body mass. In girls from age 10 to 17, the increase is 24 kg (53 lb), accounting for 42% of their young-adult weight. The duration of this weight gain in boys and girls is similar to that for height, though wide variations exist among normal teenagers in both rate and amount of height and weight increases.

Body Fat

From infancy and childhood, girls have more adipose tissue than boys.[16] After the rapid body changes of adolescence, the body fat component in girls is about twice that in boys, expressed as a percentage of total body weight. Adipose cell (adipocyte) size increases at puberty, with gradual growth throughout adolescence into young adulthood. By the end of the rapid changes of adolescent growth, both sexes have about the same number of fat cells. However, the fat cells of females are larger than those of males. This helps to account for the larger body fat component in women than in men.

Body Mineral Mass

The rate of increase in bone mass is rapid during the accelerated growth of adolescence. With the rapid linear growth and increasing height comes lengthening of long bones and increased skeletal mineral mass. The obvious characteristics in boys are greater stature, muscular torso, and broad shoulders. In girls the distinctive feature is wider hips. From birth, in the female skeletal pattern the pelvic outlet is larger than that of males. Over the adolescent growth period, this difference increases. In girls pelvic growth both in absolute amount and in relation to stature results in a broadened pelvic girth and a much greater hip width. Adequate mineral intake is essential in the adolescent diet to sustain this growth in density of body mineral mass.

Body Water

As percentages of total body weight, both total body water and extracellular water gradually decrease with age. However, since muscle tissue contains a relatively large amount of cell water, the proportion of water outside of cells declines more than that of total body water. Studies of body water content in childhood and adolescence indicate that by age 16 the total body water averages 58.4% of the total body weight.[5] Of this total water, the larger amount—38.5% of body weight—is inside of cells. The other 19.9% is outside of cells.

ADULT BODY COMPOSITION CHANGES

At a certain point of "chemical maturity," overall childhood body growth is achieved and a general pattern of relative adult body composition is set for maintaining the physically mature individual. Adults change very slowly over the remaining years of the life cycle from young adulthood through old age. As in younger years, there is also great variability in individual response to the process of aging. Genetic heritage lays the foundation; life situations influence the outcome.

Young Adults (18-40 Years)

At the end of adolescence, as indicated, the physically mature body is set. Young women have larger fat cells resulting in a larger body fat mass, as well as a wider pelvic girth, to support reproduction. They are generally smaller in body size, with less weight and height. Young men have a larger skeletal muscle mass. They are generally larger in body size, with more weight and height.

Middle Adults (40-60 Years)

During the middle adult years, there is a gradual decrease in lean body mass and a relative increase in body weight due to fat. In mid-life, as an indication of the related fat component, triceps skinfold thicknesses increase for both sexes. In middle-aged men, this increase is usually slight, but in women it is greater and fluctuates more. Studies have shown that with each decade after age 30 there is a 6.3% decrease in lean body mass.[17]

Older Adults (60-80+ years)

The changing pattern of adult body composition continues and becomes more marked in aging. Potassium-40 isotope measures of lean body mass show a continuous age-related decline that accelerates in later life.[17] For example, an average loss of 1 kg of lean body mass between ages 70-75 years has been reported, and at about age 70 the skeletal muscle in protein g per kg body weight returns almost to the level it was at birth. The newborn level of approximately 200 g protein per kg body weight rises to about 450 g between ages 21-30 years. Then it gradually decreases until at age 70 it is nearly to the beginning infant value of about 200 g again. Skinfold measures in older adults become less accurate to indicate body fat stores because of changes in skin compressibility and the pendulous and redundant fat folds.

Reference Body Composition Standards

It is evident that body composition changes widely with age and sex during the adult years. Frame size also helps to account for some of this variability. Using a measure of elbow breadth to determine skeletal breadth, Frisancho[18] has provided more comprehensive standards of weight and body composition by frame size and height. These recent standards provide more realistic references for assessment of nutritional status of adults aged 25-54 years, and for older adults aged 55-74 years.

EFFECT OF WEIGHT CHANGES AND PHYSICAL TRAINING ON BODY COMPOSITION

Obesity and Weight Reduction

As obesity develops and a person grows fatter, the skeletal mineral mass remains fairly constant. However, to carry the increasing weight, adjustments must be made in other body compartments. More muscle is needed, more blood vessels are required to serve the increasing tissue, more skin must develop to cover the larger body surface area.

Concepts of Reference Body and Obesity Tissue

To meet practical needs for estimating the body fat and other tissue changes with weight gains and losses, Grande and Keys[5] developed the concepts of "reference body" and "obesity tissue." The reference body used for comparison is that of a healthy man aged 25 with height and weight corresponding to those of the U.S. standard height-weight tables. Obesity tissue refers to the sum of the various body tissues gained or lost by healthy men during experimental periods of 6 months. These researchers found that this obesity tissue is not all fat. It is composed of 14% extracellular fluid (ECF), 62% fat, and 24% cell residue. When a person gains weight, fat deposits as measured by skinfolds seem to be larger in the abdominal area. But when an obese person loses weight on a reduction diet the fat changes tend to be distributed proportionally in all parts of the body. During the weight-loss process, body water and fat decrease first, and a following loss in lean body mass is avoided by increasing physical exercise. Gradually such a person may maintain a healthy weight with a changed body composition of smaller fat and ECF components and increased lean body mass. Athletes develop similar body composition patterns during training and competition.

Abnormal Weight Loss and Rehabilitation

For some persons, excessive and compulsive fixation on lean body mass and loss of body fat can become obsessive and enduring. For example, a compulsive runner's ideal of 5% body fat may lead him to seek even lower levels, despite physical indications against it. Such striving has even resulted in some persons suffering permanent disabilities and death, sometimes from cardiac arrest caused by a prolonged deficiency of linoleic acid, the essential fatty acid preferred as fuel by the heart muscle.[19] Similar compulsive ideals of 5% body fat are regularly found in ballet dancers, gymnasts, models, and victims of anorexia nervosa. Young women and adolescent girls suffering from anorexia nervosa, an increasingly common form of malnutrition in Western society, experience a reduction in both lean body mass and body fat. The wasting process is not limited to the body fat stores. Hence, recovery must involve increases in both the lean and fat components of the body. But such rehabilitation does not necessarily require a high-protein diet. Forbes and associates[20] studied patients with anorexia nervosa using two different diets, one providing 20% of the daily energy from protein and the other 10%. In all the subjects, ages 13-22, there was no significant difference in body composition measures used to monitor progress. During recovery about two-thirds of the weight gained in each case was lean tissue, regardless of which diet was used.

BODY COMPOSITION CHANGES IN DISEASE

In varying degrees, numerous diseases alter body composition during the life cycle. Hypermetabolic conditions, tumor-host imbalances, deficient immune system syndromes, or diseases affecting body organ systems that control body composition balances can create life-threatening effects on various body components. Three examples are used here to illustrate these effects:

Cancer Cachexia

Although decreased food intake plays a role, the syndrome of cancer cachexia is not merely the result of progressive starvation in the affected person. Rather, it is a far more complex metabolic problem resulting from complications of the disease and its treatment.[21] There is a progressive depletion of body fat as adipose tissue mobilizes its fatty acids to be used as sources of energy. There is also a progressive loss of muscle mass from both increased breakdown and decreased synthesis of protein tissue. Total body water, both ICF and ECF, increase. The only effective treatment is the control and cure of the cancer by surgery, radiation, or chemotherapy. However, vigorous personalized nutritional management can provide needed support for these medical treatments and increase successful results.

Acquired Immunodeficiency Syndrome (AIDS)

The devastating effects of this newly described disorder of immune function may bring infections or tumors, rapid deterioration, or chronic and relentless wasting of the body. Studies by Kottler[22] and his research associates, measuring a number of body composition variables in AIDS patients, demonstrated the extent of losses in body fat and lean body mass, without repletion, over times of apparent clinical stability. Total body water was affected, with a decrease in ICF and increase in ECF. These studies indicate that severe progressive malnutrition occurs in AIDS patients, and a key question is the effect that this malnutrition has on the underlying immune deficiency. While the vital search continues for control of the AIDS virus, nutritional therapy of the malnutrition may play an important role in treatment since malnutrition from any cause is an insult to the immune system.

Renal Disease

Through its destructive effect on the kidneys' nephrons, renal disease decreases the body's ability to maintain normal water and nutrient balances. In nephrosis there is massive protein loss and body water imbalance, with evidence of the grossly distorted increase in ECF in abdominal ascites. In advancing chronic renal failure, catabolism decreases the lean body mass. Osteodystrophy from loss of the kidneys' role in activating vitamin D causes bone calcium loss and diminishes body mineral mass. Water and electrolyte losses bring dehydration.

Summary

Throughout the human life cycle, body composition is a basic reflection of nutritional status. Its ideal maintenance during the early growth and development years, as well as in aging through the adult years, is a primary health goal. This ideal body composition is sustained by body balances in energy, water, and nutrients. The gross components of body composition are lean body mass, fat, water, and mineral mass. These components can be measured directly by postmortem examinations, but current study uses a variety of indirect measures including differing responses to light and radiation by tissues of different densities. The most common method used in general health care practice is anthropometrics.

Body composition changes during the life cycle in ways that both support and reflect the needs of normal growth and development. From the rapid fetal changes that sustain the beginning of life to the gradual changes of aging that signal the decline of life, nutritional intake provides vital life supports, which are conditioned by weight changes and state of physical fitness. Abnormal changes result from various diseases that interfere with these life supports.

Review Questions

1. Describe four basic forms of the body's physiologic balance. What does the term "homeostasis" mean? Relate the concepts of change and balance to this term.
2. Identify the four gross components of body composition. Identify and describe three indirect methods of measuring body composition. Evaluate their use in health care work in general practice.
3. Define the biologic terms "compartment" and "pool." How do they apply to body composition?
4. Compare body composition changes at each stage of the life cycle in terms of growth velocity and acceleration.
5. Identify ways in which body composition changes are influenced by weight gains and losses, and by disease.

REFERENCES

1. Editorial: Lancet **2**:1017, November 3, 1984.
2. Greenleaf, J.E., Brock, P.J., Keil, L.C., and others: Drinking and water balance during exercise and heat acclimation, J. Appl. Physiol. **54**(2):414, 1983.
3. Stein, T.P.: Nutrition and protein turnover: a review, J. Parenteral Enteral Nutr. **6**(5):444, 1982.
4. Holliday, M.A.: Body composition and energy needs during growth. In Falkner, F., and Tanner, J., editors: Human growth, vol. 2: postnatal growth, New York, 1978, Plenum Press.
5. Grande, F., and Keys, A.: Body weight, body composition, and calorie status. In Goodhart R.S., and Shils, M.E., editors: Modern nutrition in health and disease, ed. 6, Philadelphia, 1980, Lea & Febiger.
6. Mattila, K., Haavisto, M., and Rajala, S.: Body mass index and mortality in the elderly, Br. Med. J. **292**:867, March 29, 1986.
7. Conway, J.M., Norris, K.H., and Bodwell, C.E.: A new approach for the estimation of body composition: infrared interactance, Am. J. Clin. Nutr. **40**:1123, December 1984.
8. McBride, J.: The light way to measure body fat—with infrared interactance technology, J. Am. Diet. Assoc. **86**(9):1216, September 1986.
9. Mazess, R.B., Peppler, W.W., and Gibbons, M.: Total body composition by dual-photon (153-Gd) absorptiometry, Am. J. Clin. Nutr. **40**:834, October 1984.
10. Davies, R., and Saba, S.: Osteoporosis, Am. Fam. Physician **32**:107, November 1985.
11. Napoli, M.: Disease of the week, The New Republic **195**(22):17, December 1, 1986.
12. Cummings, S.R., and Black D.: Should perimenopausal women be screened for osteoporosis? Ann. Intern. Med. **104**(6):817, June 1986.
13. King, J.C.: Dietary risk patterns during pregnancy. In Weininger, J., and Briggs, G., eds.: Nutrition Update, **1**:206, 1983.
14. Rosso, P.: Nutritional needs of the human fetus, Clin. Nutr. **2**(5):4, September-October 1983.
15. Paige, D.M.: Infant growth and nutrition, Clin. Nutr. **2**(5):14, September-October 1983.
16. Heald, F.P.: Nutrition in adolescence, Clin. Nutr. **2**(5):19, September-October 1983.
17. Russell, R.M.: Evaluating the nutritional status of the elderly, Clin. Nutr. **2**(6):4, November-December 1983.

18. Frisancho, A.R.: New standards of weight and body composition by frame size and height for assessment of nutritional status of adults and the elderly, Am. J. Clin. Nutr. **40**:808, October 1984.
19. Yates, A., Leehey, K., and Shisslak, C.M.: Running—an analogue of anorexia? N. Engl. J. Med. **308**:251, February 3, 1983.
20. Forbes, G.B., Kreipe, R.E., Lipinski, B.A., and Hodgman, C.H.: Body composition changes during recovery from anorexia nervosa: comparison of two dietary regimens, Am. J. Clin. Nutr. **40**:1137, December 1984.
21. Theologides, A.: The pathogenesis of cancer cachexia. In Redfern, D.E., ed.: Nursing care of the cancer patient with nutritional problems, Columbus, Ohio, 1981, Ross Laboratories.
22. Kotler, D.P., Wang, J. and Pierson, R.N., Jr.: Body composition studies in patients with the acquired immunodeficiency syndrome, Am. J. Clin. Nutr. **42**:1255, December 1985.

FURTHER READING

Fomon, S.J., Haschke, F., Ziegler, E.E., and Nelson, S.E.: Body composition of reference children from birth to age 10 years, Am. J. Clin. Nutr. **35**:1169, 1982.

This article provides a comprehensive reference of standards reflecting the body composition changes through the first decade of childhood growth.

Garrow, J.S.: New approaches to body composition, Am. J. Clin. Nutr. **35**:1152, May 1982.

A good description is provided here of the principles and procedures involved in the water displacement method of measuring body composition.

Widdowson, E.M.: Changes in body composition during growth. In Davis, J.A., and Dobbing J., eds.: Scientific foundations of pediatrics, ed. 2, London, 1981, William Heinemann.

This chapter provides a comprehensive comparative review of body composition changes during the growth years with helpful explanations of the physiologic principles involved.

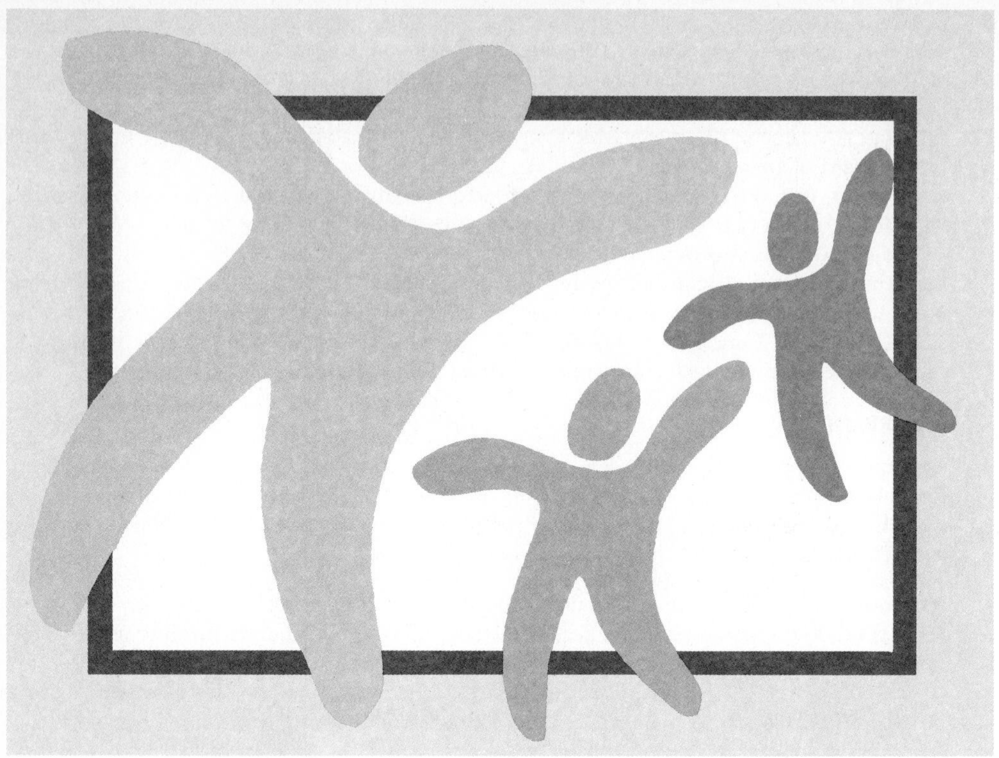

Basic Concepts

1 Both health promotion and treatment of disease require fundamental attention to nutritional status of individuals and population groups.

2 Community nutrition assessment, from national to local levels, identifies nutritional needs of population groups and provides the necessary information for planning relevant public healthcare programs.

3 Personal nutrition assessment identifies nutritional needs of individuals and provides the necessary information for planning personal nutritional care.

4 Modern health care in a changing, complex society is best provided by informed consumers educated in sound self-care and skilled health care professionals all working together as a team.

5 Comprehensive nutrition assessment helps ensure quality standards of nutritional care for all persons of any age.

Chapter Three

Nutrition Assessment

Sue Rodwell Williams

Wherefore, I say, that such constitutions as suffer quickly and strongly from errors in diet are weaker than others who do not; and that a weak person is in a state very nearly approaching to one in disease. . . . Whoever pays no attention to these things or, paying attention, does not comprehend them, how can he understand the diseases which befall a man? For, by every one of these things a man is affected and changed this way or that, and the whole of his life is subjected to them, whether in health, convalescence, or disease. Nothing else, then, can be more important or more necessary to know than these things.—*Hippocrates*

About 2500 years have passed since Hippocrates, the "father of medicine," admonished us to pay closer attention to the significant connection between nutrition and disease. Although we have begun to heed his advice in more recent times, we can hardly say yet that we have a full understanding of these things. However, we are beginning to see more clearly the essential relation of nutrition to health, thus to understand that nutrition must be an essential component of health and health care. Assessment of nutritional status and needs, therefore, provides the foundation for planning health care, for both individuals and population groups of all ages, throughout the human life cycle.

In this chapter we focus on assessment and care of persons' nutritional needs, in population groups or as individuals, in any care setting—public health or other community agency, home, office, clinic, or hospital. Wherever the place of health care and whatever the need, health-care providers and those they seek to serve—the public, families, clients, patients alike—all work together to promote health and support the healing process.

Nutrition Assessment in Health and Health Care

As students, teachers, and providers of good nutrition, both for ourselves and for others, we are engaged in important study and work. Our premise is simple but far more significant than may appear on the surface—good nutrition is essential to good health. This is the fundamental concept of this book, that nutrition is an integral component of both health and health care—for all ages. All effective community and personal nutrition must be solidly rooted here. And nutrition assessment is where we must begin.

Here we will see what nutrition assessment is, why it is a necessary starting point to meet health needs, and how it is applied in the process of health care, both for persons and for populations. Then in following chapters you will see these principles and procedures used in nutritional care for different age groups throughout the life cycle.

NUTRITIONAL STATUS OF PERSONS AND POPULATIONS

What Nutrition Assessment Is

The term "assessment" comes from a Latin word, *assessare,* which means "to sit by" or "watch over." It was applied to the making of a valuation or official estimate of goods and lands, usually for tax purposes, as it is today. In health care the term describes the process of collecting all pertinent information about the health status of a person or group of persons as the basis for determining health needs and goals and for planning health care to meet those identified needs and goals. *Nutrition assessment,* then, refers to the process of collecting all pertinent information about the nutritional status of a person or group of persons as the basis for determining nutritional needs and goals and for planning nutritional care to meet those identified needs and goals.

Why Nutrition Assessment Must Come First

The answer is obvious—if you don't know where you're going you won't know when you've arrived, if you arrive at all. Simple as that may sound, many perhaps well-intentioned people plunge ahead with a plan for nutrition education or care without first checking to see what is needed or will even work. All persons are unique. Each one of us has special needs and goals. If the vital component of nutrition in health and health care is to be fulfilled, it must meet individual human need, both physically and personally.

THE PROCESS OF HEALTH CARE

Role of Nutrition in Health

Nutrition is essential to health on two levels: (1) **Tissue level**—nutrients and energy from the food we eat build and maintain body tissues, and it is on the fundamental integrity of these body tissues that the physiologic functioning and health of the body depend. (2) **Personal level**—food has many meanings and helps fulfill many personal needs, and it is on the integrity of these personal psychosocial and cultural values that one's health as a human being depends. Both of these roles of nutrition in health must be considered in assessing needs and goals.

Community Needs and Programs

In community nutrition, assessment of groups of people helps public health officials determine health goals and allocation of resources according to priority of need. Often the focus of this nutrition and health assessment is on high-risk populations, such as those described in Chapter 11: pregnant women, infants and children, adolescents, and elderly persons, especially those under the added stress of poverty, malnutrition, and illness.

Personal Needs and Care Plans

In personal health care or clinical nutrition, assessment of individuals helps health-care providers and the person determine nutritional and health status, and plan nutritional care according to personal needs and goals. The overall goal is health promotion. If an underlying chronic disorder such as diabetes mellitus is present, or if risk factors for potential health problems such as heart disease have begun to develop, the goal is healthy control of the disorder or prevention of the health problem by reduction of risks. All of these nutrition and health goals involve personal health and nutrition education and skills in self-care, as well as collaboration of a skilled and sensitive team of health care professionals, including the nutritionist or registered dietitian. A number of such health promotion programs are described in Chapter 12 on nutrition education.

Our Changing Society

All of these approaches to health assessment and care reflect rapid and far-reaching changes in our society. It is in this context of change that we must identify nutritional needs and plan care. Our concepts of health and disease are changing, and with them our health care practices. So we turn now to this changing scene to seek our direction.

Changing Concepts of Health and Disease

The modern world is rapidly changing. As a result concepts of health and disease are also changing, profoundly affecting all persons, the public and health-care providers alike. In modern societies, as scientific knowledge has increased, the biologic basis for disease has become well established. Thus in developed countries both public and personal hygiene has improved, treatment of disease has become more scientific and skilled, and many of the once lethal diseases of childhood have been virtually eliminated. Now residents of industrialized nations live longer lives and must deal with a changing environment, as well as with the process of aging and its changing health needs. And these needs must be met in terms of changing human values, social influences, and health practices.

HUMAN VALUES AND HEALTH CARE

Health Promotion

Faced now with the so-called gift of longer life, health is viewed increasingly in more qualitative human terms. Health concepts are moving from the wholly negative view of absence of disease—the traditional *curative approach*—to a more positive view of optimal human fulfillment, function, and productivity—the modern *preventive approach*—of health promotion. This changing view has given rise to the current mode of providing health care through health maintenance organizations—HMOs. Actually this positive view was written into the preamble of the World Health Organization's constitution in 1946: "Health is a state of complete physical, mental, and social well-being, and not merely the absence of disease or infirmity." On the face of it, this sounds like a noble goal for persons of all nations, but it is not totally realistic in all cases. In fact, health is a relative concept in any culture and must be viewed in relation to a person's total wants and needs in his particular situation. Health competes with other values and is relative to a culture's way of life.

Health Care: Assessment of Needs

This recognition of cultural diversity and of different needs extends the concept of health to include moral, philosophical, and religious dimensions, as well as physical and psychosocial aspects. Perhaps a more realistic goal would be a functional one, a level of physical and mental health, based on a comprehensive assessment of personal needs, that would make for social well-being within the social system the individual must live in. Such a goal must be one that provides opportunity for personal self-fulfillment and productivity. This is our broader challenge as individuals and as health workers today.

SOCIAL INFLUENCES

A number of factors in our rapidly evolving society have contributed to changes in health values and practices. These include our advancing scientific knowledge, our increasing and diverse population, a veritable social revolution, and the rapidly developing social sciences.

Scientific Knowledge Expansion

The accelerated rate at which modern science is expanding challenges the medical profession's capacity to integrate and use it. American medical care involves cures for specific diseases, a wide variety of therapeutic techniques, numerous drugs, increasing knowledge of the body's intricate chemistry, and use of many delicate electronic and other instruments for diagnosis and treatment. This growing knowledge in each field means that few persons can gain an adequate comprehension of more than one specialty. Now the benefits of specialization are obvious. But as anyone who has ever visited a large clinic knows, it means that services are fragmented. Clients and patients feel more and more removed from their physicians and allied-health professionals. Sometimes they feel that no one member of the health team sees them as total persons. Comprehensive assessment and communication of needs is increasingly essential to apply scientific knowledge to meet human health goals.

Population Increase

Population expansion has been occurring in many nations of the world, especially in those that can least afford to feed such increased numbers. The U.S. population continues to increase, though the rate of growth has slowed somewhat during the last three decades. The 1980 census indicated that the total U.S. population had grown at that time to 232.6 million.[1] However, the baby-boom generation of the 1940s continues to create a demographic bulge that affects everything from job competition, income, and the housing market to Social Security payments. Nor is it conforming to previous patterns of American life: people are marrying later and divorcing more frequently, postponing childbirth if electing to have children at all, and setting up smaller households.

Also, recent immigration patterns are affecting the nature of the population. The number of persons admitted to the U.S. in the past few years has exceeded that of all prior years since the early 1920s. The number of U.S. residents of Asian origin has increased as thousands of refugees and immigrants have poured in. The 1980 census revealed an increase in Asian immigration during the past decade of 127.6%. Most of these persons have settled in the West, helping to give California the largest population among the states of 23.7 million and making it the most urban of the states.[1] With this population influx of Indochinese, as well as Mexican immigrants, attendant health-care needs have grown, many of them nutrition-related, making nutrition assessment increasingly important in identifying these needs.

In general this American population reflects not only total numbers and ethnic diversity, but also percentage shifts in age and location. There is an increasing percentage of older people and greater overall mobility. It is estimated that this increased movement of individuals and families covers about 20% of the total population. Also, urban-suburban trends have created changes in individual psychosocial patterns, in family settings, and in community and national social frameworks. All these changes affect health needs, lifestyles, and social values.

Social Changes

Radical changes in family and community life have come with the development of the urban-suburban complex in the highly industrial technologic society. Crowded, low-income housing in the cities contrasts with sprawling, affluent suburbs that consume, at an alarming rate, open land that was once used for agriculture. Economic affluence, higher living costs, and more emphasis on higher education, all in the face of increasing poverty in urban and rural areas, have changed human goals, health values, and health-care programs.

Development of the Social Sciences

The behavioral sciences—psychology, sociology, and anthropology—are contributing insights into human behavior and response to illness, and there is renewed effort within the health professions to understand and help the total person. More time is devoted to assessment and analysis of the effect of changing social and cultural factors on human life. The functional illness is recognized as a very real phenomenon, and the medical profession is beginning to realize that an individual's life situation and reaction to stress must be considered if total health needs are to be met.

EFFECTS OF CHANGE ON HEALTH-CARE PRACTICES

Basic Changes in the Health Care System

These scientific and social developments, together with changing attitudes toward health and disease and a more positive recognition of the role of nutrition in health care, have had some profound effects on the kind of health services provided. Assessment of needs is a fundamental health care activity for persons of all ages throughout the life cycle. Four basic changes in our health-care system are evident:

1. **Focus of care.** Primary attention focuses more on the social issues that lie at the root of many diseases and are involved in health status. Often these issues breed personal stress, poor living situations, and malnutrition. Without this focus a viable system cannot exist. This goal emphasizes preventive health maintenance and health promotion rather than the exclusive traditional medical approach of crisis intervention and curative practice alone.
2. **Systems for providing care.** Changes in health care delivery are increasingly based on two ideas: (1) *a health care team for primary care,* which includes family physician, nurse-practitioner, nutritionist (registered dietitian), with other persons such as social worker and psychologist brought in as needed; and (2) *variety of settings,* or stations for service, such as satellite community clinics or health centers, as well as home visits, surrounding a central core community hospital for special services.
3. **Role of consumer.** Changes in relations with users of health care, whether in clinical or health promotion work with individuals or community group encounters, reflect greater involvement of individuals in planning and decision-making for their own health care. The traditional medical model made "patients" of every person, passively "following orders" without questions. Now many consumers seek a more active role in personal health care, in partnership with their professional team. Such an active role requires a full assessment of needs, more health and nutrition education for self-care,[2] and full information for weighing options in care and personal decision-making.
4. **Payment for services.** Changes in payment practices, a concern in the face of increasing costs and an aging population, are moving toward a variety of plans to supplement limited help, especially for elderly persons, from Medicare. These plans of care include prepaid group medical practice, various forms of health maintenance organizations (HMOs), and individual and group health insurance. More nutritionists (registered dietitians) are in private practice or associated with a variety of community health agencies or industries interested in providing health promotion services for their employees. They are becoming licensed practitioners, with nutrition assessment and care being increasingly recognized as the essential component of health that it is.

Changing Roles of Health Care Providers

In response to these basic changes in the health care system, the work of health care providers, especially in relation to nutrition, is also changing. On the health-care team, the nutritionist (registered dietitian) carries the primary responsibility, but works closely with the other team members. This work is both a science and an art. *Science* is a body of systematic knowledge, facts, and principles born of controlled research that shows the operation of natural law. The rapid advances in scientific knowledge have provided all health workers with a stronger base on which to build professional practice. *Art* is an exceptional ability to conduct any human activity. All of us, in whatever manner we apply our nutrition knowledge, must base our work on sound science. But we must also know and care about people and their needs, because we are dealing with *human* nutrition and *human* health. Scientific knowledge has little significance apart from application to human need. In each aspect of health care we function as catalysts that bring scientific knowledge and skills to bear on persons' needs at particular points in their lives. This role is illustrated in Fig. 3-1.

Community and Personal Nutrition Assessment

In the context of these far-reaching changes in health care, then, comprehensive nutrition assessment assumes a primary role. To be valid, nutrition education and care must be based on identified needs, either for groups or for individuals, with particular attention to nutrition-risk periods during the life cycle. In community nutrition work, the needs of population groups are assessed as a base for planning nutrition programs. In personal nutrition work, the needs of individuals are assessed as a base for planning person-centered care. These two interfacing areas of nutrition assessment activities are discussed here.

Community Nutrition Assessment

With the changing health-care system currently evolving, the traditional divisions of public health and private medicine are increasingly interfacing their respective health activities. Public and private sectors of health care in any community are less distinct than in past years. Concern for the health of the community is shared. Here the term *community nutrition* is used in its broad sense to refer to nutrition activities conducted by a variety of health-related community agencies, with particular reference to traditional public health divisions and their nutrition assessment activities at national, state, and local levels.

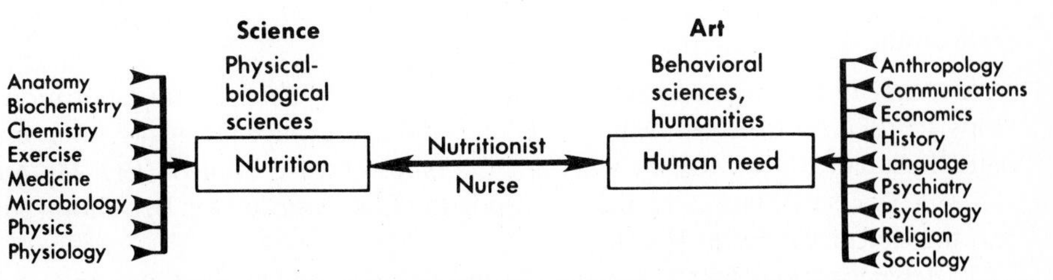

FIG. 3-1 The science and art of nutrition applied to human need.

FOCUS: POPULATION GROUPS

National Surveys

Because of their broad scope of health-related activities and network of agencies throughout the country, national government divisions are able to conduct large nutrition assessment surveys and surveillance of the overall U.S. population. Nutrition survey data describing the nutritional status of the general U.S. population and specific subgroups provide much information that is useful in general practice.[3] These data are available from two major survey programs:

1. **National Health and Nutrition Examination Surveys (NHANES).** Data from these surveys provide the most comprehensive source of nutrition assessment information available about the nutritional status of the general population. These surveys, conducted by the National Center for Health Statistics (NCHS), collect data from dietary intake studies, biochemical tests, physical measures, and clinical assessments from a cross-sectional sample selected to be representative of the U.S. population. Three surveys have been completed, one covering the years 1971-1974 (NHANES I); another covering the years 1976-1980 (NHANES II); and a recent special Hispanic survey covering the years 1982-1984 (Hispanic HANES I). (See Further Reading, p. 66, for these references.)
2. **Nationwide Food Consumption Survey (NFCS).** This survey program, conducted by the U.S. Department of Agriculture, collects information from a representative cross-sectional sample of U.S. households about food use, individual dietary intake, and demographic data related to food consumption. The two most recent surveys were completed over the years 1965-1966 and 1977-1978. Unlike the NHANES surveys, the NFCS does not collect nutritional status and health data, but it does provide nutrient intake analyses and can indicate trends in dietary practices. The NFCS has been conducted at roughly 10-year intervals since the mid-1930s. (See Further Reading, p. 66, for references.)
3. **Continuing Survey of Food Intakes by Individuals (CSFII).** The USDA began this additional survey of individuals in 1985 to study more closely particular groups of persons shown by previous surveys to be more likely than other population groups to have diets low in certain nutrients. It is the first nationwide dietary intake survey designed to be conducted year by year, and will complement the larger NFCS conducted by the USDA about every 10 years. The 1985 CSFII surveyed low-income women 19-50 years of age and their children 1-5 years of age. (See Further Reading, p. 66, for references.)

State Studies

A variety of nutrition-related assessment studies are done by state nutrition divisions, focused on different health problems and age groups. They are often coordinated by a national agency such as the Centers for Disease Control (CDC) in Atlanta, Georgia. Two such state assessments include the CDC coordinated behavioral surveys and the cancer studies in Hawaii:

1. **Behavioral Risk Factor Surveys (BRFS).** Coordinated by the CDC, these surveys were completed in 27 states plus the District of Columbia during the years 1981-1983.[3] State-specific behavioral risk factors included exercise and weight-

height, as well as alcohol use, smoking, and stress. In 1984, 20 states started an on-going system for regular assessment of these risk factors. (See Further Reading, p. 66, for references.)

2. **Hawaii Diet-Cancer Studies**. Conducted by the University of Hawaii, School of Public Health, these studies of the associations of diet and cancer in Hawaii assessed the use of selected food items as measured by a specially structured diet history.[4] Such epidemiologic studies (p. 50) provide important data relating diet and disease in multi-ethnic populations.

Local Community Studies

In local communities, many smaller population groups are assessed by community health agencies. Nutrition assessment may be a component of a comprehensive health survey, or it may be a specific nutrition program study for departmental program-planning purposes. Often such nutrition assessment is focused on specific high-risk age groups, such as pregnant women, infants, children, adolescents, or elderly persons.

GOALS: POPULATION NEEDS AND PROGRAMS

The national health goals, as well as those at state and local levels, are designed to promote positive health and prevent disease. In contrast to traditional treatment-oriented approaches to health care, health promotion supports community and individual efforts to develop lifestyles that maintain and enhance health and well-being. Owen[5] reviews the nutrition intervention activities designed to meet this basic health promotion goal and indicates that screening and assessment must come first.

Public Health Service Reports

In 1979, the Public Health Service (PHS) published the first of several reports outlining the nation's public health objectives: "Healthy People—The Surgeon General's Report on Health Promotion and Disease Prevention." This was followed in 1980 by a second PHS report using 15 specific areas of need as framework for 226 contributory objectives for improving the health of Americans: "Promoting Health, Preventing Disease: Objectives for the Nation." In 1983, a third report provided plans by which various federal agencies could implement the national health objectives: "Promoting Health, Preventing Disease: Implementation Plan for Attaining the Objectives for the Nation." (See Further Reading, p. 67, for references to all of these PHS reports.) The timeframe for meeting these national health objectives is 1990. Nutrition components are involved throughout the overall plan of action. They include nutrition objectives that cover the entire life cycle and address major U.S. health problems.

Nutrition Component: Program-Planning Process

At whatever level of community nutrition work—national, state or local—nutrition is an integral component of health and health care. The program planning process to meet these needs involves four basic areas of activity:

1. **Assessment**. The two-fold process of assessment includes: (1) data collection about the population of concern, and (2) analysis of the information to identify nutrition needs and problems.

2. **Objectives.** In relation to the identified needs or problems, both general goals and specific contributory objectives are determined to meet these needs. These goals involve decisions about what actions are to be accomplished and a projected timeline for doing the work.
3. **Program plan.** To reach the established objectives, a specific plan of action is developed and carried out as projected. The program plan must consider such items as staff, tools and documents required, source of funding, and budget for cost control.
4. **Evaluation.** Assessment of program activities and results continues throughout the nutrition project for health promotion or disease prevention. On the basis of this monitoring information, revisions may be made for study purposes or for conversion to regular, ongoing program status.

SPECIAL LIFE CYCLE ASSESSMENT NEEDS

Pregnant Women

During a woman's pregnancy, she must meet increased nutrient and energy needs to support the pregnancy during this period of rapid fetal growth and bring it to a successful outcome. At best this period is one of physiologic stress. In poor circumstances this normal stress is compounded by inadequate nutrition, bringing increased stress to both mother and baby. Ongoing nutrition assessment can identify specific needs, help prevent problems and complications, and promote a healthy pregnancy for both mother and baby.[6]

Infants and Children

The highest requirements for nutrients per kg body weight during the entire life cycle occur in infancy, when rates of growth and metabolism are at their highest point. Because of this direct relation between growth and nutritional status, close nutrition assessment is required to monitor progress. Over the slowed, erratic growth pattern of young childhood, continued assessment of progress is essential to promote health.

Adolescents

With puberty comes the second large growth spurt for the child. In both sexes intensive growth and hormonal changes profoundly affect nutritional needs. Continued monitoring of growth, changing body composition (p. 31), and nutritional status helps ensure foundations for a healthy adulthood.

Brown has provided a helpful summary of nutrition assessment and intervention guidelines for population groups from pregnancy, through infancy, childhood, and adolescence.[6]

Adults and the Elderly

With our increasing life-span, the gradual aging process through adulthood requires a sound nutritional base to maintain health and prevent or control chronic disease. Chronic diseases account for 75% of all deaths in the United States. Moreover, nutritional risk factors are related to 6-10 leading causes of death.[7] Thus nutrition assessment is a significant part of community health services. However, general procedures may need to be adapted because many assessment procedures developed for young or middle-aged adults are unreliable when applied to older persons.[8] Lee has provided helpful summaries of nutrition assessment and guidelines for both groups: adults and the elderly.[9] She also gives referral sources for agencies supplying the various types of nutrition assessment.

Methods of Community Nutrition Assessment

Assessment measures used in community nutrition center mainly on dietary intake surveys and nutrient analyses. Comparative data from biochemical tests, anthropometric measures, and clinical evaluations provide an appraisal of the individual's nutritional status, as well as practical information on response to nutrition intervention programs.

FOOD AND NUTRITION SURVEYS

Dietary Intake Surveys

Methods for assessing dietary intake of population groups take many forms, depending upon such factors as the nature and size of the group, the objectives of the survey, available staff, and funds. At best, however, our methodology is imperfect for two reasons: (1) By heritage Americans are a multi-ethnic and multi-racial population with great diversity in cultural food patterns that are influenced further by economic, psychologic, and physiologic factors. (2) Dietary surveys can only attempt to describe food intake behavior, and that behavior is constantly changing.[10] To know better what Americans are eating, special sub-group sampling is needed for some of the racial and ethnic groups. This is especially true for groups such as the homeless and migrant workers who are not included in present national surveys and are of special concern.[11] Nonetheless, traditional population assessment methods briefly described here have been used in various combinations to give some indication of nutrition and health needs.

Methods of Intake Assessment

Information about food intake of different groups of people is usually gathered by use of several basic tools:

1. **24-hour recall.** Individuals are asked to recall the specific food items they ate during the previous day, describing the nature and amount of each. Sometimes this method is used because it is simpler and less costly than some of the others, but it has disadvantages in some groups such as elderly persons whose memory may be limited. Also there are measurement problems in determining correct portion sizes.[12]
2. **Food records.** Individuals are asked to record their food intake for a brief period of time, such as 1-3-7 days, or on certain days periodically. Each person is taught how to describe food items used singly and in combination, and how to measure

amounts consumed. Studies indicate that a 1-day record gives a meaningless estimate of one individual's usual food habits, but may provide a reasonable estimate, within 15%, of the usual intake of a group of individuals.[12,13] A 3-day intake record provides information that is more accurate and that helps account for daily variation, and a combination of methods may be used. For example, the Nationwide Food Consumption Survey (NFCS) combines data from day 1 (24-hour recalls) and days 2 and 3 (written food records) to obtain more accurate population information. However, a study comparing the 1-day record with the 24-hour recall in an older adult sub-sample population of the NFCS indicated that either method provides reliable estimates, nearly as reliable as 3-day records, for a population with more stable day-to-day food habits.[14]

3. **Food frequency questionnaire (FFQ).** The purpose of this assessment tool is to help determine food intake over an extended period of time, providing useful data for investigating the relation of individual diets in a group of persons to disease risk and incidence.[4,15] The FFQ has two basic parts: (1) a list of foods, and (2) a scale for checking frequency of use over a given period of time. The food list may be comprehensive to assess overall food habits, or a specific selection to focus on use of particular food sources of nutrients related to the disease under study. Quantitative FFQs also include a means of measuring portions of food used.[4] Diet diversity indices have been developed on the basis of food-frequency data. These give descriptive information to help measure cultural aspects of diet rather than specific nutrient intakes.[16]
4. **Diet history.** The diet history as a valid nutrition assessment tool requires the skills and time of trained nutrition professionals. The classic in-depth diet history technique, for example, requires a highly trained nutritionist or dietitian who determines a comprehensive picture of the usual total diet and interprets its nutritional significance. Thus it is a costly procedure, especially for a large population group. However, study of group nutritional needs today uses adapted diet history methods to obtain valid information with the assistance of trained support-level staff or lay interviewers. Hankin[4] developed and used such an adapted diet history tool in a number of cancer epidemiologic studies in Hawaii with multi-ethnic population groups. She successfully combined FFQ techniques with methods of measuring accurate food portions, producing a questionnaire to obtain a valid and reliable diet history by trained lay interviewers. A similar method can be used to obtain information about past food habits to compare with current intake. Such information is often needed in epidemiologic surveys to study the development history of a given disease. For this information, current diet history is combined with information on frequency of use of particular disease-related foods and nutrients at designated times in the past.[17]

Nutrient Analysis

Once food intake data have been collected by any of the methods described above, a nutrient analysis of the food consumed follows. Wotecki[11] rightly points out that population diet surveys are limited by the extent of the food composition databases available. The largest such computer database is maintained by the U.S. Department of

Agriculture. Constant revision and addition of items as new food-composition data are developed help to improve the usefulness of this resource.

RELATED POPULATION ASSESSMENT ACTIVITIES

Biochemical Evaluation

Health survey data also include information from biochemical tests relating to nutritional status. For example, since anemia is a major U.S. and world health problem, iron stores are measured in national population studies by use of such tests as hemoglobin, hematocrit, and serum ferritin or transferrin levels (p. 57).[18] Biochemical assessment of nutritional status is especially important in elderly populations because they are at higher risk for developing nutrient deficiencies.[19]

Clinical Examination

Assessment methods used in nutrition- and health-related surveys include some form of physical examination for any evidence of nutritional deficiency or toxicity (p. 60). The national population studies (NHANES) include such evaluations, plus a medical history for prior or current disease.

Anthropometric Measures

Basic body measurements, such as weight-height, skinfolds, and circumferences, are standard procedures in some form in various population studies to assess body composition and nutritional status. These assessment methods are described in detail below (p. 54).

Screening and Assessment

Population screening processes identify persons at risk for various health problems. Then more comprehensive assessment and evaluation can follow to determine nutritional needs and care plans for these persons. Owen[5] outlines these relationships that guide development of nutrition components of community health-promotion programs.

Clinical Nutrition Assessment

At times during the life cycle, through growth periods or the aging process of adulthood, persons experience acute illness or injury or develop risk factors for certain chronic diseases. At such times these persons need individual clinical assessment and a personal plan for nutrition education and care.

FOCUS: INDIVIDUAL NUTRITIONAL STATUS AND NEEDS

Health Promotion

Increasing public interest in health and physical fitness, as well as changes in the health care system described here, have led to the development of a strong health-maintenance goal for persons of all ages. This is especially true for children in high-risk families with histories of conditions such as heart disease, hypertension, and diabetes mellitus, as well as for adults developing risk factors for chronic diseases of aging. Legislation has established health maintenance organizations (HMOs) as a model setting for individual health care. Numerous programs are available for health promotion and disease prevention through assessment and self-care monitoring, along with education and support for developing healthier lifestyles. A number of these programs are described in Chapter 12 on nutrition education.

Persons at Malnutrition Risk

The high risk of malnutrition in low income families caught in a cycle of poverty, as well as among the "new poor," is well known and documented, as described in Chapter 11. Now there is also a growing awareness of the extent of various degrees of malnutrition among persons in hospitals, rehabilitation centers, and other long-term care facilities. For example, a large collaborative study[20] involving 33 hospitals in the greater Chicago area with nutrition screening of 3047 patients revealed that more than 50% of the final subjects had below-normal values for one or more of the assessment measures used (serum albumin, hemoglobin, and total lymphocyte count), and a large number, 40%, were at risk by weight-height status. It is clear that nutrition assessment at admission to any health-care facility, or initial visit to any health office or clinic, is a vital first step in establishing a person's nutritional status and need for nutritional care.

Special Needs

Persons suffering hypermetabolic disease or injury are in special need of nutrition assessment, vigorous nutritional support, and continued monitoring of nutritional status. Individuals in special need of such nutrition assessment and support include those with a debilitating disease such as cancer, or severe injury such as extensive burns.[21]

THE THERAPEUTIC PROCESS

Person-Centered Care

The primary principle in nutrition practice, too often overlooked in many routine procedures, should be self-evident: to be valid, nutritional care must be *person-centered.* It must be based on initial and continuing assessment of needs and updated constantly with the person involved. A second fundamental fact also needs emphasis: despite all methods, tools or technologies described here or elsewhere, *the most therapeutic tool you will ever use is yourself.* It is to this seemingly simple yet profound human healing encounter that you bring yourself.

The Health Care Team

In the setting of the individual health center, with its strengths and despite its shortcomings, and within the essential team care provided, the nutritionist-dietitian is responsible for monitoring each person's nutritional needs, working closely with the other health team members. Thus assessing individual nutritional care needs will be the initial task in each case.

Phases of the Care Process

Five distinct yet interactive phases are essential in the therapeutic care process:

1. **Assessment.** A broad base of information about the person's body composition, nutritional status, food habits, and living situation provides necessary knowledge for assessing initial status and needs. Useful background information will come from various sources, primarily the individual and family, as well as health-care records and other team members.
2. **Analysis.** The data collected must be analyzed carefully to determine specific needs. Some will be evident immediately. Others will develop as the situation unfolds. On the basis of this analysis, a list of problems forms.
3. **Planning care.** As problems are identified, valid care can be planned with the individual and family to solve them. This plan must always be based on personal needs and goals, as well as any health problem involved.
4. **Implementing the plan.** Realistic and appropriate actions planned are carried out. In nutritional care and education this will involve decisions and actions about the diet, mode of feeding as needed, and training of the person, staff, and family to carry out the plan.
5. **Evaluating and recording results.** As the plan is carried out, results are monitored carefully to see if the needs are being met, or if revisions in the plan must be made. Records of plans, procedures, and progress guide actions and instructions for continuing self-care.

Methods of Clinical Nutrition Assessment

The basic methods used in clinical aspects of any nutrition assessment may be grouped in four types of activities: (1) dietary evaluation, (2) body measures, (3) biochemical tests, and (4) physical observations. The procedures briefly outlined here provide a good base in general practice for assessing and monitoring nutritional status, planning care, and promoting health.

DIETARY EVALUATION

The dietary evaluation methods described for use in community nutrition assessment may also be adapted for use in individual nutrition work. Of these assessment tools, two are of particular use in clinical situations: (1) food records, and (2) comprehensive nutrition history. Also, to meet increased energy and protein needs in catabolic situations, special assessments and calculations may need to be made.

Food Records

At times a full dietary analysis of all nutrient and energy values is needed and a 3-7 day food record supplies the detailed information. Obtaining accurate information about actual food intake is difficult at best. Thus careful discussion about the purpose and method of recording is essential. Nutritional analysis is usually done by computer. At other times, special assessment tests may require a specific 24-hour food record. For example, during the 24-hour period of urine collection for the creatinine and urea nitrogen excretion tests (p. 58, 60), a specific, detailed record of all food intake is required to calculate and interpret nitrogen balances involved.

Comprehensive Nutrition History

A comprehensive investigative interview and follow-up is required for person-centered care. In addition to knowledge of basic food habits, other nutrition-related information is needed: (1) living situation and other personal and family history, psychosocial and economic problems; and (2) medical history, nature, course and treatment of any prior or current health problems, including all current drugs in terms of possible drug-nutrient interactions and education about their action, side effects, and use. A helpful means of jogging memory about food habits is to lead the individual through a "typical" day of usual work or school routines and attach questions and follow-up probes about food intake to where they are and what they're doing from the time they get up to the time they go to bed. A general form for such an activity-associated day's food intake pattern is given here (see box opposite).

ANTHROPOMETRIC MEASURES

Anthropometry is the process of measuring various dimensions of the body. A number of these anthropometric measures provide basic valid estimates of muscle and fat components of body composition.[22] Further, they have the advantage of being inexpensive and simple to obtain. Skill gained through accurate practice will minimize the margin of error in making measurements. Selection and maintenance of proper equipment and attention to technique are essential. The commonly used measures for individual nutrition assessment are briefly described here.

Weight

Regular clinic beam balance scales with nondetachable weights give the most accurate measurement. An additional weight attachment is available for use with very obese persons. All scales should be checked frequently and calibrated every few months for continued accuracy. After careful reading and recording of the person's weight, obtain information about the usual body weight and check standard weight-height tables for comparison. But approach these tables with caution in applying them to individuals as specific ideals. (See Further Reading, p. 67.) In his "state of the art" review of clinical nutrition assessment, Grant[23] states that use of the so-called "ideal" weight-height tables for medium-frame adults ignores the wide *normal* variations in healthy bodies, a reminder that would apply to individuals of all ages. Keeping this in mind, interpret present weight in terms of percentage of the person's usual body weight, with general reference to standard tables (see inside book covers and Appendix). Check for any significant weight loss (Table 3-1).

Height

Use a true vertical bar, such as a flat wall-attached measuring stick or the movable measuring rod on the platform clinic scales. Have the person stand as straight as possible, without shoes or hat, heels together, and looking straight ahead. The heels, buttocks, shoulders, and head should be touching the flat wall measure or the vertical

TOOL A NUTRITION HISTORY: ACTIVITY-ASSOCIATED GENERAL DAY'S FOOD PATTERN

Name ______________________________ Date ____________

Height ________ Weight (lb) ________ (kg) ________ Age ________

Ideal weight ________

Referral

Diagnosis

Diet order

Members of household

Occupation

Recreation, physical activity

Present food intake	Place	Hour	Frequency, form, and amount checklist
Breakfast			Milk Cheese Meat Fish
Noon meal			Poultry Eggs Cream Butter, margarine
Evening meal			Other fats Vegetables, green
Extra meals			Vegetables, other Fruits (citrus) Legumes
Summary			Potato Bread—kind Sugar Desserts Beverages Alcohol Vitamins Candy

TABLE 3-1. Indications of Severe Protein-Calorie Malnutrition According to Percentage of Recent Weight Loss

% Body Weight Loss	Time Period
2%	1 week
5%	1 month
7.5%	3 months
10%	6 months

surface of the measuring rod. Read and record the measure carefully. Compare it with previous recordings to detect possible errors, and to note growth of children or diminishing height of adults.

Mid-Upper-Arm Circumference (MAC)

Use a centimeter tape made of nonstretchable material such as metal, plastic, or fiberglass, not cloth or paper. On the nondominant arm, unless it is affected by edema, locate the midpoint of the upper arm: (1) have person bend the arm at the elbow, at a 90 degree angle with palm up; (2) place the tape vertically on the posterior arm surface; and (3) mark upper arm midpoint between the acromial process of the scapula (bony protrusion on the posterior side of the upper shoulder) and the olecranon process of the elbow (bony part of the elbow). Measure upper-arm circumference at this midpoint, securing tape snugly but not so tight as to make an indentation. Read and record the measure accurately to the nearest tenth of a centimeter. Compare with standard tables and with previous individual measures to note possible changes.

Triceps Skinfold Thickness (TSF)

This measure provides an estimate of subcutaneous fat. Together with the MAC at the same spot, described above, the mid-arm muscle circumference can be calculated to give a good estimate of skeletal muscle mass. Use a standard millimeter skinfold caliper, such as the Lange caliper. If possible have the person stand with nondominant arm previously measured hanging loosely. With thumb and forefinger, grasp a vertical pinch of the skin and subcutaneous fat about 1 to 2 cm from the previously marked mid-upper-arm midpoint. Pull the skinfold gently away from the underlying muscle. Place the caliper jaws over the lifted skinfold midpoint mark while maintaining the skinfold grasp. Release the caliper extender and quickly, within 2 or 3 seconds, read the measure of the compressed skinfold to the nearest full or fraction of a millimeter. Avoid excessive pressure or delayed reading. For increased accuracy take three measures and use the mean for calculations. Record results, compare with standards and with previous individual measures to note changes.

Mid-Upper-Arm Muscle Circumference (MAMC)

As indicated, this derived value gives a good indirect measure of the body's skeletal muscle mass. First, convert the TSF mean value (millimeters), as measured, to centimeters to match the other two measuring units (divide millimeter value by 10). Then calculate the MAMC by the following formula:

$$\text{MAMC (cm)} = \text{MAC (cm)} - [3.14 \times \text{TSF (cm)}]$$

If desired, the TSF can be left in millimeters as measured and the value of the mathematical factor π in the formula changed to 0.314.

To interpret these anthropometric measures for persons of different ages and sex, compare the individual's measures as percentages of standards provided in reference tables (see Appendix). Some examples of these standards for adults at the mean values are shown in Table 3-2.

TABLE 3-2 Standards of Anthropometric Measures of Adults (50th percentile)

	Male	Female
Arm circumference (cm)	29.3	28.5
Triceps skinfold (mm)	12.5	16.5
Arm muscle circumference (cm)	25.3	23.2

Data from Jelliffe, D.B.: The assessment of the nutritional status of the community, Geneva, 1966, World Health Organization.

BIOCHEMICAL TESTS

A number of biochemical tests are available for assessing nutritional status. The most common ones used in general nutrition practice are listed here in three categories according to what they are measuring: (1) measures of the plasma protein compartment; (2) measures of the immune system's integrity (anergy); and (3) measures of protein metabolism and protein balance. In the first two categories, regularly used tests are listed first, then an additional one is used if needed. (See Further Reading references.)

Measures of Plasma Protein Compartment

1. **Basic: serum albumin, hemoglobin, and hematocrit.** These three major protein substances in the blood are early mirrors of nutritional deficiency, especially in protein, iron, and other nutrients involved in their synthesis. **Albumin** is the major blood protein; it controls the capillary fluid shift mechanism and hence water balance in the body. **Hemoglobin** is a conjugated protein in the blood; its nonprotein part, the red pigment **heme**, carries vital oxygen to the cells for cell metabolism functions. **Hematocrit** is a measure of packed red blood cell volume, the blood cells that carry the hemoglobin. Thus, low values of hemoglobin and hematocrit reflect impending or frank anemia, the world's most common nutritional deficiency symptom. Studies indicate that plasma protein values easily drop in hospitalized patients and require nutritional support. For example, serum albumin values in newly admitted patients have shown an 82% decline within three days.[24] An estimate of protein-energy malnutrition by values for serum albumin and other plasma proteins is given in Table 3-3.

TABLE 3-3 Determination of Protein-Calorie Malnutrition by Plasma Values

		Degree of Malnutrition	
Laboratory Data	Normal Values	Moderate	Severe
Serum albumin (g/dl)	3.5	2.1-3.0	<2.1
Serum transferrin (mg/dl)	180-260	100-150	<100
Total lymphocyte count			
Per mm^3	1500-4000	800-1200	<800
% of WBC	20%-53%		

2. **Additional: serum transferrin or total iron-binding capacity (TIBC).** The plasma protein transferrin also relates to anemia in its iron transport function. **Transferrin** is the plasma protein beta-globulin that binds iron and carries it to its storage sites in the bone marrow, spleen, and liver, where the iron is transferred to its storage protein *ferritin.* **TIBC** values indicate how much iron the available transferrin is carrying. Normally, only about 20% to 35% of the iron-binding capacity of transferrin is filled, leaving an unsaturated latent reserve in the plasma for handling variances in iron intake. But if the transferrin level falls, there is less total transport capacity and the cells' source of iron diminishes. Given either value by blood test, the other may be derived by the following formula:

$$\text{Transferrin} = (\text{TIBC} \times 0.76) + 18$$

Measures of Immune System Integrity

1. **Basic: lymphocytes.** Lymphocytes are special white blood cells that attack "alien invaders" in the body—bacteria, viruses, tumor cells, and other such "non-body" substances called *antigens,* partly by forming *antibodies* against them or killing them. It is evident that these special white cells are major components of the immune system, which protect the body from disease. They are made up of basic tissue protein substances. Low blood values of these special cells indicate that the immune system is weakened and the individual is more vulnerable to the effects of a disease. A total lymphocyte count (TLC) can be derived from the values for percent lymphocytes (percentage of the total white-blood-cell count that are lymphocytes) and the white-blood-cell (WBC) count, using the following formula:

$$\text{TLC} = (\%\ \text{lymphocytes} \times \text{WBC})/100$$

2. **Additional: skin testing.** The reaction of the skin to small bits of disease-causing antigens, in a similar fashion to use of a vaccine, can indicate how strong the body's antibody reaction to those antigens is, and hence serve as an indicator of the immune system's functional integrity. These skin tests use common recall antigens such as mumps, *Candida,* or purified protein derivative of tuberculin (PPD). Skin test reactions are read at 24 and 48 hours, with greater than 5 mm considered positive and the presence of one such positive result indicating intact immunity.

Measures of Protein Metabolism

1. **Urinary creatinine.** Creatinine is a metabolic product of protein tissue breakdown. The amount excreted indicates the extent of tissue catabolism. The total 24-hour excretion is interpreted in terms of ideal creatinine for height. Height is used as a basic indicator of body protein mass. The creatinine-height index (CHI) can be calculated by the following formula, using the actual 24-hour urinary creatinine excretion value (AUC) and the individual's ideal urinary excretion for height (IUC):

$$\text{CHI} = [\text{AUC}/\text{IUC}] \times 100$$

   Some standard ideal creatinine values, in relation to height and weight, are given in Table 3-4.

TABLE 3-4 Ideal Weight and Urinary Creatinine Values for Height (adults)

	Females		Males	
Height (cm)	Weight (kg)	Creatinine (mg)	Weight (kg)	Creatinine (mg)
140	44.9			
141	45.4			
142	45.9			
143	46.4			
144	47.0			
145	47.5		51.9	
146	48.0		52.4	
147	48.6	828	52.9	
148	49.2		53.5	
149	49.8		54.0	
150	50.4	852	54.5	
151	51.0		55.0	
152	51.5		55.6	
153	52.0	878	56.1	
154	52.5		56.6	
155	53.1	901	57.2	
156	53.7		57.9	
157	54.3	922	58.6	1284
158	54.9		59.3	
159	55.5		59.9	
160	56.2	949	60.5	1325
161	56.9		61.1	
162	57.6		61.7	
163	58.3	979	62.3	1362
164	58.9		62.9	
165	59.5	1005	63.5	1387
166	60.1		64.0	
167	60.7	1040	64.6	1421
168	61.4		65.2	
169	62.1		65.9	
170		1075	66.6	1465
171			67.3	
172			68.0	
173		1111	68.7	1516
174			69.4	
175		1139	70.1	1552
176			70.8	
177		1169	71.6	1589
178			72.4	
179			73.3	
180		1204	74.2	1639
181			75.0	
182			75.8	
183		1241	76.5	1692
184			77.3	
185			78.1	1735
186			78.9	
187				1776
188				
189				
190				1826

1959 Metropolitan Life Insurance Company Standards corrected for nude weight without shoe heels. Data from Jelliffe, D.B.: The assessment of the nutritional status of the community, Geneva, 1966, World Health Organization.

2. **Urinary urea nitrogen.** Urea is the chief end product of protein metabolism, so its urinary excretion rate in relation to protein intake is a basic measure of the body's protein balance. This balance is expressed in terms of nitrogen balance, the unique constituent element in protein. A 24-hour urinary urea nitrogen (UUN) excretion is used with the calculated dietary nitrogen intake (6.25 g dietary protein has a nitrogen value of 1 g) over the same 24-hour period to determine the person's nitrogen balance:

   $$\text{Nitrogen balance} = [\text{diet protein divided by } 6.25] - [\text{UUN} + 4]$$

   The formula factor of *4* above represents additional nitrogen loss through feces and skin.

OBSERVATION OF PHYSICAL SIGNS

Careful observations of physical signs of possible malnutrition provide an important added dimension to the overall individual assessment of general nutritional status. To guide a general examination for such signs, an outline is provided in Table 3-5.

TABLE 3-5 Clinical Signs of Nutritional Status

Body Area	Signs of Good Nutrition	Signs of Poor Nutrition
General appearance	Alert, responsive	Listless, apathetic, cachexic
Weight	Normal for height, age, body build	Overweight or underweight (special concern for underweight)
Posture	Erect, arms and legs straight	Sagging shoulders, sunken chest, humped back
Muscles	Well developed, firm, good tone, some fat under skin	Flaccid, poor tone, undeveloped, tender, "wasted" appearance, cannot walk properly
Nervous control	Good attention span, not irritable or restless, normal reflexes, psychological stability	Inattentive, irritable, confused, burning and tingling of hands and feet (paresthesia), loss of position and vibratory sense, weakness and tenderness of muscles (may result in inability to walk), decrease or loss of ankle and knee reflexes
Gastrointestinal function	Good appetite and digestion, normal regular elimination, no palpable (perceptible to touch) organs or masses	Anorexia, indigestion, constipation or diarrhea, liver or spleen enlargement
Cardiovascular function	Normal heart rate and rhythm, no murmurs, normal blood pressure for age	Rapid heart rate (above 100 beats/minute tachycardia), enlarged heart, abnormal rhythm, elevated blood pressure
General vitality	Endurance, energetic, sleeps well, vigorous	Easily fatigued, no energy, falls asleep easily, looks tired, apathetic

TABLE 3-5 Clinical Signs of Nutritional Status—cont'd

Body Area	Signs of Good Nutrition	Signs of Poor Nutrition
Hair	Shiny, lustrous, firm, not easily plucked, healthy scalp	Stringy, dull, brittle, dry, thin and sparse, depigmented, can be easily plucked
Skin (general)	Smooth, slightly moist, good color	Rough, dry, scaly, pale, pigmented, irritated, bruises, petechiae
Face and neck	Skin color uniform, smooth, pink, healthy appearance, not swollen	Greasy, discolored, scaly, swollen, skin dark over cheeks and under eyes, lumpiness or flakiness of skin around nose and mouth
Lips	Smooth, good color, moist, not chapped or swollen	Dry, scaly, swollen, redness and swelling (cheilosis), or angular lesions at corners of the mouth or fissures or scars (stomatitis)
Mouth, oral membranes	Reddish pink mucous membranes in oral cavity	Swollen, boggy oral mucous membranes
Gums	Good pink color, healthy, red, no swelling or bleeding	Spongy, bleed easily, marginal redness, inflamed, gum receding
Tongue	Good pink color or deep reddish in appearance, not swollen or smooth, surface papillae present, no lesion	Swelling, scarlet and raw, magenta color, beefy (glossitis), hyperemic and hypertrophic papillae, atrophic papillae
Teeth	No cavities, no pain, bright, straight, no crowding, well-shaped jaw, clean, no discoloration	Unfilled caries, absent teeth, worn surfaces mottled (fluorosis), malpositioned
Eyes	Bright, clear, shiny, no sores at corner of eyelids, membranes moist and healthy pink color, no prominent blood vessels or mount of tissue or sclera, no fatigue circles beneath	Eye membranes pale (pale conjunctivas), redness of membrane (conjunctival injection), dryness, signs of infection, Bitot's spots, redness and fissuring of eyelid corners (angular palpebritis), dryness of eye membrane (conjunctival xerosis), dull appearance of cornea (corneal xerosis), soft cornea (keratomalacia)
Neck (glands)	No enlargement	Thyroid enlarged
Nails	Firm, pink	Spoon shaped (koilonychia), brittle, ridged
Legs, feet	No tenderness, weakness, or swelling, good color	Edema, tender calf, tingling weakness
Skeleton	No malformations	Bowlegs, knock-knees, chest deformity at diaphragm, beaded ribs, prominent scapulas

Williams, S.R.: Nutritional guidance in prenatal care. In Worthington-Roberts, B.S., Vermeersch, J., and Williams, S.R., eds.: Nutrition in pregnancy and lactation, St. Louis, 1985, The C.V. Mosby Co.

ANALYSIS AND HEALTH CARE PLANNING

Assessment Data Analysis

All of the assessment information collected must be carefully analyzed to determine needs and plan care. Nutritional deficiencies will need to be replenished. Any degree of underlying malnutrition can contribute to health problems. These deficiencies may be primary or secondary, depending on the cause. *Primary* deficiency results from lack of particular nutrients in the diet, for whatever reason. *Secondary* deficiency results from barriers that interfere with normal use of the nutrients after they are consumed. This inability to use a given nutrient may stem from digestive or malabsorption problems, such as in inflammatory bowel disease or in chemotherapy or radiation treatments, or from metabolic problems, as in some genetic diseases. In the final analysis, the nutritional diagnosis will require information about all aspects related to the individual's needs (see box). These areas of need include nutritional status, underlying disease or risk factors requiring modified nutrient or food plan, any personal, cultural, ethnic, or economic need, as well as mode of feeding required, dietary management, and nutrition education for self-care. To meet individual needs and goals in all these nutrition-related areas, continuing assessment is essential to valid health care throughout.

Problem List

On the basis of this careful analysis, a problem list is usually developed, around which realistic care may be planned. The health care team, together with the individual and family, determine positive health goals. These goals will establish priorities for immediate and long-term care.

PLANNING AND IMPLEMENTING NUTRITIONAL CARE

Food Plan

Based, then, on the comprehensive assessment of nutritional needs, decisions about the food plan are made. If a modified diet is needed, it is based on the normal nutritional needs of the individual. The diet may need to be modified in one or more nutrients, in energy value (kilocalories), or in texture. The assessment process enables the nutritionist to adapt the food plan to meet the individual's own personal needs also. It must be a workable plan adapted to individual needs and desires.

Special Needs or Resources

Any special needs or resources are included in the health-care plan. Instruction is provided for food selections, preparation or seasoning, amounts, or supplements. Special help for using self-care eating devices may be needed. Resources for group support or fitness programs may be planned. Food assistance programs, such as food stamps, WIC program for women and their infants and young children, or nutritional support for elderly or disabled persons may be secured. Such programs for high-risk groups throughout the life cycle are described in Chapter 11. Resources and programs for ongoing nutrition education needs for all ages, especially for health promotion and disease prevention, are discussed in Chapter 12.

TOOL B GUIDE FOR ASSESSMENT AND CARE OF NUTRITION NEEDS

I. Assess nutrition needs
  A. Define the person
    1. Who the person is: age, sex, family, occupational role, cultural background, socioeconomic status, personal characteristics, limitations, strengths
    2. Where the person is: physical setting—place of care, its possibilities and limitations and personal setting—mental, psychological, emotional, and physical, in relation to health or disease, adaptation
    3. Nutritional status: food habits and general nutritional analysis; clinical observations and signs
  B. Determine the disease or normal physiologic stress (such as pregnancy and growth)
    1. The general disease or physiologic process: anatomy and physiology, signs and symptoms, general treatment or management, pathology, course, prognosis
    2. Patient's unique experience with the disease or physiologic stress: duration, intensity, medical management, prior diet therapy, adaptation, problems and solutions, knowledge of disease and its care—source, form, attitude, behavior response

II. Identify and define problems and develop plan of care
  A. Explore present needs
    1. Day-to-day nutritional support: maintenance, optimal intake, basic nutritional requirements
    2. Nutritional therapy: treatment by modified diet
    3. Teaching: basic nutrition knowledge or principles of special diet modification
  B. Explore future needs
    1. Continuity of care: home, responsible significant others, extended-care facility
    2. Plan for medical management: health team conferences, nursing team conferences
    3. Plan for nutritional care: diet modifications, practical food management (family situation, living alone, degree of disability, etc.), follow-up diet counseling and nutrition education, community resources

III. Carry out plan of care
  A. Physical, psychosocial responses: diet and its meaning
  B. Teaching plan: materials needed, content, sequence, methods, approaches, plan for evaluation
  C. Records of action for study

IV. Check results
  A. Follow-up care: planned with patient, family, and health team
  B. Reinforcement to strengthen learning
  C. Revision: as needed

EVALUATION AND QUALITY CARE

Assessment in Terms of Objectives

When the nutritional health-care plan is carried out, assessment in terms of the identified personal needs and goals, and the extent to which the planned actions helped solve the nutrition-related health problems, is essential to ongoing health care. This evaluation is continuous. It seeks to validate care throughout. Various areas need to be investigated: (1) estimate the achievement of any treatment goals; (2) judge the accuracy of intervention actions; and (3) determine the person's ability to follow the prescribed care plan.

Quality Care Standards

Since the establishment of Professional Standards Review Organizations (PSROs) in 1972, there has been increased emphasis on the setting of practice standards to ensure the delivery of quality personal health care. In addition, current focus on cost control in health-care settings requires that mechanisms be developed for effectively assessing health care programs on the basis of: (1) cost effectiveness, and (2) provision of nutritional services by the most qualified personnel. Within dietetics, standards for both professional and support level staff have been developed in a number of settings and applied to quality assurance of nutritional care for all persons, particularly those with special needs.[25] In each case, these models of quality care have established specific standards for: (1) identifying through careful assessment individuals who require increased nutritional support or nutrition education, (2) determining personal care priorities and spelling out the degree of care required, and (3) defining role responsibilities for carrying out each part of the plan.

The growing interface between private and public nutrition services focuses increased attention on nutrition assessment. It plays a vital role in meeting human needs. It helps meet health-promotion and disease-prevention goals for persons and populations of all ages throughout the life cycle.

Summary

Nutrition is an integral component of both health and health care. And nutrition assessment is basic to meeting these nutritional needs. Changing concepts of health and disease have developed with the changes in society and technology. As a result, the health-care system has begun to focus more on the social roots of disease and personal needs, to provide care in expanded settings and to expand the roles of health-care providers, to recognize the active role of the consumer in health-care decisions and self-care activities, and to seek ways of meeting the increased costs of modern health for all persons in varieties of economic situations.

With these changing health-care values and practices has come an increased interest in positive approaches to health and health care. National health objectives center upon health promotion and disease prevention, in which both community and individual nutrition are important parts. In meeting these health goals, nutrition assessment plays a fundamental role in identifying nutritional needs and carrying out nutrition programs and plans successfully. Community nutrition assessment methods identify needs of population groups and provide the basis for nutrition programs to meet them. Personal nutrition assessment methods identify needs of individuals and provide the basis for health care plans to meet them. Both services interface and depend on constant assessment to provide valid nutritional care.

Review Questions

1. What is the basic role of nutrition in health and health care?
2. Describe changes occurring in the health-care system and account for them in terms of human needs.
3. What role does nutrition play in meeting current national health goals? Why is nutrition assessment an essential process in this nutrition-health relation?
4. What is the function of community nutrition assessment? Describe methods used to achieve this assessment.
5. What is the function of individual nutrition assessment in health care? Describe methods used to achieve this assessment.
6. Identify phases of the health-care process and relate nutrition assessment activities to each phase.

REFERENCES

1. Sheils, M.: A portrait of America, Newsweek, January 17, 1983, p. 20.
2. Dismuke, S.E., and Miller, S.T.: Why not share the secrets of good health? The physician's role in health promotion. J.A.M.A. **249**(23):3181, 1983.
3. Wong, F.L., and Trowbridge, F.L.: Nutrition surveys and surveillance: their application to clinical practice, Clin. Nutr. **3**(3):94, May-June 1984.
4. Hankin, J.H.: A diet history method for research, clinical, and community use, J. Am. Diet. Assoc. **86**(7):868, July 1986.
5. Owen, A.L.: Community nutrition: an integral component of health and health care, Clin. Nutr. **3**(3):88, May-June 1984.
6. Brown, J.E.: Nutrition services for pregnant women, infants, children, and adolescents, Clin. Nutr. **3**(3):100, May-June 1984.
7. National Center for Health Statistics: Births, marriages, divorces, and deaths, United States, 1982. In Monthly vital statistics, vol. 31, no. 12, DHS pub. no. (DHS) 83-1120, Washington, D.C., U.S. Government Printing Office.
8. Ross Roundtable Conference Proceedings: Assessing the status of the elderly: state of the art, Columbus, Ohio, 1982, Ross Laboratories.
9. Lee, S.L.: Nutrition services for adults and the elderly, Clin. Nutr. **3**(3):109, May-June 1984.
10. Dwyer, J.T.: Diverse American eating styles, Clin. Nutr. **5**(1):2, January-February 1986.
11. Woteki, C.E.: Methods for surveying food habits: how do we know what Americans are eating? Clin. Nutr. **5**(1):9, January-February 1986.
12. Todd, K.S., Hudes, M., and Calloway, D.H.: Food intake measurement: problems and approaches, Am. J. Clin. Nutr. **37**(1):139, January 1983.
13. Guthrie, H.A.: Variability of nutrient intake over a 3-day period, J. Am. Diet. Assoc. **85**(3):325, March 1985.
14. Fanelli, M.T., and Stevenhagen, K.J.: Consistency of energy and nutrient intakes of older adults: 24-hour recall vs. 1-day food record, J. Am. Diet. Assoc. **86**(5):665, May 1986.

15. Sampson, L.: Food frequency questionnaires as a research instrument, Clin. Nutr. 4(5):171, September-October 1985.
16. Campbell, C., Roe, D.A., and Eickwort, K.: Qualitative diet indexes: a descriptive or an assessment tool? J. Am. Diet. Assoc. **81**(6):687, December 1982.
17. van Steveren, W.A., West, C.E., Hoffmans, M.D.A.F., and others: A comparison of contemporaneous and retrospective estimates of food consumption made by a dietary history method, Am. J. Epidemiol. **123**:884, May 1986.
18. Cook, J.D., and Skikne, B.S.: Serum ferritin: a possible model for the assessment of nutrient stores, Am. J. Clin. Nutr. **35**:229, May 1982.
19. Morrow, F.D.: Assessment of nutritional status in the elderly: application and interpretation of nutritional biochemistries, Clin. Nutr. **5**(3):112, May-June 1986.
20. Kamath, S.K., Lawler, M., Smith, A.E., and others: Hospital malnutrition: a 33-hospital screening study, J. Am. Diet. Assoc. **86**(2):203, February 1986.
21. Jensen, T.G., Long, J.M., III, Dudrick, S.J., and Johnson, D.A.: Nutritional assessment indications of postburn complications, J. Am. Diet. Assoc. **85**(1):68, January 1985.
22. Dixon, J.K., Validity and utility of anthropometric measurements: a survey of cancer outpatients, J. Am. Diet. Assoc. **85**(4):439, April 1985.
23. Grant, J.P., Nutritional assessment in clinical practice, Nutr. Clin. Practice **1**(1):3, February 1986.
24. Courtney, M.E., Greene, H.L., Folk, C.C., and others: Rapidly declining serum albumin values in newly hospitalized patients: prevalence, severity, and contributory factors, J. Parenter. Enteral Nutr. **6**(2):143, March-April 1982.
25. Oberfell, M.S., and Ometer, J.L.: Quality assurance. II. Application of oncology standards against a levels-of-care model, J. Am. Diet. Assoc. **81**(2):132, 1982.

FURTHER READING

Centers for Disease Control: Behavioral Risk Factor Surveillance—Selected states, surveillance summaries, M.M.W.R. **32**:155, February 1983. Prevalence surveys—U.S.:
1st quarter, 1982, M.M.W.R. **32**:10, March 8, 1983.
2nd quarter, 1982, M.M.W.R. **32**:28, July 22, 1983.
3rd quarter, 1982, M.M.W.R. **32**:46, November 25, 1983.

These reports provide information from the special behavioral risk factor surveys being conducted by the Centers for Disease Control, Atlanta, Ga.

Food consumption: households in the U.S., Spring, 1977. USDA pub. H-1, Hyattsville, Md., 1982, Human Nutrition Information Service.

Food intakes: individuals in 48 states, year 1977-78, USDA pub. I-1, Hyattsville, Md., 1983 Human Nutrition Information Service.

These reports provide information from National Food Consumption Surveys (NFCS) conducted by the U.S. Department of Agriculture.

Plan and operation of the Health and Nutrition Examination Survey, 1971-73, DHHS pub. (PHS) 79-1310. (Vital and health statistics; series 1; no. 10a) Hyattsville, Md., 1973, National Center for Health Statistics.

Plan and operation of the second National Health and Nutrition Examination Survey, 1976-80. DHHS pub. (PHS) 81-1317. (Vital and health statistics; series 1; no. 15) Hyattsville, Md., 1981, National Center for Health Statistics.

Plan and operation of the Hispanic Health and Nutrition Examination Survey, 1982-84, DHHS pub. (PHS) 85-1321. (Vital and health statistics; series 1; no. 19) Hyattsville, Md., 1985, National Center for Health Statistics.

These three reports provide information from the three NHANES studies: I, II, and the most recent one covering Hispanic populations.

Public Health Service: Healthy people: the Surgeon General's report on health promotion and disease prevention, pub. no. 79-5507, Washington, D.C., 1979, U.S. Department of Health and Human Services.

Public Health Service: Promoting health, preventing disease: objectives for the nation, Washington, D.C., 1980, U.S. Department of Health and Human Services.

Public Health Service: Promoting health—preventing disease: implementation plan for attaining the objectives for the nation, Public Health Reports, September-October (Suppl.), 1983.

These three reports provide information about the current national health program being conducted by the Public Health Service division of DHHS. These goals for health promotion and disease prevention have been scheduled to run from 1980-1990, with evaluation of progress in 1990.

Nutrition Monitoring Division, Human Nutrition Information Service: Report: national food consumption survey, continuing survey of food intakes by individuals (CSFII)—1985, Nutrition Today **21**(3):18, May-June 1986.

This is a summary of the first report of the new ongoing survey of the USDA, designed to provide regular continuous information on the nutritional status of the U.S. population, supplementing the large NFCS every 10 years. The full report (NFCS, CSFII, Report no. 85-1) may be obtained from the Government Printing Office, Washington, D.C., 20402. ($4.25)

Nutrition Monitoring Division, Human Nutrition Information Service: Report: national food consumption survey, continuing survey of food intakes by individuals (CSFII)—1985, Nutrition Today **21**(6):31, November-December 1986.

This is a summary of the second report of the new ongoing CSFII project of the USDA above, providing summary statistics. This full report (NFCS, CSFII, Report no. 85-2) may also be obtained as indicated above.

Rizek, R.L., and Posati, L.P.: Continuing survey of food intake by individuals, Fam. Econ. Rev. **1**:16, 1985.

This article provides significant background on this same project above concerning nutritional deficiencies in low-income, high-risk populations.

Simko, M.D., Cowell, C., and Gilbride, J.A.: Nutrition assessment: a comprehensive guide for planning intervention, Rockville, Md., 1984, Aspen Publishers.

This book provides a wealth of information for comprehensive clinical nutrition assessment as a basis for planning nutritional aspects of health care for individuals.

Weigley, E.S.: Average? Ideal? Desirable? A brief overview of height-weight tables in the United States, J. Am. Diet. Assoc. **84**(4):417, 1984.

This excellent article tells the story of standard height-weight tables, their development and why they should be approached with caution and good sense for individual assessments.

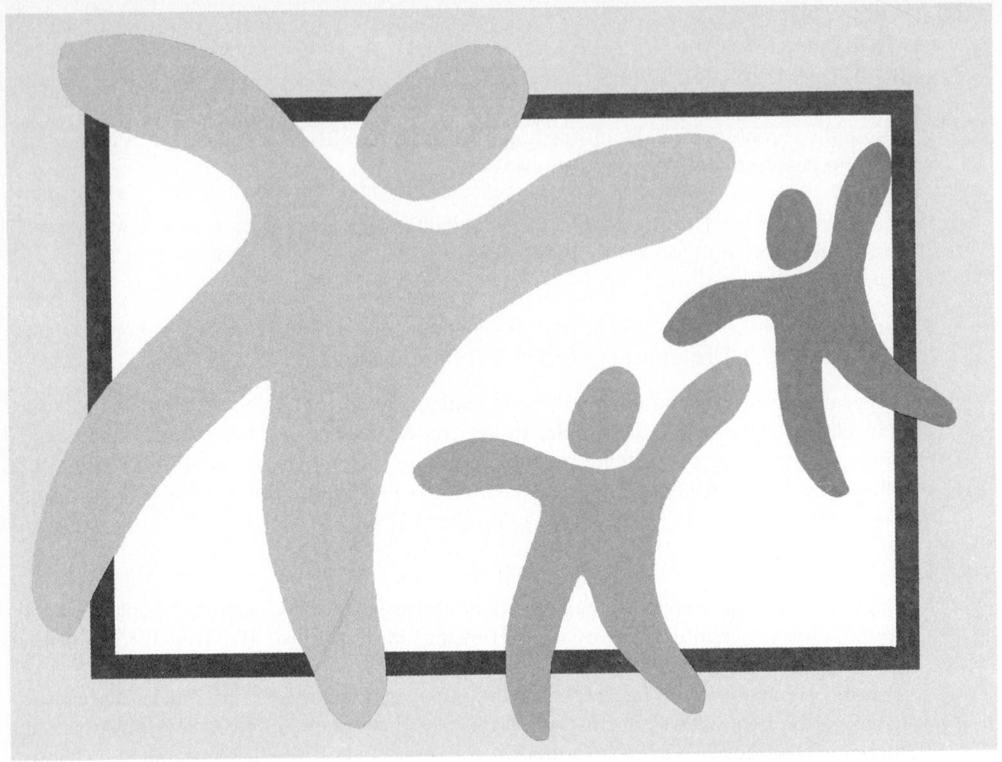

Basic Concepts

1. Data about nutritional influences on fetal growth guide sound maternal nutrition.
2. The physiology of pregnancy determines answers to maternal nutritional issues.
3. Specific nutritional deficiencies and excesses affect fetal development.
4. Prenatal weight gain follows varying individual patterns.
5. Unusual eating behaviors that occur during pregnancy require evaluation.
6. Non-nutrient dietary components affect pregnancy outcome.

Chapter Four

Maternal Nutrition and the Course and Outcome of Pregnancy

Bonnie S. Worthington-Roberts

Food is essential to life and growth. Without an adequate supply of food, and the nutrients it contains, an organism cannot grow and develop normally. Eventually it dies.

In spite of these simple and well-established facts, the role that nutrition plays in the course and outcome of pregnancy has not always been recognized. In the controlled conditions of the laboratory, researchers have been able to demonstrate harmful effects of deficient diets on pregnant animals and their offspring in a number of species. However, when studies are made on free-living human populations, direct relationships between what a mother eats during the 9 months of gestation and the course and outcome of her pregnancy are not always evident. Consequently, the emphasis that nutrition has received in prenatal care has varied over the years. At times, when researchers have been able to show positive effects, nutrition has received a great deal of attention. At other times, when studies produced equivocal results, nutrition has slipped to a position of indifference and neglect.

Part of the problem is that the changes occurring during pregnancy, their influence on nutritional needs, and the effects of long-term nutritional status on reproductive performance are not fully understood. The application of nutrition principles to pregnancy has had to depend on progress in scientific knowledge about reproduction itself, and as in any science, one of the most important advances is simply learning to ask the right questions. The emphasis of research has changed as more has become known about nutrition, reproduction, and human growth. Thus it is possible to gain a sense of perspective that helps in understanding why different dietary recommendations for pregnant women have been made.

Nutrition and Pregnancy: Historical Development

EARLY BELIEFS AND PRACTICES

During the nineteenth century much of what was known and recommended about diet during pregnancy was based on casual observation rather than controlled studies. Little information was available on the nutrient composition of foods or their biologic values. Dietary advice was influenced by belief in imitative magic: belief that the mother or child would acquire the attributes of the foods in the mother's diet. For example, pregnant women were sometimes forbidden to eat salty, acidic, or sour foods for fear the infant would be born with a "sour" disposition. The beliefs were often colored by the emotional and mystical aura surrounding the pregnant state. Eggs were sometimes restricted because of their association with the reproductive function. On the other hand, certain foods were encouraged for their presumed beneficial effects. Pregnant women were often advised to eat broths, warm milk, and ripe fruits to soothe the fetus and ease the birth process.

Obstetrical Problems

Problems in nineteenth-century obstetrical practice also influenced dietary recommendation. During the Industrial Revolution children in Europe had poor diets and worked long hours in dark factories. Rickets, which impaired normal bone formation during the growth years, was a common disorder. A contracted pelvis resulting from rickets was a major obstetrical risk. Physicians did not have the modern means of delivering infants from these mothers that are available today. Death of both mother and child during childbirth was common.

Prochownick Diet

Experience with his own patients in the 1880s led a German physician, Prochownick, to advocate a fluid-restricted, high-protein, low-carbohydrate diet for women with contracted pelvises to be followed for 6 weeks before birth. Women using such a diet produced smaller infants and had easier deliveries. The diet may have had some justification in the 1880s, but it later gained in popularity and became a standard recommendation throughout pregnancy, even when the original rationale no longer applied. Remnants of the Prochownick diet, restricting fluid and carbohydrate intake, persist today.

Early Studies and Opinions

There is very little specific information available about diet and pregnancy before the 1930s, other than reports on the effects of food shortages during and after World War I. After the war there was much effort to relate food shortages to the size of the baby, but most of the evidence presented was inconclusive and even contradictory.

RE-EVALUATION AND REDIRECTION

It was not until the mid-1960s that renewed interest in infant mortality and morbidity rates led to a reappraisal of the influence of diet on pregnancy. Once attention was redirected toward this problem, a number of significant steps were taken. The resulting progress has been so rapid that we can hardly grasp it. First, two important events occurred in rapid succession.

The White House Conference

The White House Conference on Food, Nutrition, and Health was held in Washington in December of 1969. The immediate stimulus was the nationwide shock at the disclosures of widespread hunger and malnutrition in the United States. The determination to do something about it produced the Conference as the first organizational step. Many experts there, involved in the Panel on Pregnancy and Very Young Infants, were also involved with the soon-to-be-published National Research Council (NRC) report on maternal nutrition and the course of pregnancy. They saw the Conference as a priceless opportunity to address the applied issues of diet and pregnancy within the context of their needed health services.

Benchmark NRC Report

The NRC report, *Maternal Nutrition and the Course of Pregnancy,*[1] was issued in 1970. It remains today the major source of research information on the role of nutrition in human reproduction. One of the principal findings of that report was the limited and fragmentary nature of studies on diet and pregnancy. The report singled out the need for long-term longitudinal studies on women and their families. This need still remains.

FOLLOW-UP GUIDELINES AND PROGRAMS

Initial Guidelines for Practice

In 1973, two sets of guidelines appeared as a direct outgrowth of the stimulus given to nutrition services at the White House Conference: (1) the American Public Health Association[2] guidelines and standards primarily for public health workers as an aid to assessments and program planning; and (2) the NRC[3] guidelines for uses and limitations of supplementary food provided during pregnancy. The technical issues, practical problems, and political realities were explored, along with the inherent difficulties involved in multidisciplinary and multifactorial studies.

WIC Program

In 1978, the now well-known WIC program—Special Supplementary Food Program for Women, Infants, and Children[4]—was initiated under court order. The expressed purpose of the WIC program was to provide food as an adjunct to health care during critical times of growth and development. WIC has grown from a pilot program costing $40 million in 1973 to one costing over $1 billion in 1986. Many of the same problems addressed in the 1969 White House Conference are still being encountered in the WIC program today, leading to questions of what the program is accomplishing.

ACOG-ADA Guidelines

In 1981, the American College of Obstetricians and Gynecologists (ACOG) and the American Dietetic Association (ADA) issued a joint publication, *Guidelines for Assess-*

ment of Maternal Nutrition.[5] This was indeed a milestone. The report produced the first national consensus on the relevant risk factors before and during pregnancy. This original listing has been updated by the more recent material in the NRC perinatal guide.

NRC Perinatal Guide

In 1981, the NRC produced the highly useful guide, *Nutrition Services in Perinatal Care.*[6] This report was particularly timely because it was designed for use with the rapidly growing regional networks for maternal and perinatal services. It is most helpful because it addresses the nutritional issues of infant feeding and the increasingly important concerns about substance abuse—cigarettes, drugs, and alcohol.

Continued Needs

There is increasing realization of the seamless web of variables that together influence the outcome of a pregnancy. Within the constellation of income, health, education, family and fertility, food and nutrition are just one part, but an important and modifiable one. As one recent observer stated, "Special efforts to improve prenatal, child, and maternal health showed clear evidence that the services did make a difference. . . . No one has yet teased out the relative effects of different variables."[7] This is the clearest statement of the nature of the problems that need to be addressed in the years ahead.

Nutritional Influences on Fetal Growth

It is not possible, for obvious reasons, to examine maternal-fetal relationships directly at the cellular and molecular levels in humans. Consequently, work toward understanding how maternal nutrition influences growth and development in utero must be done on animals. The technique has usually been to manipulate the diets of pregnant animals and study the effects on cellular morphology and physiology in the offspring at various stages of gestation. Over the past few years much information has accumulated from studies of this type.

EXPERIMENTS IN ANIMALS

Energy and Nutrient Restriction

Two types of dietary restrictions have been imposed on laboratory animals to study the effects of maternal nutrition on fetal growth and development. One restriction is simply not giving the animals enough food so that the diet is low in kilocalories. The other restriction holds kilocalories at an adequate level but reduces or completely eliminates one or more essential nutrients. The effects of deficiencies of almost all of the known nutrients have been studied this way, but restrictions of protein and kilocalories have more relevance to humans than restrictions of vitamins or minerals. All animals need energy and use protein in essentially the same way, but the need for vitamins and minerals and their specific functions differ from species to species.

A number of investigators have demonstrated what can happen to fetuses when pregnant animals are fed kilocalorie- or protein-restricted diets. Maternal malnutrition can interfere with the ability of the mother to conceive, it can produce death and resorption or abortion of the fetuses, and it can produce malformations or retarded growth. Of course, the more severe the dietary restrictions are, the more serious the effects will be. A reduction of as little as 25% of the total kilocalories without an imbalance in the quality of the maternal diet in rats can reduce both the number of pups born and their ability to survive.

Biochemical studies show why this occurs. One effect of protein-kilocalorie malnutrition is an impairment of cell energy metabolism by interfering with the enzymes involved in glycolysis and the citric acid cycle. Without adequate supplies of amino acids and energy, cell functions break down, and normal processes of growth cannot occur. The effects would be most damaging when cells are normally undergoing rapid division. This implies that the timing of the dietary deficiency, as well as its severity, is important.

Stages of Cell Growth

Animals grow in two ways. They get larger because their cells increase in number or because the cells they already have increase in size. Winick[8] has identified a sequence of cell growth common to all organs of the body (Fig. 4-1). In the first stage growth

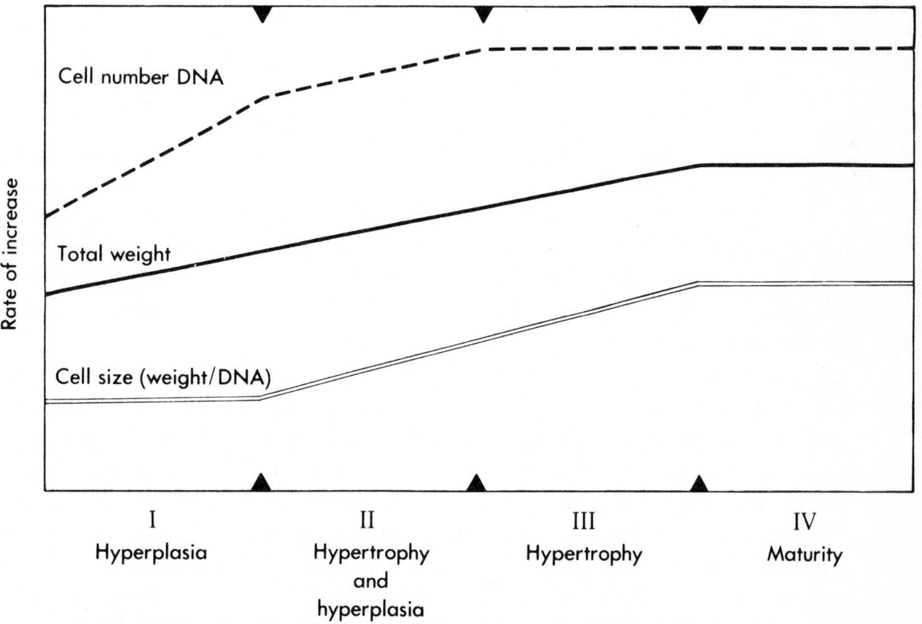

FIG. 4-1 Stages of cell growth.
(Modified from Winick, M.: Nutr. Rev. 26:195, 1968.)

takes place only by an increase in the number of cells; that is, cells are replicating and all are about equal in size. This first stage of cell growth is called *hyperplasia.* In the second stage new cells continue to be made, but the ones already present now begin to increase in size, a process called *hypertrophy.* Thus this second stage is both hyperplastic and hypertrophic. The third stage is totally hypertrophic. Here growth is taking place only by increases in cell size and no new cells are being formed. The fourth stage is *maturity,* in which all cell growth stops. In this stage there is further development as enzyme systems are elaborated and cell functions are integrated.

These stages of cell growth are not really discrete processes but merge into one another. The length of each stage and the periods of maximum cell proliferation differ according to the species and in various parts of the body. In most regions there is continuous increase until equilibrium is reached as old cells die and new ones are made. However, in nonregenerating organs such as the brain, the number and size of cells present at the end of hyperplasia must last a lifetime. For this organ in particular, any interference with normal cell growth may have consequences that cannot be repaired.

The consequences of any interference with normal cell growth would depend not only on the tissue but also on the time at which it occurs. Interference in the hyperplastic phase would result in a decrease in the number of cells. Interference at the hypertrophic phase would result in reduction of cell size. Both types of interference would cause the animal to experience growth failure. However, "catch-up growth" is possible if the insult occurred during the period of hypertrophy. This is not the case if the deficit occurred during hyperplasia.

Types of Growth Failure

It is now clear that a number of things can produce growth failure in utero. The cause can be either "intrinsic" or "extrinsic." In differential diagnosis the condition of the placentas of animals born small for gestational age is considered. In intrinsic intrauterine growth failure placentas are usually of normal size. This implies that fetal growth retardation was not caused by inadequate maternal-fetal transport but was the result of other factors. Some examples include chromosomal abnormalities and maternal infections. Extrinsic intrauterine growth failure is usually manifested by placentas that are reduced in size. This indicates that they were incapable of supplying the fetus with adequate nutrition.

The principal feature of intrinsic growth failure is the presence of multiple malformations in the fetuses. These are absent in growth failure produced experimentally by ligation of blood vessels supplying the placenta. They are variable in maternal malnutrition, depending on the timing of the restriction. In both vascular and nutritional failure, placentas are reduced in proportion to fetal weight. In the ligated animals and in late maternal malnutrition, the reduction is caused by a decrease in the average size of the cells. Maternal protein restriction maintained throughout most of gestation, however, decreases both the number and size of placental cells.

The fetuses themselves also show different patterns of growth retardation. Those subjected to vascular insufficiency show an asymmetrical retardation. The fetuses have relatively normal brain sizes and head circumferences, but their livers are greatly reduced in size, by as much as 50%, and glycogen reserves are completely absent. Proportionally these animals have bigger brains and heads compared to the rest of their bodies. They are extremely hypoglycemic at birth.

When maternal protein restriction is limited to the last few days of gestation, the fetuses show a pattern of growth retardation similar to that produced by vascular insufficiency—proportionally big heads and small bodies. However, when the restriction is imposed throughout most of the gestation period, the pattern of fetal growth retardation becomes more symmetrical. There is a 15% to 20% decrease in cell number in all organs including the brain. Head circumference is also reduced. The reduced cell number is greatest in those regions of the brain that are undergoing the most rapid rates of cell division.

Consequences of Growth Failure

These findings make it obvious that fetuses are *not* perfect parasites that can survive intrauterine insults without adverse effects. Data suggest that inadequate maternal nutrition can affect the fetus in ways that coincide with the stages of cell growth, and that the body reserves of the mother cannot always insulate the fetus from dietary deficiencies. What happens to animals whose mothers were nutritionally deprived during pregnancy depends to a great extent on how they are fed after birth.

Perhaps the finding of most concern is the effect of continued deprivation on the growth of brain cells. If prenatally malnourished pups are restricted after birth by feeding them in litters of 18 pups per dam, they demonstrate a *60%* reduction in brain cell number by the time they are weaned. This contrasts with the 20% to 25% reduction seen in either prenatal or postnatal malnutrition alone. Thus it seems that continued malnutrition throughout the entire time the brain cells are dividing produces greater deficits than would be expected if the separate effects were simply added together. Experiments have shown that nutritional rehabilitation will not enable these animals to recover their normal size once the period of cell proliferation has passed. They will continue to be small no matter how well fed they are after weaning. Other data suggest that maternal malnutrition may even have an intergenerational effect; brain cell numbers were reduced in rats whose mothers were prenatally malnourished, even though these mothers had adequate diets during lactation and after weaning.

These studies would not be so disturbing if size were not related to function. The fact is, however, that alterations in normal biochemical and developmental processes accompany fetal and neonatal malnutrition in several species of animals. Changes in the usual constituents of cells are observed, as well as the delayed appearance of specific enzyme systems. Depending on the timing of the dietary deficiency, degeneration of the cerebral cortex, the medulla, and the spinal cord occurs. Muscular development is also impaired because of a reduced number of muscle cells and fibers.

What Has Been Learned from Animal Research

Much can still be learned from experiments with animals about the processes of fetal growth and development and the consequences of maternal malnutrition. But the work to date has produced important results. General conclusions can be summarized:

1. **Growth failure.** Although a number of prenatal influences affect fetal growth, maternal malnutrition can be one cause of growth failure that results in low birth weight.
2. **Nature of tissue effects.** Animals malnourished from restrictions of their mothers' diets throughout most of gestation are characterized by: (1) reduced number and size of cells in the placenta, (2) reduced brain cell number and head size, (3) proportional reductions in the size of other organs, and (4) alterations in normal cell constituents and biochemical processes.
3. **Influencing factors.** The fetal consequences of malnutrition depend on the timing, severity, and duration of the maternal dietary restriction. These consequences may be reversible if the restriction primarily affects growth in cell size. But a reduction in the number of cells may be permanent if the restriction is maintained throughout the entire period of hyperplastic growth.

HUMAN EXPERIENCE IN FETAL GROWTH

Low Birth Weight

In view of the risks of early death or permanent disability associated with low birth weight, it is apparent that the animal research on intrauterine failure may have great implications for human problems. Of the annual incidence of low-birth-weight infants, it is estimated that 10% to 20% result from intrauterine growth failure. This means that 80,000 to 120,000 infants who have experienced malnutrition in utero are born each year in the United States. An important thing to understand when interpreting these statistics is that there is no one cause—a number of factors can retard fetal growth. When the term *fetal malnutrition* is applied to human infants, it simply means that there was a reduction in the maternal supply or placental transport of nutrients so that fetal growth is retarded significantly below genetic potential. It does not necessarily mean that the mother's nutrition was at fault. At present there is no way to judge how many growth-retarded infants are the result of maternal malnutrition.[9]

Relation of Animal Studies

Although the animal experiments are highly suggestive, be cautious in making direct applications to humans. A primary reason for doing animal research is to find out what can *possibly* happen when certain conditions are imposed. The findings do not guarantee that these things *actually* happen in the course of human events. There are a number of reasons why the dramatic results of maternal malnutrition demonstrated in animals may not occur as readily in human beings. In effect the consequences of maternal malnutrition on fetal growth and development are all magnified in the animal studies. This is because: (1) relative rates of growth and development are much slower in humans compared with laboratory animals; (2) the timing of maximal growth also differs; (3) the number and size of fetuses a mother must nourish in utero compared with her own body size and nutritional reserves are much smaller in humans than in laboratory animals; and (4) the magnitude of dietary deprivation used for experimentation is rarely encountered in human populations under ordinary circumstances.

Stages of Human Fetal Growth

Techniques for measuring cell number and size are now being used to determine the stages of maximum cell growth and development in humans, Although data are at present incomplete, a picture that generally parallels the sequence outlined for animals emerges (Fig. 4-2). After the ovum is released from the mature follicle in the ovary, it enters the Fallopian tube. It moves slowly through the tube toward the uterus, encountering potentially fertilizing sperm along the way. Fertilization usually occurs in the Fallopian tube within 48 hours, after which cell division rapidly proceeds. The resulting solid ball of cells, the *morula,* enters the uterus where it undergoes reorganization into a hollow ball, the *blastocyst.* The blastocyst ultimately buries itself in the endometrial lining of the uterus (5-7 days post-ovulation). Here the precursor cells of the placenta begin to arrange themselves into a functioning placental unit. Nutritional support for the embryo at this time comes from the endometrial lining of the uterus. After its initial development, the placenta grows rapidly throughout gestation. By 34-36 weeks it has completed cell division. From that time until term, growth continues only by increase in size of existing cells.

Embryologic studies indicate three stages of fetal growth:

1. **Blastogenesis stage.** The fertilized egg divides into cells that fold in on one another. An inner cell mass evolves, giving rise to the embryo and an outer coat, the *trophoblast,* which becomes the placenta. This process is complete about 2 weeks after fertilization.
2. **Embryonic stage.** This is the critical time when cells differentiate into three germinal layers. The *ectoderm,* outer layer, gives rise to the brain, nervous system, hair, and skin. The *mesoderm,* middle layer, produces all of the voluntary muscles, bones, and components of the cardiovascular and excretory systems. The *endoderm,* inner layer, forms the digestive and respiratory systems, and glandular organs. By 60 days' gestation all of the major features of the human infant are achieved.
3. **Fetal stage.** This is the period of most rapid growth. From the third month until term, fetal weight increases nearly 500-fold from 6 g (0.2 oz) to 3000-3500 g (6.5-7.5 lb) at birth. The average weight curve from 10 weeks to term is shown in Fig. 4-3.

Measurements of DNA and protein in embryonic and fetal tissues show that embryonic growth occurs only by increase in number of cells. Fetal growth continues in cell number, but now also involves increase in cell size.

Growth-Retarded Infants

From the sequence described, it is possible to estimate the effects of malnutrition on growth at different stages of gestation. In the early months of pregnancy a severe limit on supply or transport of nutrients would have to occur to cause retarded growth because the quantitative requirements of the embryo are extremely small. Nevertheless, a restriction of materials and energy needed for cell synthesis and cell differen-

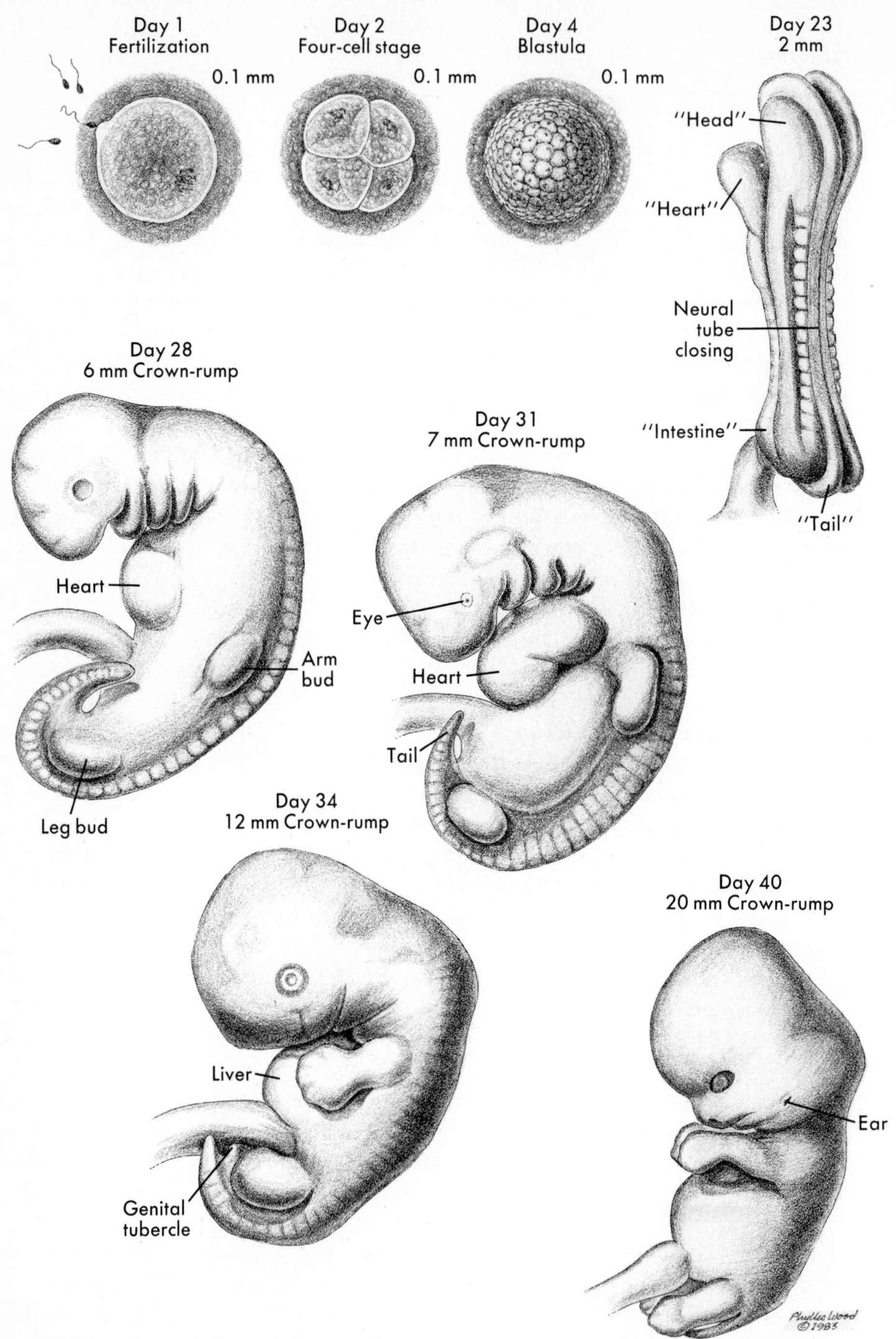

FIG. 4-2 Stages of fetal development.

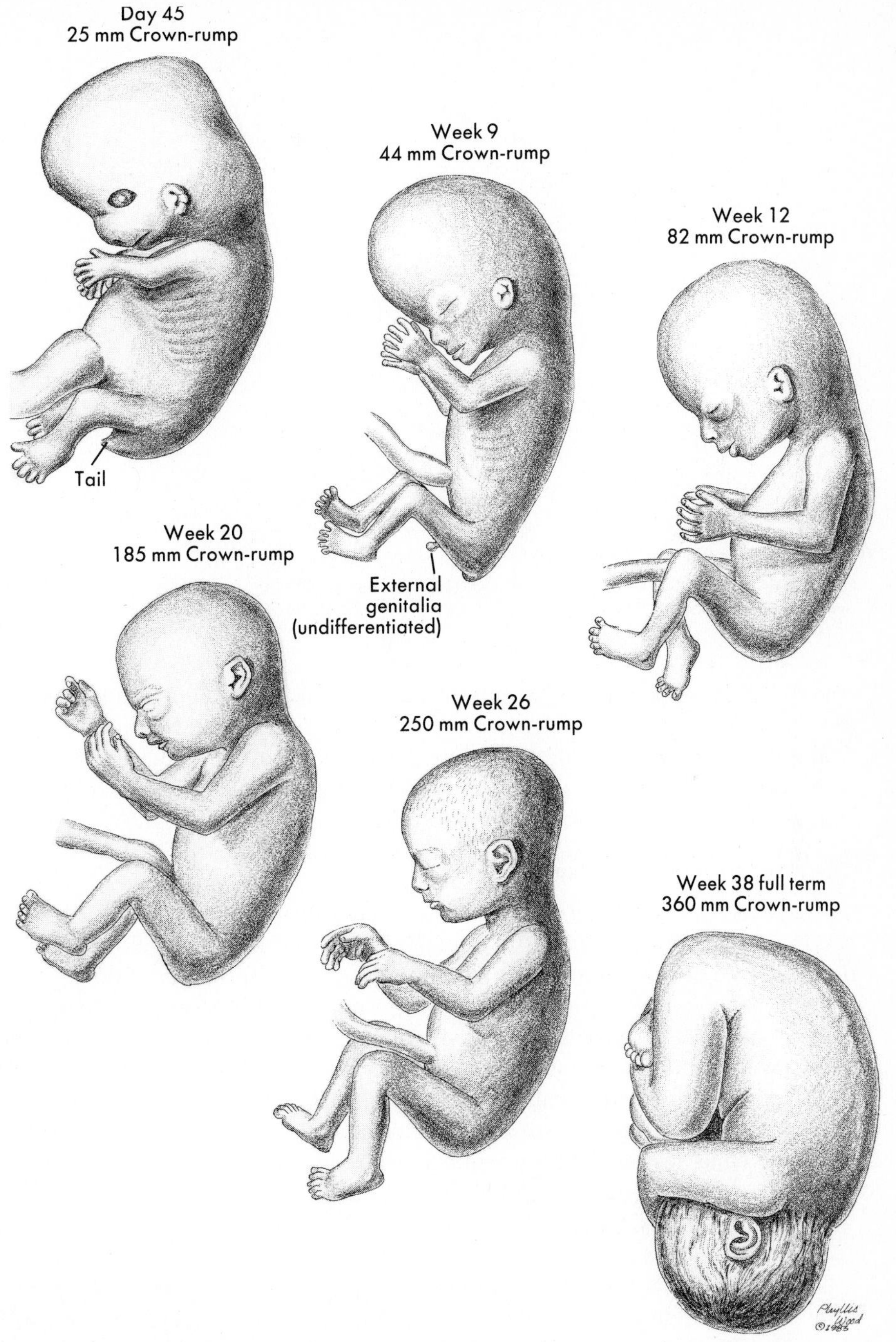

FIG. 4-2 Stages of fetal development—cont'd.

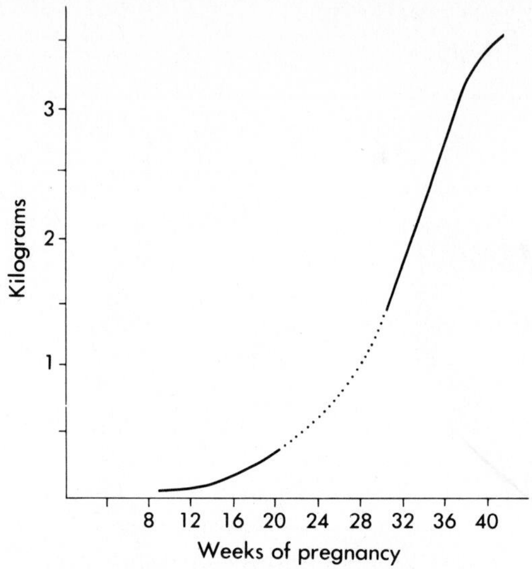

FIG. 4-3 Average curve of fetal growth.
(From Hytten, F.E., and Leitch, I.: The physiology of human pregnancy, ed. 2, Oxford, 1971, Blackwell Scientific Publications.)

tiation could produce malformations or cause the embryo to die. Malnutrition after the third month of gestation would not have teratogenic effects, but it could interfere with fetal growth. Nutrient requirements are greatest in the last trimester of pregnancy, when cells are increasing rapidly in both number and size. Even a relatively mild restriction could have serious effects at this time.

Characteristics of SGA Infants

The effects of fetal malnutrition are reflected in the characteristics of *small-for-gestational-age (SGA)* infants, who though full term are poorly developed. Their conditions are variable, suggesting the multiple causes and importance of timing shown in animals. Among those SGA infants that do not have birth anomalies, there are two patterns of growth retardation. One type affects weight more than length; the other affects weight and length equally:

1. **Type I: Growth retardation primarily affecting weight.** Head size (circumference) and skeletal growth are about normal, but the infants have poorly developed muscles and almost no subcutaneous fat. The resemblance of these infants' characteristics to the large head, small body features of animals malnourished during the last weeks of gestation, either by maternal dietary restrictions or uterine ligation, is remarkable.
2. **Type II: Growth reduction in both weight and height.** Size of all parts of the body, including head circumference and skeleton, is reduced proportionally. The physical characteristics of these infants are similar to those of rat pups whose mothers had deficient diets throughout all of gestation.

EFFECTS OF MATERNAL MALNUTRITION

Observations described above provide fertile grounds for speculation, but what is the evidence in human populations that maternal malnutrition causes fetal malnutrition? Of necessity much of the information is incidental. Nonetheless, there have been three kinds of studies that have addressed this question with highly significant results: (1) natural experiments in which birth statistics before, during, and after periods of acute famine are studied and compared: (2) measurements of organ size and cell numbers in stillbirths and neonatal deaths in which all causes not related to maternal malnutrition have been ruled out; and (3) epidemiologic studies of the nutritional correlates of birth weights.

Natural Experiments

The hardships of war afford researchers an opportunity to study the effects of severe dietary restrictions during pregnancy under conditions that fortunately are seldom duplicated. Throughout most of Europe at various times during World War II, food shortages were common. Reports were made on the effects of these shortages during the 1940s, but they are being considered with renewed interest today in light of the findings from animal research. Experiences in Russia and Holland provide examples of these effects:

1. **Russia.** During the siege of Leningrad in 1942 and its immediate aftermath, there was an 18-month period of severe starvation. Comparison of statistics for infants born before, during, and after the siege revealed an expected toll in the course and outcome of pregnancy under such desperate conditions. During the famine period there was a twofold increase in fetal mortality, as well as an increase in the number of infants weighing less than 2500 g (5.4 lb) at birth.
2. **Holland.** Similar findings were reported from Holland. Here the results are more insightful because the famine began suddenly and was limited to about 6 months during the winter of 1944-1945. It was not accompanied by other deprivations as severe as those experienced during the siege of Leningrad, and the women of Holland had fairly good diets before the food shortage. During the famine period dietary intake dropped to less than 1000 kcal a day, and protein was limited to 30 to 40 g. Since the famine lasted only 6 months, babies conceived before and during that period were exposed for varying lengths of time, but none was exposed for the entire course of gestation. On the average, birth weights of infants exposed to the famine were reduced by 200 g (7 oz). Weights were lowest for babies exposed to the famine during the entire last half of the pregnancy. Added exposure before that time did not reduce birth weights further. In fact, babies exposed to the famine during the first 27 weeks of gestation, but finishing their terms after the famine ended, had higher average birth weights than those who were only exposed during the last 3 weeks of gestation. The data for stillbirths and congenital malformations followed a different pattern. The rates were lowest for infants conceived before the famine and highest for those conceived during it.

   The findings are in line with what is expected from knowledge of the stages of human growth. Poor nutrition in the latter part of pregnancy affects fetal growth, whereas poor nutrition in the early months affects development of the embryo and its capacity to survive.

3. **Great Britain.** It is interesting to note that, in contrast with the experiences in Russia and Holland, the prenatal mortality rate in Great Britain, which had been fairly constant before the war, actually declined between 1940-1945 despite the poor environmental conditions and no discernible improvements in prenatal care. One possible explanation is that pregnant and lactating women were given priority status for food in Britain as a matter of national policy.

Organ Studies

Studies that attempt to relate the size of organs in human infants to maternal nutrition must control for other conditions known to affect fetal growth. One group of researchers looked at the organs of 252 American stillborn infants and infants dying in the first 48 hours of life, excluding all multiple births, maternal complications, and congenital defects. The infants were grouped as coming from poor or nonpoor families according to income. Comparisons of organs between the two groups showed that the mass of adipose tissue and the size of individual fat cells were smaller in the poor infants. These infants also had smaller livers, adrenal glands, thymuses, and spleens. Heart, kidney, and skeleton were also reduced, but the differences were not as great. The ranking in organ size is consistent with reductions noted in animals who have been prenatally malnourished and in humans who have experienced uterine or placental disorders. Since the last two conditions were ruled out of the study, the investigators concluded that undernutrition could be responsible for prenatal growth retardation in infants from low-income families.

The organs in infants who survive intrauterine malnutrition cannot be studied to see if cells are reduced in number or size, but one organ is available. This is the placenta. One scientist[10] reported that the size of placentas and the number of placental cells are 15% to 20% below normal when infants experience growth failure. By comparing placentas from different sources, he has shown that those from indigent populations in developing countries have reductions in cell numbers similar to the reductions noted in placentas from American infants with intrauterine growth failure. In one interesting U.S. case a mother who was severely undernourished from anorexia nervosa during pregnancy gave birth to an infant weighing less than 2500 g (5.4 lb). When the placenta was examined, it was found to have only 50% of the normal number of cells.

Nutritional Correlates of Birth Weight

Studies of the relationship between maternal nutrition and the birth weight of the infant have tended to focus directly on the nutrient composition of the diet during pregnancy. Because of variations in the nutritional requirements of individuals, these studies have produced conflicting results. However, there are two indicators of long-term and immediate nutritional status that have shown consistent associations with birth weight. These are: (1) *maternal body size,* height and prepregnancy weight of the mother; and (2) *maternal weight gain,* the amount of weight gained by the mother during the pregnancy itself.

Maternal Body Size

It should not be surprising that big mothers have big babies. What is less often appreciated is that the size of the infant at birth largely depends on the size of the mother and is not influenced to a great degree by the size of the father. This was shown years ago in a classic experiment in which Shire stallions were bred with Shetland mares and Shetland stallions with Shire mares. The newborn foals were always an appropriate size to the mother's breeds. No intermediate sizes were ever produced. The same effects have been demonstrated in a number of animals, and there is indirect evidence for the same phenomenon in humans.

It has been further demonstrated in humans that height and prepregnancy weight of the mother have independent and additive effects on the birth weight of a child. In an analysis of 4095 mothers in Aberdeen, Scotland,[11] it was found that, on average, the tallest and heaviest mothers had babies who weighed 500 g (1 lb) more at birth than babies of the shortest and lightest mothers. It is postulated that maternal size is a conditioning factor on the ultimate size of the placenta and thus controls the blood supply of nutrients available to the fetus.

This idea has support in findings from the Collaborative Perinatal Project of the National Institutes of Health. In this project, Naeye[12] analyzed data from nearly 60,000 pregnancies to discover causes of fetal and neonatal mortality among different racial groups. He found that Puerto Ricans experience a higher rate of placental growth retardation than whites. However, this difference disappears when women with prepregnancy weights of 45 kg (101 lb) or less are excluded from the analysis. Naeye concludes that the high rate of placental growth retardation in Puerto Ricans is a result of the greater proportion of women who enter pregnancy with low body weights. Further data from Naeye's study show that, regardless of race or ethnic origin, mothers with low prepregnancy weights have much lighter placentas than heavier mothers.

Maternal Underweight

Infants of underweight women show several kinds of morbidity. Edwards and colleagues[13] compared outcomes for women who entered pregnancy at 10% or more below standard weight for height with outcomes for women who entered pregnancy at normal weight. The women were matched for age, race, parity, and socioeconomic status. The incidence of both low birth weight and prematurity was significantly higher among the underweight mothers. Infants of underweight women also scored lower on the Apgar scale. This scale measures the general condition of the neonate as evidenced by heart rate, respiration, muscle tone, reflex irritability, and color at delivery. Differences in Apgar scores were even greater when only those infants of women who were excessive cigarette smokers were compared. Underweight women who smoked more than one pack of cigarettes a day during pregnancy had three times the number of infants with low Apgar scores compared with their normal weight controls.

Underweight women were also subject to different rates of pregnancy complications.[13] Anemia occurred more frequently in the underweight group, and those who were both underweight and anemic had an incidence of low birth weight of 17.4%, compared to 3.6% among women who were anemic but of normal weight. The investigators point out that underweight status and iron deficiency anemia both reflect long-term suboptimal nutritional intake. They suggest this as a possible explanation for the apparent influence of anemia and underweight in mothers on the incidence of low birth weight.

Maternal Weight Gain

International surveys support the view that mature women from developed countries gain about 10.8-15.7 kg (24-35 lb) during the course of a "typical" 40-week pregnancy. The normal pattern of weight gain is illustrated in Fig. 4-4. Less than half the total weight gain resides in the fetus, placenta, and amniotic fluid. The remainder is found in maternal reproductive tissues, fluid, blood, and "stores." The weight component labeled "maternal stores" is largely composed of body fat, although some increase in the lean body mass, other than reproductive tissue, may also occur. The action of progesterone in the pregnant woman promotes the development of a fat pad that serves as a caloric reserve for both pregnancy and lactation. Fatfold measurements from 10 to 30 weeks' gestation have shown gradual increases in subcutaneous fat at the abdomen, back, and upper thigh.[14] The pregnant woman who attempts to restrict

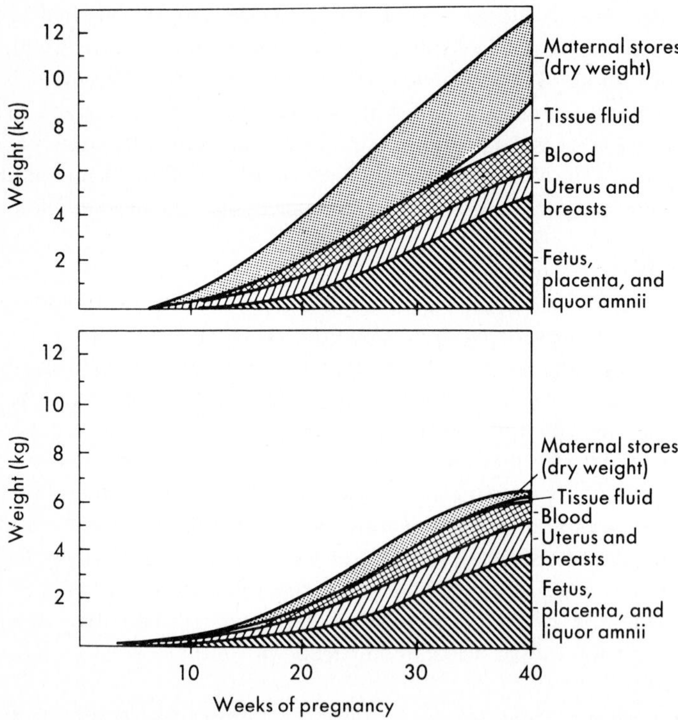

FIG. 4-4 Estimated composition of weight gain during pregnancy for a normal, healthy, Northern European woman (above) and a poor, underfed woman from India (below). (Modified from Hurley, L.S.: Developmental nutrition, Englewood Cliffs, N.J., 1980, Prentice-Hall, Inc.)

weight gain to avoid development of the fat pad will simultaneously affect to some degree normal development of the other products of pregnancy.

SUPPLEMENTATION TRIALS

It is also apparent from the research on infant birth weight that special dietary management for low-income women and others who are known to be at risk of reproductive problems could produce highly beneficial results.[15,16] A number of supplementation studies have been conducted around the world; the reported outcomes in Guatemala and Canada provide documentation of benefit.

Guatemala Study

The study in Guatemala is one of the most comprehensive investigations of the relationship between maternal nutrition and the outcome of pregnancy that has ever been undertaken. It involves all women of childbearing age in four villages in a long-term, prospective study to see what effects nutrition has on physical growth and mental development of their offspring.[17] Before beginning their study the investigators collected a great deal of information about birth statistics, dietary practices, and nutritional status of the women in the four villages. They found evidence of chronic but moderate malnutrition by measuring heights, weights, and head circumferences. During pregnancy, women averaged a weight gain of only 6.7 kg (15 lb). They typically consumed about 1500 kilocalories and 40 g of protein per day. This protein-kilocalorie ratio is adequate. The moderate degree of malnutrition was primarily the result of insufficient food consumption. Mean birth weights in the population were between 3000 and 3200 g (6.5-7 lb), but about one-third of the infants carried to term were of low birth weight.

The plan of the study included the provision of dietary supplements to all pregnant women who would voluntarily accept them. In two of the villages the supplement "Atole" contained both protein and kilocalories. The supplement "Fresco" was given to women in the other two villages. It contained kilocalories but no protein. Both supplements had approximately equal amounts of vitamins and minerals.

Intakes from the supplements and home diets were recorded in each trimester of pregnancy to make sure that the women were not substituting the supplements for their usual food. The records showed that the supplements did, in fact, increase the total intake by an average of 26,820 kilocalories during the entire course of pregnancy. However, since consumption of the supplements was voluntary, there were wide ranges of intakes. The researchers were therefore able to divide the women into a low supplement group and a high supplement group according to the total number of additional kilocalories they consumed. The level of 20,000 kilocalories were chosen as the dividing line because this was the median value for all the women. When the women were divided this way, there was a difference of 34,000 kilocalories between the mean supplemental intakes of the high and low groups.

During the first 4 years of the study, complete data on maternal supplementation and birth weight were available for 405 infants born in the 4 villages. The first thing to be noted in the results is that for full term infants there was a consistent increase in birth weight as the total supplemental kilocalories of the mother increased. The distribution was such that for each 10,000 kilocalories ingested by the mother during pregnancy, birth weight of the infant increased 50 g (1.7 oz). The greatest difference in birth weight was observed between infants whose mothers consumed less than 20,000 supplemental kilocalories and those whose mothers consumed 20,000 supplemental kilocalories or more. The significance of this is shown by the percent of low birth weight babies born to high- and low-supplemented mothers (Fig. 4-5). The rate of low birth weight was roughly two times lower when the mothers consumed 20,000 supplemental kilocalories or more throughout gestation.

The investigators also examined weights of the placentas. They found, on the average, that the group with low maternal supplementation had placentas weighing 11%

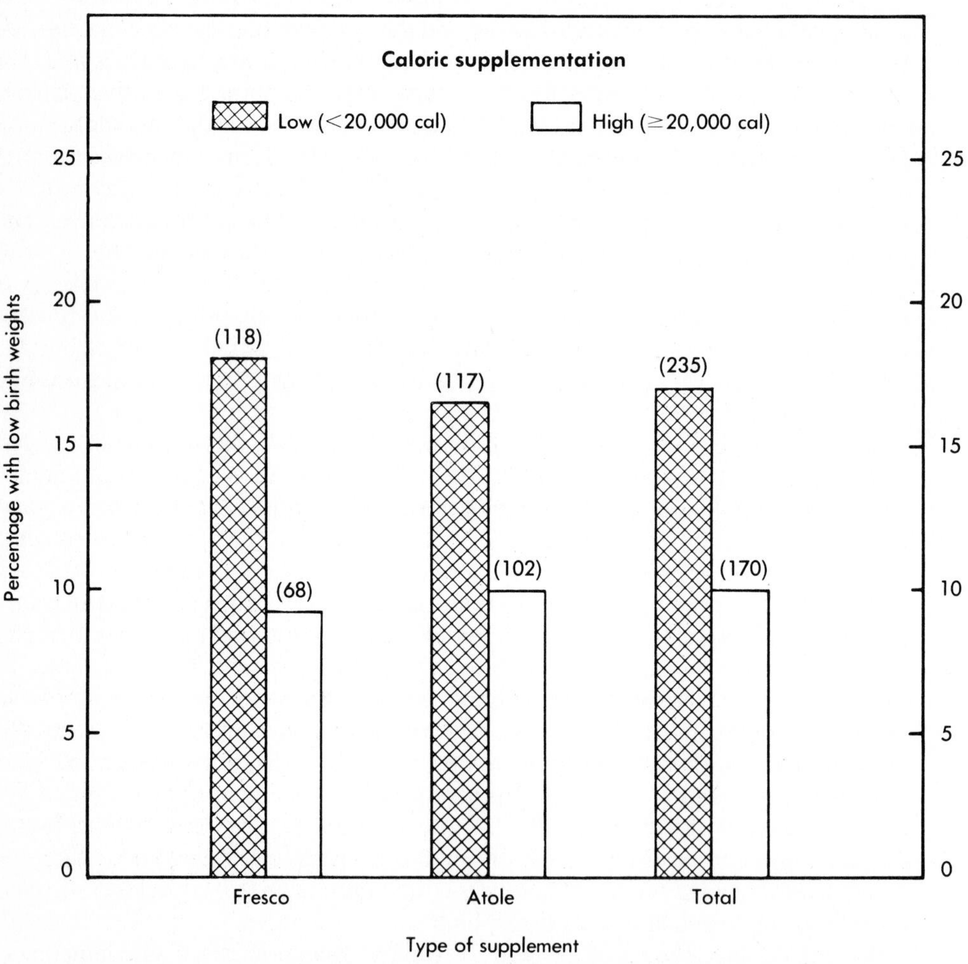

FIG. 4-5 Relationship between supplemented calories during pregnancy and proportion of low-birth-weight babies (≤2500 g). Numbers in parentheses indicate number of cases.
(From Lechtig, A., and others: Effect of food supplementation during pregnancy on birthweight, Pediatrics 56:508-519, 1975. Reprinted with permission.)

less than the group with high maternal supplementation. Further analysis showed that most of the association between maternal supplementation and birth weight could be explained statistically by the difference in placental weight. This supports the earlier observation that the size of the placenta may be the means by which maternal nutrition affects birth weight.

An interesting aspect of these findings is that there was no difference in placental weight, mean birth weight, or the percent of low-birth-weight babies associated with the *type* of supplement used. As long as the kilocalories were equivalent, it did not matter whether the supplement contained protein. This may seem surprising in view of the emphasis people tend to place on the importance of protein in the diet and the research that has been done on the effects of protein restriction in animals. The authors of this study concluded that in a population experiencing chronic but moderate malnutrition the limiting factor in the diet is kilocalories—energy, not protein. The amount of protein may actually be higher than that needed to maintain tissue synthesis, but the women simply do not consume enough kilocalories to spare protein from meeting energy needs. For infants of these women the increment in birth weight from the consumption of additional kilocalories is mostly caused by the accumulation of fetal adipose tissue. The benefits are that the entire birth weight distribution is shifted upward. Low-birth-weight infants still have greater risks, but the fact that fewer of them are born causes a reduction in the overall rate of neonatal death.

Canadian Study

The experiences of Primrose and Higgins[18] at the Montreal Diet Dispensary in Canada show that the benefits of extra kilocalories and special dietary management during pregnancy are not confined to chronically malnourished women in developing countries. They can also improve the pregnancy performance of high-risk mothers in more affluent nations. Knowing the risk of reproductive problems associated with low income, these investigators selected the hospital handling the highest percentage of poor patients in Montreal. All patients from two of the hospital's public maternity clinics enrolled, a total of 1544 women between 1963 and 1970. A unique feature was that dietary needs for kilocalories and protein were individually calculated for each woman based on her body weight for height with adjustments for protein deficiency, underweight, and other stress conditions. Women whose family incomes fell below specified levels, 70% of all women in the study, were given supplies of milk, eggs, and oranges every 2 weeks. All of the women received counseling on food selection to meet their individual needs every time they visited the clinic, and nutritionists visited them at home at least once during their pregnancies.

Such intensive nutritional care enabled the women to average 93% of their total kilocalorie needs and 96% of their total protein requirements throughout gestation. Since the majority started out with large average daily deficits, they all showed significant improvements in the quality of their diets. Birth statistics indicate how the mothers and their infants benefited from these measures. The incidence of low birth weight in this high-risk study group was brought down to the all-Canada rate and was lower than the rate for Quebec province. Stillbirths, neonatal mortality, and perinatal mortality were also lower than the rates prevailing in Canada and Quebec.

In this study, Primrose and Higgins found a direct relationship between maternal weight gains and birth weights, which were in turn directly related to the length of time the women had received Diet Dispensary services. No such relationship between birth weights and service was observed for other public patients who were not part of the study but who received prenatal care and gave birth at the same hospital.

It is impossible to know how much of the improvements in pregnancy performance and outcome demonstrated in this study can be attributed to the diets of the women, the food supplements, or the special attention they received. What is important about the study is that it shows how high-risk mothers, against all odds, can experience successful pregnancies when superior nutritional guidance is a part of their prenatal care.

Conclusions

Not all supplementation programs provided to high-risk pregnant women have demonstrated the degree of positive impact that was shown in Guatemala and Montreal. This varied response should certainly be expected, given the different populations served, the different supplements employed, the various methods of supplement administration, and a variety of other differing variables. Overall, the findings appear to suggest that *the worse the nutritional condition of the mother upon entering pregnancy, the more valuable the prenatal diet and nutritional supplement will be in improving her pregnancy course and outcome.*

A general conclusion after review of all published reports on prenatal supplementation studies is that whereas poor women in developing countries often suffer some degree of malnutrition before and during pregnancy, only a minority of women in developed countries are truly undernourished.[16] Diet counseling and nutritional supplementation of the latter group will clearly yield less dramatic measurable improvements in outcome. As yet undefined improvements in outcome may actually occur, but existing methodologies prevent their definition. In developed countries it would seem, however, that nutrition intervention should focus on those women whose prepregnancy status is inferior. Refined processes of clinical assessment and monitoring will help identify these women and establish a nutritional milieu that supports an optimal pregnancy course and outcome for them.

Physiologic Basis for Nutritional Needs During Pregnancy

GENERAL PHYSIOLOGIC CHANGES

Normal pregnancy is accompanied by anatomic and physiologic changes that affect almost every function of the body. Many of these changes are apparent in the very early weeks. This indicates that they are not merely a response to the normal physiologic stress imposed by the fetus, but are also an integral part of the maternal-fetal-placental system which creates the most favorable environment possible for the developing child. The changes are necessary to regulate maternal metabolism, promote fetal growth, and prepare the mother for labor, birth, and lactation. These changes are too complex to be given full treatment here. However, a look at some that have effects on general metabolism will lay the foundation for interpreting nutritional requirements and dietary allowances.

ROLE OF THE PLACENTA

The placenta is not a passive barrier between the mother and the fetus. Rather it plays an active role in reproduction.[19] Here we will look at its finely developed structure for support of the fetus, its capacity for nutrient transfer that ensures fetal nourishment, its delivery of oxygen and both respiratory and excretory exchanges, and its hormonal controls. The placenta is the principal site of production for several important hormones that regulate maternal growth and development. And for the fetus it is a true "life line"—the only way that nutrients, oxygen, and waste products can be exchanged.

Structure and Development

Evolving from a tiny mass of cells in the first weeks of pregnancy, the placenta becomes a complex network of tissue and blood vessels weighing about 650 g (1.4 lb) at term. The vital role it plays as a link between mother and child is represented by the two principal parts of the placenta—one uterine and the other fetal. On the maternal side the placenta is part of the uterine mucosa. When the tiny blastocyst implants itself in the uterus 6 to 7 days after fertilization, the uterine tissue and blood vessels break down to form small spaces called *lacunae* that fill with maternal blood. These spaces are eventually bounded on the maternal side by the *decidua* or basal plate. Blood begins to circulate in the spaces at about 12 days gestation.

Meanwhile the trophoblast grows and sends out rootlike villi into the pools of maternal blood. The villi contain capillaries, which will exchange nutrients and metabolic waste products between the mother and the fetus. In the early weeks of pregnancy the villi are thick columns of cells. But as they subdivide throughout gestation the villi become thinner and produce numerous branches. Some branches become anchored in the maternal tissue, and others remain free or floating in the intervillous spaces. The multiple villous branches provide a large surface membrane area for efficient exchange of nutrients and metabolic waste products between mother and fetus (Fig. 4-6). Even though uterine and embryonic tissues are intermingled, the blood of the mother and the embryo-fetus never mix because they are always separated by two cell layers (Fig. 4-7).

Mechanisms of Nutrient Transfer

The efficiency of placental nutrient transfer is a determinant of fetal well-being. Reduced surface area of the villi, insufficient vascularization, or changes in the hydrostatic pressure in the intervillous space can limit the supply of nutrients available to the fetus and inhibit normal growth.

Nutrient transfer in the placenta is a complex process. It employs all the mechanisms used for the absorption of nutrients from the gastrointestinal tract: simple diffusion, facilitated diffusion, active transport, and pinocytosis. However, the placenta maintains two completely separate blood supplies. The maternal circulation remains in the intervillous space. The fetal capillaries are separated from the maternal blood by two layers of cells. Their thickness is approximately 5.5 μm (Fig. 4-7).

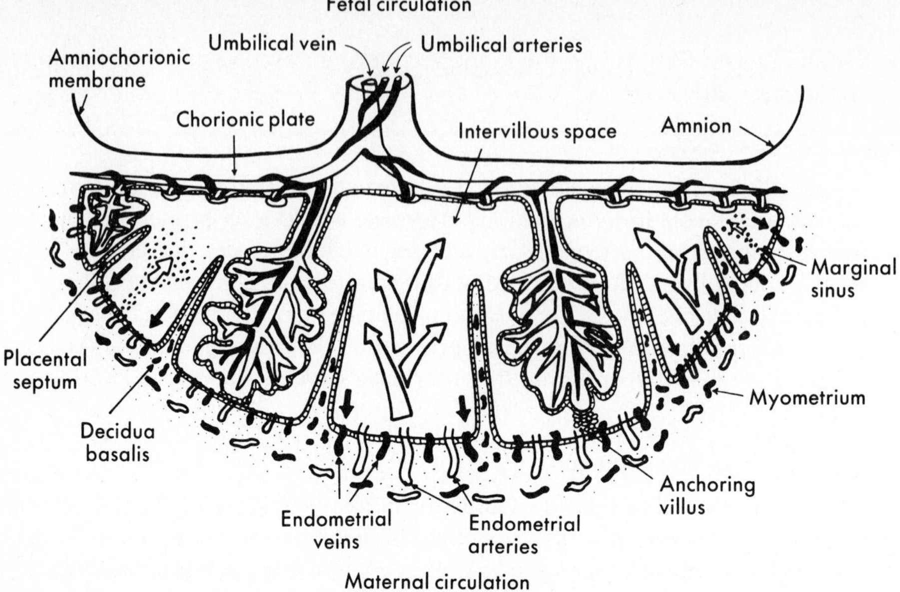

FIG. 4-6 Diagrammatic representation of a section through a mature placenta showing the relationship of the fetal placenta (villous chorion) to the maternal placenta (decidua basalis), fetal placental circulation, and maternal placental circulation. Maternal blood is forced into the intervillous space, and exchanges occur with the fetal blood as the maternal blood flows around the villi. Incoming arterial blood pushes venous blood into the endometrial veins, which are scattered over the surface of the maternal placenta. Umbilical arteries carry deoxygenated fetal blood to the placenta, and the umbilical vein carries oxygenated blood to the fetus.

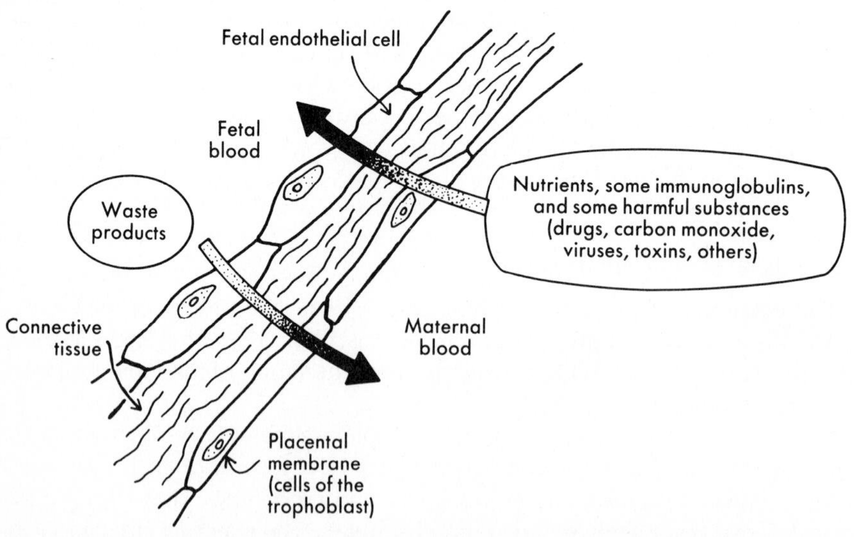

FIG. 4-7 Nutrients, waste products, and other transportable compounds must cross two layers of cells in the process of movement through the placenta.

Although the same nutrient may be simultaneously transferred by more than one mechanism, the major means of transport can be estimated by comparing nutrient concentrations in maternal and cord blood. If the concentrations are equal, the transfer has most likely occurred by simple or facilitated diffusion. Simple diffusion is a passive process in which nutrients move from high concentrations in the maternal blood to lower concentrations in fetal capillaries until equilibrium is reached. Facilitated diffusion differs from simple diffusion in that the rate of transfer is faster than would be expected. The mechanism of facilitated diffusion is not established, but it is thought that a carrier in the membrane is employed. Active transport requires both a carrier protein and metabolic energy to move a nutrient against an electrochemical gradient. The substances cross the placenta via specified mechanisms.[20] Various materials transported by different mechanisms are shown in Table 4-1.

Most proteins do not cross the placenta, since their molecular size is too big to allow penetration through the cells of the villi. This protects the fetus from acquiring harmful agents of high molecular weight. But it also means that the fetus must synthesize its own proteins from its supply of amino acids. An exception is the maternal immunoglobulin IgG. It is not known why this particular protein crosses the placenta, but it appears that the selectivity is related to the structure and not to the size of the molecule. IgG is probably transported by pinocytosis. The benefits to the fetus are that it has the same resistance to infectious diseases as the mother has. This resistance lasts from 6 to 9 months after birth, until the infant can manufacture antibodies.

The placenta also acts to assure that once nutrients are transported to the fetus, they do not "slide back down" the concentration gradient into the mother's blood. Ascorbic acid, for example, crosses the placenta in its oxidized form as dehydroascorbic acid. Once inside the fetus, it is converted back to active L-ascorbic acid, to which the

TABLE 4-1 Placental Transport Mechanisms and Materials Transported by Each Mechanism

Transport Mechanism	Substance Transported
Passive diffusion	Oxygen
	Carbon dioxide
	Fatty acids
	Steroids
	Nucleosides
	Electrolytes
	Fat-soluble vitamins
Facilitated diffusion	Most monosaccharides
Active transport	Amino acids
	Some cations (calcium, iron)
	Iodine
	Phosphate
	Water-soluble vitamins*
Solvent drag†	Electrolytes

*At very high concentrations vitamin C has been shown to cross the placenta via diffusion.
†Movement of ions with water as it flows back and forth across the membrane.

placenta is impermeable. Calcium transport is subject to similar protection through the mediation of hormones. Active transport of calcium makes the mother hypocalcemic compared with the fetus. Her response is to secrete parathyroid hormone (PTH) to favor bone resorption and increase serum calcium levels. If PTH reached the fetus, the effect would be to reverse the normal process of bone development. The relative impermeability of the placenta to maternal PTH prevents this from happening. Instead, the fetus responds to its own high blood calcium levels by secreting endogenous calcitonin, the hormone that enhances the deposition of calcium in bone. Meanwhile the placenta is freely permeable to vitamin D, favoring calcium retention in both the mother and the fetus.

The placenta not only transports nutrients but also in some cases has been known to store them. The placenta can store most vitamins depending on their availability to the mother. Heightened release of these vitamins to the fetus generally depends closely on saturation of vitamin reserves in the placenta. Much remains to be learned about modifiability of placental vitamin transfer by placental abnormalities. In any event, it appears that adequate vitamin nutrition of the fetus is assured only when placental vitamin binders are saturated.

Respiratory and Excretory Exchange

Besides serving as a lifeline for nutrients, the placenta functions in the exchange of respiratory gases and waste products between the mother and fetus. The delivery of oxygen to the fetus is just as important to proper metabolism as an adequate supply of nutrients. The mother makes adjustments in her breathing to meet fetal oxygen needs, but the amount of oxygen that reaches the fetus ultimately depends on the blood flow through the uterus to the placental villi. Near term the rate of flow through the intervillous space is 375 to 560 ml per min. Exchange is made between maternal red cells, which characteristically have a lower affinity for oxygen during pregnancy, and fetal red cells, which have a high affinity.

Maternal nutrition can influence oxygen exchange through the production of hemoglobin. Each gram of hemoglobin carries 1.34 ml of oxygen. In normal concentrations it can deliver up to 16 ml of oxygen per 100 ml of blood to the placenta. If maternal hemoglobin levels are depressed from iron deficiency, the supply of oxygen per 100 ml of blood is reduced. Since the fetus can tolerate little variation in the rate at which oxygen is supplied, the mother must compensate by increasing her cardiac output.

Another function of the placenta is to rid the fetus of metabolic wastes. The placenta is freely permeable to carbon dioxide, water, urea, creatinine, and uric acid. Hyperventilation by the mother reduces her PCO_2 so that carbon dioxide exchange from the fetus is accomplished by simple diffusion. Urea, creatinine, and uric acid, which are the wastes of fetal amino acid metabolism, move through the placenta by diffusion and active transport.

Placental Hormones

The production of hormones to regulate the activities of pregnancy is one of the most interesting special functions of the placenta. From the earliest days of pregnancy the cells of the trophoblast and their successors in the placenta manufacture a large variety of hormones. The first to be manufactured in appreciable amounts is the protein hormone *human chorionic gonadotropin (HCG).* Early in the differentiation of the trophoblast this hormone is found coating the trophoblast's outer cell surfaces, where it is believed to act as an immunologically protective layer, preventing the rejection of the blastocyst and thereby facilitating implantation. HCG also stimulates the synthesis of *estrogen* in the placenta. Synthesis of estrogen actually begins in the free-floating blastocyst where it acts to facilitate implantation. The fact that the cells of the small, primitive blastocyst are already equipped to conduct complex steroid manipulation is a measure of the importance of these hormones at this early stage.

As pregnancy proceeds, large amounts of *progesterone* are synthesized in the placenta, principally from maternal cholesterol. In addition to sustaining pregnancy, this hormone serves as a raw material for the production of estrogens, mainly *estrone, estradiol, and estriol,* which in turn act on many organs and tissues of both the mother and fetus. Interestingly, the human placenta lacks the enzymes needed for converting the large amounts of progesterone it makes into certain essential estrogens and other steroids. Consequently, these synthetic events are carried out in the "fetal zone" cells. These cells are clusters of transient cells found in the developing adrenal glands of the fetus. They lack the enzymes necessary to manufacture progesterone but possess the requisite ones for its conversion. In this way the fetal and placental tissues complement each other. When the fetus endocrine glands become sufficiently mature to take over the manufacture of steroid hormones, the fetal zone cells gradually diminish and eventually disappear. Presumably this sophisticated collaboration is organized and timed by precise genetic instructions and is regulated by equally precise releasing hormones.

Because a great variety of regulatory hormones are synthesized in the placenta, including HCG, human placental lactogen (HPL), chorionic somatomammotropin, and human chorionic thyrotropin (HCT), the placental control during pregnancy must be as comprehensive as that maintained by the pituitary gland throughout life. By means of these hormones the placenta not only carries out the functions of the fetus' pituitary until the organ is ready to perform on its own, but also conducts the entire "endocrine orchestra of pregnancy," which performs largely in the placenta itself.

IMMUNOLOGIC PROTECTION

During pregnancy it is absolutely vital that the embryo be protected from immunologic rejection by maternal tissue. This vital task is accomplished in two ways, by suppressing normal lymphocyte action and forming barriers to other rejection actions:

Lymphocyte Suppression

One of the mechanisms that plays a part in this task is the nonspecific suppression of lymphocytes, the cells that normally mediate the rejection of a graft. Experiments have shown that lymphocytes can be suppressed by HCG, HPL, prolactin, cortisone, progesterone, the estrogens, and a variety of proteins and glycoproteins.

Barrier Protection

It is also likely that the embryo is protected by the large, tightly packed decidual cells that enclose it soon after the implantation of the blastocyst. This protective barrier prevents the drainage of lymphocytes to maternal tissues. In addition, the maternal blood vessels do not invade the trophoblast of the placenta, so this potential means of graft rejection is blocked. In the early days of the development of the trophoblast further protection is provided by the absence of the expression of antigens. So even though the embryonic tissue is "foreign," it manages to conceal the fact, at least for a while.[21]

CHANGES IN BLOOD VOLUME AND COMPOSITION

Plasma Volume Increase

Plasma is the fluid component of blood; serum is the part of plasma that remains after its coagulation factors have been removed. Total plasma volume in a nonpregnant woman averages 2600 ml. Near the end of the first trimester of pregnancy, plasma volume begins to increase, and by 34 weeks it is about 50% greater than it was at conception. There is considerable variation from these averages. Women who have small volumes to begin with usually have a greater increase, as do women who have had multiple pregnancies and multiple births. Research has shown that the increase in plasma volume is correlated with obstetrical performance. A British group found that women who have a small increase when compared with the average are more likely to have stillbirths, abortions, and low-birth-weight babies. Clearly the restriction of a normal expansion of plasma volume is undesirable in pregnancy.

Levels of Blood Constituents

If the availability of nutrients or the synthesis of normal blood constituents does not keep pace with the expansion of plasma volume, their concentrations per 100 ml of blood will decrease, even though the total amount may rise. This is apparently what happens with red blood cells, serum proteins, minerals, and water-soluble vitamins.

1. **Red blood cells.** Red cell production is stimulated during pregnancy so that their numbers gradually rise, but the increase is not as large as the expansion of plasma volume. The hematocrit, which is normally around 35% in women, may be as low as 29% to 31% during pregnancy. The amount of hemoglobin in each red blood cell does not change, but because there are fewer red blood cells per 100 ml of blood, *hemodilution* occurs. Nonpregnant hemoglobin values of 13 to 14 g per 100 ml can drop as low as 10 or 11 g per 100 ml in the early months.
2. **Major nutrients.** Serum levels of the major nutrients typical for pregnant and nonpregnant women are compared in Table 4-2. The values for pregnant women must be interpreted with caution. Investigators have obtained different values depending on the laboratory methods used. Moreover, levels of certain nutrients can be influenced by a number of maternal factors such as age, parity, smoking, and the use of various medications before or during pregnancy. Even the sex of the fetus can influence the mother's blood levels of some nutrients. The levels will also fluctuate at different times during gestation.

TABLE 4-2 Serum Nutrient Levels in Pregnant and Nonpregnant Women

Nutrient	Normal Nonpregnancy Range	Values in Pregnancy
Total protein	6.5-8.5 g/100 ml	6.0-8.0
Albumin	3.5-5.0 g/100 ml	3.0-4.5
Glucose	<110 mg/100 ml	<120
Cholesterol	120-190 mg/100 ml	200-325
Vitamin A	20-60 μg/100 ml	20-60
Carotene	50-300 μg/100 ml	80-325
Ascorbic acid	0.2-2.0 mg/100 ml	0.2-1.5
Folic acid	5-21 ng/100 ml	3-15
Calcium	4.6-5.5 mEq/L	4.2-5.2
Iron/iron-binding capacity	>50/250-400 μg/100 ml	>40/300-450

Modified from Aubry, R.H., Roberts, A., and Cuenca, V.: Clin. Perinatol. **2:**207, 1975.

3. **Serum protein.** Total serum protein gradually decreases during pregnancy, leveling off at about 28 weeks. Most of the reduction in serum proteins is a result of a sharp decline in the *albumin* fraction. Alpha and beta globulins show a progressive increase. The reduction in serum albumin changes colloidal osmotic pressure of the blood, a major force operating the capillary fluid shift mechanism for circulation of tissue fluids. This serum albumin reduction, in conjunction with the expanded plasma volume, is another factor responsible for the tendency of pregnant women to accumulate extracellular fluid.
4. **Fat-soluble nutrients.** In contrast to the water-soluble nutrients, those that are fat-soluble show increased serum concentrations during pregnancy. There are also progressive increases in serum triglycerides, cholesterol, and free fatty acids. These higher lipid levels are reflected in the higher concentrations of most of the lipoproteins in the serum.
5. **Cholesterol.** Cholesterol is a precursor for the synthesis of progesterone and estrogen in the placenta. Most of the increased cholesterol is in very low-density lipoproteins (VLDL). Lesser increases are seen in low-density lipoproteins (LDL) and high-density lipoproteins (HDL) cholesterol. However, in pregnancy HDL cholesterol is always higher or unchanged but never lower than values for nonpregnant women. This pattern is opposite to that found in atherosclerosis-related hyperlipoproteinemia where HDL cholesterol is usually reduced.

CHANGES IN RENAL FUNCTION

To facilitate the clearance of creatinine, urea, and other waste products of fetal and maternal metabolism, blood flow through the kidneys and the nephrons' glomerular filtration rate are increased during pregnancy. This is one adaptation that appears to be purely mechanical, since no effects of hormones on this aspect of kidney function have been shown. However, there are consequences for nutrition.

According to researchers,[22] "The kidney during pregnancy shows an astonishing profligacy with nutrients." Normally most of the glucose, amino acids, and water-soluble vitamins that are filtered by the nephrons are reabsorbed in the tubules to preserve the body's balance. However, in pregnancy substantial quantities of these nutrients appear in the urine. The most satisfactory explanation at present is that the higher glomerular filtration rate offers the tubules greater quantities of nutrients than they can feasibly reabsorb. Because the change in filtration rate is largely mechanical, there may not be an accompanying mechanism by which the tubules can readjust.

Nutrient Functions and Needs

The nutrients enter into all of the major metabolic processes involving the production of energy, synthesis of cells, maintenance of their structure and function, and the regulation of body processes. We will look first at the basis for the RDA nutrient and energy standards for pregnancy. Then, in considering each of these nutrient functions, emphasis is given to those nutrients that have major roles in pregnancy and why their requirements during pregnancy increase.

RECOMMENDED DIETARY ALLOWANCES (RDA)

The Food and Nutrition Board of the National Research Council is well aware of the problems of determining nutrient requirements during pregnancy and considers them when setting dietary allowances and making recommendations about the need for supplementation. Recommended Dietary Allowances (RDA) are based on the best available evidence from metabolic balance studies and from indirect estimates.[23]

The 1980 edition (the most recent issue to date) of the RDA standards for pregnant and nonpregnant adult women is presented in Table 4-3. The figures in the table indicate the needs of a "reference" woman who is 25 to 50 years of age, 160 cm (64 in) tall, and weighs 54 kg (120 lb) when she conceives. Women may need more or less of the amounts listed for kilocalories and protein depending on body size, activity, and health status. The allowances for vitamins and minerals provide sufficient room for individual variation, an important consideration, so that they can be applied to all healthy women. They may not be adequate for women who enter pregnancy in poor nutritional status or who suffer from chronic disease or other complicating conditions. They may not be appropriate for the young pregnant adolescent or the "elderly primigravida" who conceives for the first time after age 35.

ENERGY

Pregnancy Requirements

During pregnancy, two factors that determine energy requirements are: (1) changes in the mother's usual physical activity, and (2) increase in her basal metabolism to support the work required for growth of the fetus and the accessory tissues. The cumulative energy cost of pregnancy has been estimated at 80,000 kilocalories.[24] This amount is derived from the kilocalorie equivalents of protein and fat stored in the products of conception and from increased oxygen consumption of the mother. The total 80,000 kilocalories break down to an addition of only 300 extra kilocalories to the daily allowance of the nonpregnant reference woman. A portion of the energy increment may be offset by the tendency of pregnant women to reduce their physical activity in the last trimester.

TABLE 4-3 Recommended Dietary Allowances for Adult Women (ages 23 to 50 years)*

	Nonpregnant	Pregnant
Energy (kcal)	1600-2400	+300
Protein (gm)	44	+30
Vitamin A (RE)	800	+200
Vitamin D (μg)	5	+5
Vitamin E (mg)	8	+2
Vitamin C (ascorbic acid) (mg)	60	+20
Folic acid (μg)	400	+400
Niacin (mg)	13	+2
Riboflavin (mg)	1.2	+0.3
Thiamin (mg)	1.0	+0.4
Vitamin B_6 (mg)	2.0	+0.6
Vitamin B_{12} (μg)	3.0	+1.0
Calcium (mg)	800	+400
Phosphorus (mg)	800	+400
Iodine (μg)	150	+25
Iron (mg)	18	*
Magnesium (mg)	300	+150
Zinc (mg)	15	+5

From Food and Nutrition Board, National Research Council, National Academy of Sciences: Recommended dietary allowances, ed. 9, Washington, D.C., 1980, U.S. Government Printing Office.
*30-60 mg of supplemental iron per day is recommended.

Issue of Energy Requirement

The traditional explanation for increased energy needs during pregnancy has recently been challenged.[23-25] Durnin and associates[25] monitored food intake of sixty-seven pregnant women in Glasgow using an individual weighed food inventory technique. They found that total pregnancy energy requirements appeared to be closer to 20,000 kilocalories than 80,000. On this basis, these researchers proposed that the real requirements seem to be no more than about 50–100 extra kilocalories per day for the first 34-36 weeks, and about 200-300 extra kilocalories per day for the final few weeks. Needless to say, this issue of energy needs for the pregnant woman will continue to be explored. Until more information is available, individual energy needs can be calculated by allowing approximately 40 kilocalories per kg of pregnant body weight, or about 18 kilocalories per lb. However, appetite and weight gain are the best indicators that energy needs are being met.

Dieting, Fasting, and Food Restriction

The degree to which the mother is parasitized by the fetus has been debated for many decades. Although it is known that the fetus can draw on maternal stores when maternal food intake is restricted, the extent and duration of this process is unknown. Several effects of food restriction need to be considered.

1. **Body composition.** Studies on the effect of food restriction on the body composition of pregnant and nonpregnant rats have provided new insights into the nature of maternal-fetal interactions during reduced availability of nutrients.[28] This work

showed that at term, pregnant rats fed 50% of the amount of food fed to control animals had a similar body composition as pair-fed nonpregnant rats, but the mean body weight of the fetus was significantly reduced. These results support the idea that the pregnant food-restricted rat is not extensively parasitized by the fetus. Important metabolic adjustments must occur to allow the mother to prevent fetal parasitism.

2. **Dutch famine experience.** Human data are obviously limited, but the Dutch famine experience during World War II supports the idea that the malnourished mother is able to protect her body stores of nutrients from fetal parasitism. Mean infant birth weight was reduced by 10%, but most mothers were estimated to have lost less than 3% of their initial body weight during the stress of famine during pregnancy. The mothers appeared to be less affected than their infants, an observation consistent with that from animal data. Thus optimal fetal growth occurs only when the mother is able to accumulate a critical amount of extra body stores during pregnancy. Evidence clearly contradicts the concept that the fetus is protected by the mother when nutritional status is less than optimal or that the fetus can protect itself by parasitizing the mother.
3. **Maternal adaptation.** The fact that nature protects the mother more than the fetus seems reasonable from the point of view of survival of the species. During a famine caused by a serious crop failure, for example, a normal-sized newborn delivered by a nutritionally depleted mother would have little chance to survive if the mother could not initiate lactation, protect herself and her young, and cover enough ground during the day to secure food. A stronger and healthier mother who produces a small baby or few offspring probably has a better chance to survive and conceive again. Although the food-restricted mother adapts to her unfortunate predicament, the metabolic and physiologic mechanisms that allow for this adaptation are largely unknown. Major adaptations are known to occur in protein and amino acid metabolism, but the mechanism involved is still unknown. Many other factors are probably important, such as modified expansion in blood volume or deposition in maternal stores. It is possible that the normal sequence of physiologic adjustment to pregnancy is retarded in the face of the nutrient deficit. The ultimate result might well be suboptimal completion of the final stages of adjustment such that adequate growth of the conceptus is prevented.
4. **Increased ketones.** One recognized consequence of food restriction is the increased production of ketone bodies and their ultimate spillage into the urine. Although the fetus can metabolize ketones to some degree, the results of maternal ketosis are unclear. Data collected from both animals and humans indicate that ketones are probably normally presented to the fetal brain at various times during pregnancy. After an overnight fast, maternal ketone concentrations are about three times greater in pregnant than in nonpregnant women and ketonuria will often be seen. Coetzee and colleagues[29] found that urine concentrations of ketones may abruptly increase in the presence of less than a twofold increase in blood concentrations, and that blood levels generally fall within the upper limit of the normal range. These researchers conclude that acetonuria in normal pregnancy "probably does not usually signify that any abnormality is present." More serious conditions of ketoacidosis, however, should be viewed as more hazardous.

Carbohydrate Kilocalories

Carbohydrate is the body's primary fuel. During pregnancy, for optimal protein use in tissue building and to prevent ketosis, *at least* 5 g of carbohydrate for every 100 kilocalories of food should be provided. This would amount to a *minimum* of 20% of the total kilocalories or about 115 g daily for the pregnant reference woman. Ideally, however, to make the diet palatable and to meet vitamin and mineral needs, it is usual that 50% to 55% of the total kilocalories come from carbohydrate foods.

PROTEIN

Pregnancy Requirements

Requirements for protein during pregnancy are based on the needs of the nonpregnant reference woman plus the extra amounts needed for growth. The easiest way to determine how much extra protein is needed daily to support the synthesis of new tissue is to divide the amounts contained in the products of conception and maternal body by the average length of gestation. About 925 g of protein are deposited in a normal-weight fetus and in the maternal accessory tissues.[24] When this is divided by the 280 days of pregnancy, the average is 3.3 g of protein that must be added to normal daily requirements. The rate at which new tissue is synthesized, however, is not constant throughout gestation. Maternal and fetal growth do not accelerate until the second month, and the rate progressively increases until just before term. The need for protein follows this growth rate. Only about an extra 0.6 g of protein is used each day for new tissue synthesis in the first month of pregnancy, but by 30 weeks gestation protein is being used at the rate of 6.1 g per day. If this is added to the normal maintenance needs of the reference woman, 18.6 to 24 g of protein per day are required.

Protein Utilization

These calculations of protein need would equal dietary allowances if 100% of the protein eaten could be used in the body. Actually, however, the efficiency of protein utilization depends on its digestibility and amino acid composition. Proteins that do not contain all eight essential amino acids in amounts proportional to human requirements are utilized less efficiently. Even a high-quality protein, such as that in eggs, is utilized much less than 100%. Protein utilization from a mixed diet is about 70% and from a totally vegetarian diet it is even less efficient. Protein utilization also depends on kilocalorie intake. It has been shown that an extra 100 kilocalories during pregnancy will have the same effect on nitrogen retention as an additional 0.28 g of nitrogen itself. This means that kilocalories from nonprotein sources, that is, carbohydrates and fats, have a sparing effect. If these kilocalories are inadequate, protein requirements would increase. Finally, the trials that measure nitrogen loss are conducted on a limited number of subjects. There is much variation from the averages obtained. Since a dietary allowance must cover the needs of all healthy women, room for individual differences must be built in.

RDA Standard

Because of these considerations, RDAs for protein are set much higher than calculated requirements of 18.6 to 24 g per day. The National Research Council allows 44 g of protein a day for the nonpregnant reference woman with an extra 30 g per day starting in the second month of pregnancy. If individual allowances are calculated on the basis of body weight, daily need would be about 1.3 g per kg of pregnant body weight or about 0.6 g per lb. The RDA standard is based on a mixed diet in which at least one third of the protein comes from high-quality animal foods. Thus vegetarian diets that exclude all animal products can only be made adequate when more total protein is consumed, or when foods are selected so that those low in a particular amino acid are complemented by foods in which that amino acid is high.

Protein Deficiency

Adverse consequences of protein deficiency during pregnancy are difficult to separate from the effects of kilocalorie deficiency in real-life situations. Almost all cases of limited protein intake are accompanied by limitation in availability of kilocalories. Under such circumstances decreased birth weight and greater incidence of preeclampsia have been reported. As indicated previously in discussion of the Guatemala study,[17] provision of supplemental kilocalories alone to pregnant women with deficient levels of protein intake was just as effective as provision of both protein and kilocalories in influencing birth weight of babies. Zlatnik and Burmeister[30] also reported that birth weight and other anthropometric indices of the newborn infant were not related to the level of dietary protein during pregnancy.

Protein Excess

Adverse effects of excessive protein during pregnancy are poorly understood at the present time. The New York supplementation study[31] has provoked much discussion of this issue, since use of the high-protein supplement was associated with an increased number of very prematurely born infants and excessive neonatal deaths. In light of these findings other data have been reviewed. Analysis of a number of past supplementation studies in human populations[32] has suggested that providing a supplement with more than 20% of the kilocalories from protein is associated with retarded fetal growth, whereas supplements providing less than 20% of the kilocalories from protein yield increments in birth weight of offspring. Although these data suggest that too much protein, presented in an unbalanced nutritional package, may have adverse effects on pregnancy course and outcome, data are limited and the debate continues about the relevance of the observations.

VITAMINS

Folic Acid and Vitamin B_{12}

Both folic acid and vitamin B_{12} are required for cell division to proceed. If either vitamin is lacking, detrimental effects are especially great in the tissues that have high turnover rates in the body. One of the first signs of folic acid or B_{12} deficiency is megaloblastic anemia, caused by the production of abnormal red blood cells. These cells are arrested in their development, so bone marrow contains a large number of immature megaloblasts and hemoglobin levels are reduced. Anemia is associated with increased risk of adverse pregnancy course and outcome. Although folic acid deficiency effects are debated, a supplement is nonetheless recommended.

1. **Folic acid deficiency**. The consequences of folic acid deficiency during pregnancy are controversial. Maternal folic acid deficiency in experimental animals is associated with increased incidence of problems related to pregnancy and increased delivery of abnormal offspring.[33] Fetal malformations have been described in offspring of women using drugs that are folate antagonists (Table 4-4). Evidence in humans suggests that deficiency of this vitamin may be associated with abruptio placentae, spontaneous abortion, pre-eclampsia, fetal malformations, and subnormal infant development (Table 4-4). Such reports, however, are not direct proof of association.
2. **Neural tube defect**. The biggest controversy relates to the role of folic acid deficiency in the etiology of neural tube defects. The work of Smithells[34-37] and Laurence[38] in northern Europe suggests that multivitamin or folic acid supplementation of women with previous neural tube defect offspring is associated with significant reduction in second occurrence of the problem. Since methodologic details of these projects have been heavily criticized, the merit of these reports has been questioned. A controlled supplementation trial currently under way in northern Europe may never be successfully completed.[39] A retrospective study in progress in the U.S. addressing supplementation practices around the time of conception may not yield reliable data.[40] A new report by Malloy and associates[41] found no differences in serum folate or B_{12} concentrations in early pregnancy between 32 mothers of infants with neural tube defects and 395 randomly selected pregnant controls. The role of folic acid deficiency in the etiology of neural tube defects in humans may never be clarified.
3. **Justification for folate supplement**. However, folate supplementation may be justified on the basis of increased needs of pregnancy in the face of marginal dietary supply. Although wise meal planning and appropriate cooking methods may meet daily folate needs, many American women don't follow these recommended practices. Thus attitudes vary about use of supplements in routine prenatal management. Supplements are clearly justified in instances of low intake or in circumstances of unusually high requirements, such as multiple pregnancy or chronic hemolytic anemia. Some drugs, such as anticonvulsant agents, may impair folate metabolism and in so doing increase the requirement for the vitamin. Supplements are considered justified in these cases, but possible interference of folate with the action of the drug should be determined in all cases before therapy is instituted. Women with a history of long-term use of oral contraceptive agents should have careful assessment of folic acid status. Then supplementation should be started before or very soon after conception has occurred. At the present time the National Research Council recommends that an oral folic acid supplement of 400 μg per day be given in the last half of pregnancy.[23]

TABLE 4-4 Vitamin and Mineral Deficiencies and Excesses and Human Pregnancy Course and Outcome*

	Deficiency	Excess
VITAMIN A	Indian woman, blind from vitamin A deficiency, gave birth to premature infant with microcephaly and anophthalmia Prenatal vitamin A deficiency has been related in several instances to eye abnormalities and impaired vision in children	Congenital renal anomalies in infant whose mother consumed high doses of vitamin A during pregnancy. Multiple malformations, esp. involving CNS, in infant whose mother consumed 150,000 IU of vitamin A from day 19 through day 40 of pregnancy Higher concentrations of vitamin A found in blood of mothers of infants with CNS anomalies vs. mothers of normal infants. Liver vitamin A levels from abortuses and/or malformed fetuses were higher than in normal fetal liver Amnionic fluid conc. of vitamin A in 2nd trimester were significantly higher in mothers of infants with neural tube defects vs. controls Prominent frontal bossing, hydrocephalus, microphthalmia, and small, malformed, low-set, undifferentiated ears in two infants whose mothers had taken isotretinoin (a vitamin A analogue) in the first trimester of pregnancy. Also microcephaly, hypertelorism, small ear canals, cleft palate, small mouth, and congenital heart disease. One child did not survive FDA 17 reported cases of birth defects and 20 reported instances of spontaneous abortions in women receiving isotretinoin
VITAMIN D	Fetal rickets: mother had low serum vitamin D, developed osteomalacia some months after delivery Neonatal rickets: mother suffered from osteomalacia during pregnancy Low levels of 25-OH-D seen in hypocalcemic premature infants and their mothers Enamel hypoplasia of the teeth seen in infants with neonatal tetany; maternal vitamin D deficiency was associated Babies with vitamin D-resistant or vitamin D-dependent rickets demonstrate growth failure, convulsions, and rickets in the neonatal period Vitamin D supplementation of pregnant Asian women was associated with improved maternal weight gain, normal	Infants of mothers treated with high doses of vitamin D for hypoparathyroidism show no evidence of cardiovascular or craniofacial abnormalities, although mothers do not develop hypercalcemia Excessive intake of vitamin D or unusual sensitivity to the vitamin might be related to mild idiopathic hypercalcemia in infants Supravalvular aortic stenosis with elfin facies and mental retardation appeared in Gottingen, Germany, where rickets prophylaxis (consisting of huge doses of vitamin D) was begun

	25-OH-D levels in mothers and infants at term, reduced incidence of SGA babies and neonatal hypocalcemia Neonatal hypocalcemia is more common during months when daily sunlight is least	
VITAMIN E	Correlation noted between birthweight and cord blood levels of vitamin E, but gestational age and other variables not controlled for	Comparison of 50 spontaneously aborting women with 50 women with normal pregnancies showed a significantly higher percentage of aborting women with serum α-tocopherol above normal limits; a causal association was not proposed
VITAMIN K	Some evidence that use of dicumarol during pregnancy is associated with increased fetal mortality and morbidity. Cases reported of fetal abnormalities in infants of mothers treated with anticoagulants. Prenatal vitamin K deficiency caused by dicumarol drugs known to produce coumadin syndrome unless dosage properly controlled	Parenteral administration of menadione to the mother has been associated with hyperbilirubinemia and kernicterus of premature infants and severe hyperbilirubinemia in term infants
THIAMIN	If severe deficiency, congenital beriberi. If mild to moderate deficiency, no reported complications	
RIBOFLAVIN	In study of 900 pregnant women, 190 were riboflavin deficient. These women had higher incidence of vomiting during pregnancy, premature delivery, stillbirths. No increased incidence of malformations seen. Unsuccessful lactation more common Among middle-class European women, biochemical evidence of riboflavin deficiency not associated with abortion, hydroamnios, preeclampsia, stillbirth or low birthweights	
ASCORBIC ACID	Vanderbilt study of over 2000 pregnant women assessed diet and serum vitamin C; frequency of congenital malformations no higher in women with lowest serum levels, but increased frequency of premature births in women with lowest intake; these women also had lowest serum concentrations of vitamin C Similar findings reported by Wideman et al. Several reports indicate low serum vitamin C levels associated wtih threatened abortion or history of previous abortions Other studies found no relation	In one study, women took large doses (6 g/day for 3 days) of ascorbic acid to terminate suspected pregnancies; each had 10- to 15-day delay in onset of menstrual period. In 16 of 20, menstrual bleeding occurred within 1 to 3 days after starting the treatment. Results interpreted as indicating that large doses of ascorbic acid interrupted pregnancies. Since pregnancies were not initially confirmed, conclusion must be questioned Several infants have been reported to develop "conditioned scurvy" in neonatal period due to excessive ascorbic acid catabolism following high prenatal acid exposure

Continued.

TABLE 4-4 Vitamin and Mineral Deficiencies and Excesses and Human Pregnancy Course and Outcome—cont'd

	Deficiency	Excess
FOLATE	Humans treated with folate antagonists (methotrexate, aminopterin, chlorambucil) during early pregnancy often suffer spontaneous abortion Some cases reported of severe congenital anomalies in term infants associated with use of these drugs during pregnancy While naturally occurring folate deficiency in pregnant women has not been *proven* to have an adverse effect on pregnancy outcome, correlations have been reported between red cell folate level and incidence of congenital malformations, SGA babies, and third trimester bleeding Observation questioned by others and relationship between folate deficiency and abruptio placentae is equally controversial Most folate supplementation studies report no effect on pregnancy outcome but several reports from Africa and India indicated that rate of prematurity was significantly reduced Prospective study of 800 women indicated low red cell folate level associated with increased incidence of SGA infants and congenital malformations Large prospective study showed significantly lower levels of red cell folate in mothers who subsequently bore infants with neural tube defects vs. controls Several reports from northern Europe showed that women previously delivering babies with neural tube defects showed reduced incidence of same problem when multiple-vitamin supplementation (rich in folic acid) or pure folic acid supplementation was provided instead of no supplement at all. These highly controversial reports are currently being evaluated	
VITAMIN B_{12}	Pernicious anemia rare in women of childbearing age but generally is accompanied by infertility Human fetus with vitamin B_{12} dependency successfully treated by feeding high doses of vitamin B_{12} to mother	
VITAMIN B_6	Low maternal blood levels of B_6 have not generally been associated with neonatal clinical sequelae. Several stud-	

	ies reported that women with low dietary and/or serum levels of B_6 produced more babies with low Apgar scores than comparable mothers with good B_6 status
	Supplementation of pregnant women with B_6 has not been found to reduce any clinical complication of pregnancy except pregnancy sickness
	Maternal serum levels of B_6 were inversely correlated with degree of pure pregnancy depression
	Pregnant women in low socioeconomic group showed biochemical evidence of B_6 deficiency and orolingual lesions (e.g., glossitis, angular stomatitis); both responded positively to B_6 supplementation
	Pyridoxine supplementation of nonsupplemented pregnant women during labor (100 mg IM) appeared to favorably influence oxygen transport to newborn
IRON	Mean hemoglobin level of fetus is unaffected by maternal iron levels, unless deficiency is severe
	Infants of anemic mothers showed reduced iron stores and greater tendency to develop anemia in first year of life
	Effect of maternal iron deficiency on birthweight of infant is controversial
	Increased incidence of prematurity reported with maternal iron deficiency
	No evidence links iron deficiency with congenital malformations
CALCIUM	Mean bone densities of malnourished mothers and their neonates were lower vs. well-nourished counterparts
	Study of Indian women with low daily intake (~400 mg/day) indicated that daily supplementation during the third trimester was associated with increased bone density in infants
	Calcium deficiency proposed to be major etiologic factor in toxemia of pregnancy. Data indicate that in populations with low intake, incidence of eclampsia is higher. Supplementation of pregnant women also associated with reduced incidence of pre-eclampsia. Also noted that individuals with high intake have lower blood pressure and rats with restricted intake develop hypertension that is reversible with calcium administration. Furthermore, eclampsia syndrome is quite similar to that of tetany caused by hypocalcemia.

Continued.

TABLE 4-4 Vitamin and Mineral Deficiencies and Excesses and Human Pregnancy Course and Outcome—cont'd

	Deficiency	Excess
IODINE	Cretinism first described in 16th century; association with goiter was recognized in 19th century although cretinism does not always occur where there is a high incidence of endemic goiter. Cretinous children show mental and physical retardation with potbelly, large tongue and facial characteristics like Down's syndrome. Iodine prophylaxis has reduced the incidence of cretinism and goiter dramatically New Guinea reported the most recent outbreak of cretinism, related to substituting local iodine-rich salt with imported rock salt low in iodine. Intramuscular iodized oil injections to women prior to pregnancy were later shown to markedly reduce incidence of cretinism. In addition offspring of injected women were significantly faster and more accurate in tests of manual function than children without cretinism from non-injected mothers	Women provided large amounts of iodides during pregnancy (often as treatment for asthma or bronchitis) have had infants with congenital goiter and hypothyroidism. Neonatal mortality was high; infants were mentally retarded. Radioactive sodium iodide use during pregnancy is associated with the same outcome
SODIUM	Hyponatremia has been reported in offspring of women who rigorously restricted sodium during pregnancy Sodium restriction does not help prevent or alleviate toxemia of pregnancy	
POTASSIUM	Human embryonic kidney development in culture is abnormal. Suggests that potassium insufficiency in fetal plasma may cause abnormal development of the kidney in humans	
COPPER	Menkes kinky hair syndrome demonstrates impact of prenatal copper deficiency in humans. Abnormalities seen in development of brain, hair, bones, and blood vessels Woman treated with penicillamine during pregnancy bore infant with connective tissue defects including lax skin, hyperflexibility of joints, fragility of veins, varicosities, impairment of wound healing. Copper deficiency proposed to be of possible etiologic importance	Small amounts of metallic copper from IUDs can prevent mammalian embryogenesis; teratogenicity not established

ZINC	Epidemiologic data may support relationship between zinc deficiency and CNS malformations; significant zinc deficiency found in Egypt, Turkey, and Iran where high rates of CNS anomalies are seen Women with acrodermatitis enteropathica (a genetic disorder of zinc metabolism now treated with supplemental zinc) have shown very poor pregnancy outcome in the past when zinc therapy was not used; miscarriage and malformations were much higher than in general population Alcohol-abusing mothers show reduced serum levels of zinc and are known to demonstrate higher than normal incidence of poor pregnancy outcome. Relationship proposed but not proven Among 272 pregnant adolescent women in Belfast, 2 aborted spontaneously; these two women had serum zinc levels in the lower range and hair zinc values in the higher range Leukocyte zinc levels were significantly lower in mothers giving birth so SGA babies vs. mothers of normal babies or mothers of infants who were small but appropriate for gestational age Plasma zinc concentration was significantly lower in the maternal blood of 54 mothers of congenitally abnormal babies either within 24 hours or 24 months previously when compared with control mothers	Zinc supplements given to pregnant women (100 mg zinc sulfate, three times daily) during third trimester; in four consecutive subjects, three delivered prematurely and one gave birth to a stillborn infant
FLUORIDE	None known, although one report suggests that prenatal fluoride supplements were associated with reduced incidence of dental caries in offspring	Mothers using well water containing 12 to 18 ppm fluoride produced offspring with significant mottling of the deciduous teeth

*For references to specific studies cited in this table, see: Worthington-Roberts, B. Nutritional deficiencies and excesses: impact on pregnancy, part 2. J. Perinatol. **5**:12-21, 1985.

Vitamin B_6

Vitamin B_6, or pyridoxine, is concerned with amino acid metabolism and protein synthesis. In its active form of pyridoxal phosphate the vitamin is a cofactor in reactions involving a group of enzymes known as transaminases. Vitamin B_6 requirements increase in pregnancy not only because of the greater need for nonessential amino acids in growth but also because the body is making more niacin from tryptophan.

1. **Fetal needs.** Urinary excretion of vitamin B_6 metabolites during pregnancy is ten to fifteen times higher than in nonpregnant women, but blood values are typically reduced. Investigators are not sure what the clinical significance of this is. There is evidence that the placenta concentrates vitamin B_6 and that levels in cord blood are much higher than in the maternal circulation. This could mean that the reduced maternal blood levels are simply the result of physiologic adjustments. On the other hand, there is also evidence that the fetus takes up more vitamin B_6 and that maternal levels increase when oral supplements are used.[42] Limited animal data suggest adverse pregnancy outcome in the presence of vitamin B_6 deficiency.[43] In addition, European researchers[44] observed that the depth of pregnancy depression correlated negatively with serum vitamin B_6 concentration. Roepke and Kirksey[45] and Schuster's group[46] observed significantly lower Apgar scores in newborns of mothers with evidence of vitamin B_6 deficiency when compared with offspring of controls. The meaning of these observations remains to be determined.
2. **Maternal nausea and vomiting.** While the precise etiology of nausea and vomiting during pregnancy remains unknown, interest continues in the possibility that vitamin B_6 status may be important. Vitamin B_6 is known to catalyze a number of reactions involving neurotransmitter production and in that capacity could conceivably affect an assortment of physiologic states. However, a clear connection between vitamin B_6 and pregnancy nausea remains to be observed.[47,48] In one small study[49] relief of symptoms of pregnancy sickness appeared to be superior in women using Bendectin (an anti-nausea drug now off the market) with added vitamin B_6, as compared with women using Bendectin alone. Additional controlled double-blind studies are required to draw any firm conclusions about the value of vitamin B_6 supplements in the management of pregnancy nausea.
3. **Vitamin B_6 supplement.** Whether or not routine supplementation with vitamin B_6 is justified during pregnancy remains to be determined by additional observations in human subjects. The tendency at the moment is to regard the apparent alterations in B_6 status as an indication of some poorly understood physiologic adjustment to pregnancy. Supplementation is therefore not routine, but pregnant women will need some guidance in selecting foods to meet their allowances.

Vitamin C

Vitamin C deficiency has not been shown to affect the course or outcome of pregnancy in humans (Table 4-4). But questions have arisen about its possible association with several specific conditions made known through isolated clinical observations.

For example, low plasma levels of vitamin C have been reported in association with premature rupture of the membranes[50] and pre-eclampsia.[51] An extra 15 mg of vitamin C a day is recommended for the pregnant woman. This total recommendation of 60 mg a day is easily met by the U.S. diet. Large intakes of vitamin C supplements may adversely influence fetal metabolism. Metabolic dependency on high doses may develop in the fetus, bringing possible scurvy in the neonatal period.[52,53]

Thiamin, Riboflavin, and Niacin

Since thiamin, riboflavin, and niacin are all part of the reactions that produce energy in the body, requirements are related to caloric intake. The adult RDA are 0.5, 0.6, and 6.6 mg per 1000 kilocalories for thiamin, riboflavin, and niacin respectively. Since kilocalorie allowances increase during pregnancy, the allowances for thiamin, riboflavin, and niacin automatically increase also. In addition, evidence from urinary excretion studies indicates that pregnant women have higher requirements for thiamin and riboflavin than nonpregnant women. The RDAs for these two nutrients therefore include additional adjustments.

In animals, severe deficiencies of thiamin, riboflavin, or niacin during pregnancy have resulted in fetal death, reduced growth, and congenital malformation. The skeleton and organs that arise from the ectoderm appear to be especially susceptible to riboflavin deficiency. Lack of riboflavin in the mother's diet was once thought to be a cause of prematurity in humans, but recent studies have failed to find a correlation.

Researchers have evaluated the thiamin status of pregnant women at various stages of gestation and have found that 25% to 30% have values that would be considered deficient by nonpregnant standards. Although there have been some reported cases of congenital beriberi from maternal thiamin deficiency, there is no evidence of impairment at the levels consumed by women in developed countries. The niacin status of pregnant women has been inadequately investigated. However, there are no cases indicating that niacin deficiency in humans produces the malformations noted in experimental animals.

Vitamin D

This vitamin has long been appreciated for its positive effects on calcium balance during pregnancy. Recent evidence suggests that vitamin D may be involved in neonatal calcium homeostasis. Observations in Great Britain indicate that the peak season for neonatal hypocalcemia coincides with the time of least sunlight.[54] In addition, serum vitamin D levels are often low in such infants, suggesting that some cases of neonatal hypocalcemia and enamel hypoplasia may relate to maternal vitamin D deficiency and subsequent limitation in placental transport of vitamin D to the fetus.[55] A recent study of pregnant Asian women showed that vitamin D supplementation during the third trimester was associated with an improved rate of maternal weight gain, higher maternal and newborn serum 25(OH)D levels at term, a reduced incidence of symptomatic hypocalcemia in newborns, and a lower percentage of small-for-gestational-age infants.[56] But excessive amounts of vitamin D may be harmful during gestation. Severe infantile hypercalcemia and associated problems have been reported in newborn animals and in human infants. (See Table 4-4.)

Vitamin A

Both vitamin A and carotene cross the placenta, and fetal storage of vitamin A accounts in part for the recommendation that pregnant women consume an extra 1000 IU of this vitamin daily. An intake of this level can readily be provided by dietary sources, and there appears to be no need for routine supplementation. Although vitamin A deficiency is teratogenic in lower animals, confirmatory evidence in humans is lacking.[33,57] Excessive use and the toxic effects have posed problems:

1. **Megadose toxicity.** Excessive vitamin A consumption is believed to be teratogenic in humans (Table 4-4), but most scientific evidence describes developmental anomalies in animals. However, one report has described a human infant with congenital renal anomalies associated with maternal ingestion of large doses of vitamin A, about ten times the RDA, during pregnancy.[58] Another report[59] from Scandinavia indicated that a microcephalic child with multiple malformations of the central nervous system was born to a mother who consumed 150,000 IU of vitamin A daily during gestation days 19 to 40.
2. **Vitamin A analog.** The adverse effects of excessive vitamin A intake in early pregnancy have been dramatically illustrated by the recent introduction of *isotretinoin* (Accutane) into the marketplace.[60-62] The drug isotretinoin, used for the treatment of cystic acne, is an analog of vitamin A. Since its first appearance on pharmacy shelves in the early 1980s, more than seventeen cases of birth defects and twenty instances of spontaneous abortion have been associated with its use. This toxicity syndrome has been called the *Isotretinoin Teratogen Syndrome* and described by Benke.[60] Major features include prominent frontal bossing, hydrocephalus, microphthalmia, and small, malformed, low-set, undifferentiated ears. More cautionary labeling has now been provided with the product and physicians are warned about the possible dangers of prenatal exposure.[63]

Vitamin E

Requirements for this vitamin are believed to increase somewhat during pregnancy, but deficiency in humans rarely occurs and has not been linked with either reproductive disorders or reduced fertility. Since vitamin E deficiency in experimental animals has long been associated with spontaneous abortion, interest in the use of vitamin E for prevention of abortion has been a popular idea. In general, however, studies in humans have not supported this preventive measure. Several studies have shown, however, that the fetal vitamin E level is one-third to one-fourth the maternal concentration in both premature and term infants. Maternal levels of vitamin E rise during pregnancy such that by the third trimester these levels become 60% greater than in the nonpregnant controls. It has been found, however, that the maternal level must be from 150% to 500% of the value of the nonpregnant controls if the cord blood values are to reach the low-normal adult vitamin E concentrations.

Although the vitamin E level in the infant at birth is significantly less than in the mother, the infant's level has been shown to correlate directly with the maternal concentration.[64] Attempts to raise the fetal level by supplementing the mother with vitamin E during the last trimester confirmed the direct correlation of fetal and maternal vitamin E concentrations. It has been concluded, however, that parenteral vitamin

E administration to the mother before delivery is not enough to prevent the hemolytic anemia of vitamin E deficiency in the infant. Since this problem develops within 6 weeks after birth, it can best be prevented by oral supplementation of the infant during the postnatal interval.

Other Vitamins

Little is known about the dietary requirements for vitamin K, biotin, and pantothenic acid. Safe and adequate dietary intakes for these vitamins were suggested in the 1980 edition of the RDA (Table 4-5).

MINERALS

Iron

During pregnancy, iron is needed for the manufacture of hemoglobin in both maternal and fetal red blood cells. The fetus accumulates most of its iron during the last trimester. At term a normal-weight infant has about 246 mg of iron in blood and body stores. An additional 134 mg are stored in the placenta. About 290 mg are used to expand the volume of the mother's blood.

Maintenance of erythropoiesis is one of the few instances during pregnancy when the fetus acts as a true parasite. It assures its own production of hemoglobin by drawing iron from the mother. Maternal iron deficiency, therefore, does not usually result in an infant who is anemic at birth. The most common cause of iron deficiency anemia

TABLE 4-5 Estimated Safe and Adequate Daily Dietary Intakes of Additional Selected Vitamins and Minerals for Adolescents and Adults

	Age Group	
	Adolescents	**Adults**
Age	11+	
Vitamins		
Vitamin K (μg)	50-100	70-140
Biotin (μg)	100-200	100-200
Pantothenic acid (mg)	4-7	4-7
Trace elements (mg)		
Copper	2.0-3.0	2.0-3.0
Manganese	2.5-5.0	2.5-5.0
Fluoride	1.5-2.5	1.5-4.0
Chromium	0.05-0.2	0.05-0.2
Selenium	0.05-0.2	0.05.0.2
Molybdenum	0.15-0.5	0.15-0.5
Electrolytes (mg)		
Sodium	900-2700	1100-3300
Potassium	1525-4575	1875-5625
Chloride	1400-4200	1700-5100

Modified from Food and Nutrition Board, National Research Council, National Academy of Sciences: Recommended dietary allowances, rev. 1980, Washington, D.C., U.S. Government Printing Office.

in the infant is prematurity. The infant who has a short gestation simply does not have time to accumulate sufficient iron during the last trimester.[65]

Iron deficiency in the mother may have adverse effects on her obstetrical performance.[66] A reduction in hemoglobin concentration means that the mother must increase her cardiac output to maintain adequate oxygen use by placental and fetal cells. This extra work fatigues the mother and makes her more susceptible to other sources of physiologic stress. A very low maternal hemoglobin level places the mother at risk of cardiac arrest and leads to a poor prognosis for survival should she hemorrhage on delivery.

Setting requirements for iron during pregnancy is complicated by changes in the erythropoiesis system. Even when women have adequate iron status at conception, the plasma volume increases faster than the number of red blood cells so that ***hemodilution*** occurs. However, erythropoiesis is stimulated in the last half of pregnancy, and the rate of red blood cell production goes up. If sufficient iron is available, hemoglobin levels should rise to at least 12 mg per 100 ml by term.

Generally, the initial drop in hemoglobin is a normal physiological phenomenon, but there is concern that the usual iron intakes of pregnant women may not support increased erythropoiesis and fetal demands in the last half of pregnancy.[67] Iron absorption increases during pregnancy to as much as 30% compared with the usual 10% absorption from the diet. Also working in the mother's favor is the 120 mg or so that she saves over the course of gestation because she is not menstruating. However, even when these adjustments are taken into account, the pregnant woman still may need to consume about 18 to 21 mg of iron each day to maintain iron reserves (Fig. 4-8). This amount could be supplied if large servings of iron-rich foods are eaten, but

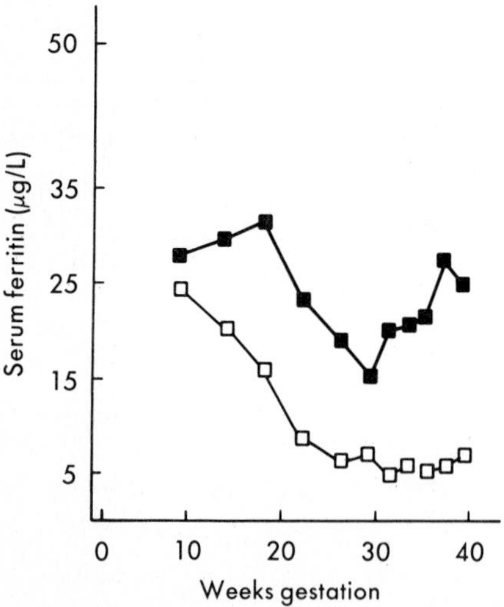

FIG. 4-8 Changes in serum ferritin during pregnancy in women treated with (■) and without (□) oral iron supplementation. Results are given as means.

(Modified from Romslo, I., et al.: Br. J. Obstet. Gynaecol. 90:101, 1983.)

unfortunately, such foods are limited to organ meats, oysters, clams, and prune juice. These are not foods that make up a large part of a typical diet. From an average mixed diet, about 6 mg of iron are obtained from each 1000 kilocalories of food. At this rate a pregnant woman would have to eat 3000 to 5000 kilocalories of food per day to meet her iron needs. Furthermore, studies have shown that most women enter pregnancy with low iron stores so they have little to draw on to maintain normal hemoglobin.

For these reasons the National Research Council does not set a dietary allowance during pregnancy. Instead, it recommends that pregnant women receive an oral iron supplement of 30 to 60 mg per day.[23] This amount should maintain hemoglobin levels in normal pregnant women, but those who are anemic when they enter pregnancy will need a larger dose. Simple ferrous salts should be used. There are no advantages in using compounds with claims of unique properties that increase absorption or enhance erythropoiesis. The best prenatal supplements provide iron in a form that demonstrates good bioavailability.

Calcium

The fetus acquires most of its calcium in the last trimester when skeletal growth is maximum and teeth are being formed. Widdowson[68] has calculated that the fetus draws 13 mg per hour of calcium from the maternal blood supply, or 250-300 mg per day. At birth the infant has accumulated approximately 25 g. Additional calcium is stored in the maternal skeleton as a reserve for lactation.

Extensive adjustments in calcium metabolism are routinely observed in the pregnant woman.[69] Hormonal factors are largely responsible:

1. **Human chorionic somatomammotropin** (from placenta). Progressively enhances the rate of bone turnover throughout pregnancy.
2. **Estrogen** (largely from placenta). Inhibits bone resorption and thus provokes a compensatory release of PTH, which maintains the serum calcium level while enhancing intestinal calcium absorption and decreasing its urinary excretion.

The net effect of this hormonal action is the promotion of progressive calcium retention. The prenatal changes begin well ahead of the time when fetal mineralization starts. It thus appears that anticipatory adjustments prepare the maternal organism for the increased calcium demands later on. Mineralization of the fetal skeleton is ultimately stimulated, largely through active placental calcium transport leading to fetal hypercalcemia and subsequent endocrine adjustments. Vitamin D and its metabolites also cross the placenta and appear in fetal blood in the same concentration found in maternal circulation.

The current RDA standard for calcium during pregnancy is 1200 mg daily, a level 400 mg higher than recommended for the nonpregnant woman. Some argue that this allowance is set too high, since apparently successful pregnancies occur in many other cultures with calcium intakes substantially below those recommended. The explanation likely relates to the large calcium reservoir in the maternal skeleton, of which the total requirements of pregnancy (30 g) amount to about 2.5%. Also, in many other cultures diets contain less protein and this factor might serve to reduce the degree of calcium loss in the urine. Researchers[70] have reported data from balance studies suggesting that if maternal intake of calcium is low, stores of calcium will be depleted to meet fetal needs. If this is the case, frequent pregnancies and consistently low calcium intakes throughout the childbearing years could contribute to suboptimal bone density in later life. Clinical osteomalacia in multiparous women has been observed.[71]

Phosphorus

The RDA standard for phosphorus is the same as that for calcium, 800 mg with an extra 400 mg during pregnancy. It is so widely available in foods that a dietary deficiency is rare. In fact, it is possible that the problem may be too much phosphorus rather than too little. Most adults can tolerate relatively wide variation in dietary calcium-phosphorus ratios when vitamin D is adequate. To protect the pregnant woman, a dietary intake of 10 μg of vitamin D per day is advised. However, pregnancy is a time when calcium reserves are severely stressed. Lowered concentrations of serum calcium and the mild alkalosis from the mother's reduced P_{CO_2} tend to increase muscular irritability. When this is compounded by high phosphorus intakes, an imbalance of the body calcium-phosphorus ratio could result.

Calcium-phosphorus balance relates to maintenance of normal neuromuscular action. Twenty years ago it was suggested that sudden clonic or tonic contractions of the gastrocnemius muscle (posterior "calf" muscle that flexes knee and ankle joints), occurring often at night, was caused by a decline in serum calcium. Prevention or relief was proclaimed to come from reduction of milk intake, a high phosphorus and calcium beverage. Supplementation with nonphosphate calcium salts was also recommended, along with regular use of aluminium hydroxide to form insoluble aluminum phosphate salts in the gut. While anecdotal reports have suggested benefit of these measures,[72] several controlled and double-blind studies have failed to show any correlation between leg cramps and either intake of dairy products or the type of calcium supplement used.

Magnesium

Magnesium is much like calcium and phosphorus in that most of it is stored in the bones. The amounts that are biochemically active are concentrated in nerve and muscle cells. Deficiencies of magnesium produce neuromuscular dysfunction characterized by tremors and convulsions. Magnesium-deficient pregnant rats show impaired abdominal contractions during parturition. Not a great deal is known about the need for magnesium during pregnancy. The RDA standard is based on estimates of the amounts accumulated by the mother and the fetus.

Zinc

This mineral has an active role in metabolism for several reasons: (1) it is a component of insulin; (2) it is part of the carbonic anhydrase enzyme system that helps maintain acid-base balance in the tissues; and (3) it acts in the synthesis of DNA and RNA, which gives it a very important role in reproduction.

Much recent interest has centered on the significance of zinc deficiency in adversely affecting pregnancy course and outcome.[73-76] Zinc is a known constituent of a number of important metalloenzymes and a necessary cofactor for other enzymes. Zinc deficiency is highly teratogenic in rats and leads to development of congenital malformations.[77] Nonhuman primates also are affected. Abnormal brain development and behavior have been described in offspring of zinc-deficient monkeys.[78] Evidence from human populations suggests that the malformation rate and other poor pregnancy outcomes may be higher in populations where zinc deficiency is recognized.[79-81] For example, Jameson[82] observed in Scandinavia that women with low serum levels of zinc had higher incidence of abnormal deliveries, including congenital malformations. However, since conflicting reports also appear in the literature[83-85] and questions remain about satisfactory measures of zinc status, the true role of zinc deficiency in adverse course and outcome of human pregnancy remains unknown. The potential hazard of prenatal zinc supplements has not been determined in human populations. Haphazard use of such supplements, however, has no role in wise prenatal care.

Iodine

For many years it has been understood that maternal iodine deficiency leads to cretinism in offspring. It is still seen in some parts of the world today. Recent data also suggest that suboptimal iodine nutrition of the mother may compromise development of her fetus, even when cretinism does not occur. Connolly and colleagues[86] evaluated motor performance of children born to mothers living in an iodine-deficient region of New Guinea. Some mothers received iodized oil and others received a placebo. Children born to mothers given iodine were significantly faster and more accurate in tests of manual function than children of control mothers. These findings indicate that iodine deficiency may lead to a spectrum of subclinical deficits that place children at a developmental disadvantage.

Fluoride

The role of fluoride in prenatal development is poorly understood at present. Some questions have existed over the past 50 years about the degree of fluoride transport across the placenta. Should it cross the placenta, questions still remain about its value in the development of caries-resistant permanent teeth. Researchers in Florida[87] examined nearly 500 women (and their offspring) who were given varying levels of fluoride during the last two trimesters of their pregnancies. About half of the women received fluoridated water only, and the other half received not only the fluoridated water but also a sodium fluoride supplement of 1 mg fluoride daily. When the offspring were examined at 5 to 9 years of age, the following observations were made:

1. **Children with prenatal fluoride supplement**: 0.17 + 0.07 decayed and filled surfaces; 97% were caries free.
2. **Children without prenatal fluoride supplement**: 8.70 + 0.60 decayed and filled surfaces; 15% were caries-free.

Development of the primary dentition begins at 10–12 weeks of pregnancy. From the sixth to ninth months of pregnancy, the first four permanent molars and eight of the permanent incisors begin to form. Thus 32 of the ultimate teeth are forming and developing during human pregnancy. Since there is no indication that color of the teeth is adversely affected and some evidence that caries resistance and morphologic characteristics are improved, prenatal fluoride supplementation may be justified. *It should be recognized, however, that this issue is highly controversial and to date for-*

mal support for routine prenatal fluoride supplementation has not been voiced by any established medical or dental organization.

Sodium

The metabolism of sodium is altered during pregnancy under the stimulus of a modified hormonal milieu. Glomerular filtration increases markedly over time to "clean up" the increased maternal blood volume. An additional filtered sodium load of 5000 to 10,000 mEq daily is typically seen during pregnancy. Compensatory mechanisms come into play to maintain fluid and electrolyte balance.

Restriction of dietary sodium has been common in the past among pregnant women with edema, but moderate edema is normal during pregnancy and should not be combated with diuretics and low-sodium diets. The increased fluid retained normally during pregnancy actually somewhat increases the body's demand for sodium. Rigorous sodium restriction in pregnant animals stresses the renin-angiotensin-aldosterone system to the point of breakdown. Such animals show reduced weight gain and altered fluid consumption patterns.[88] They also tend to develop water intoxication along with renal and adrenal tissue degeneration.[89] Neonatal hyponatremia (low blood sodium) has been observed in offspring of women who unduly restricted sodium intake before delivery.[90] The damage potential to the maternal renin-angiotensin-aldosterone system also exists. Although moderation in the American habit of excessive salt use is appropriate for all people, aggressive restriction is unwarranted during pregnancy. No less than 2-3 g of sodium should be consumed daily.

Other Minerals

One of the more recent advances in nutrition research is the discovery that many other trace elements are necessary for human growth, general health, and reproduction. Chromium, manganese, copper, selenium, molybdenum, vanadium, tin, nickel, and silicon have all been shown to be needed by the body. Like iodine, calcium, and phosphorus, these elements (and likely others as well) participate in reactions that control body processes. Studies in animals have revealed that deficiencies produce widespread and serious metabolic defects. Limited knowledge of requirements in humans makes it impossible to establish RDA standards for the majority of these minerals. The current RDA does, however, list estimated safe and adequate daily dietary intakes for copper, manganese, fluoride, chromium, selenium, and molybdenum (Table 4-5). No figures are available for pregnant women. Since toxic levels for many of the trace elements may not be much higher than usual intakes, pregnant women should not take supplements that would greatly exceed the upper limits recommended.

Positive Teaching to Correct Nutrient Deficiencies

GENERAL COUNSELING APPROACH

Reinforcing Good Habits

On the basis of detailed diet history, identify first the mother's good food habits and the nutrient contributions these habits make toward meeting her increased needs for pregnancy. Explain why these increased nutrients help her have a healthy pregnancy and a healthy baby. Reinforce these good food habits and encourage her to continue them.

Encouraging Needed Changes in Food Practices

To help correct inadequate food practices, provide positive teaching to help the mother change those food habits that need improving. Basic counseling actions reviewed here will support the mother's efforts to make these needed habit changes.

BASIC COUNSELING ACTIONS

Identify Unmet Needs

Help the mother relate her food habits to unmet nutrient needs of her pregnancy. Guide her to identify for herself the instances in which her particular food intake fails to meet specific nutrient demands of pregnancy. Tool A on page 118 may be useful to help her see some key nutrients she needs and some specific foods that can supply them.

Clarify Reasons for Increased Nutrient Needs

Discuss the reasons for these increased needs of pregnancy. Here you are trying to build motivation for making the desired behavior change by helping the mother see *why* it is important for her to do so. Point to the positive results for her baby's health, as well as her own, from such changed food behavior.

Identify Reasons for Dietary Deficiencies

What are her problems in obtaining appropriate foods? What limiting factors exist in her personal living situation? What personal reasons are there for her usual food choices? A variety of factors may be involved and they are all interrelated. On the whole, problems hindering the mother from getting the food she needs relate to three basic areas: (1) the nature of the available food supply; (2) the physical status and personal characteristics of the woman; or (3) the nature of her personal environment. Some of these factors may be simple things of which the mother is aware and can readily change. Others, however, may be larger problems requiring team help from the nutritionist, social worker, nurse, and physician, as well as any needed outside resources. In any event, consider these three basic problem areas in analyzing needs:

1. **Food supply**. There may be a lack of food available because of poor resources, insufficient funds for a large family or lack of money in general to sustain even minimal needs, inadequate food storage facilities with food spoilage and waste, or lack of skills in general food management and preparation.
2. **The person herself.** Physical problems may be present, such as underlying disease, food intolerances or aversions, poor appetite or low energy level, and generally low nutritional reserves. Personal problems may include ignorance of food needs or food values, special beliefs about food, lack of education, illiteracy, language barrier, carelessness, lack of concern or general apathy, and under-

TOOL A NUTRITIONAL ANALYSIS SHEET

Food Groups	Major Nutrient Contributions	Recommended Daily Intake (Number of Servings)	My Intake	Analysis of Food Needs
Protein-rich Foods				
Milk-cheese	Protein (complete, high biological value); Ca, P, Mg; vitamin D; riboflavin	1 qt milk 2 oz cheese or ½ cup cottage cheese		
Egg-meat	Protein (complete, high biological value); B complex vitamins; folic acid (liver); vitamin A (liver); iron (liver especially)	2 eggs 2 servings meat (3-4 oz each) Liver once a week at least		
Vitamin- and Mineral-rich Foods				
Grains, whole or enriched, breads or cereals, legumes	Protein (incomplete, supplementary); B complex vitamins; iron, Ca, P, Mg; energy (protein sparing)	4 or more servings		
Green and yellow vegetables	Vitamin A; folic acid	1-2 servings		
Citrus fruits and other vitamin C–rich fruits and vegetables	Vitamin C	2 servings		
Potatoes and other vegetables and fruits	Energy (protein sparing); added vitamins and minerals	1 serving or as needed for calories		
Fats—margarine, butter, and oils	Vitamin A (butter, fortified margarine); vitamin E (vegetable oils); energy (protein sparing)	1-2 tbsp as needed for calories		
Iodized salt	Iodine	Use with food to taste		

From Williams, S.: Handbook of maternal and infant nutrition, Berkeley, Calif., 1976, SRW Productions, Inc.

underlying psychosocial or emotional needs. In many of these situations there may be a pride that resents disclosure of problems related to personal needs.

3. **Environment.** Too often, problems attributed to personal factors are in reality the result of overwhelming environmental factors and the woman needs assistance. She may not be living in a home of her own and has little control over food selection and preparation. Also, there may be cultural or family food customs, especially during pregnancy, that limit food choices. Further, there may be socioeconomic problems from low income, unemployment, or frank poverty. Moreover, in some communities there may be attitudes and political influences that limit the availability of food assistance programs for pregnant adolescents and young women.

Explore Possible Solutions

Discuss possible solutions to problems or alternative practices available. Whatever the situation discovered, identify any problems, needs, or limitations on the woman's ability to make the desired changes, and explore with her possible solutions:

1. **Low income.** Lack of money for food may be a fundamental problem. Depending on degree of need, two areas of assistance may be discussed: (1) economical buying practices to help her spend her limited budget as wisely as possible; or (2) food assistance programs available in her community, such as food stamps and WIC. Consultation with the health team social worker will help provide guidance.
2. **Food aversions or intolerances.** Review the basis of the rejection as a means of securing acceptance of the food, if possible, or a reasonable alternative to supply the nutrients needed, or determining another form of the food in question.
3. **Cultural food pattern.** Nutrient needs should be related to a variety of acceptable food forms and preparations within the appropriate cultural food pattern. However, within one general cultural group, individual food habits can vary widely, so careful exploration of individual needs, desires, and possibilities during pregnancy is necessary.
4. **Vegetarian food patterns.** Explore first the type or level of vegetarian pattern the woman may be following. Many vegetarian food plans exclude only meat, some even allowing fish. Here ample primary protein may be obtained from dairy foods and eggs. However, if a strict vegetarian pattern is followed, more careful planning is necessary.
5. **Strict vegetarian pattern.** Persons who consume no animal protein are sometimes called *vegans.* Pregnant women must seek the best possible combinations of complementary protein foods to obtain an adequate amount of essential amino acids. Since vegans do not use dairy products, low intakes of calcium and vitamin B_{12} may result. Also, high fiber and phytate intake, common to vegan diets, may reduce calcium bioavailability. Alternative sources of calcium and B_{12} might include calcium-fortified soy milk, vitamin B_{12}-fortified soy products, nutritional yeasts, or vitamin-mineral supplements. These strict diets may also be low in iron and zinc since the richest sources of these minerals are animal products. Good sources of zinc such as soy products, whole grains, legumes,

nuts, and seeds can be used. There is a biologic competition for absorption between zinc and iron, so iron supplementation during pregnancy when zinc intakes are marginal may compromise zinc status further. Both minerals will be needed in adequate, not excessive, amounts.

Weight Gain During Pregnancy

HEALTHY WEIGHT GAINS

Importance of Adequate Weight Gain

The studies reviewed earlier in this chapter point to the importance of maintaining an adequate weight gain during pregnancy. By this time it should be apparent that the weight gained in a normal pregnancy is the result of physiologic processes designed specifically to foster fetal and maternal growth. Much of the weight gain can be accounted for by the products of gestation (Fig. 4-4).

Individual Needs

The total number of pounds gained in pregnancy will vary among individual women (Fig. 4-9).[91-95] Young mothers and primigravidae usually gain more than older mothers and multigravidae. A usual gain for most healthy women is about 20-30 lbs (9-13 kg). Those who are underweight at conception will need to gain more. Those who are obese may demonstrate good pregnancy course and outcome with a weight gain less than 9 kg. Adolescents and women carrying more than one fetus typically gain substantially more than 11 kg.

COMPONENTS OF WEIGHT GAIN

Focus of Positive Growth

Much of the past confusion about weight gain during pregnancy and the misguided attempts to restrict it result from the failure to appreciate that the components and rate of weight gain are more important than the actual number of pounds a woman puts on. Pregnancy should be a positive period of growth in which most of the gain is in lean body (protein) tissue. A gain from too much fluid or too much fat is not conducive to good health.

Growth Components

Table 4-6 shows how weight gain is usually apportioned in a normal pregnancy from conception to term. Almost 7.3 kg (16 lb) of a typical weight gain consists of the fetus, placenta, amniotic fluid, and growth of the uterus and breasts. Another 4.9 kg (11 lbs) is from general growth of the mother's body and storage of nutrient reserves.

QUALITY AND RATE OF WEIGHT GAIN

Pattern of Growth

Note that the weight gain in the first 10 weeks is small and that much of it is caused by the growth of the uterus and expansion of the mother's blood. At this time the fetus

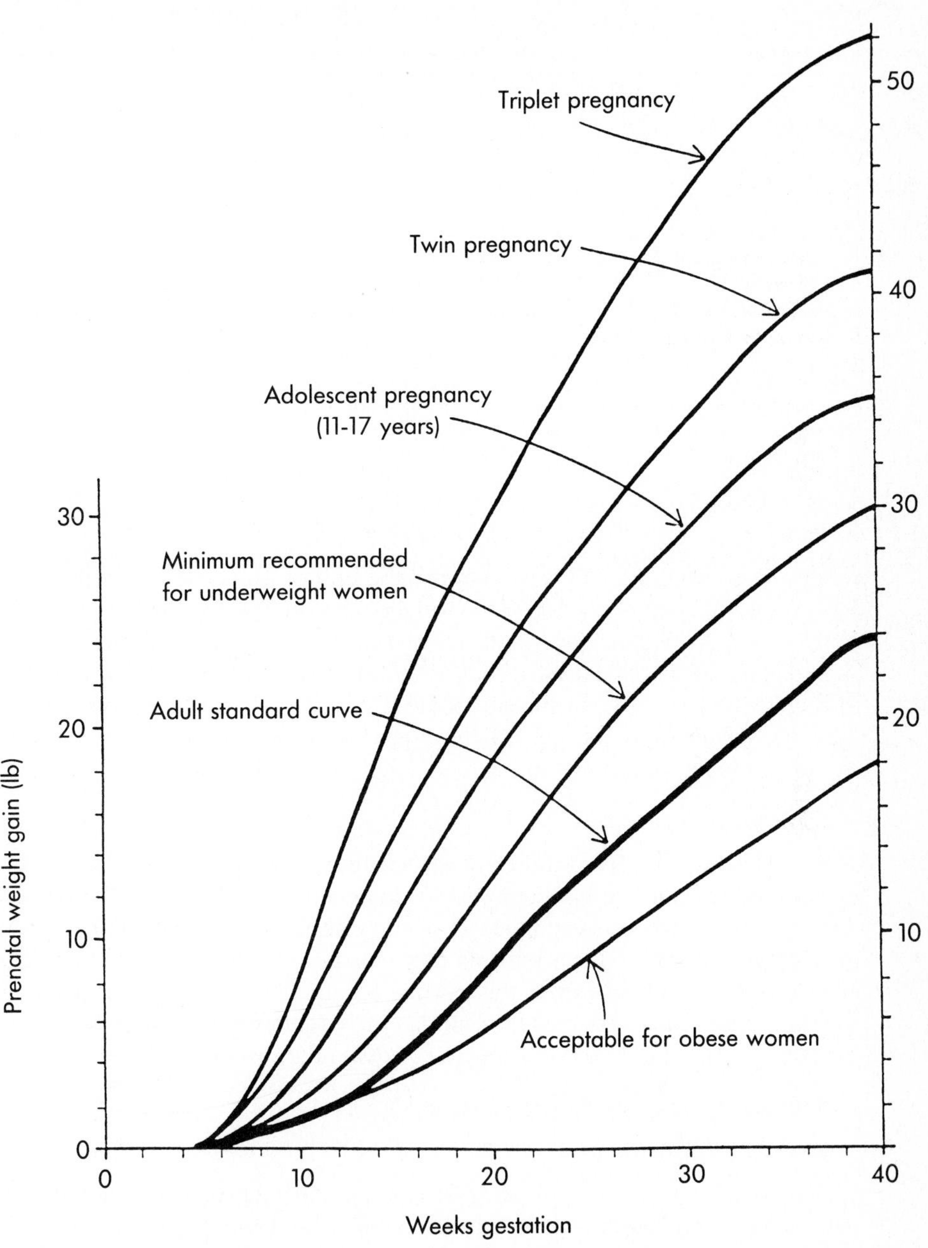

FIG. 4-9 Weight gain during pregnancy for selected subgroups of women.

TABLE 4-6 Components of the Average Weight Gained in Normal Pregnancy

Component	Amount (gm) Gained at			
	10 Weeks	20 Weeks	30 Weeks	40 Weeks
A. Total gain of body weight	650	4,000	8,500	12,500
Fetus	5	300	1,500	3,300
Placenta	20	170	430	650
Amniotic fluid	30	250	600	800
Increase of				
Uterus	135	585	819	900
Mammary gland	34	180	360	405
Maternal blood	100	600	1,300	1,250
B. Total (rounded)	320	2,100	5,000	7,300
C. Weight not accounted for (A − B)	330	1,900	3,500	5,200

From Committee on Maternal Nutrition; Food and Nutrition Board, National Research Council, National Academy of Sciences: Maternal nutrition and the course of pregnancy, Washington, D.C., 1970, U.S. Government Printing Office.

weighs only about 5 g (0.17 oz). Toward the end of pregnancy, growth of the fetus accounts for the largest portion of the weight increase. This pattern explains why many of the RDAs do not increase until the second trimester. The mother's rate of gain should generally parallel these trends. If she eats to appetite, the mother should gain a total of 0.9-1.8 kg (2-4 lb) by the end of the first trimester and about 0.45 kg (1 lb) each week thereafter. If pounds gained are plotted over the weeks of gestation, the curve would resemble that shown in Fig. 4-9 (Adult Standard Curve).

Sudden Weight Gain

A sudden weight gain that greatly exceeds the usual rate is likely to be caused by excess fluid retention. It has been repeatedly stated throughout this chapter that mild generalized edema and accumulation of some fluid in the lower limbs is not detrimental. Women with edema can gain as much as 9 L of fluid and still have clinically normal pregnancies. However, this normal accumulation of fluid is gradual. A large shift in water balance reflected by a sudden increase in weight is usually an indication of toxemia, particularly if it occurs after the twentieth week.

RECOMMENDATIONS FOR WEIGHT MANAGEMENT

Goal: Optimal Nutrition

The fundamental goal of weight management during pregnancy should be to promote optimal nutrition for the mother and child. Available data suggest that a gain of approximately 9 to 13 kg (20 to 30 lb) produces the most favorable outcome. Naeye[96] reported that the best obstetrical outcomes occur among normal-weight women who gain from 80% to 120% of this amount.

Underweight Women

Women who are underweight at conception will need to gain more to accommodate both "catch up" growth and adequate growth to support the pregnancy. In Naeye's report, the best outcomes among underweight women occurred when they gained approximately 13 kg (30 lb) during pregnancy. This important gain cannot be achieved if deliberate efforts are made to restrict food intake.

Obese Women

At the same time, obesity is *not* one of the outcomes of pregnancy that health professionals should promote. Excessive weight gain and obesity in pregnancy also carry risks.[92,93] In Naeye's study,[95] it was found that regardless of pre-conceptional weight status, women who gained over 14.4 kg (32 lb) during pregnancy had higher rates of perinatal mortality than mothers with weight gains in the 80% to 120% range of 12 kg (27 lb). This difference persisted when nonnutritional factors that could influence obstetrical outcomes were controlled. Mothers who were quite overweight had the best outcomes when they gained 6 to 7 kg (15 to 16 lb). This gain accounts for the weight of the products of gestation without the additional accumulation of maternal fat. Morbidly obese women represent a unique high-risk group. Optimal weight gain during pregnancy has not been defined for this population.[91,92]

These findings do *not* mean that overweight women should be placed on rigorous kilocalorie-restricted diets during pregnancy. In Naeye's study,[96] overweight women who gained less than 6 kg (15 lb) had a perinatal mortality rate two times higher than normal weight women who also had low weight gains. What these findings do imply is that being overweight during pregnancy can potentially be as great a problem as being underweight.

Individual Needs

Again, the individual pregnant women and her needs are the focus of care. Since each woman is a unique individual with her own history and needs, weight management should be flexible and *personalized*. Every woman should have an evaluation of her weight status at conception as part of her total nutrition assessment. An analysis of her usual dietary and activity patterns, along with her weight history, will help determine the weight gain that is best for *her*. The recommendation that pregnant women should "eat to appetite" must not be taken as a license to overeat or to indulge in "empty kilocalorie" foods. To achieve the desired intake, guidance should be given in the selection of foods that are nutritious, appealing, and conducive to weight gain within the optimal range.

Food Beliefs, Cravings, Avoidances, and Aversions

Most women change their diets during the course of pregnancy. Some changes are based on medical advice, others on folk medical beliefs, and others on changes in preference and appetite that may be idiosyncratic or culturally patterned. Since those changes that are culturally sanctioned will affect a woman's willingness to follow prescribed dietary regimens, the health care provider should be sensitized to their existence.

FOOD BELIEFS AND FOOD BEHAVIORS

Food Effects on Fetus

Many beliefs have been recorded about prenatal diet, such as the idea that the mother can mark her child before birth by eating specific foods. Overuse of a craved food during pregnancy is thought to explain physical or behavioral peculiarities of the infant. More often, unsatiated cravings are thought to explain birthmarks that mimic the shape of the desired food (such as strawberry- or drumstick-shaped marks). Behavioral markings have also been thought to derive from the prenatal diet; that is, the mother's consumption of many foods has been said to cause the child to like such foods after birth.

Food Effects on Delivery

Another important group of beliefs concerns dietary means by which the mother can ensure an easier delivery. Most important, from the biomedical viewpoint, are beliefs that lead a woman to avoid animal protein foods or to avoid "excessive" weight gain. Most lay people know very well that a smaller weight gain during pregnancy produces a smaller infant. Thus, since a smaller baby may be "easier to deliver," low weight gain has been proposed as desirable, especially since it is commonly believed that the baby can "catch up" after birth.

Food Aversions and Cravings

Food avoidances are those foods that the mother consciously chooses not to consume during her pregnancy, usually for a reason she can articulate and that seems reasonable to her. The four most commonly avoided foods are sources of animal protein: milk, lean meats, pork, and liver. Cravings and aversions are powerful urges toward or away from foods, including foods about which women experience no unusual attitudes outside of pregnancy. The most commonly reported craved foods are sweets and dairy products. The most common aversions are reported to be alcohol, caffeinated drinks, and meats. However, cravings and aversions are not limited to any particular foods or food groups.

NUTRITIONAL SIGNIFICANCE

General Effects

The nutritional significance of these food-related behaviors is difficult to evaluate. Available information has often been collected in an anecdotal or one-sided manner. Thus there is limited detailed information on dietary alterations that appear to be detrimental but little knowledge of total subcultural prenatal dietary intakes. As a result, it is difficult to quantify the nutritional effect of restrictive beliefs, avoidances, cravings, or aversions. The nutritional importance of such practices cannot be assessed without reference to the rest of the woman's diet. Overall, however, most cravings result in increased intakes of calcium and energy, whereas aversions often result in decreased intake of animal protein. Such cravings and aversions are not necessarily deleterious.

The Practice of Pica

One type of compulsive food behavior or craving during pregnancy, however, does carry potential danger.[97] This practice is termed *pica* (from the Latin word for magpie, with reference to the bird's omnivorous appetite). Human pica refers to the compulsion for persistent ingestion of unsuitable substances having little or no nutritional value. Pica of pregnancy[98] most often involves consumption of dirt or clay (geophagia) or starch (amylophagia). However, compulsive ingestion of a variety of nonfood substances has been noted, such as ice, burnt matches, hair, stone or gravel, charcoal, soot, cigarette ashes, mothballs, antacid tablets, milk of magnesia, baking soda, coffee grounds, and tire inner tubes. The practice of pica is neither new nor limited to any one geographical area, race, creed, culture, sex, or status within a culture.

Nutritional and Medical Implications

The medical implications of pica are not well understood, although several speculations have been made. The displacement effect of pica substances could result in reduced intake of nutritious foods, leading to inadequate dietary intakes of essential nutrients. Alternatively, substances that provide kilocalories, for example, starch, could lead to obesity if ingested in large amounts above the usual dietary intakes. Some pica substances may contain toxic compounds or quantities of nutrients not tolerated in disease states. Some pica substances interfere with the absorption of certain mineral elements, such as iron. Other less commonly reported complications of pica include:

1. **Lead poisoning.** Congenital lead poisoning secondary to maternal pica for wall plaster.
2. **Irritable uterus.** Tender, irritable uterus with dystocia associated with fecal impaction from clay ingestion.
3. **Anemia.** Fetal hemolytic anemia caused by maternal ingestion of mothballs and toilet air fresheners.
4. **Obstruction.** Parotid enlargement and gastric and small bowel obstruction from ingestion of excessive amounts of laundry starch.
5. **Infection.** Parasitic infection from ingestion of contaminated soil or clay.

Pica Cases

Two cases of pica and its consequences during pregnancy are summarized here as examples:

Case 1. In England a 21-year-old woman was hospitalized at 38 weeks gestation because of severe anemia. She was generally tired, occasionally dizzy, and had edema of the ankles and mild anorexia. After 3 weeks of concentrated treatment with iron and folic acid she showed no improvement. Through further questioning it was found that throughout her pregnancy, she had been eating toilet air freshener blocks at the rate of 1 to 2 per week. Cessation of this practice led to immediate improvement.

Case 2. A 31-year-old black woman was admitted to a rural emergency room with extreme weakness, severe nausea and vomiting, and fever. The patient reported no bowel movements during the preceeding 2 weeks. On examination she was lethargic and appeared critically ill. Within 10 minutes of arrival she experienced a grand mal seizure followed by cardiorespiratory arrest. Efforts at resuscitation were unsuccessful and the woman died. Autopsy findings included 3 L of pus within the peritoneal cavity and a 4 cm perforation of the sigmoid colon. Free within the cavity were stones measuring 2.5 cm in diameter and a clay ball measuring 5 cm in diameter. Near the site of perforation, the colon was impacted with hardened claylike material. Subsequent inquiry of the family revealed that clay ingestion in the rural area was commonplace, and the husband noted that three of the patient's four children occasionally ate clay from the same bank their mother had used.

Etiology of Pica

The etiology of pica is poorly understood, although several proposals have been made. One theory suggests that the ingestion of nonfood substances relieves nausea and vomiting. Another theory suggests that a deficiency of an essential nutrient such as calcium or iron results in the eating of nonfood substances that contain these nutrients. When pregnant women were questioned about the practice of pica, they gave a variety of answers:

- A taste for clay
- Clay kept the baby from being marked at birth
- Nervous tension was relieved
- Starch made the newborn lighter in color
- Starch helped the baby "slide out" more easily during delivery
- Clay quieted hunger pains
- Clay and starch were pleasant to chew
- Social approval of pica

Many of these reasons given are based on superstition, customs and tradition, or practices passed from mother to daughter over generations.

Effects of Potentially Harmful Food Components

A number of food components have shown harmful effects on the course and outcome of pregnancy.[97] Several of these agents and their effects are described here, including alcohol, caffeine, food additives, and food contaminants:

ALCOHOL

Fetal Alcohol Syndrome (FAS)

During the past 15 years health researchers have become aware of the adverse effect of excessive consumption of alcohol on fetal development. In 1973 pediatricians in Seattle, Washington, described a unique set of characteristics of infants born to women who were chronic alcoholics. These infants exhibited specific anomalies of the eyes, nose, heart, and central nervous sytem that were accompanied by growth retardation, small head circumference, and mental retardation. The investigators named the condition "fetal alcohol syndrome" (FAS) (Table 4-7). The condition is compatible with life but is associated with permanent disabilities (Fig. 4-10).

There is a high rate of prenatal mortality among infants with FAS. Those infants who survive are generally irritable and hyperactive after birth. These symptoms are attributed to alcohol withdrawal. Physical and mental development is impaired. FAS infants exhibit poor rates of weight gain and failure to thrive despite concerted efforts at nutritional rehabilitation. The following case illustrates the occurrence of FAS due to maternal ingestion of alcohol, in this instance in the unusual form of large amounts of cough syrup:

Case: Fetal Alcohol Syndrome. An infant with typical features of FAS, including a head circumference below the 10th percentile on the National Center for Health Statistics growth chart, was born at term to a 24-year-old mother who reported consumption of 480 to 840 ml per day of a nonprescription cough syrup. The alcohol content of the syrup was 9.5%, which amounted to 36.5 to 63.8 g of alcohol per day, equivalent to the alcohol content of 1 to 2 L of 4% beer or 0.5 to 1.0 L of wine. Intensive prenatal care had been instituted with entry into an addiction treatment program at an undefined point in pregnancy. No evidence of distortion of truth was found with urinary test for substance abuse. Whether pregnancy outcome was related to alcohol, to other drugs, or to their interactive effects is not clear. The case emphasizes the need for awareness of the full content of over-the-counter drugs used in pregnancy.

Fetal Alcohol Effects

The impact of more moderate levels of alcohol consumption on fetal development has been the focus of much research during the past decade. It is now well recognized that moderate drinkers may produce offspring with "fetal alcohol effects" showing

TABLE 4-7 Facial Characteristics in Fetal Alcohol Syndrome

	Features Necessary to Characteristic Face	Associated Features
Eyes	Short palpebral fissures	
Nose	Short and upturned in early childhood; hypoplastic philtrum	Flat nasal bridge; epicanthal folds
Maxilla	Flattened	
Mouth	Thinned upper vermilion	Prominent lateral palatine ridges; cleft lip with or without cleft palate; small teeth
Mandible		Retrognathia in infancy; micrognathia or relative prognathia in adolescents
Ears		Posterior rotation; abnormal concha

From Clarren, S.K.: Recognition of fetal alcohol syndrome, J.A.M.A. **245**:2436, 1981. Copyright 1981, American Medical Association.

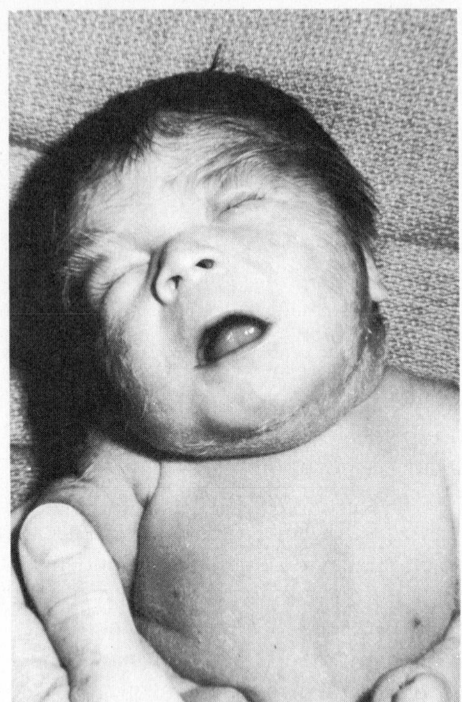
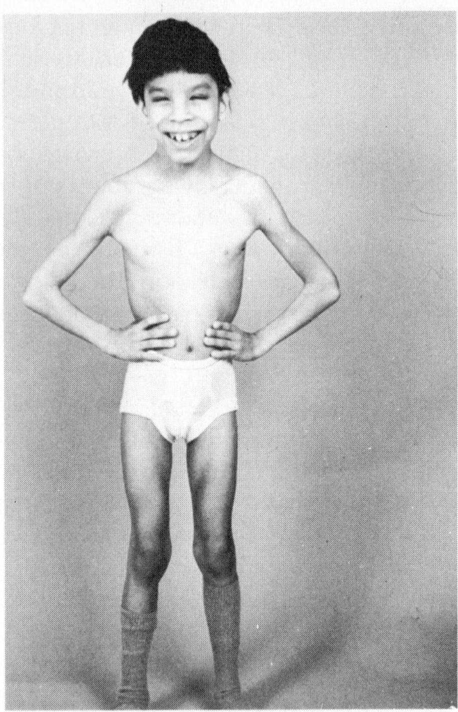

FIG. 4-10 Child with FAS at day 1 and 8 years of age. This child was diagnosed at birth and has spent all his life in a foster home where the quality of care has been excellent. His IQ has remained stable at 40-45. Although he is more seriously retarded than most children with FAS, he demonstrates the resistance of the disability to environmental intervention. (Courtesy of Dr. Ann P. Streissguth, University of Washington, Seattle.)

more subtle features of FAS. Such women also demonstrate a higher rate of spontaneous abortion, abruptio placentae, and low-birth-weight delivery.

General Actions of Alcohol

At present, the mechanisms by which alcohol produces such widespread effects on the fetus are not completely understood. Since alcohol can cross the placenta, the current hypothesis is that high alcohol levels build up in the fetus and produce direct toxic effects that are most severe in the early phases of pregnancy during blastogenesis and cell differentiation. Another theory is that some of the effects of alcohol may be caused by maternal malnutrition. We may not think of alcohol as a food, but it yields 7 kilocalories per gram. Alcohol is considered an "empty kilocalorie" food because most alcoholic beverages supply little or no nutrients. Women who derive a substantial portion of their daily caloric needs from alcohol may not have an appetite for more nutritious foods. Deficiencies of folic acid, magnesium, and zinc have been shown to be highly teratogenic in animals, so it is reasonable to suspect that deficiencies of these nutrients could play a role in FAS.

Alcohol Use by Pregnant Women

Although the adverse effects of maternal alcohol consumption on fetal development have been known for over a decade, a significant number of women still choose to drink alcohol while they are pregnant. One research team[99] reported that among women delivering in a large urban hospital in Massachusetts, 82% had consumed alcohol during pregnancy: 3% consumed alcoholic beverages more than 20 times per month, and 3% consumed more than 20 oz (600 ml) per month. Streissguth and coworkers[100] reported patterns of alcohol use among pregnant women in a large urban area who had been exposed to a heavy media campaign aimed at preventing fetal alcohol effects. Looking at precampaign and postcampaign data (1974-1975 and 1980-1981), the number of women who reported any alcohol use around the time of the first prenatal visit dropped from 81% to 42%, but among drinkers, there was no decrease in the proportion of women who reported heavier drinking. As these authors suggest, the relative constancy in the proportion of "heavier" drinkers and binge drinkers, particularly around the time of conception, indicates the need for more attention to this important period of gestation in advice to women who are planning a pregnancy.

Prenatal Care for Alcoholic Mothers

According to Rosett and colleagues,[101,102] pregnancy course and outcome can be significantly improved if problem drinkers agree to change their habits after conception has occurred. These workers reported that infants born to women who reduced their heavy drinking did not differ in growth from offspring of rare and moderate drinkers. They did, however, show a higher frequency of abnormalities. This group urges that facilities providing routine prenatal care integrate therapy for heavy drinking into their counseling sessions. Since the desire to have a healthy baby is a powerful motivating force, therapeutic success can be achieved with some of the heaviest drinkers.

CAFFEINE

Animal Studies

The danger of caffeine to the developing fetus has been studied in several animal models. Massive doses appear to be teratogenic in mice, but the effects of smaller quantities have not been satisfactorily examined. One research group[103] did observe that offspring of rats fed coffee during pregnancy had reduced body, liver, and brain weight at birth. By 39 days, these animals had recovered in size but demonstrated increased locomotion, decreased grooming time, and decreased time spent with a novel object. Another research team[104] reported that when caffeine was introduced into the diet of rats throughout pregnancy and lactation, offspring of successive pregnancies showed growth reductions, although teratogenic effects were not seen with this moderate level of caffeine exposure.

A 1980 report from the Food and Drug Administration (FDA) suggested that rather modest amounts of caffeine provided to pregnant rats may increase the incidence of defects in development of the digits.[105] Pregnant rats provided an amount of caffeine (per unit size) the equivalent of about 12 to 40 cups of coffee per day for humans produced offspring with an increased incidence of partial or complete absence of the digits of the paws. A Virginia woman subsequently claimed that her 15-year-old child with no fingers or toes was damaged in utero by her daily consumption of 10 to 12 cups of coffee. Although data were limited in relation to human use of caffeine in pregnancy, a general warning was voiced to the public in 1981 to avoid unnecessary caffeine consumption during pregnancy.

Conclusions

Since this warning was released in the early 1980s, three systematic observations of large groups of pregnant women have not provided cause for alarm.[106-108] However, one recent report suggested that a rather low level of daily caffeine consumption (about 150 mg) is associated with greater risk of late first and second trimester spontaneous abortion.[109] Since available data from observations of human populations are inconclusive, common sense suggests that caution should be exercised and pregnant women should be advised to use caffeine in moderation, if at all.

FOOD ADDITIVES

The teratogenicity of common food additives is largely unknown in human situations. Metabolism of cyclamate and red dye no. 2 reportedly damages developing rat embryos,[110] but both of these additives have now been banned for use in the U.S. food supply. Saccharin, mannitol, xylitol, aspartame, and other artificial sweeteners have come under careful scrutiny in the last few years. Kline and coworkers[111] have reported, however, that incidence of spontaneous abortion in a human population was not associated with ingestion of any sugar substitute.

Saccharin

Because saccharin has been shown to be weakly carcinogenic in rats, however, moderation in its use seems appropriate. This is especially true for women of reproductive age, since studies in rats indicate that saccharin can most effectively initiate bladder cancer when the mother is exposed to high doses before pregnancy and the offspring are exposed in utero and throughout their lives. Saccharin can also markedly promote or enhance the potential of other carcinogens in rats, providing another reason for moderation in use.[112]

Aspartame

The increasing use of aspartame in the American food supply has been associated with outcries from a minority of scientists who propose that one or more of the breakdown products of aspartame may interfere with normal fetal development. Chemically, aspartame is L-aspartyl-L-phenylalanine methyl ester. The dipeptide ester is metabolized into three moieties in the small intestine, so that studies of the safety of aspartame are essentially studies of aspartic acid, phenylalanine, and methanol.

1. **Human studies with pregnant women.** Human subjects have been fed up to 6 times the 99th percentile of the projected daily intake ($6 \times 34 = 200$ mg per kg). No evidence of risk to the fetus has been observed. Aspartame does not readily cross

the placenta. Small elevations of blood methanol following such abusive doses of aspartame have not led to measurable increases in blood formic acid, which is the product responsible for the acidosis and ocular toxicity of methanol poisoning. Phenylalanine is concentrated on the fetal side of the placenta.

2. **Phenylalanine and PKU.** The phenylalanine component of aspartame has raised the most concern due to the known damaging impact of phenylalanine on brain tissue of children with phenylketonuria (PKU). Individuals with this genetic disease lack the liver enzyme that converts phenylalanine to tyrosine. Thus, blood levels of phenylalanine rise to high levels and mental retardation is the ultimate result. Aspartame in abusive doses up to 200 mg per kg in normal subjects, or to 100 mg per kg in PKU heterozygotes (carriers of the gene for PKU), have not been found to raise blood phenylalanine levels to the range generally accepted to be associated with mental retardation in the offspring.
3. **Conclusions.** One might conclude that, under foreseeable conditions of use, aspartame poses no risk for use in pregnancy. However, since limited data are available to date on pregnancy course and outcome in heavy aspartame users, it may be wise to recommend moderation in aspartame use during pregnancy, especially in women known to be PKU heterozygotes.[113]

FOOD CONTAMINANTS

General Toxicity

A number of "contaminants" are found in food. Some of these may adversely affect pregnancy course and outcome if consumed in sufficient amounts.[114] Most heavy metals are embryotoxic but only mercury, lead, cadmium, and possibly nickel and selenium have been implicated in this regard. Lead toxicity has long been known to be associated with abortion and menstrual disorders.[115,116] Evidence as to whether lead is teratogenic is conflicting.[117] Some authors report a correlation between atmospheric lead levels and congenital malformations, whereas others deny these associations. In sheep, prenatal lead exposure has also been shown to affect the offspring's learning ability.

Mercury Poisoning

Probably the earliest instance of massive, unplanned exposure of a local population to an environmental toxicant occurred in 1953 in and around Minamata, a town located on a bay in southern Japan. Unusual neurologic problems (for example, mental confusion, convulsions, and coma) began afflicting villagers. Over a third of the affected individuals died, and many infants and children suffered permanent brain damage from prenatal and neonatal exposure. Mercury was transported across the placenta and also appeared in breast milk of mothers consuming contaminated fish. Eventually the source of the mercury was traced to the effluent discharged from a local plastics factory into Minamata Bay. A similar incident occurred in Niigata, Japan in 1964.

Another massive methylmercury disaster occurred in Iraq during the winter of 1971-1972. In this case barley and wheat grain treated with methylmercury as a fungicide had been purchased from Mexico. The grain sacks carried a written warning—

but only in Spanish. Thirty-one pregnant women who ate the grain were hospitalized with methylmercury poisoning. Almost half of them died. Infants born to surviving mothers showed evidence of cerebral palsy, blindness, and severe brain damage. Similar outbreaks have occurred in Russia, Sweden, and elsewhere.[118]

Other Heavy Metals

Several other heavy metals probably affect the fetus and infant. Cadmium, which is derived accidently from tobacco smoke, the electroplating industry, and deterioration of rubber tires, is a known cause of developmental malformations in rodents. In rats nickel in low doses causes embryotoxicity and eye malformations in the progeny. Selenium is also a suspect teratogen.

Pesticides

A number of pesticides have been a major concern among public health professionals for quite some time. The Environmental Protection Agency reports that about one-third of the 1500 active ingredients in registered pesticides are toxic, and one-quarter are mutagenic and carcinogenic. Although the agency has established limits on the amounts of pesticide residues that are allowed in foods, it has restricted the use of only five: heptaclor, chlordane, DDT, Mirex, and DBCP. Once deposited in the food chain, they are almost impossible to eliminate. The effects of exposure to low concentrations of these toxins are not only unknown but also difficult to investigate because of the problem of finding pesticide-free control populations.

PCBs

Polychlorinated biphenyls (PCBs), used as plasticizers and heat exchange fluids, comprise another group of chemicals that endanger health. In Kyushu, Japan in 1968, a number of pregnant and lactating women ingested cooking oil contaminated with PCBs. As a result, they had small-for-gestational-age infants with dark skin, eye defects, and other abnormalities. Although prenatal exposure was probably significant, evidence indicated that transfer of PCBs through breast milk was the most significant route of exposure. Polybromated biphenyl (PBB), produced commercially as a fire retardant, also provoked attention after its accidental entry into cattle feed in Michigan in 1973-1974. Over 30,000 cattle and many sheep, swine, and poultry died or were slaughtered. Contaminated meat, milk, and eggs were identified in local food supplies, and stillbirths among affected cattle increased. Adverse effects in human pregnancy have not yet been reported, but considerable concern still exists.

Effects of Rigorous Physical Activity

For many years questions have been raised about the effect of heavy maternal physical activity during pregnancy on fetal growth. Some insight may be gained from studies related to both heavy physical labor and modern fitness programs, as well as to athletic training.

HEAVY PHYSICAL LABOR

Ethiopian Study

In a study conducted in Ethiopia, trained nutritionists visited pregnant women in their homes for a period of three consecutive days. During this time dietary surveys were conducted. Two groups of women who had similar energy and protein intakes during pregnancy were then compared. One group of mothers was forced by circumstances beyond their control to engage in hard physical work throughout pregnancy. The second group of mothers had servants to do such physical labor. Mothers in both groups ate on the mean about 1550 kilocalories a day.

Study Results

When the two groups of Ethiopian women were compared, the women who engaged in hard physical labor had significantly lower pregnancy weight gains and smaller babies than did mothers who did not have to engage in such work. Kilocalorie deficiency was likely involved in the etiology of fetal growth retardation that was seen. In addition, however, the oxygen debt incurred by moderate exercise is increased in human pregnancies, and this may lead to fetal hypoxia. This response is also evident in animal studies where uterine blood flow decreases during maternal exercise.

FITNESS PROGRAMS

The circumstances of mandatory physical labor described above, further imposed on an underlying state of moderate undernutrition, may seem far removed from today's modern fitness-conscious woman who opts to engage in a rigorous exercise program during pregnancy. But some useful comparisons can be made.

Conflicting Advice

The fitness-conscious pregnant woman often gets conflicting advice from her physician and other health professionals. The obstetrical textbooks rarely offer more than a single paragraph concerning physical activities during pregnancy. Obstetricians tend to form their own philosophies about athletic participation or various physical activities during pregnancy, and their recommendations often are based on their own (or their wives') experiences.

Effect of Physical Training

Physical training during pregnancy has been examined in normal Finnish primigravidae who were randomly divided into training and nontraining groups. In the experimental group an exercise program of 1 hour per day, 3 days per week, was instituted in the first trimester. During this exercise period the subjects were instructed to maintain their pulse rate over 140 beats per minute. These pregnant women in the training group showed a work capacity that was 17.6% higher than comparable pregnant and nonpregnant groups.

Aerobic Exercise Effect

In a similar study in Wisconsin, the effects of an aerobic exercise program were observed in a group of pregnant women.[119] Twelve women participated in an aerobics class during the second and third trimesters, whereas eight control women did not perform any regular exercise. On the basis of submaximal exercise test results, an 18% improvement and a 4% decline in absolute aerobic capacity was observed in the exercise and control groups respectively. Functional aerobic capacity rose 8% in the exercise group and declined 10% in the control group. A comparison of pregnancy outcome of the two groups showed no difference in labor duration, Apgar scores, or fetal growth.

Athletic Training Effect

Studies of Olympic athletes who trained while they were pregnant have failed to show any deleterious effects on their offspring. First stage labor was slightly prolonged, but total labor was shortened because of a more rapid second stage. This shortened second stage of labor was attributed to their capacity to raise intra-abdominal pressure more effectively. Other researchers have also shown no adverse fetal effects in women who strenuously trained during a pregnancy and participated in stress testing up to submaximal effort. Pomerance and Gluck[120] found no relation between physical fitness scores during pregnancy and birth weight, birth length, head circumference, or Apgar scores of the offspring.

GENERAL EXERCISE LEVELS DURING PREGNANCY

Basic Recommendation

It is the general feeling among experienced clinicians that pregnant women should continue to do things they do well, and are accustomed to doing, but in moderation. Obviously, some reservations exist about complete endorsement of continuing all athletic activities during pregnancy.

Complications

In conditions such as pre-eclampsia, abruptio placentae, and placenta previa, in which fetal-maternal circulation may be impaired, the fall in uterine blood flow with exercise will not be well tolerated. Also, regulation of the level of physical activity may be necessary in women with diabetes, cervical defects, or a history of spontaneous abortion. Increased ligamentous relaxation and increased joint mobility may predispose the mother to injury in such activities as gymnastics.

Heavier Exercise

Common sense should be used in considering involvement in heavier exercise and sports, especially where risk of injury is increased. These activities would include such events as contact sports, scuba diving, alpine and water skiing, and high altitude climbing.

Energy Intake

In the final analysis, the more active woman will need to remember that higher energy expenditure levels require higher energy intakes to maintain nutritional support of the pregnancy. Since birth weight is strongly related to both prepregnancy weight and weight gain, the pregnant athlete must have counseling on proper kilocalorie intake.

Effects of Cigarette Smoking

FETAL GROWTH RETARDATION

Fetal growth retardation is often seen in offspring of cigarette smokers. It has been postulated that this condition is due to the reduced food intake of the mother. But observations have shown that this is not true. Women who smoke often consume more kilocalories per day than women who do not smoke.[121]

EFFECTIVE CAUSE

The growth-retarding impact of smoking relates to the effects of carbon monoxide, nicotine, and possibly other compounds on placental perfusion and oxygen transport to the fetus. It is also likely that efficiency of kilocalorie utilization is reduced in women who smoke. Whether or not encouraging greater weight gain among smoking mothers will increase the infant's size is as yet an unanswered question. However, several reports have suggested that greater weight is directly related to greater infant birth weight in this population.[121,122] In any event, the wisest counsel to mothers who smoke is to stop—at least during the pregnancy.

Common Complaints with Dietary Implications

General nutritional guidance may also be needed during pregnancy for common functional gastrointestinal difficulties encountered. These complaints are highly individual in form and extent. They will, therefore, require individual counseling and assurances for control. Usually these difficulties are relatively minor. But if they persist or become extreme, they will need medical care. In most cases general investigation of food practices will reveal some areas where diet counseling may help relieve them. Some of the more common difficulties include nausea, constipation, hemorrhoids, or heartburn.

NAUSEA AND VOMITING

Difficulty with nausea and vomiting is usually mild and limited to early pregnancy. It is commonly called "morning sickness" because it tends to occur early in the day, but it can come at any time of day. Usually it lasts only a brief period at the beginning of the pregnancy, but in some women it may persist longer.

In the usual mild condition, a number of factors may contribute. Some are physiologic, based on normal hormonal changes that occur early in pregnancy. Other factors may be psychologic, such as various tensions and anxieties concerning the pregnancy itself. Simple treatment generally improves food toleration. Small frequent meals, fairly dry and consisting chiefly of easily digested energy foods such as carbohydrates, are more readily tolerated. Cooking odors should be avoided as much as possible. Liquids are best taken between meals instead of with food. If the condition persists and develops into *hyperemesis*—severe, prolonged, persistent vomiting—medical attention is required to prevent complications and dehydration. However, such an increase in symptoms is rare. Most conditions pass early in the pregnancy and respond to the simple dietary remedies given here. Women should be reassured that mild short-term nausea is common in early pregnancy and will not harm the fetus.

CONSTIPATION

The condition of constipation is seldom more than minor. Hormonal changes in pregnancy tend to increase relaxation of the gastrointestinal muscles. Also, the pressure of the enlarging uterus on the lower portion of the intestine, especially during the latter part of the pregnancy, may make elimination somewhat difficult at times. Increased fluid intake, use of naturally laxative foods and fiber, such as whole grains with added bran, fibrous fruits and vegetables, dried fruits (especially prunes and figs), and other fruits and juices generally induce regularity. Laxatives should be avoided. They should only be used in special situations under medical supervision.

HEMORRHOIDS

A fairly common complaint during the latter part of pregnancy is that of hemorrhoids. These are enlarged veins in the anus, often protruding through the anal sphincter. This vein enlargement is usually caused by the increased weight of the fetus and the downward pressure it produces. The hemorrhoids may cause considerable discomfort, burning, and itching. Occasionally they may rupture and bleed under the pressure of a bowel movement, therefore causing more anxiety. The difficulty is usually remedied by the dietary suggestions given above to control constipation. Also, observing general hygiene recommendations concerning sufficient rest during the latter part of the day may help to relieve the pressure of the uterus on the lower intestine.

HEARTBURN OR FULL FEELING

The related complaints of "heartburn" or "full feeling" are sometimes voiced by pregnant women. These discomforts may occur especially after meals, usually caused by the pressure of the enlarging uterus crowding the stomach thereby causing some difficulty after eating. Food mixtures may sometimes be pushed back into the lower part of the esophagus, causing a "burning" sensation from the gastric acid mixed with the food mass. This burning sensation is commonly called heartburn simply because of the proximity of the lower esophagus to the heart. It has nothing to do with the heart and its action. A full feeling comes from general gastric pressure, caused by a lack of normal space in the area, and is accentuated by a large meal or gas formation. These complaints are generally remedied by dividing the day's food intake into a number of small meals during the day. Attention may also be given to relaxation, adequate chewing, eating slowly, and avoiding tensions during meals. Comfort is also improved by wearing loosefitting clothing.

Improving the Outcome of Pregnancy

GENERAL NUTRITION RELATIONSHIPS

Birth Weight

There are sufficient parallels between animal and human research to conclude that maternal nutrition can influence reproductive performance, especially of women who have a high risk of giving birth to low-birth-weight infants. Birth weight reflects intrauterine growth. It is a determinant of the child's potential for survival and future health. This is true of both physical and mental performance.

Brain Development and Learning Ability

There has been much discussion about the possible effects of prenatal nutrition on intelligence and learning ability. Whether an infant whose size and number of brain cells are reduced at birth from maternal malnutrition is going to have a permanent mental disability is not currently known. Given the understanding of growth and development, however, it is reasonable to suppose that the consequences will depend to some extent on the child's nutrition in postnatal life, as well as the physical and social environment in which he or she is born. A follow-up study of children born during the World War II famine in Holland could find no evidence of lower-than-average intelligence or a higher incidence of mental retardation. It is possible that acute dietary deprivation during pregnancy of previously well-nourished women can be compensated by adequate nutrition later on.

Lifetime Nutrition

However, the situation in Holland is not what typically occurs. Most women in good nutritional status before conception do not suddenly have poor diets during pregnancy and then try to make up for it by feeding their children well after they are born. The factors that place a pregnant woman at nutritional risk typically have operated over her *lifetime* and will continue to affect the nutritional status, growth, and development of her child (Fig. 4-11). These influences include poverty, poor education, a deprived environment, and poor health. Surveys have shown clear associations between these factors and the nutritional status of infants, children, and women of childbearing age. All women need nutritional guidance during pregnancy. But those who conceive in poor nutritional status, and whose life circumstances impair their ability to secure adequate diets for themselves and their families, require very special care.

IMPLICATIONS FOR PRACTICE

Optimal maternal weight gain

The studies on weight gain during pregnancy have great importance for clinical practice. There must surely be an upper limit to birth weight that will not be exceeded despite progressively higher maternal weight gains. Further, obesity engenders its own health risks and should not be encouraged. However, a number of studies clearly show that pregnancy is no time for women to try to lose weight. The common practice

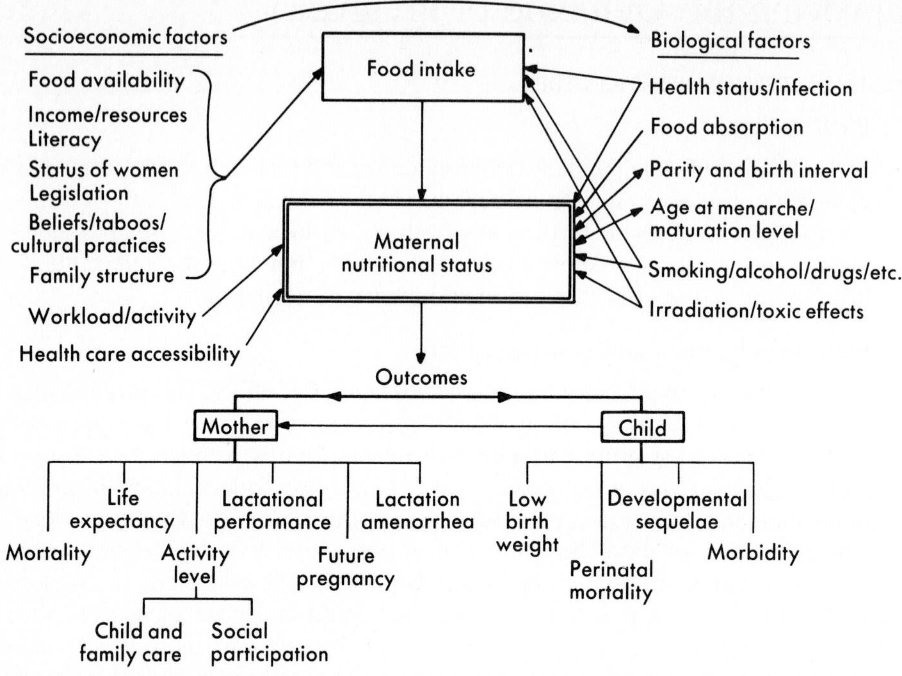

FIG. 4-11 Influences on and outcomes of maternal nutritional status.
(Modified from Hofvander, Y.: Maternal and young child nutrition, Paris, 1983, United Nations Educational, Scientific and Cultural Organization.)

of restricting weight gain by placing pregnant women on low kilocalorie diets must be discouraged. There are public health implications that can be shown not only for low-income mothers but also for those from the upper socioeconomic strata.

Optimal Infant Birth Weight

A vast body of information on the distribution of birth weights around the world has been summarized by Hytten and Leitch.[24] Data on American infants show that average birth weights range from 3000 to 3500 g (6.5 to 7.6 lb). However, when perinatal mortality rates are examined, the lowest rates occur when newborns weigh between 3500 and 4000 g (7.6 and 8.7 lb). In other words, it would appear that the optimal birth weight for the lowest risk of mortality is somewhat higher than the average birth weight.

Optimal Maternal Nutrition

Intrauterine growth for nonwhites declines during the last trimester of pregnancy, and growth curves for even the more affluent white infants are lower in the United States than in Scandinavian countries. When this is compared with the demonstrated effects of maternal height, prepregnancy weight, and weight gain on the size and weight of infants carried to term, there is reason to believe that improving maternal nutrition before and during pregnancy is one of the most practical steps that can be taken toward improving birth weights and the rate of perinatal death.

Summary

The relative importance of nutrition in prenatal development has been studied and debated for a number of years. Available evidence strongly supports a key role for maternal nutritional status in significantly affecting the fate of both mother and child. Animal data and human observations clearly suggest that human maternal prepregnancy weight and weight gain during pregnancy positively correlate with birth weight of the offspring.

Supplementation programs for pregnant women are successful when they are properly administered and focused on needy populations. The benefit of such programs may also be substantial even when health-care workers or food-program administrators are unable to measure that benefit with available tools. With limited time and resources in prenatal settings, priority should be given to those women with greatest need. Dietary recommendations must be tailored to meet the specific needs of each woman served.

Review Questions

1. Describe significant historical observations about the relationship between maternal diet and pregnancy outcome.
2. Discuss current dietary recommendations during pregnancy and justify each of them.
3. Define appropriate weight gain guidelines for pregnancy.
4. Define known effects of specific nutrient deficiencies and excesses in human pregnancy.
5. Summarize current information about the impact of alcohol, caffeine, and other food substances on pregnancy course and outcome.
6. Outline appropriate management recommendations for the common gastrointestinal complaints of pregnancy.

REFERENCES

1. Committee on Maternal Nutrition, Food and Nutrition Board, National Research Council: Maternal nutrition and the course of pregnancy, Washington, D.C., 1970, National Academy of Sciences.
2. Christakis, G., ed.: Maternal nutrition assessment, Am. J. Public Health 63(Suppl.):1, 1973.
3. Committee on Maternal Nutrition, Food and Nutrition Board, National Research Council: Nutritional supplementation and the outcome of pregnancy, Washington, D.C., 1973, National Academy of Sciences.

4. Select Panel for the Promotion of Child Health, U.S. Department of Health and Human Services: Better health for our children: a national strategy, vols. 1–3, pub. no. (PHS) 79-55071, Washington, D.C., 1981, U.S. Government Printing Office.
5. Task Force on Nutrition: Assessment of maternal nutrition, Chicago, 1978, American College of Obstetricians and Gynecologists.
6. Committee on Nutrition of the Mother and Preschool Child: Nutrition services in perinatal care, Washington, D.C., 1981, National Academy Press.
7. Starr, P.: The social transformation of American medicine, New York, 1982, Basic Books, Inc.
8. Winick, M., Brasel, J.A., and Rosso, P.: Nutrition and cell growth. In Winick, M., ed.: Nutrition and development, New York, 1972, John Wiley & Sons.
9. Stevenson, R.E.: The fetus and the newly born infant, St. Louis, 1973, Times Mirror/Mosby College Publishing.
10. Winick, M.: Fetal malnutrition, Clin. Obstet. Gynecol. **13**:526, 1970.
11. Thomson, A.M., Bellewicz, W.Z., and Hytten, F.E.: The assessment of fetal growth, J. Obstet. Gynaecol. Br. Commonw. **75**:903, 1968.
12. Naeye, P.L.: Causes of fetal and neonatal mortality by race in a selected U.S. population, Am. J. Public Health **69**:857, 1979.
13. Edwards, L.E., and others: Pregnancy in the underweight woman: course, outcome, and growth patterns of the infant, Am. J. Obstet. Gynecol. **135**:297, 1979.
14. Viegas, O., Cole, T.J., and Wharton, B.A.: Impaired fat deposition in pregnancy: an indicator for nutritional intervention, Am. J. Clin. Nutr. **45**:23, 1987.
15. Caan, B., Horgen, D.M., Margen, S., King, J.C., and Jewell, N.P.: Benefits associated with WIC supplemental feeding during the interpregnancy interval, Am. J. Clin. Nutr. **45**:29, 1987.
16. Paige, D.M., and Davis, L.R.: Fetal growth, maternal nutrition, and dietary supplementation, Clin. Nutr. **5**:191, 1986.
17. Lechtig, A., and others: Effect of food supplementation during pregnancy on birth weight, Pediatrics **56**:508, 1975.
18. Primrose, T., and Higgins, A.: A study of human antepartum nutrition, J. Reprod. Med. **7**:257, 1971.
19. Munro, H.N.: Role of the placenta in ensuring fetal nutrition, Fed. Proc. **45**:2500, 1986.
20. Hill, E.P., and Longo, L.D.: Dynamics of maternal-fetal nutrient transfer, Fed. Proc. **39**:239, 1980.
21. Beaconsfield, P., Birdwood, G., and Beaconsfield, P.: The placenta, Sci. Am. **243**:95, 1980.
22. Hytten, F.E., and Thomson, A.M.: Maternal physiological adjustments. In Committee on Maternal Nutrition, Food and Nutrition Board, National Research Council, National Academy of Sciences: Maternal nutrition and the course of pregnancy, Washington, D.C., 1970, U.S. Government Printing Office.
23. Food and Nutrition Board, National Research Council, National Academy of Sciences: Recommended dietary allowances, ed. 9, Washington, D.C., 1980, U.S. Government Printing Office.
24. Hytten, F.E., and Leitch, I.: The physiology of human pregnancy, ed. 2, Oxford, 1971, Blackwell Scientific Publications, Inc.
25. Durnin, J.V.G.A., Grant, S., McKillip, F.M., and Fitzgerald, G.: Is nutritional status endangered by virtually no extra intake during pregnancy? Lancet **2**:823, 1985.
26. McNeil, G., and Payne, P.R.: Energy expenditure of pregnant and lactating women, Lancet **2**:1237, 1985.
27. Saha, N.: Energy equation in pregnancy, Lancet **1**:102, 1986.
28. Rosso, P.: Nutrition and maternal-fetal exchange, Am. J. Clin. Nutr. **34**:744, 1981.

29. Coetzee, E.J., Jackson, W.P.U., and Berman, P.A.: Ketonuria in pregnancy with special reference to caloric-restricted food intake in obese diabetics, Diabetes **29**:177, 1980.
30. Zlatnick, F.J., and Burmeister, L.F.: Dietary protein in pregnancy: effect on anthropometric indices of the newborn infant, Am. J. Obstet. Gynecol. **146**:199, 1983.
31. Rush, D., Stein, Z., and Susser, M.: A randomized controlled trial of prenatal supplementation in New York City, Pediatrics **65**:683, 1980.
32. Rush, D., Stein, Z., and Susser, M.: Controlled trial of prenatal nutrition supplementation defended, Pediatrics **66**:656, 1980.
33. Giroud, A.: Nutritional requirements of the embryo, World Rev. Nutr. Diet. **18**:195, 1973.
34. Smithells, R.W., Sheppard, S., and Schorah, C.J.: Vitamin deficiencies and neural tube defects, Arch. Dis. Child. **51**:944, 1976.
35. Smithells, R.W., Sheppard, S., Schorah, C.J., and others: Possible prevention of neural tube defects by periconceptional vitamin supplementation, Lancet **1**:339, 1980.
36. Smithells, R.W., Sheppard, S., Schorah, C.J., and others: Apparent prevention of neural tube defects by periconceptional vitamin supplementation, Arch. Dis. Child. **56**:911, 1981.
37. Smithells, R.W., Seller, M.J., Harris, D.W., and others: Further experience of vitamin supplementation for prevention of neural tube defect recurrences, Lancet **1**:1027, 1983.
38. Laurence, K.M., James, N., Miller, M.H., and others: Double-blind randomized controlled trial of folate treatment before conception to prevent recurrence of neural tube defects, Br. Med. J. **282**:1509, 1981.
39. Wald, N.J.: Neural tube defects and vitamins: the need for a randomized clinical trial, Br. J. Obstet. Gynaecol. **91**:516, 1984.
40. U.S. Department of Health and Human Services: Vitamins: are they the key to preventing neural tube defects? NICHD New Notes, March 18, 1985.
41. Molloy, A.M., Kirke, P., and others: Maternal serum folate and vitamin B_{12} concentrations in pregnancies associated with neural tube defects, Arch. Dis. Child. **60**:660, 1985.
42. Ejderjamm, J., and Hamfelt, A.: Pyridoxal phosphate concentration in blood in newborn infants and their mothers compared with the amount of extra pyridoxal taken during pregnancy and breast-feeding, Acta Paediatr. Scand. **69**:327, 1980.
43. Worthington-Roberts, B., Vermeersch, J., and Williams, S.R.: Nutrition in pregnancy and lactation, ed. 3, St. Louis, 1985, Times Mirror/Mosby College Publishing.
44. Pulkkinen, M.O., Salminen, J., and Virtanen, S.: Serum vitamin B_6 in pure pregnancy depression, Acta Obstet. Gynecol. Scand. **57**:471, 1978.
45. Roepke, and Kirksey, A.: Vitamin B_6 nutriture during pregnancy and lactation. I. Vitamin B_6 intake, levels of the vitamin in biological fluids, and conditions of the infant at birth, Am. J. Clin. Nutr. **32**:2249, 1979.
46. Schuster, K., Bailey, L.B., and Mahan, C.S.: Vitamin B_6 status of the low-income adolescent and adult pregnant women and the condition of their infants at birth, Am. J. Clin. Nutr. **34**:1731, 1981.
47. Schuster, K., Bailey, L.B., and Mahan, C.S.: Effect of maternal pyridoxine HCl supplementation on the vitamin B_6 status of mother and infant and on pregnancy outcome, J. Nutr. **114**:977, 1984.
48. Schuster, K., and Bailey, L.B., Dimperio, D., and Mahan, C.S.: Morning sickness and vitamin B_6 status of pregnant women, Hum. Nutr. Clin. Nutr. **39C**:75, 1984.
49. Wheatley, D.: Treatment of pregnancy sickness, Br. J. Obstet. Gynaecol. **84**:444, 1977.
50. Wideman, C.L., Baird, G.H., and Bolding, O.T.: Ascorbic acid deficiency and premature rupture of fetal membranes, Am. J. Obstet. Gynecol. **88**:592, 1964.
51. Clemetson, C.A.B., and Anderson, L.: Ascorbic acid metabolism in pre-eclampsia, Obstet. Gynecol. **24**:774, 1964.

52. Cochrane, W.A.: Overnutrition in prenatal and neonatal life: a problem? Can. Med. Assoc. J. **93**:893, 1965.
53. Norkus, E.P., and Rosso, P.: Effects of maternal intake of ascorbic acid on the postnatal metabolism of this vitamin in the guinea pig, J. Nutr. **111**:624, 1981.
54. Roberts, R.A., Cohen, M.D., and Forfar, J.O.: Antenatal factors in neonatal hypocalcemic convulsions, Lancet **2**:809, 1973.
55. Purvis, R.J., and others: Enamel hypoplasia of the teeth associated with neonatal tetany: a manifestation of maternal vitamin D deficiency, Lancet **2**:811, 1973.
56. Brooke, O.G., Brown, I.R.F., Bone, C.D.M.R., and others: Vitamin D supplements in pregnant Asian women: effects on calcium status and fetal growth, Br. Med. J. **1**:751, 1980.
57. Hurley, L.S.: Developmental nutrition, Englewood Cliffs, N.J., 1980, Prentice-Hall.
58. Bernhardt, I.R., and Dorsey, D.J.: Hypervitaminosis A and congenital renal anomalies in a human infant, Obstet. Gynecol. **43**:750, 1974.
59. Strange, L., Carlstrom, K., and Eriksson, M.: Hypervitaminosis A in early human pregnancy and malformations of the central nervous system, Acta Obstet. Scand. **57**:289, 1978.
60. Benke, P.I.: The isotretinoin syndrome, J.A.M.A. **25**:3267, 1984.
61. de la Cruz, E., Vangvanichyakern, K., and Desposito, F.: Multiple congenital malformations associated with maternal isotretinoin therapy, Pediatrics **74**:428, 1984.
62. Lammar, E.J., and others: Retinoic acid embryopathy, New Engl. J. Med. **313**:837, 1985.
63. Marwick, C.: More cautionary labeling appears on isotretinoin, J.A.M.A. **251**:3208, 1984.
64. Haga, P., Ek, J., and Kran, S.: Plasma tocopherol levels and vitamin B-lipoprotein relationships during pregnancy and in cord blood, Am. J. Clin. Nutr. **36**:1200, 1982.
65. Sisson, T.R.C., and Lund, C.J.: The influence of maternal iron deficiency on the newborn, Am. J. Clin. Nutr. **6**:376, 1958.
66. McFee, J.G.: Anemia: a high-risk complication of pregnancy, Clin. Obstet. Gynecol. **16**:153, 1973.
67. Romslo, I., and others: Iron requirement in normal pregnancy assessed by serum ferritin, serum transferrin saturation and erythrocyte protoporphyrin determinations, Br. J. Obstet. Gynaecol. **90**:101, 1983.
68. Widdowson, E.M.: Growth and composition of the fetus and newborn. In Assali, N.S., ed.: Biology of gestation, vol. 2, New York, 1968, Academic Press.
69. Villar, J., and Belizan, J.M.: Calcium during pregnancy, Clin. Nutr. **5**:55, 1986.
70. Duggin, G.G., and others: Calcium balance in pregnancy, Lancet **2**:926, 1974.
71. Felton, D.J.C., and Stone, W.D.: Osteomalacia in Asian immigrants during pregnancy, Br. Med. J. **1**:1521, 1966.
72. Hammar, M., Larsson, L., and Tegler, L.: Calcium treatment of leg cramps in pregnancy, Acta Obstet. Gynecol. Scand. **60**:345, 1981.
73. Allen, L.H.: Trace elements and outcome of human pregnancy, Clin. Nutr. **5**:72, 1986.
74. Apgar, J.: Zinc and reproduction, Annu. Rev. Nutr. **5**:43, 1985.
75. Solomons, N.H., Helitzer-Allen, D., and Villar, J.: Zinc needs during pregnancy, Clin. Nutr. **5**:63, 1986.
76. Soltan, M.H., and Jenkins, M.H.: Maternal and fetal plasma zinc concentration and fetal abnormality, Br. J. Obstet. Gynaecol. **89**:56, 1982.
77. Hurley, L.S.: Trace metals in mammalian development, Johns Hopkins Med. J. **148**:1, 1981.
78. Sandstead, H.H., and others: Zinc deficiency in pregnant rhesus monkeys: effects on behavior of infants, Am. J. Clin. Nutr. **31**:844, 1978.
79. Bergmann, K.E., Makosch, G., and Tews, K.H.: Abnormalities of hair zinc concentration in mothers of newborn infants with spina bifida, Am. J. Clin. Nutr. **33**:2145, 1980.

80. Cherry, F.F., Bennett, E.A., Bazzano, G.S., and others: Plasma zinc hypertension-toxemia and other reproductive variables in adolescent pregnancy, Am. J. Clin. Nutr. **34**:2367, 1981.
81. Meadows, N.J., Ruse, W., Smith, M.F., and others: Zinc and small babies, Lancet **2**:1135, 1981.
82. Jameson, S.: Effects of zinc deficiency in human reproduction, Acta Med. Scand. **593**(Suppl.):1976.
83. Ghosh, A., Fong, L.Y.Y., Wan, C.W., and others: Zinc deficiency is not a cause for abortion, congenital abnormality, and small-for-gestational-age infant in Chinese women, Br. J. Obstet. Gynecol. **92**:886, 1985.
84. Hunt, I.F., Murphy, N.J., Cleaver, B., and others: Zinc supplementation during pregnancy: effects on selected blood constituents and on progress and outcome of pregnancy in low-income women of Mexican descent, Am. J. Clin. Nutr. **40**:508, 1984.
85. Mukherjee, M.D., Sandstead, H.H., Ratnaparkhi, L.K., and others: Maternal zinc, iron, folic acid, and protein nutriture and outcome of human pregnancy, Am. J. Clin. Nutr. **40**:496, 1984.
86. Connolly, K.J., Pharoah, P.O.D., and Hertzel, B.S.: Fetal iodine deficiency and motor performance during childhood, Lancet **2**:1149, 1979.
87. Glenn, F.B., Glenn, W.D., and Duncan, R.C.: Fluoride tablet supplementation during pregnancy for caries immunity: a study of the offspring produced, Am. J. Obstet. Gynecol. **143**:560, 1982.
88. Bursey, R.G., and Watson, M.L.: The effect of sodium restriction during gestation on offspring brain development in rats, Am. J. Clin. Nutr. **37**:43, 1983.
89. Pike, R.L., Miles, J.E., and Wardlaw, J.M.: Juxtaglomerular degranulation and zona glomerulosa exhaustion in pregnant rats induced by low sodium intakes and reversed by sodium load, Am. J. Obstet. Gynecol. **95**:604, 1966.
90. Lelong-Tissier, M.C., and others: Hyponatremie maternofetale carentielle par regime desode, Arch. Fr. Pediatr. **34**:64, 1977.
91. Abrams, B.F., and Laros, R.K.: Prepregnancy weight, weight gain, and birth weight, Am. J. Obstet. Gynecol. **154**:503, 1986.
92. Garbaciak, J.A., Richter, M., Miller, S., and Barton, J.J.: Maternal weight and pregnancy complications, Am. J. Obstet. Gynecol. **152**:238, 1985.
93. King, J.C.: Obesity in pregnancy. In Frankle, R., Dwyer, J., Moragne, L., and Owen, A., eds.: Dietary treatment and prevention of obesity, London, 1985, John Libbey.
94. National Center for Health Statistics: Maternal weight gain and the outcome of pregnancy, United States, 1980, DHHS pub. no. (PHS) 86-1922, Hyattsville, Md., 1986, U.S. Public Health Service.
95. Villar, J., and Cossio, T.G.: Nutritional factors associated with low birth weight and short gestational age, Clin. Nutr. **5**:78, 1986.
96. Naeye, R.L.: Weight gain and the outcome of pregnancy, Am. J. Obstet. Gynecol. **135**:3, 1979.
97. National Research Council, Food and Nutrition Board: Alternative dietary practices and nutritional abuses in pregnancy, Washington, D.C., 1982, National Academy of Sciences.
98. Lackey, CJ: Pica—Pregnancy etiological mystery. In National Research Council: Alternative dietary practices and nutritional abuses in pregnancy, Washington, D.C., 1982, National Academy of Sciences.
99. Lillien, L.J., Huber, A.M., and Rajala, M.M.: Diet and ethanol intake during pregnancy, J. Am. Diet. Assoc. **81**:252, 1982.
100. Streissguth, A.P., and others: Comparison of drinking and smoking patterns during pregnancy over a six-year interval, Am. J. Obstet. Gynecol. **145**:716, 1983.

101. Rosett, H.L., and others: Patterns of alcohol consumption and fetal development, Obstet. Gynecol. **61**:539, 1983.
102. Rosett, H.L., Weiner, L., and Edelin, K.C.: Treatment experience with pregnant problem drinkers, J.A.M.A. **249**:2029, 1983.
103. Groisser, D.S., Rosso, P., and Winick, M.: Coffee consumption during pregnancy: subsequent behavioral abnormalities of the offspring, J. Nutr. **112**:829, 1982.
104. Dunlop, M., and Court, J.M.: Effects of maternal caffeine ingestion on neonatal growth in rats, Biol. Neonate **39**:178, 1981.
105. Collins, T.F.X., Welsh, J.J., Black, T.N., and Ruggles, D.I.: A study of the teratogenic potential of caffeine ingestion in drinking water, Food. Chem. Toxicol. **21**:763, 1983.
106. Kurppa, K., and others: Coffee consumption during pregnancy, New Engl. J. Med. **306**:1548, 1982.
107. Linn, S., and others: No association between coffee consumption and adverse outcomes of pregnancy, New Engl. J. Med. **306**:141, 1982.
108. Rosenberg, L., and others: Selected birth defects in relation to caffeine-containing beverages, J.A.M.A. **247**:1429, 1982.
109. Furuhashi, N.: Effects of caffeine consumption during pregnancy, Gynecol. Obstet. Invest. **19**:187, 1985.
110. Streitfeld, P.P.: Congenital malformation: teratogenic foods and additives, Birth Fam. J. **5**:7, 1978.
111. Kline, J., and others: Spontaneous abortion and the use of sugar substitutes, Am. J. Obstet. Gynecol. **130**:708, 1978.
112. Hoover, R.: Saccharin—bitter aftertaste? New Engl. J. Med. **302**:573, 1980.
113. Sturtevant, F.M.: Use of aspartame in pregnancy, Int. J. Fertil. **30**:85, 1985.
114. Hickey, P.J.: Ecological statistical studies concerning environmental pollution and chronic disease. In Digest of Technical Papers, Second International Geological Science Electronics Symposium, Washington, D.C., April 14-17, 1970.
115. Rom, W.N.: Effect of lead on the female and reproduction: a review, Mt. Sinai J. Med. **43**:542, 1976.
116. Stofen, D., and Waldron, H.A.: Subclinical lead poisoning, New York, 1974, Academic Press.
117. Clayton, B.E.: Lead: the relation of environment and experimental work, Br. Med. Bull. **31**:236, 1975.
118. Koos, B.J., and Longo, L.D.: Mercury toxicity in the pregnant woman, fetus, and newborn infant: a review, Am. J. Obstet. Gynecol. **126**:390, 1976.
119. Collings, C.A., Curet, L.B., and Mullin, J.P.: Maternal and fetal responses to a maternal aerobic exercise program, Am. J. Obstet. Gynecol. **145**:702, 1983.
120. Pomerance, J., and Gluck, L.: Physical fitness in pregnancy: its effects on pregnancy outcome, Am. J. Obstet. Gynecol. **119**:867, 1975.
121. Picone, T.A., Allen, L.H., Schramm, M.M., and Olsen, P.N.: Pregnancy outcome in North American women, I. Effects of diet, cigarette smoking, and psychological stress on maternal weight gain, Am. J. Clin. Nutr. **36**:1205, 1982.
122. Papoz, L., and others: Maternal smoking and birth weight in relation to dietary habits, Am. J. Obstet. Gynecol. **142**:870, 1982.

FURTHER READING

Brown, J.E.: Nutrition for your pregnancy, Minneapolis, 1983, University of Minnesota Press.

This well-written popular book on diet and nutrition during pregnancy provides an excellent resource for the general public.

Committee on Maternal Nutrition, Food and Nutrition Board, National Research Council, National Academy of Sciences: Maternal nutrition and the course of pregnancy, Washington, D.C., 1970, U.S. Government Printing Office.

This classic benchmark publication summarizes known data on nutrition and pregnancy outcome.

Committee on Nutrition of the Mother and Preschool Child, Food and Nutrition Board, National Research Council, National Academy of Sciences: Nutritional services in perinatal care, Washington, D.C., 1981, U.S. Government Printing Office.

This consensus statement of an expert committee summarizes recommendations for appropriate nutritional management of high-risk perinatal patients.

Hess, M.A., and Hunt, A.E.: Pickles and ice cream, New York, 1982, McGraw-Hill Book Co.

This is an award-winning book on diet and pregnancy written for the general public.

Hytten, F.E., and Leitch, I.: The physiology of human pregnancy, ed. 2, Oxford, 1971, Blackwell Scientific Publications, Ltd.

This classic work describes physiologic phenomena in normal pregnancy.

Worthington-Roberts, B., Vermeersch, J., and Williams, S.: Nutrition in pregnancy and lactation, St. Louis, 1985, Times Mirror/Mosby College Publishing.

This book provides a much more detailed discussion of issues related to nutrition during pregnancy and lactation.

CASE STUDY

A professional woman 35 years of age visits her health-care provider for advice. She and her husband are planning a pregnancy and she wishes to approach this project systematically. An interview and physical examination reveals that she:

has been using oral contraceptives for 10 years
smokes
is 10 lb underweight
enjoys wine with her meals
has a family history of diabetes
has a typical 60-hour work week
intends to continue her career during and after pregnancy

1. Outline appropriate recommendations for the pre-conception period.
2. Define those issues that require discussion about the pregnancy period itself.
3. Summarize appropriate anticipatory guidance for the postpartum period.

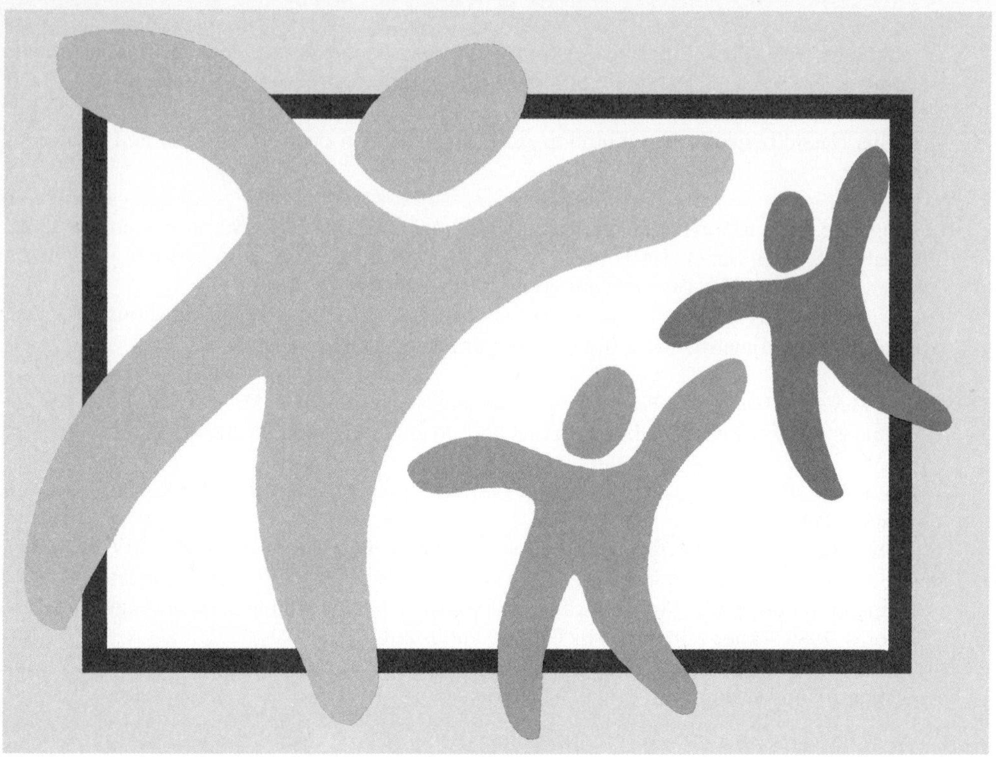

Basic Concepts

1. Specific female anatomy and physiology provide the required structures and functions for normal postpartum lactation.
2. Human milk is specially adapted to meeting human infants' needs.
3. Successful lactation requires nutritional support.
4. Breast-feeding provides the primary means of supporting growth and development of young infants.
5. Physiologic knowledge and personal skills underlie sensitive counseling for the breast-feeding mother.

Chapter Five

Lactation and Human Milk

Bonnie S. Worthington-Roberts

Lactation is an ancient physiologic process accomplished by females since the origin of mammals. Today, as in times past, the process of breast-feeding is successfully initiated by at least 99% of women who try. All that is required of the lactating mother is an intact mammary gland (or preferably two) and the presence and operation of appropriate physiologic mechanisms that allow for adequate milk production and release.

From this basic physiologic view, the establishment and maintenance of human lactation are determined by at least three factors:

1. The anatomical structure of the mammary tissue and the development of alveoli, ducts, and nipples to produce and then deliver the milk
2. The initiation and maintenance of milk secretion
3. The ejection or propulsion of milk from the alveoli to the nipple

But the operational term above is the word "human." This brings an added personal dimension to the physiologic process. Breast-feeding is a very personal process for a mother.

In this chapter, then, we will look at lactation, human milk, and breast-feeding in both physiologic and human terms. We will see that clear knowledge of the physiologic factors listed above, and of nutritional needs, is essential for effective lactation management. But further, we will also see that sensitivity to the personal needs involved is essential for helping mothers to have satisfying breast-feeding experiences. We will use both of these aspects as we provide individual support for today's largely inexperienced breast-feeding mother.

Breast Anatomy and Development

ANATOMY OF THE MAMMARY GLAND

Basic Structure

The mammary gland of the human female consists of glandular epithelium and a duct system embedded in interstitial tissue and fat (Fig. 5-1).[1] The size of the breast is

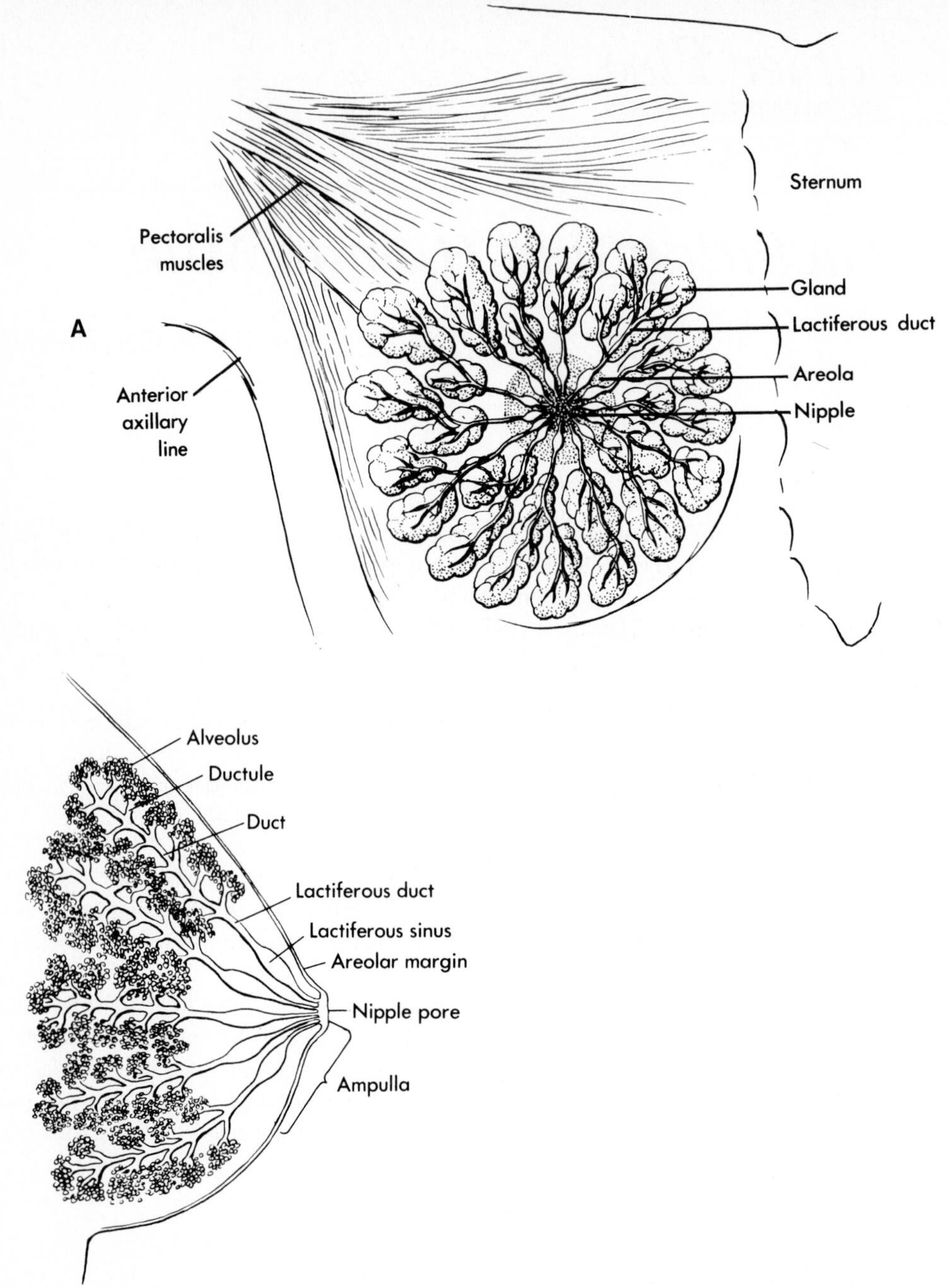

FIG. 5-1 A, General anatomical features of the human breast showing its location on the anterior region of the thorax between the sternum and the anterior axillary line. **B**, Detailed structural features of the human mammary gland showing the terminal glandular (alveolar) tissue of each lobule leading into the duct system, which eventually enlarges into the lactiferous duct and lactiferous sinus. The lactiferous sinuses rest beneath the areola and converge at the nipple pore.

variable, but in most instances it extends from the second through sixth ribs and from the sternum to the anterior axillary line. The mammary tissue lies directly over the pectoralis major muscle and is separated from this muscle by a layer of fat, which is continuous with the fatty stroma of the gland itself.

Areola

The center of the fully developed breast in the adult woman is marked by the areola, a circular pigmented skin area from 1.5 to 2.5 cm in diameter. The surface of the areola appears rough because of the presence of large, somewhat modified sebaceous glands, which are located directly beneath the skin in the thin subcutaneous tissue layer. The fatty secretion of these glands is believed to lubricate the nipple. Bundles of smooth muscle fibers in the areolar tissue serve to stiffen the nipple for a better grasp by the sucking infant.

Nipple and Duct System

The nipple is elevated above the breast and contains 15 to 20 lactiferous ducts surrounded by fibromuscular tissue and covered by wrinkled skin. Partly within this compartment of the nipple and partly below its base, these ducts expand to form the short lactiferous sinuses in which milk may be stored. The sinuses are the continuations of the mammary ducts, which extend radially from the nipple toward the chest wall with numerous secondary branches. The duct system ends in epithelial masses, which form lobules of the breast (Fig. 5-1).

Adolescent-Adult Development

During adolescence the female breasts enlarge to their adult size. Frequently, one breast is slightly larger than the other, but this difference is usually unnoticeable. In a nonpregnant woman the mature breast weighs approximately 200 g, the left being somewhat larger than the right. During pregnancy there is some increase in size and weight such that by term the breast may weigh between 400 and 600 g. During lactation this weight increases to between 600 and 800 g.

Variation after Childbirth

Wide variation in the structural composition of the human breasts has been observed in women after childbirth. Some breasts contain little secretory tissue; some large breasts contain less glandular tissue than much smaller organs. It is well known, however, that neither size nor structural composition of the breast significantly influences lactation success in the average woman. Almost all woman who want to breastfeed find that they can.

BREAST DEVELOPMENT

Infancy and Childhood

In the human newborn the mammary glands are developed sufficiently to appear as distinct, round elevations, palpable as moveable soft masses. Histologically the future milk ducts and glandular lobules can be recognized easily. In many infants an everted nipple is seen, and in about 10% a greatly enlarged gland can be palpated. These early glandular structures can produce a milklike secretion ("witch's milk") 2 or 3 days after birth. All of these neonatal phenomena related to the mammary glands probably result from the intensive developmental processes that occur in the last stages of intrauterine life. Usually they subside in the first few weeks after birth. Some involution in the breast takes place by the time the infant is several weeks old, and this is followed by the "quiescent" period of mammary growth and activity during infancy and childhood.

Adolescence

With the onset of puberty and during adolescence, an increased output of estrogenic hormone accomplishes ovarian maturation and follicular stimulation in the female. As a result of this response, the mammary ducts elongate, and their lining epithelium reduplicates and proliferates. The growth of the ductal epithelium is accompanied by growth of periductal fibrous and fatty tissue, which is largely responsible for the increasing size and firmness of the female adolescent gland. During this period the areola and nipple also grow and become more heavily pigmented.

BREAST MATURATION

Hormonal Effects

As the developing woman matures and ovulation patterns become established, the regular development of progesterone-producing corpora lutea in the ovaries promotes the second stage of mammary development. Lobules gradually appear, giving the mammary glands the characteristic lobular structure found during the childbearing period. This differentiation into a lobular gland is completed about 12 to 18 months after the first menstrual period, but further development continues in proportion to the intensity of the hormonal stimuli during each menstrual cycle and especially during pregnancies.

Functional Mammary Tissue

Some young women enter reproductive life with insufficient functional mammary tissue to produce enough milk for their baby's total nourishment. In some cases this relates to underdevelopment of the mammary ductwork associated with periodic amenorrhea or very late menarche. In addition, there are women who have had surgery to remove cysts, tumors, or other growths; others have undergone surgery for breast reduction or reconstruction. For whatever reason, circumstances exist in which functional mammary tissue is insufficient to fully support a nursing infant. *Fortunately these situations are rare.*

Preparation During Pregnancy

The mammary gland of a nonpregnant woman is inadequately prepared for secretory activity. Only during pregnancy do these changes occur that make satisfactory milk production possible. In the first trimester of pregnancy the terminal ductules sprouting from the mammary ducts proliferate to create a maximal number of epithelial elements for future alveolar cell formation. In the mid-trimester the reduplicated terminal ductules group together to form large lobules. Their lumina begin to dilate, and the alveoli thus formed are lined with cuboidal epithelium. In the last trimester the existent alveoli progressively dilate in the final preparation for the lactation process.

Role of the Placenta

The placenta plays an important role in mammary growth in pregnancy. In some animals hypophysectomy, ovariectomy, or both can be performed after a certain stage of gestation without interrupting pregnancy and mammary development. The placenta secretes ovarian-like hormones in large quantities. Placental lactogen, prolactin, and chorionic gonadotropin have been identified as contributing to mammary gland growth. Human chorionic somatomammotropin promotes mammary growth and lactation in experimental animals and presumably is secreted in sufficient amounts to act with placental progesterone and estradiol to stimulate breast development in pregnancy.

Antepartum Preparation

Although mammary growth and development occur rapidly throughout pregnancy, additional proliferation of parenchymal cells takes place shortly before parturition. The proliferation of epithelial cells that begins just before parturition in response to increasing titers of prolactin results in daughter cells with a new complement of enzymes.

The Physiology of Lactation

GENERAL ACTIVITY

Initial Postpartum Secretions

Full lactation does not begin as soon as the baby is born. During the first 2 or 3 days after birth, a small amount of *colostrum* is secreted. In subsequent days a rapid increase in milk secretion occurs, and in usual cases lactation has become reasonably well established by the end of the first week. In primiparas, however, the establishment of lactation may be delayed until the third week or even later. Generally, therefore, the first 2 or 3 weeks are a period of lactation initiation, and this is followed by the longer period of maintenance of lactation.

Milk Production Stages

Initiation and maintenance of lactation comprises a complex neuroendocrine process. It involves the sensory nerves in the nipples, the spinal cord, the hypothalamus, and the pituitary gland with its various hormones. The process of milk production occurs in two distinct stages: (1) secretion of milk into the alveolar lumen, and (2) propulsion or ejection whereby the milk passes along the duct system. The two events are closely related and often occur simultaneously in the nursing mother.

The secretion of milk involves both the synthesis of the milk components and the passage of the formed product into the alveolar lumen (Fig. 5-2). These events may be under independent control, since the accumulation of both lipid and protein reaches a

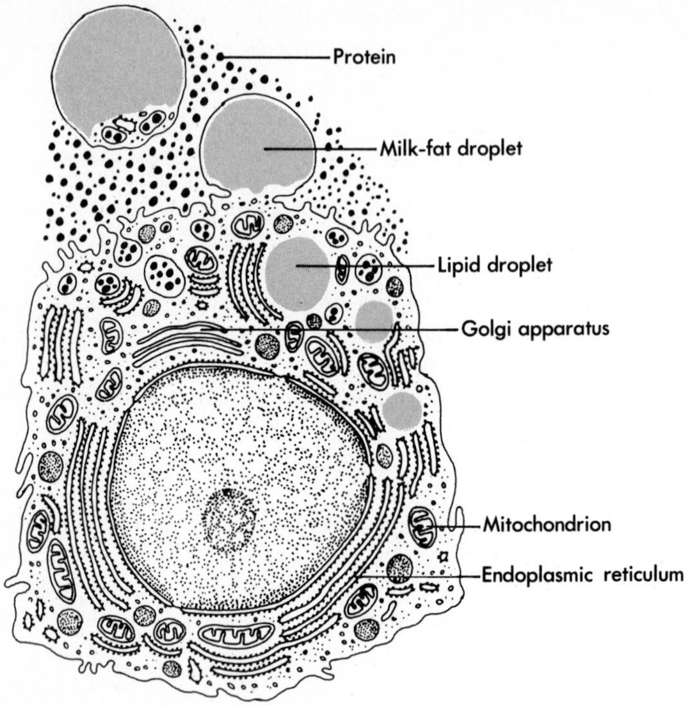

FIG. 5-2 Diagrammatic representation of a mammary gland cell showing the basic cuboidal shape with typical microvillus border and basal nucleus. Cytoplasmic organization is characteristic of cells undergoing active protein synthesis and secretion. The synthetic apparatus consists of many free ribosomes and an extensive system of rough endoplasmic reticulum. A large Golgi body is located above the nucleus, and associated with it are some vacuoles containing fibrillar or particulate material that condenses into a central core or granule. Toward the apex the granules become progressively larger and contain more dense protein granules. The vacuoles fuse with the surface membrane and liberate their contents intact into the lumen. Fat droplets are found throughout the cell but are largest near the apex. They protrude into the lumen and appear to pinch off from the cell proper along with a small bit of cytoplasm. Other cytoplasmic structures include large mitochondria with closely packed cristae, lysosomes, and a small number of smooth membranous tubules and vesicles.

(Modified from Lentz, T.L.: Cell fine structure: an atlas of drawings of whole cell-structure, Philadelphia, 1971, W.B. Saunders Co.)

high level during the latter part of pregnancy. Shortly before parturition the accumulated secretory products begin to pass into the lumen. The secretory process is activated again by the sucking stimulus of the infant.

In general, each milk-producing alveolar cell proceeds through a secretory process that is preceded and followed by a resting stage (Fig. 5-3). Milk synthesis is most active during the suckling period but occurs at lower levels at other times. The secretory cells

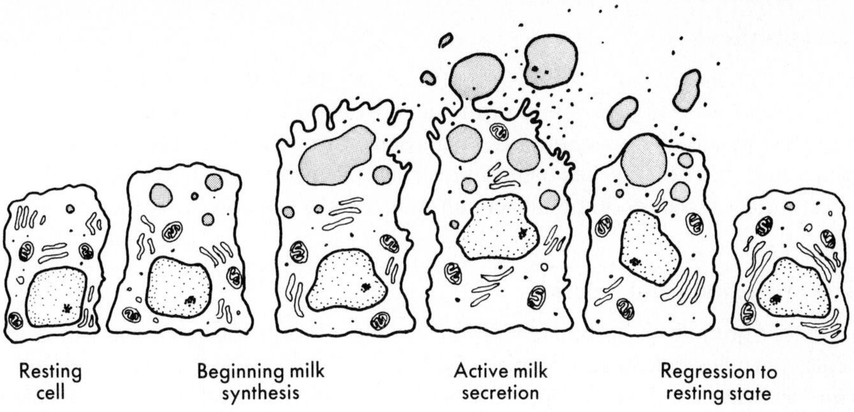

FIG. 5-3 Diagrammatic representation of the cycle of changes that occur in secretory cells of the alveoli from resting stage through milk production and secretion with eventual return to the resting stage.

are cuboidal but change to a cylindrical shape just before milk secretion while cellular water uptake is increased. As secretion commences, the enlarged cell with its thickened apical membrane becomes clublike in shape. The tip pinches off, leaving the cell intact. The milk constituents are then free in the secreted solution, and the cell retains a cap of membrane. Between periods of active milk secretion, alveolar cells return to their characteristic resting state.

FAT SYNTHESIS AND RELEASE

Initial Synthesis

Fat synthesis takes place in the endoplasmic reticulum from precursor compounds synthesized intracellularly or imported from the maternal circulation. Alveolar cells are able to synthesize short-chain fatty acids, which are derived predominantly from available acetate. Long-chain fatty acids and triglycerides are derived from maternal plasma; these fatty acids are predominantly used for the synthesis of milk fat. Synthesis of triglyceride from intracellular carbohydrate also plays a predominant role in fat production for human milk.

Final Preparation and Release

The process of esterification of fatty acids takes place in the endoplasmic reticulum. The resultant triglycerides accumulate as small fat droplets in the cisternae of the endoplasmic reticulum but eventually coalesce in the basal region of the cell to form large droplets that migrate toward the cell apex. Ultimately these droplets bulge into the alveolar lumen for eventual discharge via apocrine secretion. Apocrine secretion involves the protrusion of the cell surface into the lumen with eventual pinching off of the protruded unit. This discharged material usually contains fat globules, protein, and a small amount of cytoplasm, all of which will appear in human milk.

PROTEIN SYNTHESIS AND DISCHARGE

Initial Synthesis

The vast majority of proteins present in normal milk are specific to mammary secretions and are not identified in any quantity elsewhere in nature. The formation of milk protein and mammary enzymes is induced by prolactin and further stimulated by insulin and cortisol. Studies using ultrastructural techniques have clearly shown that the abundant rough endothelial reticulum is the site of protein synthesis in the secretory cell.

Final Preparation and Release

Protein granules accumulate within the Golgi complexes in the form of macromolecular particles before transport through the cell and release into the lumen by apocrine secretion or reverse pinocytosis. The proteins in milk are derived from two sources: (1) some are synthesized *de novo* in the mammary gland, and (2) others are derived as such from plasma. Inclusion of plasma-derived proteins in the milk secretion occurs primarily in the early secretory product colostrum. Thereafter the three main proteins in milk—casein, alpha-lactalbumin, and beta-lactalbumin—are synthesized within the gland from amino acid precursors. All of the essential and some of the nonessential amino acids are taken up directly from the plasma, but some of the nonessential amino acids are synthesized by the alveolar cells of the gland.

CARBOHYDRATE SYNTHESIS AND RELEASE

Lactose Synthesis

The predominant carbohydrate in milk is lactose. Its synthesis occurs within the Golgi apparatus of the alveolar cell. The synthesis of lactose combines glucose and galactose. Most of the intracellular glucose is derived continually from circulating blood glucose; galactose is synthesized from glucose.

Final Preparation and Release

Once synthesized within the Golgi complex, lactose is attached to protein and carried to the cell surface in a vesicle. It is then released from the surface of the cell by reverse pinocytosis, as occurs with several other milk components.

THE ROLE OF HORMONES

Milk Secretion

The stimulus for milk secretion derives largely from the hormone prolactin (Fig. 5-4). This hormone acts on alveolar cells and promotes continual milk production and release. *Maintenance* of milk secretion, however, requires other hormonal factors from the anterior pituitary. If sucking is discontinued during the lactation period, pituitary release of these necessary hormones ceases and milk secretion usually stops in the following few days, with accompanying atrophy and sloughing of alveolar cells.

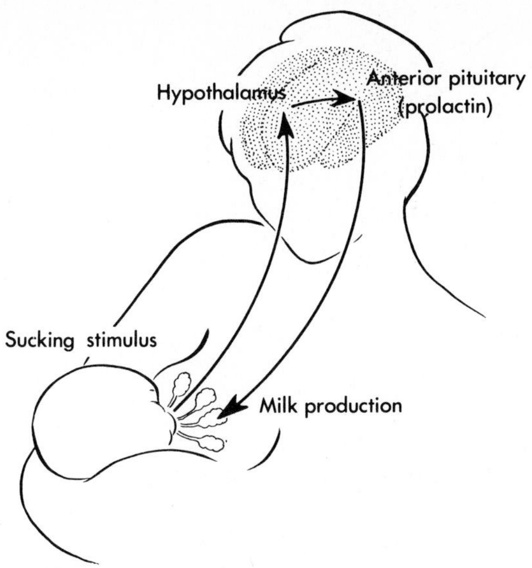

FIG. 5-4 Diagrammatic representation of the basic physiological features of milk production. The sucking stimulus provided by the baby sends a message to the hypothalamus. The hypothalamus stimulates the anterior pituitary to release prolactin, the hormone that promotes milk production by alveolar cells of the mammary glands.

Relation of Oral Contraceptive Agents

Estrogen inhibits milk production, especially in the early stage of lactation. However, studies of the use of combined estrogen-progestin oral contraceptive agents (OTA) indicate that lactation is not inhibited in women who wish to nurse their infants, as long as the pill is not used in the immediate postpartum period. Some dose-related suppression of the quantity of milk produced and the duration of lactation is found with extended use. Even though several reports suggest that measurable composition changes occur in the milk produced by women taking OTA, results are inconsistent and largely viewed as insignificant.

THE "LET-DOWN" REFLEX

Primary Stimulus

Once milk production and secretion have been accomplished, the baby may then obtain this milk by promoting its ejection from the alveoli and ducts. The milk ejection or "let-down" reflex is a neurohormonal mechanism regulated in part by central nervous system factors (Fig. 5-5). The primary stimulus is sucking on the nipple, which triggers the discharge of the hormone oxytocin from the posterior pituitary. Oxytocin is carried in the bloodstream to the myoepithelial cells around the alveoli and along the duct system, where it is easily available to the nursing baby.

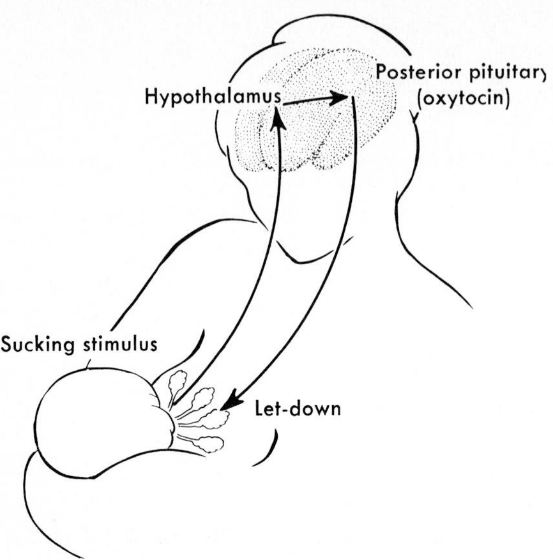

FIG. 5-5 Diagrammatic representation of the basic features of the "let-down reflex." The sucking stimulus arrives at the hypothalamus, which promotes the release of oxytocin from the posterior pituitary. Oxytocin stimulates the contraction of the myoepithelial cells around the alveoli in the mammary glands. Contraction of these musclelike cells causes the milk to be propelled through the duct system and into the lactiferous sinuses, where it becomes available to the nursing infant.

Psychologic Influences

The milk ejection reflex appears to be sensitive to small differences in circulating oxytocin level. Thus even minor emotional and psychologic disturbances can influence the degree to which breast milk is released to the baby. The significance of psychologic influences on the milk ejection reflex in humans has been demonstrated by numerous case histories. These experiences illustrate the fact that milk ejection can be inhibited by embarrassment or stress, or it can be conditioned to be set off by the mere thought of the baby or the sound of his cry. This observation has been confirmed by experimental stimulation (or inhibition) of the milk ejection reflex. Signs of successful let-down of milk are easily recognized by the nursing mother. Common and significant occurrences include: (1) milk dripping from the breasts before the baby starts nursing, (2) milk dripping from the breast opposite to the one being nursed, and (3) uterine cramps during nursing as a result of oxytocin action on the uterus.

Sucking Stimulus

Sucking stimulation is widely accepted as the most effective means of maintaining adequate lactation. There is considerable evidence in human subjects that the restriction of sucking significantly inhibits lactation. Artificial suckling stimulation in the form of manual expression or a breast pump has repeatedly been recommended as a means of increasing milk yield or maintaining yield in the absence of the baby. Evidence suggests that feeding on demand optimally stimulates the lactation process.

Duration of Lactation

Local and cultural patterns of infant feeding are of great significance in determining the duration of breast-feeding for a given mother. Although successful lactation can continue as long as sucking stimulation is maintained, a gradual fall in the amount of milk produced generally develops after 12 months. This drop in milk output largely relates to reduced demand and loss of recurrent nipple stimulation by the baby.

General Nature of Mammalian Milk

UNIQUE SPECIES VARIATION

Many investigators during the past decade have defined the biochemical and nutritional properties of different types of mammalian milk. It is clear from these studies that each type of milk is unique and consists of a highly complex mixture of organic and inorganic compounds.

Mother-Child Relation and Nature of Milk

It is likely that the characteristics of mammalian milks relate directly to variable mother-child relationships that take place in infancy. Shaul[2] found support for this idea while examining five groups of wild animals:

Group 1. Marsupials and animals that bear their young while in hibernation. In these animals the mother is available at all times and the milk is dilute and low in fat.

Group 2. Animals born in a relatively mature state that follow or are carried by their mothers at all times. Here the maternal attentiveness is high and the milk produced is rather low in fat and dilute. The low fat content is often seen in milks of animals that nurse frequently.

Group 3. Animals that leave their young in a secluded place and return to them at widely spaced intervals. The lioness is a good example of this type. But in all cases this group of animals has very concentrated milk that is high in fat.

Group 4. Animals born in a relatively immature state and that remain for a considerable time in nests or burrows. The mother must leave for several hours at a time and nursing is more "on schedule" rather than "on demand."

Group 5. Animals that spend much time in cold water or when on land are frequently made wet by the mother returning from the water. In all these cases the milk is very concentrated and has an extremely high fat content.

Comparison of Human Milk

Human milk is dilute and thus resembles the milk of the marsupials and hibernating bears whose offspring feed frequently. It is therefore not surprising that the human baby demands to be fed frequently. For this reason, in many parts of the world the mother carries the baby wherever she goes.

THE NATURE OF HUMAN MILK

Variable Basic Content

Reports during the past 15 years on the biochemical composition of human milk have included over 800 publications. Large numbers of new components continue to be characterized such that more than a hundred constituents are now recognized. Human milk consists of a solution of protein, sugar, and salts in which a variety of fatty compounds are suspended (Table 5-1). The composition varies from one human to another, from one period of lactation to the next, and even hourly during the day. The composition of a given milk sample is related not only to the amount secreted and the stage of the lactation but also to the timing of the withdrawal and to individual variations among lactating mothers. These latter individual variations may be affected by such variables as maternal age, parity, health, and social class. Gestational age of the infant also makes a difference.

Relation to Maternal Nutrition

Although many data have been recorded on the differences in samples of human milk, the general picture is the same throughout the world. Except for vitamin and fat

TABLE 5-1 Nutrient Content of Human Milk and Cow's Milk

Constituent (Per Liter)	Human Milk	Cow's Milk	Constituent (Per Liter)	Human Milk	Cow's Milk
Energy (kcal)	690	660	Minerals		
Protein (g)	9	35	Calcium (mg)	241-340	1200
Fat (g)	40	38	Phosphorus (mg)	150	920
Lactose (g)	68	49	Sodium (mg)	160	506
Vitamins			Potassium (mg)	530	1570
Vitamin A (IU)	1898	1025	Chlorine (mg)	400	1028
Vitamin D (activity)	40	14	Magnesium (mg)	38-41	120
Vitamin E (IU)	3.2	0.4	Sulfur (mg)	140	300
Vitamin K (μg)	34	170	Iron (mg)*	0.56-0.3	0.5
Thiamin (μg)	150	370	Iodine (mg)	200	80
Riboflavin (μg)	380	1700	Manganese (μg)†	5.9-4.0	20-40
Niacin (mg)	1.7	0.9	Copper (μg)	60	110
Pyridoxine (μg)	130	460	Zinc (mg)‡	4-0.5	3-5
Folic acid (μg)	41-84.6	2.9-68	Selenium (μg)	20	5-50
Cobalamine (μg)	0.5	4	Fluoride (mg)	0.05	0.03-0.1
Ascorbic acid (μg)	44	17	Chromium (μg)	4	2

Based on data from Hambraeus, L.: Pediatr. Clin. North Am. 24:17, 1977; Blanc, B.: World Rev. Nutr. Diet. 36:1, 1981; Jensen, R.G., Haggerty, M.M., and McMahon, K.E.: Am. J. Clin. Nutr. 31:990, 1978; Vuori, E., and Kuitunen, P.: Acta Paediatr. Scand. 68:33, 1978; Nayman, R., et al.: Am. J. Clin. Nutr. 32:1279, 1979; Siimes, M.A., Vuori, E., and Kuitunen, P.: Acta Paediatr. Scand. 68:29, 1979; Vuori, E.: Acta Paediatr. Scand. 68:571, 1979; Keimpulainen, J., and Vuori, E.: Am. J. Clin. Nutr. 33:2299, 1980; Jansson, L., Akesson, B., and Holmberg, L.: Am. J. Clin. Nutr. 34:8, 1981; Reeve, L.E., Chesney, R.W., and DeLuca, H.F.: Am. J. Clin. Nutr. 36:122, 1982; and Cooperman, J.M., et al.: Am. J. Clin. Nutr. 36:576, 1982.

*Median values at 2 weeks and 5 months of lactation.

†Median values at 2 weeks and 5 months of lactation, after which time the manganese content of human milk tends to increase.

‡Median values at 2 weeks and 37 weeks of lactation.

content, the composition of human milk appears to be largely independent of the state of the mother's nutrition, at least until malnutrition becomes severe. Even after prolonged lactation for 2 years or more, the quality of the milk produced by Indian and African women appears to be relatively well maintained, although the quantity may be small. Also, it is well known that severely undernourished women during time of famine often manage to feed their babies reasonably well.

COLOSTRUM

General Composition

In the first few days after birth, the mammary glands secrete a small amount of thin, milky fluid called colostrum. The volume varies between 2 and 10 ml per feeding per day during the first 3 days, related in part to the parity of the mother. Women who have had other pregnancies, particularly those who have nursed babies previously, usually demonstrate colostrum output sooner and in greater volume than other women. Colostrum is typically yellow, a feature associated with its relatively high carotene content. Also, it contains more protein and less sugar than milk produced thereafter. As might be expected from these composition differences, it is lower in kilocalories than mature milk—67 versus 75 kilocalories per 100 ml. The ash content of colostrum is high, and concentrations of sodium, potassium, and chloride are greater than in mature milk. The few composition analyses of human colostrum that have been reported show striking variability during any one day and from day to day. It is likely that these differences partially reflect the unstable secretory patterns that exist in the mammary apparatus as it begins active production, secretion, and ejection of milk.

Transitional Milk

Colostrum changes to transitional milk between the third and sixth days, at which time the protein content is still rather high. By the tenth day the major changes have been completed, and by the end of the first month the protein content reaches a consistent level that does not fall significantly thereafter. As the content of protein falls, the content of lactose progressively rises. This is also the case for fat, which increases to typical levels as lactation becomes more firmly established.

PRETERM MILK

Adaptation in Composition

With the renewed interest in the feeding of human milk to preterm infants, substantial attention has been focused on the composition of milk produced by mothers who have delivered prematurely. Early reports suggested that the protein and nonprotein nitrogen content of preterm milk was higher than that of term milk. Additional observations revealed that preterm milk might also be higher in its concentration of calcium, IgA, sodium, potassium, chloride, phosphorus, magnesium, medium-chain and polyunsaturated long-chain fatty acids, and total lipids, but lower in its lactose level than term milk. Thus the opinion developed that premature infants who are fed their mother's milk might demonstrate superior growth and development to that observed in premature infants fed banked human milk. In general this suspicion has proved to be true for very low-birth-weight infants as reported by researchers who have completed appropriate comparisons.[3,4] It appears, however, that commercial infant formulas designed for low-birth-weight infants may also be superior to banked human milk in supporting growth of these babies.[5]

Very Low-Birth-Weight Infant Issue

The controversy surrounding the nutritional adequacy of human milk for very low-birth-weight infants still exists. Although recent observations suggest that premature infants can thrive on milk from their own mothers; it is known that protein and sodium concentrations are marginal and calcium and phosphate levels are too low to support optimal development of the skeleton. In the face of immature gastrointestinal and renal function and poor nutrient stores, the very low-birth-weight infant who is provided human milk will often profit from an organized supplementation program.

Supplemented Feeding

It is even possible to supplement human milk with a powdered or liquid product designed to improve nutritional adequacy for very low-birth-weight infants.* The powdered fortifier contains protein and carbohydrate and increases the caloric density of breast milk to about 24 kilocalories per oz. The product is sold in premeasured packets; one packet is designed for addition to 25 ml of human milk. The liquid fortifier is similar in composition and is designed to be mixed with human milk or fed alternately with human milk.

Composition of Mature Human Milk

PROTEIN

Amount and Types of Protein

It is well known that different animals show different rates of growth. This fact appears to be related to their milk. The slowest rate of growth is found in humans and human milk contains the least protein. The major proteins found in breast milk are casein (curd protein) and lactalbumin (whey protein). It also contains a number of other proteins, such as lactoferrin, serum albumin, beta-lactoglobulins, immunoglobulins, and other glycoproteins. The concentration of protein found in human milk is lower than the previously accepted value of 1.5 g per 100 ml that was calculated from analyzed nitrogen content. Since human milk has been found to contain 25% of its nitrogen in nonprotein compounds, the lower protein concentration (0.8-0.9 g per 100 ml) is now accepted as the true amount.

Initial Changes

The protein content of human milk, like that of other mammals, falls rapidly over the first few days of lactation and reflects a relatively higher loss of those proteins

*Human Milk Fortifier, Mead Johnson Laboratories (powdered); Similac Natural Care, Ross Laboratories (liquid).

important in immune functions. Colostrum averages about 2% protein; transitional and mature milk average 1.5% and 1.0%, respectively.

Relation to Maternal Diet

Observations of many women in a variety of countries have shown that protein content of human milk is not reduced in mothers consuming a diet low in protein or poor in protein quality. A study in Pakistan supports this idea.[6] Here the protein quality and quantity of milk collected from women of a very low socioeconomic group in Karachi was similar to that of well-nourished women there and in other parts of the world. Of interest, however, was the observation that the concentration of lysine and methionine in the free amino acid content of milk samples from malnourished women was reduced when compared with milk from healthy, well-nourished mothers. The investigators suggest that this finding could imply a reduction in nutritional *quality* of the protein in these samples. It seems important to recognize, however, that dietary amino acid deficits may be readily subsized from maternal tissues as long as reserves are available from which to draw. Temporary fluctuations in free amino acid levels may be apparent, therefore, but alterations in quantity or quality of intact milk proteins are much less likely to occur until maternal protein stores are severely depleted.

Effect of Chronic Maternal Protein Deficit

With chronic protein undernutrition, breast milk composition may change. One study was carried out to assess the effects of prolonged lactation on the quantity of protein and patterns of free amino acids in breast milk obtained from Thai women at various times during lactation.[7] Protein levels decreased from 1.56% during the first week to a low of about 0.6% from 180 to 270 days and then rose to about 0.7%. Using these data, one can calculate that a 3-month-old infant in the 50th percentile for weight would require about 1250 ml of milk per day to meet protein needs. Since few infants in developing countries would receive this volume of milk daily and since supplemental sources of protein are scarce, the protein status of such infants could be significantly compromised.

Amino Acids

The amino acid content of human milk is recognized as ideal for the human infant. It is relatively low in several amino acids that are known to be detrimental if found in the blood at high levels (for example, phenylalanine). Also, it is high in other amino acids that the infant cannot synthesize well, such as cystine and taurine. Some of the positive features of the amino acid composition of human milk are summarized in Table 5-2. These characteristics are especially useful to infants whose biochemical capabilities are underdeveloped at birth.

Nonprotein Nitrogen

The total amount of nonprotein nitrogen in human milk averages nearly 25% of all nitrogen and is significantly higher than that found in cow's milk (about 5%). Nonprotein nitrogen sources consist of a variety of organic, and trace amounts of inorganic, compounds shed into the milk supply. Among these compounds are peptides

TABLE 5-2 Significant Features About the Amino Acid Composition of Human Milk

Characteristic	Explanation
Lower in methionine and rich in cystine	An enzyme, cystathionase, is late to develop in the fetus; this impairs optimum conversion of methionine to cystine, which is needed for growth and development; methionine may increase in the bloodstream of an infant fed cow's milk but not one fed human milk; hypermethioninemia may damage the central nervous system
Lower in phenylalanine and tyrosine	The enzymes tyrosine aminotransferase and parahydroxyphenyl pyruvate oxidase are late in developing: cow's milk-fed babies may develop hyperphenylalaninemia and hypertyrosinemia, which may adversely affect development of the central nervous system, especially in the premature; breast milk offers much less problem
Rich in taurine	Breast milk provides taurine for bile acid conjugation, and it *may* also be a neurotransmitter or neuromodulator in the brain and retina; humans cannot synthesize taurine well; cow's milk contains little taurine; the requirement for taurine in the developing neonate is uncertain

and free amino acids, the latter of which may provide a nutritional advantage to the infant. Nonprotein nitrogen sources also include urea, creatinine, and sugar amines. Since each species of mammal seems to carry a characteristic pattern of free amino acids in its nonprotein nitrogen pool, scientists have speculated that this is of nutritional significance.

Taurine

Much recent discussion has centered on the amino acid taurine. Since taurine is found in particularly high levels in fetal brain tissue, it has been proposed that it may play a role in the development of the brain. In addition, taurine is associated with bile acid and thus plays an important role in digestion and may function in the management of cholesterol in the body. Since human milk contains much more taurine than does cow's milk, it has been speculated that the breast-fed infant might profit significantly from the higher taurine intake. Interestingly, however, observations have shown that breast-fed babies maintain plasma taurine levels that are similar to those of formula-fed infants. It would appear that taurine is not an essential amino acid for infants.

LIPIDS

Amount

The total lipid content of human milk varies considerably from one woman to another and is even affected by parity and season of the year. Separate observations by different investigators around the world give the following average levels of fat in human milk: 2.02%, 3.1%, 3.2%, 3.27%, 3.95%, 4.5%, and 5.3%. Sampling methods may affect fat content, since the first milk (foremilk) is low in fat and the last milk (hindmilk) shows about a threefold increase in the fat content.

Types

Nearly 90% of the lipid in human milk is present in the form of triglycerides. But small amounts of phospholipids, cholesterol, diglycerides, monoglycerides, glycolipids, sterol esters, and free fatty acids are also found. The fatty acid composition of human milk differs greatly from that of cow's milk. The content of the essential fatty acid linoleic acid is considerably greater in human milk than in cow's milk. The content of short-chain saturated fatty acids (C_4 to C_8) is greater in cow's milk. Of equal interest is the observation that human milk contains more cholesterol than cow's milk and much more cholesterol than commercial infant formulas. A beneficial effect of this higher cholesterol level has been suggested on grounds that: (1) it is needed by the rapidly growing central nervous system for myelin synthesis, and (2) it stimulates in early life the development of enzymes necessary for cholesterol degradation.

Effect of Low Maternal Fat Resources

Evidence suggests that the fat content of breast milk may be reduced to as low as 1.0 g per 100 ml. Under these circumstances the caloric content of the milk may be decreased with significant lessening of available energy for the infant. The basis for low-fat milk composition is believed to be related not only to diet during lactation but also to inadequate energy intake in pregnancy with a resulting inadequate subcutaneous "fat bank."

Maternal Diet Effect on Composition

The composition of the fat in human milk varies significantly with the diet of the mother. Lactating women fed a diet rich in polyunsaturated fats, such as corn and cottonseed oils, produce milk with an increased content of polyunsaturated fats. This is best seen by comparing the milk of total vegetarians with that of nonvegetarians, as seen in Table 5-3. Over the years, as dietary unsaturated fat intake has increased in the United States, the fatty acid composition of breast milk samples has reflected this change (Table 5-4).

TABLE 5-3 Mean Breast Milk Fatty Acid Concentration in Vegetarians (Vegans) and Nonvegetarians (Controls)

Methyl Esters	Vegans*	Controls*
Lauric ($C_{12:0}$)	39	33
Myristic ($C_{14:0}$)	68	80
Palmitic ($C_{16:0}$)	166	276
Stearic ($C_{18:0}$)	52	108
Palmitoleic ($C_{16:1}$)	12	36
Oleic ($C_{18:1}$)	313	353
Linoleic ($C_{18:2}$)	317	69
Linolenic ($C_{18:3}$)	15	8

Modified from Sanders, T.A.B., and others: Am. J. Clin. Nutr. **31**:805, 1978.

*Mean values expressed as milligrams per gram total methyl esters detected for four vegans and four controls (nonvegetarians).

TABLE 5-4 Fatty Acid Composition of Human Milk: Past and Present

Fatty Acid	Breast Milk Content (Percent of Total Fatty Acid)	
	1953*	1977†
Lauric ($C_{12:0}$)	5.5	3.8
Myristic ($C_{14:0}$)	8.5	5.2
Palmitic ($C_{16:0}$)	23.2	22.5
Palmitoleic ($C_{16:1}$)	3.0	4.1
Stearic ($C_{18:0}$)	6.9	8.7
Oleic ($C_{18:1}$)	36.5	39.5
Linoleic ($C_{18:2}$)	7.8	14.4
Linolenic ($C_{18:3}$)	—	2.0

*Based on data from Macy, I.G., et al.: The composition of milks, Pub. No. 254, Washington, D.C., 1958, National Research Council.

†Based on data from Guthrie, H.A., Picciano, M.F., and Sheehe, D.: J. Pediatr. **90**:39, 1977.

When maternal energy intake is severely restricted, fatty acid composition of human milk resembles that of depot fat. This effect is to be expected; it represents fat mobilization in response to the reduction in energy intake. A substantial increase in the proportion of dietary kilocalories from carbohydrate will result in an increase in milk content of lauric and myristic acids, The significance of this latter observation is unknown.

Fat-Digesting Enzymes

Human milk contains several lipases. One is a serum-stimulated lipase (lipoprotein lipase) that may appear in the milk as a result of leakage from the mammary tissue. Another lipolytic milk enzyme has a similar activity to that of pancreatic lipase, breaking down triglycerides to free fatty acids and glycerol. This enzyme is present in the fat fraction and appears to be inhibited by bile salts. It probably is responsible for lipolysis of milk refrigerated or frozen for later use. Additional lipases in the skim milk fraction are inactive until they encounter bile. These lipases, the bile-salt-stimulated lipases, are believed to be present only in the milk of primates and are thought to serve some useful purpose for this species. Since the bile-salt-stimulated lipases have been clearly shown to be stable and active in the intestine of infants, they can contribute significantly to the hydrolysis of milk triglycerides and partly account for the greater ease in fat digestion that is commonly demonstrated by breast-fed babies.

Carnitine

Both human milk and cow's milk contain carnitine, which is thought to aid in the digestion of fat.[8] Evidence has been presented that supplementation of some infant formulas with carnitine may be in order. Human milk contains about 59 nmole per ml. Formula products based on milk and beef contain 50 to 656 nmole per ml. Those prepared from soy isolate, and specialized formulations from egg white and casein, carry an amount equal to or less than 4 nmole per ml. Most manufacturers of soy formulas for infants now add carnitine to their products.

CARBOHYDRATE

Lactose

Lactose is the main carbohydrate in human milk. It occurs there in two forms, alpha-lactose and beta-lactose. It is relatively insoluble and is slowly digested and absorbed in the small intestine. It is believed that the acid milieu that is created helps to check the growth of undesirable bacteria in the infant's gut and to improve the absorption of calcium, phosphorus, magnesium, and other metals. Since human milk contains much more lactose than cow's milk (7% and 4.8%, respectively), these gut-associated benefits of lactose are theoretically more significant in the breast-fed than in the bottle-fed infant.

Other Carbohydrates

For a long time it was thought that lactose was the only carbohydrate in human milk. However, chromatographic processing of human milk samples has revealed trace amounts of glucose, galactose, glucosamines, and other nitrogen-containing oligosaccharides. The role or significance of these minor carbohydrates has not been defined, but it is possible that one or more of them could contribute to the gut colonization by specific micro-organisms with potentially beneficial effects to the infant. The nitrogen-containing oligosaccharides, for example, have a *L. bifidus*-promoting activity. This organism breaks down lactose into lactic acid and acetic acid, and thus is responsible for the acid reaction of the intestinal contents of breast-fed infants that may interfere with the growth of some enteropathogenic organisms.

Amylase

Although human milk does not contain much complex carbohydrate, it does contain a starch-splitting enzyme, amylase, which is quite stable at pH levels found in the stomach and small intestine.[9] This enzyme may provide an alternative pathway for digestion of glucose polymers and starches in early infancy when pancreatic amylase is low or absent in duodenal fluid. The physiologic importance of mammary amylase may be analogous to that of the bile-salt-stimulated lipase found in human milk.

MINERALS

Comparison with Cow's Milk

One of the most striking differences between human and cow's milk lies in the mineral composition. As with protein, it is believed that this difference may be related to the rate of growth of the species that produced the milk. According to typical estimates, there is six times more phosphorus, four times more calcium, three times more total ash, and three times more protein in cow's milk than in human milk. The high mineral and protein composition of cow's milk distinctly affects the solute or osmolar load provided to the kidney. One might speculate that the kidney of the newborn infant is prepared to handle the solute load derived from breast milk but is stressed unduly by the requirements placed on it when cow's milk, especially nonfat milk, is selected as an alternate.

Major and Trace Minerals

The major minerals found in mature human milk are potassium, calcium, phosphorus, chlorine, and sodium. Iron, copper, and manganese are found in only trace amounts, and since these elements are required for normal red blood cell synthesis, infants fed too long on milk alone become anemic. Minute amounts of zinc, magnesium, aluminum, iodine, chromium, selenium, and fluoride are also found in breast milk. Infants who are not provided with fluoridated water in addition to breast milk may benefit from a daily oral fluoride supplement of regulated dosage predetermined by the physician and pharmacist. Providing the lactating woman with a fluoride supplement does not alter her milk output of fluoride (Fig. 5-6).

Varying Mineral Composition

The total mineral content of human milk is fairly constant, but the specific amounts of individual minerals may vary with the status of the mother and the stage of lactation. Observations from a number of laboratories have shown declining concentrations of several minerals over the weeks and months following the onset of lactation (Fig. 5-7). Of substantial interest are other reports in which dietary intake and supplementation habits of mothers have been compared with mineral composition of milk. In most situations no relationship has been found between maternal mineral intake and milk mineral content.

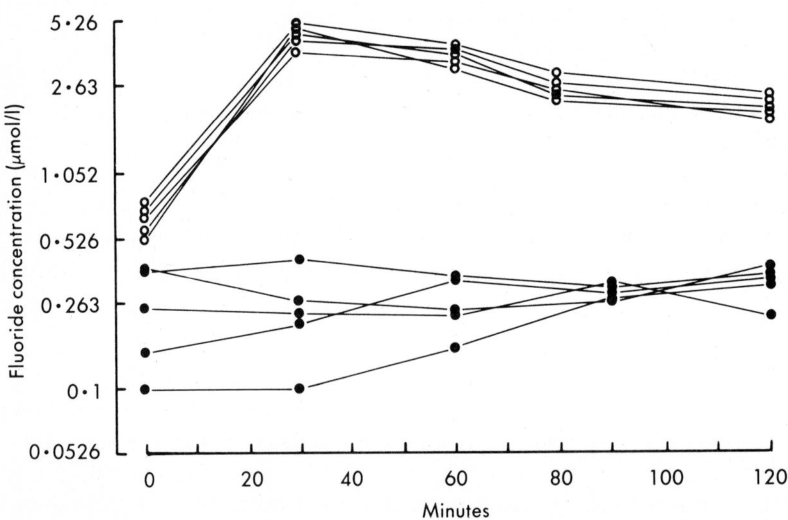

FIG. 5-6 Plasma *(open symbols)* and breast milk *(closed symbols)* fluoride concentrations in mothers after oral dose of 1.5 mg fluoride as sodium fluoride solution. (Conversion: fluoride—1 mole/l ≈ 19 ng/ml.)

(From Ekstrand, J.: No evidence of transfer of fluoride from plasma to breast milk, Br. Med. J. **283**:761, 1981.)

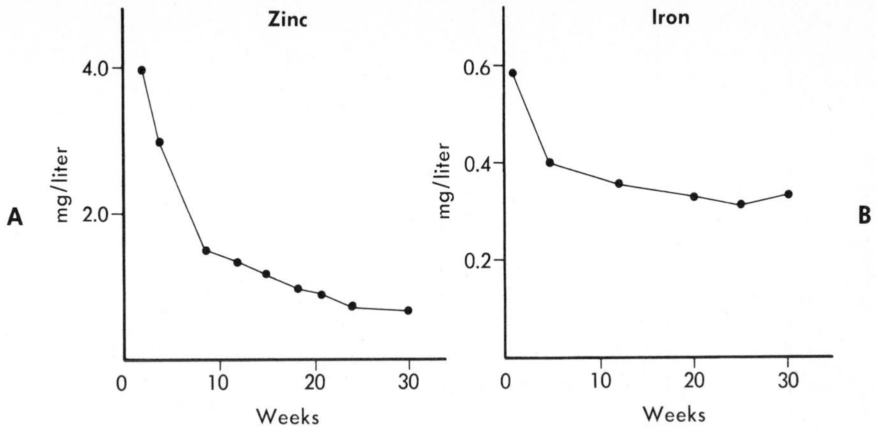

FIG. 5-7 The average zinc and iron concentrations of human milk in 229 breast milk samples from Finnish women.

(**A** modified from Vuori, E., and Kuitunen, P.: Acta Paediatr. Scand. **68**:33, 1979; **B** modified from Siimes, M.A., Vuori, E., and Kuitunen, P.: Acta Paediatr. Scand. **68**:29, 1979.)

Absorption

Some minerals are more easily absorbed from breast milk than from cow's milk or commercial formulas. McMillan and others[10,11] reported that nearly 50% of the iron in human milk is absorbed, whereas availability of iron from cow's milk and iron-fortified formulas is only 10% and 4%, respectively. More recently Garry and associates[12] found that iron absorption from human milk may be much higher than 50% during the first 3 months of life. An explanation for this improved absorption has not been found.

Iron Supplementation

Whether or not breast-fed infants should receive iron supplements is still the subject of much debate.[12,13] Several studies suggest that infants who are breast-fed during the first 6 months of life and receive little or no dietary iron other than that in human milk appear to be iron sufficient at age 6 months. However, based on changes in total body iron determined by body weights and hemoglobin and ferritin concentrations. Owen and others[13] concluded that some nonsupplemented breast-fed infants are in negative iron balance between ages 3 and 6 months. One might suggest that human milk alone cannot provide sufficient iron for optimal infant nutrition after 5 or 6 months of life.

Zinc Bioavailability

Like iron, the bioavailability of zinc is substantially better from human milk than from other alternative preparations.[14] In one study the bioavailability of zinc fed to rats in various milk solutions was 59.2% for human milk, 42% for cow's milk, and 26.8% to 39% for commercial formulas. In other work human subjects demonstrated better absorption of zinc from human milk than from cow's milk or selected infant formulas (Fig. 5-8). An explanation for the better absorption of zinc from human milk is still

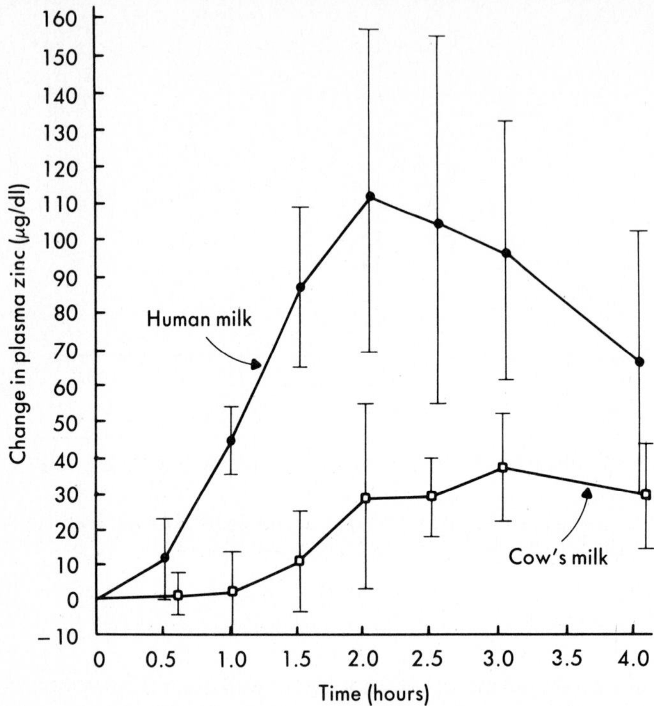

FIG. 5-8 Changes in plasma zinc concentration after ingestion of 25 mg of zinc with human milk (five subjects) and cow's milk (seven subjects). Points represent means ± SD variation from baseline value.

(From Casey, C.E., Walravens, P.A., and Hambidge, K.M.: Availability of zinc: loading tests with human milk, cow's milk, and infant formulas, Pediatrics **68**:394, 1981. Copyright American Academy of Pediatrics 1981.)

being sought. It has been suggested, however, that the unique distribution and binding of zinc, and some other elements, to high- and low-molecular-weight fractions of milk very likely are related to the differences in bioavailability that have now been demonstrated by a number of investigators.

FAT-SOLUBLE VITAMINS

General Vitamin Content

All the vitamins, both fat- and water-soluble, required for good nutrition and health are supplied in breast milk, but the amounts vary markedly from one person to another. Several reasons may account for this observation. Genetic differences likely are important, but diet and drug use by individual women also influence vitamin composition of milk. The vitamin content of human milk may be seen to change dramatically in some instances over the first few days of lactation. Generally the level of water-soluble vitamins goes up and the level of fat-soluble vitamins declines. However, exceptions exist. None of the normal variations poses any risk to the infant.

Vitamin D

The amount of biologically active vitamin D in human milk has been found to be low (40 to 50 I.U. per L). However, it is possible that maternal sunshine exposure and dietary intake may affect infant vitamin D status through their effects on breast milk vitamin D content. This possibility is supported by the recent finding that a short course of oral vitamin D (2400 I.U. per day) supplementation or exposure to ultraviolet phototherapy quickly raised the levels of antirachitic (vitamin D) sterols in the plasma and milk of three lactating women.[15] There was a peak effect after 1 week with oral vitamin D supplementation and after 2 to 3 days after ultraviolet irradiation. The levels then rapidly returned to baseline. Other reports show a direct relationship between maternal and infant levels of 25-hydroxyvitamin D, implying that maternal vitamin D intake directly affects the vitamin D concentration in breast milk.

Vitamin D Supplementation

A question remains regarding the need for vitamin D supplementation in the term, exclusively breast-fed infant. Although some clinicians do not believe it is necessary, the bulk of data support the practice. Greer and associates[16,17] found low serum 25-hydroxyvitamin D concentrations and early decreases in bone mineral content in breast-fed infants not receiving supplemental vitamin D. Ozsoylu and Hasanoglu[18] reported low serum 25-hydroxyvitamin D levels at 1 month of age in breast-fed infants not supplemented with vitamin D. In some of the sunniest parts of the world, such as the Middle East, rickets is common in certain breast-fed infants because cultural practices keep the babies well clothed and indoors for the first year.[19] Even in the United States, reports of resurgence in rickets among breast-fed infants provoke considerable concern.[20,21] Since no harm is associated with vitamin D supplementation at 400 I.U. per day and since expense and inconvenience are trivial, support of this practice seems justifiable. For light-skinned suburban populations in sunny regions and seasons, one may worry less about compliance with this recommendation.

Vitamin A

Milk is a good source of vitamin A and its precursors. Its concentration in human milk is influenced by the quality and quantity of the dietary elements consumed by the mother. The vitamin A content of breast milk is reportedly much lower in some developing countries than in the West. Maternal serum vitamin A levels in these same regions are also typically low. Vitamin A or carotene intake of some Western mothers is higher in the spring and summer months because of greater supplies of yellow and leafy green vegetables. Modern methods of preservation, however, have extended the length of seasons for many vegetables and fruits so that dietary differences from season to season may be minimal for many women with access to supermarkets, home freezers, and other such luxuries of modern society.

Vitamin E

Levels of vitamin E in human milk are substantially greater than those in cow's milk. As might be expected, serum levels of vitamin E rise quickly in breast-fed infants and are maintained at normal levels without much fluctuation. Cow's-milk-fed babies demonstrate instead depressed circulating levels of vitamin E unless supplemented. Fortunately, manufacturers of infant formulas have increased their levels of vitamin E fortification to avoid potential deficiency.

Vitamin K

In human milk vitamin K is present at a level of 15 μg per 100 ml. Cow's milk contains much more than this amount with a typical reported value of 60 μg per 100 ml. Vitamin K is produced by the intestinal flora, but it takes several days for the sterile infant gut to establish an effective microbe population. Even then, onset of hemorrhagic disease with bleeding as late as 4 weeks after delivery has been associated with breast-feeding if no vitamin K had been given at birth. It is recommended, therefore, that all newborn infants receive vitamin K.

WATER-SOLUBLE VITAMINS

Effect of Maternal Intake

The levels of water-soluble vitamins in human milk are more likely to reflect maternal diet or supplement intake more than most other ingested compounds. Maternal dietary supplementation with most of these vitamins has been shown to increase their content in breast milk. This is especially true in women whose dietary patterns or nutritional status are suboptimal. It appears that with some of these vitamins a plateau may be reached where increased intake has no further impact on milk composition. This idea was nicely demonstrated when varying levels of supplemental ascorbic acid were provided to lactating women.[22] With comparable diets, women consuming either 90 mg or 250 mg per day of ascorbic acid produced milk with similar concentrations of this vitamin. Women taking 1000 mg of ascorbic acid per day produced milk that was only slightly higher in its ascorbic acid content.

Vitamin B_6

Felice and Kirksey[23] have provided evidence that milk concentration of vitamin B_6 may be a sensitive indicator of vitamin B_6 status of the mother. They further suggest that the majority of lactating women produce milk with a vitamin B_6 content that is substantially less than that recommended for good health and growth of infants. These researchers observed that mothers receiving 2.5 mg per day of supplemental vitamin B_6 per day failed to supply their breast-feeding infants with 0.3 mg of vitamin B_6 per day, which is the RDA for young infants.[24]

Vitamin B_{12}

The vitamin B_{12} content of human milk has recently been re-evaluated.[25] The content of 19 samples of milk ranged from 0.33 to 3.2 ng per ml (mean 0.97 ng per ml), and ingestion of supplemental B_{12} did not significantly affect milk content. Human milk from well-fed mothers was found to contain adequate amounts of B_{12}. Its bioavailability, however, depends on the sufficiency of proteolytic enzymes to release it from its bound form.

RESISTANCE FACTORS

A thorough discussion of the composition of breast milk of necessity must include mention of the beneficial components of human milk that are not classified as nutrients (Table 5-5).

Bifidus Factor

One of the earliest resistance factors to be described in human milk was the bifidus factor, which may be a nitrogen-containing polysaccharide that favors the growth of *L. bifidus*. Its uniqueness to human milk has recently been confirmed.[26] *L. bifidus* confers a protective effect against invasive enteropathogenic organisms.

Immunoglobulins

Various immunoglobulins are present in human milk, including IgA, IgG, IgD, and IgE. Although IgG appears to migrate from maternal serum into milk, evidence suggests that IgA, IgD, and IgE are produced locally in mammary tissue. A variety of studies support the idea of migration of lymphoblasts from maternal gut-associated lymphoid tissue to the mammary glands followed by local production of immunoglobulins at this site and secretion of them into the milk. This mechanism allows for maternal lymphoblasts to obtain antigenic exposure from distant sites and carry this experience to the mammary tissue where synthesis of appropriate antibodies can occur for protection of the suckling infant.

Secretory IgA (sIgA) is the predominant immunoglobulin in human milk. It is found in large amounts in colostrum and in smaller, but still significant, levels in mature breast milk. Secretory immunoglobulins have been shown to be a major host resistance factor against organisms that infect the gastrointestinal tract, in particular *E. coli*

TABLE 5-5 Antiinfectious Factors in Human Milk

Factor	Function
Bifidus factor	Stimulates growth of bifidobacteria, which antagonizes the survival of enterobacteria
Secretory IgA (sIgA), IgM, IgE, IgD, and IgG	Act against bacterial invasion of the mucosa and/or colonization of the gut (show bacterial and viral neutralizing capacity; activate alternative complement pathway)
Antistaphylococcus factor	Inhibits systemic staphylococcal infection
Lactoferrin	Binds iron and inhibits bacterial multiplication
Lactoperoxidase	Kills streptococci and enteric bacteria
Complement (C_3, C_4)	Promotes opsonization (the rendering of bacteria and other cells susceptible to phagocytosis)
Interferon	Inhibits intracellular viral replication
Lysozyme	Lyses bacteria through destruction of the cell wall
B_{12}-binding protein	Renders vitamin B_{12} unavailable for bacterial growth
Lymphocytes	Synthesize secretory IgA; may have other roles
Macrophages	Synthesize complement, lactoferrin, lysozyme, and other factors; carry out phagocytosis and probably other functions

and the enteroviruses. Also, a protective effect against other organisms has been demonstrated. Human milk clearly exhibits a prophylactic effect against septicemia of the newborn.

Other Host Resistance Factors

Some of the other host resistance factors in breast milk are also worthy of mention. Lysozyme, an antimicrobial enzyme, occurs at 300 times the concentration found in cow's milk. Lactoferrin has been described recently as a compound with a "monilia-static" effect against *Candida albicans.* It inhibits the growth of staphylococci and *E. coli* by binding iron, which the bacteria require to proliferate. Lactoperoxidase, which has been shown in vitro to act with other substances in combating streptococci, is also found in human milk. Specific prostaglandins have also been defined, and these may protect the integrity of the gastrointestinal tract epithelium against noxious substances.[27]

Lymphocyte-Macrophage Activities

Of additional interest is the discovery that the lymphocytes in human milk produce the antiviral substance interferon. Macrophages are also found in colostrum and mature milk; 21,000 per mm^3 reportedly are present in a typical colostrum specimen. Macrophages are motile and phagocytic and have been shown to produce complement, lactoferrin, lysozyme, and other factors. The full role of the macrophages is still under investigation, but they undoubtedly have a protective function, both within the mammary lacteals and subsequently within the baby. A number of investigators have studied the activities of lymphocytes in human milk. Milk samples from lactating mothers have been collected at various times post partum and examined for cell types present and in vitro activities of the various identified cells. The greatest number of cells appear in colostrum with numbers dropping significantly during the following 8 weeks.

Effect of Maternal Malnutrition

As one might expect, maternal malnutrition adversely affects not only the nutritional composition of human milk but also its content of immunologic substances. Observations of malnourished Colombian women showed that colostrum contained only one-third the normal concentration of IgG and less than half the normal level of albumin. Significant reductions in colostrum levels of IgA and the fourth component of complement (C_4) were also observed.[28] These differences noted tended to disappear in mature milk, concomitant with improvement in the nutritional status of the malnourished mothers during the first several weeks post partum. The authors conclude that the protective qualities of colostrum and milk may be significantly influenced by maternal nutritional status.

CONTAMINANTS

The lactating woman is often exposed to a variety of nonnutritional substances that may be transferred to her milk. Such substances include drugs, environmental pollutants, viruses, caffeine, alcohol, and food allergens. Although moderate amounts of many of these agents are believed to pose no risk to nursing infants, some substances provoke concern because of known or suspected adverse reactions.

Drugs

Much research has focused on the release of drugs into the milk of lactating women. Whether the mother drinks it, eats it, sniffs it, inserts it as an anal or vaginal suppository, or injects it, some level of the active agents in the drug enters the maternal tissues and blood and finally migrates to the breast milk. The difference in method of administration determines the amount of drug that finally enters the blood and the speed with which it reaches the capillaries of the breast. In general the amount of a drug excreted in milk is not more than 1% to 2% of the maternal dose.[29] Although concern exists about the amount of a given drug in the breast milk, of greater concern is the amount that actually reaches the infant's bloodstream. Unfortunately, there is no accurate way to measure this because other factors also affect the level in the infant's bloodstream. The tolerance of the chemical to the pH of the stomach and the enzymatic activity of the intestinal tract is significant. The volume of milk consumed by the infant is a factor as well.

Harmful Drug Effects

Some drugs appear in human milk in sufficient quantities to be harmful to the infant (Table 5-6).[30] Sedatives used to relieve tension may produce drowsiness in the baby as well as the mother. Valium residuals in mother's milk induce lethargy in breast-fed babies. Lithium carbonate, a drug prescribed for relief of manic depression, may induce lowered body temperature, loss of muscle tone, and bluish skin in the nursing infant. Reserpine produces a bluish tint to the skin along with other disorders. Both cyclophosphamide and methotrexate cause bone marrow depression when ingested by infants. A variety of disorders follow intake by infants of breast milk contaminated with antimicrobial agents of one kind or another. Penicillin in breast milk may produce an allergic reaction in a sensitive infant. Other antibiotics may produce similar reactions, as well as sleepiness, vomiting, and refusal to eat. Radioactive iodine may damage the thyroid gland. Bowel problems in infants may result from maternal consumption of some laxatives, such as anthraquinone, aloes, cascara, emodin, and rheum (rhubarb). Safe laxatives include magnesia, castor oil, mineral oil, bisacodyl (Dulcolax), senna phenophthalein or nonprescription Ex-Lax, and fecal softeners. Heroin or the painkiller dextropropoxyphene (Darvon) can lead to infant addiction.

Maternal Adjustments for Needed Drugs

If a mother needs a specific medication and the hazards to the infant are believed to be minimal, the following important adjustments can be made to minimize the effects:

1. **Action time.** Do not use the long-acting form of the drug because the infant has even more difficulty in excreting the agents, which usually require detoxification in the liver. Accumulation in the infant is then a genuine concern.

TABLE 5-6 Abbreviated Guide to Drug Therapy in Nursing Mothers

DRUGS THAT ARE CONTRAINDICATED DURING BREAST-FEEDING:

Drug	Reported Sign or Symptom in Infant or Effect on Lactation
Amethopterin*	Possible immune suppression; unknown effect on growth or association with carcinogenesis
Bromocriptine	Suppresses lactation
Cimetidine**	May suppress gastric acidity in infant, inhibit drug metabolism, and cause CNS stimulation
Clemastine	Drowsiness, irritability, refusal to feed, high-pitched cry, neck stiffness
Cyclophosphamide*	Possible immune suppression; unknown effect on growth or association with carcinogenesis
Ergotamine	Vomiting, diarrhea, convulsions (doses used in migraine medications)
Gold salts	Rash, inflammation of kidney and liver
Methimazole	Potential for interfering with thyroid function
Phenindione	Hemorrhage
Thiouracil	Decreased thyroid function; does not apply to propylthiouracil

DRUGS THAT REQUIRE TEMPORARY CESSATION OF BREAST-FEEDING:

Drug	Recommended Alteration in Breast-Feeding Pattern
Metronidazole	Discontinue breast-feeding 12-24 hr to allow excretion of dose
Radiopharmaceuticals	Radioactivity present in milk, consult nuclear medicine physician before performing diagnostic study so that radionuclide that has shortest excretion time in breast milk can be used; prior to study mother should pump her breast and store enough milk in freezer for feeding the infant; after study the mother should pump her breast to maintain milk production but discard all milk pumped for the required time that radioactivity is present in milk.
Gallium-69 (^{69}Ga)	Radioactivity in milk present for 2 wk
Iodine-125 (^{125}I)	Risk of thyroid cancer; radioactivity in milk for 12 days
Iodine-131 (^{131}I)	Radioactivity in milk present 2-14 days, depending on study
Radioactive sodium	Radioactivity in milk present 96 hr
Technetium-99m (^{99m}Tc)	Radioactivity in milk present 15 hr to 3 days

*Data not available for other cytotoxic agents. **Drug is concentrated in breast milk.
Modified from Committee on Drugs, American Academy of Pediatrics, The transfer of drugs and other chemicals into breast milk, Pediatrics 72:375, 1983

2. **Dose schedule.** Schedule the doses so the least amount of the drug gets into the milk. Given the usual absorption rates and peak blood levels of most drugs, having the mother take the medication immediately after breast feeding is the safest time for the infant.
3. **Observations.** Watch the infant for any unusual signs or symptoms such as change in feeding pattern or sleeping habits, fussiness, or rash.
4. **Drug amount in milk.** When possible, choose the drug that produces the least amount in the milk.

Drug Information

One of the best sources of information on drugs in relation to human milk and infant health is the family pharmacist. It is also wise to read the product label to evaluate product composition and precautionary statements. Effective December 26, 1979, all drug manufacturers in the United States are required to provide relevant information on the labels of new drugs developed and marketed since that date. Whatever is known about excretion of the drug into milk and whatever is known of the effect on the infant will be indicated on the label. If nothing is known, the label will state that fact. In such a case, and in all use of drugs, the prudent mother should exercise due caution.

Environmental Contaminants

The current concern over pesticide residues, industrial wastes, and other environmental contaminants is not without cause. Many of these compounds have accidentally contaminated food and water supplies around the world. In general the chemical contaminants that appear in breast milk have high lipid solubility, resistance to physical degradation or biologic metabolism, wide distribution in the environment, and slow or absent excretion rates. Of greatest concern among such chemicals are the organohalides such as polychlorinated biphenyls (PCBs) and dichlorodiphenyltrichloroethane (DDT). Long-term low-level exposure to the organohalides results in a gradual accumulation of residues in fat, including the fat of breast milk. Lactation is the only way in which large amounts of such residues can be excreted.

Exposure Levels to Contaminants

Savage and associates[31] conducted a study of environmental contaminants that focused on levels of chlorinated hydrocarbon insecticide residues in nearly 1500 human milk samples around the United States. The majority of samples showed low but detectable levels of most of these insecticides or their metabolites, but significant differences were found among the five geographic regions. The southeastern U.S. had the highest mean residue levels, whereas the northwest has the least. Although nursing infants around the U.S. would generally receive low levels of some of these residues, a small number could be exposed to fairly high amounts.

Is There a "Safe" Level?

It is clear that human milk is a variable source of contaminants, but it is difficult to define a "safe" level of exposure to these compounds. However, both the World Health Organization and the U.S. Food and Drug Administration have set "regulatory" or "allowable" levels for daily intake of several organohalides (Table 5-7). These standards provide a large margin of safety, so the fact that a given infant exceeds the level does not mean that such exposure is toxic. Much remains to be learned about the chemical contamination of human milk. Meanwhile, it is heartening to know that very few cases of illness caused by transmission of environmental chemicals through breast milk have appeared.

TABLE 5-7 "Typical" Levels, FDA Action Levels, Allowable Daily Intake, and Calculated Daily Intake of Representative Breast-fed Infants

Substance	Typical Levels* (ppb)	FDA Action Levels for Cow's Milk† (ppb)	Allowable Daily Intake (μg/kg)	Daily Intake of Breast-fed Infants‡ (μg/kg)
Dieldrin	1-6	7.5	0.1	0.8
Heptachlor epoxide	8-30	7.5	0.5	4
PCBs	40-100	62.5	1	14
DDT (including metabolites)	50-200	50	5	28

Modified from Rogan, W.J., Bagniewska, A., and Damstra, T.: N. Engl. J. Med. **302**:1450, 1980.
*Levels considered typical in whole milk in the United States.
†Assuming 2.5% fat. FDA action levels represent the limit at or above which the FDA will take legal action against a product to remove it from the market.
‡Intake of a 5 kg infant drinking 700 ml of milk per day; levels are based on high values given under typical levels.

Heavy Metals

Lead and mercury, both heavy metals, are transferred placentally to the fetus and also to the infant via maternal milk. Rat studies have shown that lactation increases maternal lead absorption from the gut, which leads ultimately to an increased level of lead excretion via the milk. The exact mechanism for this phenomenon is not known. However, lactose may play a dominant role, since it is known to facilitate the absorption of calcium, other trace elements, and lead.

Nicotine

Nicotine enters human milk and can cause nicotine "poisoning" of the breast-fed infant. Infants 3 to 4 days of age whose mothers smoked 6 to 16 cigarettes a day were reported to refuse to suckle, to become apathetic, vomit, and retain urine and feces. In a chain-smoking mother the nicotine content of milk may reach 75 μg/L. In the case of mothers who smoke very little it is likely that the amount of nicotine the infant would get from breathing cigarette smoke in the immediate environment would be more significant than that obtained from milk.

Caffeine

Caffeine passes from the maternal bloodstream into breast milk. Although a small dose of caffeine comparable to that obtained from a cup of coffee is transported at low levels from the mother to her milk (1%), caffeine does reach the infant where it can accumulate over time. Wakeful, hyperactive infants sometimes are victims of caffeine stimulation. A mother who drinks more than 6 to 8 cups of any caffeine-containing beverage in a day's time might expect her infant to demonstrate "coffee nerves." Such an infant does not require hospitalization, and verification of blood caffeine levels is not mandatory, although it might be helpful. An elimination trial should suffice to evaluate the role of maternal caffeine ingestion, and subsequent elimination, on infant behavior.

Alcohol

Beverage alcohol also passes from the mother's bloodstream into her breast milk. Ethanol has been shown to reach human milk in a concentration similar to that in maternal blood. Interestingly, however, the major breakdown product of ethanol, acetaldehyde, does not appear in human milk even though considerable amounts may have been measured in maternal blood. The role of the mammary gland in eliminating acetaldehyde may be similar to that of the placenta. If human milk contains large amounts of ethanol, the nursing infant may develop a pseudo-Cushing syndrome as described by Binkiewicz, Robinson, and Senior.[32] The 4-month-old infant they describe (Fig. 5-9) was breast-fed by a mother who consumed at least 50 12-oz cans of beer weekly, plus generous amounts of other, more concentrated alcoholic drinks.

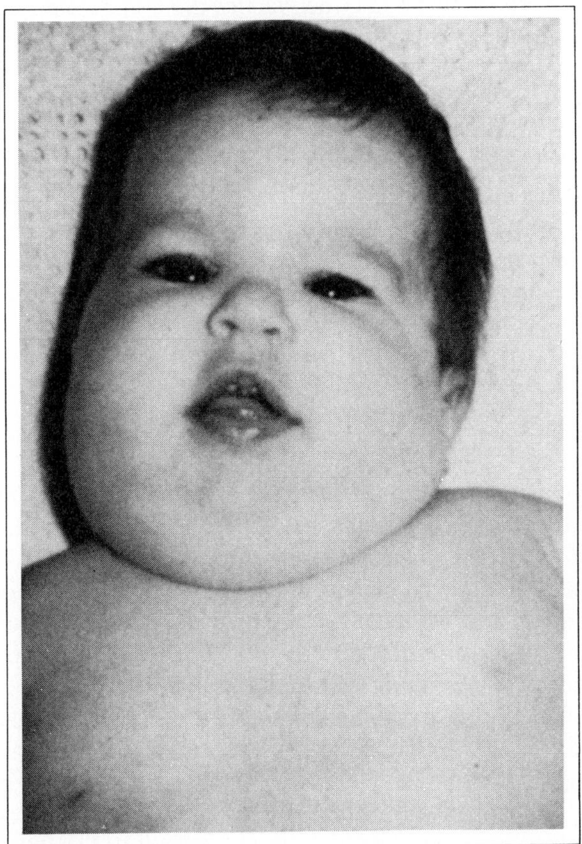

FIG. 5-9 Cushingoid appearance in a 4-month-old infant whose mother consumed at least 50 cans of beer weekly plus generous portions of other, more concentrated alcoholic beverages.

(From Binkiewicz, A., Robinson, M.J., and Senior, B.: Pseudo-Cushing syndrome caused by alcohol in breast milk, J. Pediatr. 93:965, 1978.)

When the mother stopped drinking but continued to nurse, the infant's growth rate promptly increased and her appearance gradually returned to normal. The mother also noted that she did not sleep as much as she did before.

Diet for the Nursing Mother

GENERAL RECOMMENDATIONS

Nutrients

The Committee on Recommended Dietary Allowances (RDA) of the Food and Nutrition Board considers the optimal diet for the lactating woman to be one that supplies somewhat more of each nutrient than that recommended for the nonpregnant female (Table 5-8). Obviously, the needs of individual women relate directly to the volume of milk produced daily.

Milk Volume

Observations of completely breast-fed babies who appear to be thriving suggest that daily volume of breast milk consumption ranges from 340 to over 1000 ml per day. The mean falls between 600 and 900 ml daily, at least for representative North American women. Mothers of twins may show an enhanced capacity for milk production. Hartmann,[33] in Western Australia, compared milk outputs of mothers of single infants with that of mothers of twins. The obvious difference in milk production is demonstrated in Fig. 5-10.

ENERGY

Prenatal Storage

During pregnancy most women store approximately 2 to 4 kg of body fat, which can be mobilized to supply a portion of the additional energy for lactation. It is estimated that stored fat will provide 200 to 300 kilocalories per day during a lactation period of 3 months. This amount of energy represents only part of the energy cost to produce milk. The remainder of the energy needs should be derived from the daily diet during the first 3 months of lactation. During this time lactation can be successfully supported and readjustment of maternal fat stores can take place. If lactation continues beyond the initial 3 months or if maternal weight falls below the ideal weight for height, the daily extra energy allowance may need to be increased accordingly. If more than one infant is being nursed during the first few months of life, maternal kilocalorie stores will be more quickly used, and daily supplemental energy needs may double when maternal stores are depleted.

Efficiency of Milk Production

The efficiency of milk production has been estimated by several researchers by the observation of energy intake and energy utilization of breast-feeding and non-breast-feeding mothers. English and Hitchcock[34] compared the energy intake of 16 nursing

TABLE 5-8 Recommended Daily Dietary Allowances for Lactation

	Age			
	11-14 Years	15-18 Years	19-22 Years	23-50 Years
BODY SIZE				
Weight (kg)	46	55	55	55
(lb)	101	120	120	120
Height (cm)	157	163	163	163
(in)	62	64	64	64
NUTRIENTS				
Energy (kcal)	2700	2600	2600	2500
Protein (g)	66	66	64	64
Vitamin A (RE*)	1200	1200	1200	1200
Vitamin D (μg)	15	15	12.5	10
Vitamin E activity (mgαTE)†	13	13	13	13
Ascorbic acid (mg)	90	100	100	100
Folacin (μg)	500	500	500	500
Niacin (mg‡)	20	19	19	18
Riboflavin (mg)	1.8	1.8	1.8	1.7
Thiamin (mg)	1.6	1.6	1.6	1.5
Vitamin B_6 (mg)	2.3	2.5	2.5	2.5
Vitamin B_{12} (μg)	4.0	4.0	4.0	4.0
Calcium (mg)	1600	1600	1200	1200
Phosphorus (mg)	1600	1600	1200	1200
Iodine (μg)	200	200	200	200
Iron (mg)	18§	18§	18§	18§
Magnesium (mg)	450	450	450	450
Zinc (mg)	25	25	25	25

Modified from Food and Nutrition Board, National Research Council, National Academy of Sciences: Recommended dietary allowances, ed. 9, Washington, D.C., 1980, U.S. Government Printing Office.

**RE,* Retinol equivalent.

†α-Tocopherol equivalents; 1 mg d-α-tocopherol = 1 αTE.

‡Although allowances are expressed as niacin, it is recognized that on the average, 1 mg of niacin is derived from each 60 mg of dietary tryptophan.

§Iron needs during lactation are not substantially different from those of nonpregnant women, but continued supplementation of the mother for 2 to 3 months after parturition is advisable to replenish stores depleted by pregnancy.

mothers and 10 nonnursing mothers and found that the energy intake of breastfeeders in the sixth and eighth postpartum week was 2460 kilocalories per day. The energy intake of nonnursing mothers during the same postpartum period was 1880 kilocalories per day—a difference of 580 kilocalories. In a later study lactating women were found to take in 2716 kilocalories per day and nonnursing mothers 2125 kilocalories—a difference resulting from nursing of 590 kilocalories. By adding the assumed energy equivalents of body weight being lost, total energy available to the two groups was about 2977 and 2364 kilocalories per day, respectively. If one assumes that the energy requirements for basal metabolism and activity are equivalent for the two groups, the energy needed for daily milk production is close to 560 kilocalories. The production efficiency of human milk is therefore about 90%.

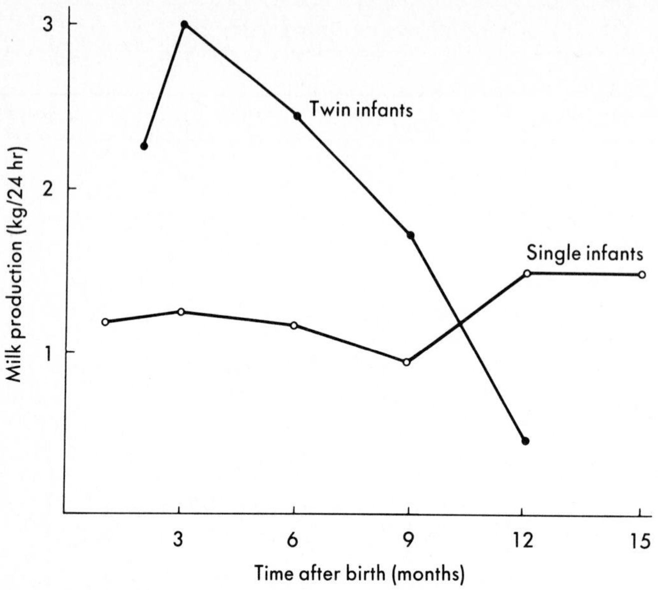

FIG. 5-10 Milk outputs of Western Australian women breast-feeding twins and exclusively breast-feeding single babies.
(Based on data from Hartmann, P.E., et al.: Birth Fam. J. **8**:215, 1981.)

Energy Needs

Recent observations of lactating women have led some researchers to propose that energy needs have been overestimated. Butte and others[35] found that typical women who were producing about 750 ml of milk per day had a mean daily energy intake of 2171 + 545 kilocalories per day. Observations of postpartum weight-loss patterns and subsequent calculations of energy balance led them to an estimation of 80% efficiency in energy utilization for milk production. When energy available from the diet (2171 kilocalories per day) was added to the energy derived from tissue mobilization (315 kilocalories per day) and the caloric equivalent of the milk was subtracted (597 kilocalories per day), a net balance of 1889 kilocalories per day was left for maintenance and activity. These findings suggest that successful lactation is compatible with gradual weight reduction and attainable with energy intakes less than current recommendations.

Similarly, Manning-Dalton and Allen[36] evaluated postpartum weight loss patterns, breast-feeding completeness, and daily kilocalorie intakes of well-nourished North American women. In spite of low mean kilocalorie intakes (2178 kilocalories per day), breast-feeding was successful, and weight loss during the 12 to 90 days post partum averaged only 2.0 kg for the entire sample and 1.6 kg for the solely breast-feeding women. These authors emphasize that almost every aspect of maternal energy balance in lactation needs further investigation. In the meantime it should be recognized that the RDA for energy in lactation is probably higher than necessary, especially for the well-nourished women with a sedentary lifestyle. It is also apparent that the commonly held belief that breast-feeding helps the mother lose weight cannot be substantiated.

Postpartum Maternal Weight Concerns

For many women the usual slow rate of weight loss after childbirth may not satisfy their desires for immediate return to prepregnancy body weight. It is therefore likely that dietary restriction may be self-imposed, even though it is discouraged by health professionals. It is important to recognize, however, that moderate to severe restriction of caloric intake during lactation will compromise the woman's ability to synthesize milk. This is especially significant in the early weeks of lactation initiation before the process is firmly established. As a result of this effect of caloric restriction on milk production, lactating women should be advised to accept a gradual rate of weight loss in the first 6 months after childbirth. Otherwise, lactation success may be limited and the infant may suffer from insufficient milk supply to meet growth needs.

PROTEIN

Basis for Protein Need

Along with the recommended energy increment, a 20 g increase in daily protein intake is advised for lactating women. The extra protein is believed to be necessary to cover the requirement for milk production with an allowance of 70% efficiency of protein utilization.

Diet Increase

The increased needs for protein, as well as energy, can be met easily by consumption of about 3 to 4 extra cups per day of whole milk. This will provide the needed protein and energy but will not cover the increased recommendations for other nutrients—ascorbic acid, vitamin E, and folic acid. Thus other foods such as citrus fruits, vegetable oils, and leafy green vegetables will also need to be added to the daily diet to supply them.

VEGETARIAN DIETS

Maintenance of lactation while consuming a vegetarian diet can be managed well, providing all the basic principles of sensible vegetarian eating are followed carefully. The nutritional needs of the lactating vegetarian woman are the same as those of the lactating woman with a more traditional diet. Appropriate extra sources of kilocalories and protein must be clearly defined. If dairy products are acceptable in the chosen dietary regimen, extra milk can be used as indicated. If dairy products are not included in the accepted list of foods, extra energy and high-quality protein must be obtained from appropriately combined vegetables, legumes, grains, nuts, and other such food sources in large amounts. Calcium needs can be met by eating large quantities of leafy green vegetables, calcium-fortified foods, and other significant sources of vegetable calcium. Dietary supplements may be unacceptable. Thus intelligent daily diet planning is essential for maintenance of successful lactation and health of the vegetarian mother.

THE QUESTION OF SUPPLEMENTATION

Dietary Supply

Although lactation increases a woman's requirement for nearly all nutrients, these increased needs can be provided by a well-balanced diet as outlined. For this reason nutritional supplements are generally unnecessary except when there is a deficient intake of one or more nutrients. It is true, for example, if the lactating woman does not tolerate milk, calcium supplementation as well as alternative energy and protein sources are needed to help prevent unnecessary calcium withdrawal from bones.

Calcium Needs

Although there is no evidence that calcium composition of human milk can be influenced by dietary intake of calcium, it is well known that dietary calcium deficiency promotes mobilization of calcium from bones to maintain milk calcium levels during lactation. Older clinical literature documents cases of osteomalacia in mothers who nursed their infants for long periods of time while on inadequate diets. Also, it has been proposed that the relatively high incidence of osteomalacia and osteoporosis in the United States is partially related to the waning intake of dairy products by adult women, particularly those who have supported multiple pregnancies and lactation experiences. Whether or not this is the case is still unknown. It stands to reason, however, that prolonged lactation accompanied by poor calcium intake may significantly compromise the calcium status of the skeletal system and increase its susceptibility to fractures and other forms of trauma.

COST OF NUTRITIONAL SUPPORT FOR LACTATION

The cost of providing adequate nutritional support for the lactating mother depends heavily upon what foods she selects to meet her nutritional needs. Some older studies suggest that human milk costs more than bottle-feeding because of the extra nutrients the mother must consume. It is clear, however, in examining the costs of appropriate extra foods for the lactating mother that human milk is cheaper than proprietary cow's milk formulas if economical food choices are made (Tables 5-9, 5-10, and 5-11). The present difference between the costs of commercially prepared cow's-milk formulas and human milk undoubtedly will continue to increase in coming years, since the price of "double cycle" animal food products, including cow's milk, continues to escalate. Beyond the price consideration, however, it is hard to justify "wastage" of human milk and the resultant unnecessary draw on the precious supply of other animal protein available to the world's population. Human milk represents a vital national resource, which if utilized to its fullest extent, could markedly improve not only the health and nutritional status of today's children but also the "natural resource base" of many underdeveloped countries.

TABLE 5-9 Nutrients, Amounts, and Estimated Cost of Foods Needed to Meet Additional Nutritional Requirements of a Lactating Woman: Standard (Nonbudget) Plan

Suggested Foods	Amounts	Cost*	Calories	Protein	A	C	B_1	B_2	B_3	Calcium	Iron
Milk, fresh, 2%	2 cups	.28	290	18	700		0.14	0.82	0.4	576	
Meat (round steak)	2 oz	.60	150	13	35		0.04	0.11	2.8	6	1.7
Vegetable, dark green or yellow (broccoli, cooked)	¾ cup	.18	20	2.5	1990	70	0.07	0.15	0.6	68	0.6
Other vegetable or fruit (grapefruit)	½	.15	45	1	10	44	0.05	0.02	0.2	19	0.5
Citrus fruit (orange juice)	½ cup	.14	60	1	275	60	0.11	0.01	0.5	12	0.1
Enriched (or whole grain) bread	1 slice	.07	65	3			0.09	0.03	0.8	24	0.8
TOTAL		1.42	630	38.5	3010	174	0.5	1.14	5.3	705	3.7

*Costs of June 1986, Seattle, Wash.

TABLE 5-10 Nutrients, Amounts, and Estimated Cost of Foods Needed to Meet Additional Nutritional Requirements of a Lactating Woman: Budget Plan

Suggested Foods	Amounts	Cost*	Calories	Protein	A	C	B_1	B_2	B_3	Calcium	Iron
Nonfat dry milk (prepared for drinking)	2 cups	.19	180	18	20		0.18	0.88	0.40	592	
Peanut butter	2 oz	.19	190	8			0.04	0.04	4.8	18	0.6
Vegetable, dark green or yellow (carrots, cooked)	¾ cup	.17	25	0.5	7610	4.5	0.04	0.03	0.04	24	0.45
Citrus fruit (tomato juice)	½ cup	.08	25	1	970	20	0.06	0.04	0.95	86	1.1
Enriched (or whole grain) bread	2 slices	.14	130	6			0.18	0.06	1.6	48	1.6
TOTAL		.77	550	33.5	8600	24.5	0.5	1.05	7.79	768	3.75

*Costs of June 1986, Seattle, Wash.

TABLE 5-11 Cost Per Day of the Most Commonly Used Prepared Formulas, Basic Equipment, and Fuel*

Formula Products and Other Expenses	Cost Per Day with Bottles and Nipples			Cost Per Day with Disposable Holders and Liners		
Dry, powdered (52 scoops per can)	$1.40			$1.40		
Double-strength liquid (13 oz. can)		1.49			1.49	
Ready-to-feed liquid (32 oz can)			2.19			2.19
Unbreakable bottles with nipples ($10.68/dozen)	.08	.08	.08			
Extra nipples ($3.32/dozen)	.02	.02	.02			
Electricity (to clean and sterilize water/bottles)	.03	.03	.03			
OR						
Disposable holders				.06	.06	.06
Liners (one used per feed)				.13	.13	.13
TOTAL	$1.53	1.62	2.32	$1.59	1.68	2.38

*Costs of June 1986, Seattle, Wash.

Advantages of Breast-Feeding

BASIC VALUES

Human milk is adapted to the needs of human infants. The process of lactation is normal for mammals. Thus it is not surprising that a number of advantages have been defined for mothers and infants who participate in the breast-feeding experience (see box, p. 185). The degree of advantage varies among mother-infant pairs, since availability of alternative foods, environmental conditions, and lifestyle characteristics are

PROPOSED ADVANTAGES OF BREAST-FEEDING

1. Breast milk is nutritionally superior to any alternative.
2. Breast milk is bacteriologically safe and always fresh.
3. Breast milk contains a variety of anti-infectious factors and immune cells.
4. Breast milk is the least allergenic of any infant food.
5. Breast-fed babies are less likely to be overfed.
6. Breast-feeding promotes good jaw and tooth development.
7. Breast-feeding *generally* costs less than the commercial infant formulas currently available.
8. Breast-feeding automatically promotes close mother-child contact.
9. Breast-feeding is *generally* more convenient once the process is established.

markedly different from one setting to another. Reviewing the issue with an open mind, however, leaves no doubt that in the majority of situations breast-feeding provides distinct benefits for both child and family.

ANTI-INFECTIVE PROPERTIES

Around the turn of the century there was little knowledge of microbiology or of immunology, and bottle-fed infants suffered from a much higher incidence of diarrhea and acute gastrointestinal tract infection. They also experienced higher mortality rates than breast-fed infants. Throughout much of the United States and the industrialized West, techniques for microbial control of the artificial diet have lessened the differences in mortality between bottle-fed and breast-fed infants. However, small differences are still apparent in the number and severity of illnesses contracted by bottle-fed and breast-fed infants.

Although the protective effect of breast milk is fully appreciated, not all studies show that breast-fed babies demonstrate reduced morbidity. It is also true that the reported morbidity among breast-fed infants may have nothing to do with the anti-infectious properties of human milk but might instead relate to different parenting strategies or lifestyle characteristics of mothers who choose to breast-feed instead of bottle-feed. Whatever the case, substantial data provide for the notion that breast-feeding reduces infant morbidity, especially in the early months of life.

OPTIMAL NUTRITION

Berger[37] suggests that one of the main advantages of breast-feeding is freedom from "formulogenic disease." The complications of improper dilutions such as incorrect caloric density and excessive renal solute load are not concerns for breast-fed babies. Colostrum and breast milk contain factors whose functions are unclear, as well as micronutrients whose value to the newborn only becomes apparent when they are omitted from infant formulas. Human milk appears to have a fat composition and protein content ideally suited to the growth rate of the human infant; it is the standard by which formulas are measured.

APPROPRIATE GROWTH AND DEVELOPMENT

Comparative Growth Curves

Bottle-fed and breast-fed infants follow similar growth curves from birth until the third or fourth month of age. From the fourth month on, the bottle-fed infant gains weight at a faster rate, especially beyond the sixth month of life. A sizable number of pediatric specialists feel that the slower rate of growth among older breast-fed infants represents the ideal pattern for optimal health. It has even been suggested that the National Center for Health Statistics standards are not appropriate for evaluating the growth performance of breast-fed infants and that growth curves based exclusively on breast-fed infants should be used for that purpose. Thus far such curves are not available, and agreement about what represents optimal growth in infancy has not yet been reached.

Efficiency of Milk Utilization

Butte and others[38] have demonstrated recently, however, the efficiency with which human milk is utilized by the young infant for maintenance and growth. Forty-five healthy, full-term infants who were exclusively breast-fed were observed for the first 4 months of life. The amount of breast milk ingested over a 24-hour period was determined by test-weighing using automatic electronic scales. At each feeding over a subsequent 24-hour period, milk samples were expressed from alternate breasts for analysis. Although adequate growth was demonstrated by the infants, this was accomplished with energy and protein intakes substantially less than that which is currently recommended. In the case of energy the following observations were recorded:

	Energy Intake (kcal/day)	Energy Intake (kcal/kg/day)
1 month	520 ± 131	110 ± 24
2 months	468 ± 115	83 ± 19
3 months	458 ± 124	74 ± 20
4 months	477 ± 111	71 ± 17

REDUCED RISK OF ALLERGY

Basis of Allergic Response

Development of food allergy has been associated with the penetration into the body of intact proteins or large peptide fragments with antigenic determinants. Under ordinary circumstances, secretory antibodies, efficient intraluminal digestion, and impermeable intestinal epithelial cells and intercellular junctions combine to form a "mucosal barrier" in the healthy intestine. Intestinal absorption of whole protein macromolecules is thought to be maximal in the newborn period and to decrease with age. Formula feeding, as opposed to breast-feeding, has been associated with increased susceptibility to food allergies. Whether this is more directly related to exposure to "foreign" antigens in commercial formulas, to differences in intestinal morphology with different food sources, to a protective action of breast milk, or to a combination of these mechanisms has not been determined. Recent studies suggest that breast milk may promote early closure of the mucosal barrier. In other studies antibodies directed toward milk components have been found in human milk, and these may be involved in the prevention of allergies by hindering the intestinal absorption of intact immunogenic food proteins by the neonate.

Family History

Although arguments against the value of breast-feeding for allergy prevention have been presented in the literature with some vigor, these contributions clearly represent the minority viewpoint. It seems appropriate, therefore, that families with a history of allergy should be counseled about the desirability of breast-feeding combined with an allergen-avoidance diet for the baby during the majority of the first year of life.

Breast Milk Allergens

Allergy to breast milk is uncommon, and some researchers question whether it exists at all. It has been shown, however, that allergens from foods that a mother consumes may enter her breast milk and occasionally promote an allergic reaction in a sensitive infant. Colic in breast-fed babies has been blamed on adverse response to cow's milk allergens in mother's milk. Although a study reported in 1978[39] provided some support for this idea, a more recent investigation in which cow's milk was withdrawn from the maternal diet did not support this practice of alleviating colic in breast-fed infants.[40] Of interest in this latter investigation was the trend of increased rates of colic associated with increased diversity of maternal diet. Similarly, rates of colic were found to be significantly higher on days that mothers reported eating chocolate or fruit. Finally, six infants were recently observed who developed inflammatory protocolitis in the first month of life while being breast-fed exclusively.[41] Rectal biopsies showed a wide spectrum of acute and chronic inflammatory changes. All infants responded clinically to initiation of feeding with either a hydrolyzed casein or soy-protein-based formula. Breast-feeding was resumed in five of the six infants; all had immediate recurrence of symptoms. Elimination of cow's milk from the maternal diet led to tolerance of breast-feeding in two infants, but there was no change in the other three.

Although adverse reactions to consumption of breast milk are uncommon, they do occur. *Sometimes* alteration of maternal diet may be useful. Gerard[42] proposes that if food allergies are present on both sides of the family, the lactating mother should vary her diet and avoid large intake of any one specific food, particularly cow's milk and egg products. If the baby later develops symptoms suggestive of allergy, the mother should modify her diet rather than feed her baby cow's milk or soy formula.

NORMAL PSYCHOLOGIC DEVELOPMENT

Breast-feeding has been referred to as the period of "exterior gestation" because it provides continuity with the intrauterine environment while providing security and nourishment. Some workers have suggested that prolactin, coupled with sensory input from the baby, produces "mothering" responses in most women. Many women who have raised both breast-fed and bottle-fed infants state that they feel a special closeness to the breast-fed child that has persisted into adult life. Much attention has been focused on what might be termed *mater-infant bonding.* Breast-feeding promotes strong emotional ties while meeting the infant's most basic physical need.

REDUCED RISK OF OBESITY

Attempts have been made to assess the value of breast-feeding as protection against the development of obesity. But present data do not allow for satisfactory assessment of the merits of these statements. Published reports have yielded conflicting findings. Thus for the time being it seems inappropriate to advocate breast-feeding as a means of protection against infantile obesity.

OTHER INFANT BENEFITS

An array of other advantages for babies has been proposed as being associated with breast-feeding. Many clinicians have suggested that low-birth-weight infants who are provided human milk are less likely to develop necrotizing enterocolitis. Auricchio and associates[43] have proposed that breast-feeding protects against the development of clinical symptoms of celiac disease. Support for these and other hypotheses is limited, but future observations may confirm their validity.

MATERNAL BENEFITS

Involution of Uterus

One of the earliest documented maternal benefits of breast-feeding is the effect of oxytocin on the involution of the uterus. Early breast-feeding, even on the delivery table, stimulates contractions of the uterus that help to control blood loss.

Suppression of Ovulation

The stimulation of the nipples and resultant secretion of prolactin suppress ovulation in many women, particularly when supplements and solids are not offered to the baby. This is believed to be of major significance in promoting short-term child spacing in the developing countries. When solid foods become a major source of nourishment for the child, nipple stimulation and prolactin levels decrease in the lactating mother, and ovulation and menstruation usually begin again.

Ease of Feeding

One of the prime benefits expressed by most women who breast-feed is the ease with which feeding is managed, particularly at night. The actual time spent nursing the infant may be greater during the first 2 weeks for the breast-feeding mother, since the infant eats more frequently to build up the mother's milk supply. More total time is spent in "nursing" by the bottle-feeding mother, however, since she must make the formula, clean the tools and bottles, and heat the feedings before serving them.

Economy

Cost can no longer be used as a *major reason* for breast-feeding in the United States, but for some women it may be a relevant factor. Although evaporated milk formula costs about the same as the additional food required by the lactating woman, proprietary formulas, especially ready-to-feed ones (the only type that rivals breast-feeding in convenience), may be more expensive than breast-feeding. For some people, both in the United States and elsewhere, the expense of a commercial formula is prohibitive.

Incidence of Breast-Feeding

GENERAL BACKGROUND

In spite of the recognized benefits of breast-feeding for the child and the mother, the number of babies in the United States who were formula-fed climbed to an estimated 82% in the two decades before 1970. Comparable statistics were reported from England and France in the period following World War II.

CURRENT TRENDS

Increased Practice

More recent reports indicate that this prior trend has reversed (Fig. 5-11).[44] More mothers are not only breast-feeding but also continuing to do so for a longer period of time throughout the months of their infants' most rapid growth and high nutritional demands. It is also apparent that the increased incidence of breast-feeding has not been limited to mothers with higher income or more education. From 1971 to 1981 the incidence at 2 months post partum more than tripled among mothers in lower income families. The incidence of breast-feeding increased fivefold among mothers whose education did not extend beyond elementary or high school. Incidence of breast-feeding among mothers on the WIC program has increased. As might be expected, breast-feeding in any one year, especially long term, is much more common among mothers who have successfully breast-fed a previous child. Even mothers of preterm infants, however, may nurse for long periods of time.

Maternal Employment

Recent surveys have considered the employment status of the mother as it relates to choices about infant feeding.[44,45] One report from a large survey in 1984 indicates that the incidence of breast-feeding among employed women is higher than among those who are unemployed. However, for infants at 5 and 6 months of age, the proportion of unemployed women breast-feeding is higher (Table 5-12).

Regional Differences

Regional differences have been reported in the current incidence of breast-feeding.[44] Among the U.S. Census regions in 1984, breast-feeding in hospitals was the least prevalent in the South East and South Central regions (46%-58%), and the most prevalent in the Mountain and Pacific regions (78%).

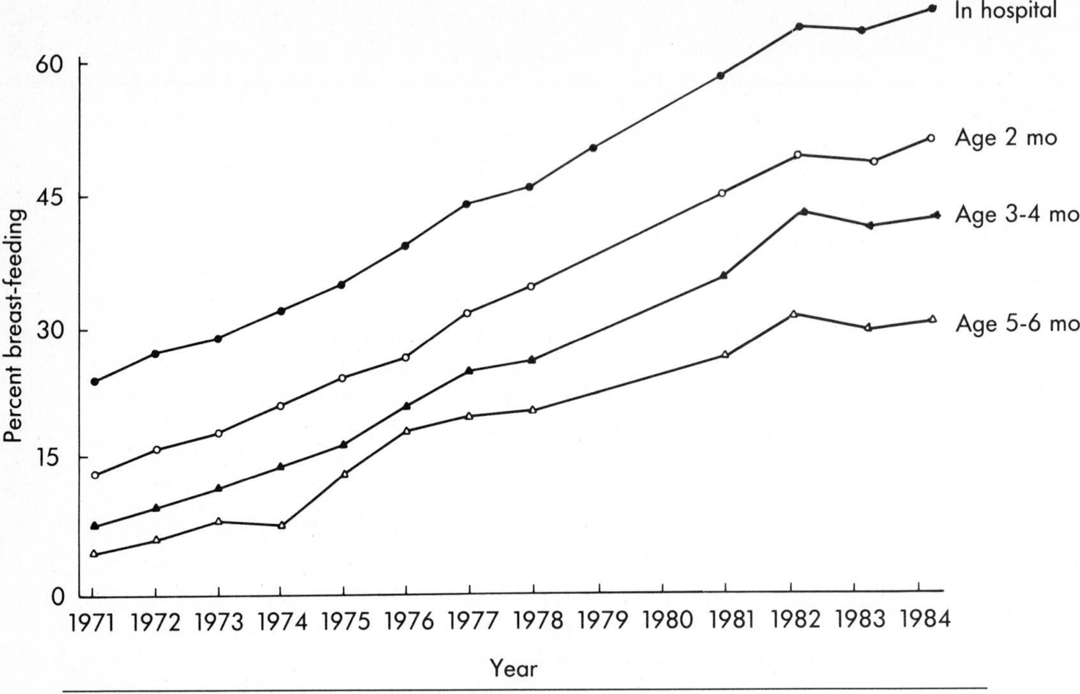

FIG. 5-11 Percent of infants in the United States breast-feeding at different ages (from 1971 to 1981).

(Based on data from Martinez, G.A., and Nalezienski, J.P.: The recent trend in breast-feeding, Pediatrics 64:686, 1979; Martinez, G.A., and Dodd, D.A.: 1981 milk feeding patterns in the United States during the first 12 months of life, Pediatrics 71:166, 1983; and Martinez, G.A., and Krieger, F.W.: 1984 milk-feeding patterns in the United States. Pediatrics 76:1004, 1985).

TABLE 5-12 Infants Breast-feeding in the Hospital and at 5 and 6 Months by Maternal Employment Status (1984)

Employment Status	In Hospital (%)	At 5-6 Months (%)
Full-time	56.2	12.3
Part-time	67.6	28.9
Total employed	60.3	18.2
Unemployed	58.6	29.2

Modified from Martinez, G.A., and Krieger, F.W.: 1984 Milk-feeding patterns in the United States, Pediatrics 76:1004, 1985.

Influence of Change in Medical Attitude

One of the greatest influences on the current trend toward breast-feeding is the change in medical attitude. Today the American Academy of Pediatrics (AAP) actively recommends breast-feeding, as indicated by the following report of its Committee on Nutrition.

Role of Health Professionals

ATTITUDE OF THE MEDICAL PROFESSION

AAP Recommendation

Beginning with its 1978 report, the American Academy of Pediatrics (AAP) has recommended that all physicians encourage mothers to breast-feed their infants.[46,47] The AAP Committee on Nutrition declared:

1. Despite technologic advances in infant formulas, breast milk is "the best food for every newborn infant."
2. All physicians need to become "much more knowledgeable" about infant nutrition in general and breast-feeding in particular.
3. Attitudes, practices, and instruction in prenatal clinics and maternity wards should be changed to encourage breast-feeding.
4. In hospitals, mothers and infants should be kept together after birth so babies can be fed on demand.
5. Not only should information about breast-feeding be supplied to all school children, but nursing should also be portrayed as natural on television and in other media.
6. To prevent conflict between breast-feeding and employment, legislation should mandate three- or four-month postdelivery leaves so that working mothers can breast-feed.

This hearty endorsement was followed in 1982[47] by a critical evaluation of how and why breast-feeding should be encouraged. The AAP again voiced its support for the promotion of breast-feeding but made note of the maternal characteristics and family circumstances that may need attention when deciding on infant feeding strategies.

Guidance and Education

The major role of the health-care provider is to educate families about the available alternatives for infant feeding. With accurate information about the advantages and disadvantages of each option, the family is then ready to make a choice. Without good justification, the clinician or teacher should not "push" a family into an infant feeding method that does not suit them. On the other hand, it is very clear that mothers who are most satisfied with the breast-feeding experience are those who have solid support within and without the home. The health care team can provide this support, and the AAP encourages this practice among its membership.

GUIDELINES FOR SUPPORT ACTIVITIES

To reinforce the needed changes in health care practices, the AAP provided specific guidelines for activities to support breast-feeding. The final recommendations of the AAP include the following practices:[47]

- Education about breast-feeding in school for boys as well as girls since later support by the father helps breast-feeding succeed
- Public education through television, newspapers, magazines, and radio to enhance the acceptability of breast-feeding

- Improved education about breast-feeding techniques in medical and nursing schools, and residency programs in obstetrics, pediatrics, and family practice
- Factual educational material designed to present advantages of breast-feeding
- Encouragement not to use breast-feeding alternatives for relief, vacation, or night feeding until nursing is well established
- Breast-feeding information provided in prenatal classes and at any prenatal contact
- Decreased sedation of the mother for labor and birth
- Extended contact between mother and infant in the first 25 hours
- Rooming-in encouraged except when specifically contraindicated
- Avoidance of routine supplemental feeding
- Lactation suppressants not given unless requested by the mother
- Discharge packs of formula given only at the descretion of the physician or at the request of the mother, not as a routine hospital practice
- Development of day nurseries adjacent to school or workplaces to encourage and support working and school-aged mothers to breast-feed
- Utilization of lay support groups such as La Leche League
- Encouragement of continued breast-feeding of the hospitalized child
- Relactation instruction when necessary

ESTABLISHING LACTATION

Need for Support and Instruction

The role of the health-care provider has become increasingly more important to successful lactation over the past few years. When most women lived in an extended family setting, there were abundant "models" for the new mother to emulate. She did not doubt that she could breast-feed her infant. Her grandmother, mother, and many friends had breast-fed children. The presence of these older women was also a source of supportive advice. Similarly, the knowledge of how to suckle the young of the species is no longer instinctive in some primates. Chimpanzees reared in captivity who have never observed a suckling pair of their species have considerable difficulty establishing lactation. In our modern society today many women live apart from their families. They may never have observed a mother breast-feeding her child. Therefore they may need considerable support and instruction from some other source if lactation is to be a successful undertaking.

Individual and Group Instruction

Most breast-feeding instruction is provided on an individual basis, counseling one mother at a time. However, larger clinics may find it beneficial to use group discussion for the prenatal and follow-up sessions. Good results have been obtained in group sessions when the teacher is skilled at managing discussion and is adequately prepared with factual material and teaching aids.

Consistent and Continuing Guidance

Rarely is the clinician who conducts the prenatal session the same one who provides instruction at the initial feeding session in the hospital. Care must be taken to provide continuity of advice and methods when many persons are involved. Contradictory information is little better than none at all. Through the use of in-service training sessions, standardized procedure manuals, and printed instructions for the new breast-feeding mother, consistent advice for mothers is assured.

Prenatal Counseling

THE DECISION TO BREAST-FEED

Parents' Attitudes

The decision to breast-feed is a significant one for the parents and is usually made relatively early in the pregnancy. Berger[37] has examined the factors that influence this decision and notes that they are complex and interrelated.

Professional Support

Where parents have not yet made a decision or have not been exposed to the advantages of breast-feeding, it is the responsibility of the health-care professionals to support lactation as the optimal method of infant feeding. Although health professionals must support the parents' ultimate decision regarding feeding method, they too often fail to take a positive stand in support of lactation early enough in the prenatal period to influence the decision-making process. It has long been recognized that physicians who support lactation have higher percentages of breast-feeding mothers among their patients.

Follow-up Instruction Opportunities

When the decision has been made to breast-feed, an individual or small group instruction session is indicated. Simply handing out pamphlets is not very effective. These sessions may be held early in the second trimester. Both parents should be included in the instruction session if possible. Fathers tend to be more supportive if they know what to expect and understand possible difficulties they may encounter. The prenatal visit provides the opportunity to get to know the parents, to find out how much they know about breast-feeding, what fears and apprehensions they may have, and to estimate how much help and support the mother is likely to need in the early weeks of breast-feeding. It is important to remember that there is a typical breast-feeding personality. Women who appear to be "nervous" can learn to breast-feed successfully if they cultivate a relaxed and confident attitude. This is best accomplished by adequate instruction along with professional and family support.

LACTATION EDUCATION PROGRAM

In the beginning of the lactation education program, the health professional should discuss the advantages of breast-feeding as outlined earlier here. He or she should listen and respond to any concerns that the parents may have. Then the physiology of lactation and the mother's diet will be discussed.

Physiology of Lactation

The general physiology of lactation should be covered, explaining briefly the structure of the breast and hormonal controls of the process. A good understanding of mammary gland physiology is a great aid in promoting confidence in the ability to lactate. Women should realize that breast size is not a factor in the success of lactation. They should be informed that the glandular structure is adequately developed in virtually all women during pregnancy and differences in breast size are mainly the result of variation in the content of adipose tissue. Simplified diagrams and explanations such as those provided here may be useful for breast-feeding education.

Diet for Lactation

A brief discussion of the dietary requirements for lactation should be included in the prenatal visits. It is usually sufficient to stress that additional amounts of the same types of foods that belong in any well-balanced diet, with special attention to good sources of calcium and vitamin C, will adequately provide the additional nutrition. Although fluid is an essential component of breast milk and its consumption should be encouraged, thirst accurately indicates fluid requirements in most women. The body's ability to conserve fluid by concentrating urine allows women to succeed in lactation with wide variations in levels of fluid intake.

NIPPLE CONDITIONING

Breast Support

Although several studies suggest that prenatal nipple conditioning does not prevent nipple soreness during early lactation, it may be useful for some women. In societies where the breast is uncovered or where clothing is loosely worn, nipple soreness is much less a problem. The woman who plans to breast-feed should purchase a nursing brassiere that will suffice for the increased size required for the last few months of pregnancy, as well as for lactation. If her breasts are very heavy, or if the woman feels uncomfortable with the weight unsupported, the brassiere can be worn day and night. One of the easiest ways to get the nipples used to tactile stimulation is to leave the flaps on the brassiere open as much as possible during the day and night. This allows the nipples to rub against clothing and gradually desensitizes them.

Salves and Soaps

No special ointments or preparations are generally required for nipple conditioning. Pure lanolin, a component of many of the breast creams on the market, appears to be harmless, but products containing alcohol or petroleum-based products are to be avoided, since they remove natural lubricants from the nipple and areola. Since soap is drying, it is advisable to wash the nipple area with water only.

Inverted Nipples

Inverted nipples occasionally occur. They can be diagnosed by pressing the areola between the thumb and forefinger. A flat or normal nipple will protrude; a truly inverted nipple will retract. Truly inverted nipples are rare. When they do occur, they can be treated by massage.

Nipple Shield

Not only may exercises be helpful in the prenatal period to prepare flat or inverted nipples for lactation, but also use of a nipple shield may be even more effective (Fig. 5-12). The rubber nipple tip of the shield should be removed and only the plastic base with the hole in the center applied over the areola inside a well-fitting brassiere. The constant even pressure will cause the nipple to evert through the hole. The shield can be worn daily for the last weeks or months of pregnancy. Only the plastic or glass ones should be used because the all-rubber shields pull on the skin, holding the moisture in.

EFFECT OF ANESTHETICS

Another major consideration to be discussed during prenatal visits is the effect of anesthetics and analgesics given during labor and delivery on early feedings. Research indicates that even the nerve conduction anesthetics affect the newborn's reflexes and may impair ability to suck well. The baby may be lethargic and disinterested in feeding or may take the breast and suck only weakly until the effects of the anesthesia have worn off. This information may be useful to the mother in selecting an anesthetic if it is to be used. The baby who is uncooperative because of sedation can still breast-feed successfully. Probably it will take just a few days longer to establish a let-down reflex and to produce an adequate milk supply. The baby who is severely affected may not suck well until after the third or fourth day of life. With the current trend toward early hospital discharges, it might be beneficial to keep mother and baby in the hospital for an extra day or two to provide good follow-up care at home to ensure that lactation gets off to a good start.

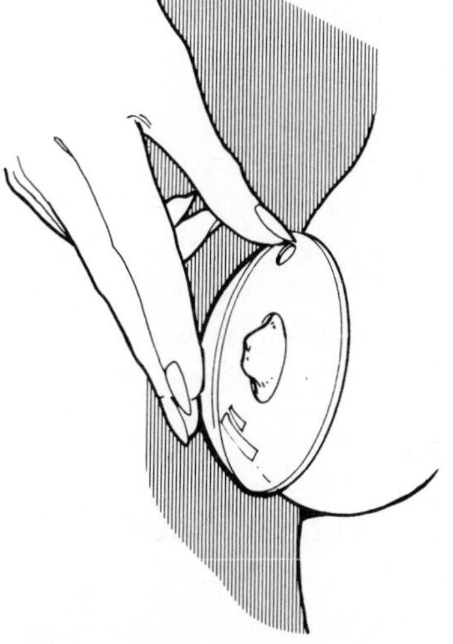

FIG. 5-12 Breast shield in place.

RESOURCES

The mother should be encouraged to jot down questions that arise. Several excellent books on breast-feeding are referenced at the end of this chapter. Most are available in paperback and from public libraries. Some large clinics have established their own lending libraries. Clients will benefit from talking with mothers who are already successfully breast-feeding. If no suitable candidates can be found from office files, local chapters of La Leche League, an international organization of mothers and professionals dedicated to spreading information about breast-feeding, will usually be able to assist the parents.

IN-HOSPITAL POSTPARTUM SUPPORT

Importance of Initial Days

The most critical period in establishing lactation is the first 7 to 10 days after birth. Fortunately, for a portion of this time, most new mothers are in a hospital and can receive almost continuous instruction and support. A follow-up call a few days after discharge is also beneficial. Early discharge with trained home-care follow-up is also an alternative.

The First Feeding

Although many hospital routines prohibit early feeding, the overwhelming bulk of recent research shows that the best time for the first feeding, providing that mother and baby are physically able, is within a half hour after birth. This can be accomplished on the delivery table.

Nature of First Feedings

The first few feedings will provide colostrum, which has been shown to be very beneficial to the infant. In addition to colostrum's nutritional bonus, drainage of this viscous material from the ducts in prelacteal feedings prevents problems of stasis and engorgement and stimulates milk production. There is little scientific support for the practice of giving glucose water for the first feeding.

Support for the New Mother

Breast-feeding will often be a new experience for the mother, as well as for the baby. She may be apprehensive and unsure of herself, and need help and guidance in handling the infant. The clinician who is to instruct the mother at the first feeding should try to make her feel as much at ease as possible. The father should be encouraged to be present at feedings and during instruction if the hospital permits it and if the mother is comfortable with his presence. The father's support, knowledge, and understanding will be valuable later on. Also, he may remember techniques and advice the mother has forgotten.

Typical Concerns of the Breast-Feeding Mother

Even though the prenatal and early postnatal assistance with lactation may have been of high quality, it is likely that mothers will have additional problems and questions during the first few weeks. A variety of concerns often develop and attention to these concerns may well determine the duration of breast-feeding for some distraught mothers.

ANXIETY OVER QUANTITY AND QUALITY OF MILK SUPPLY

Sufficient Quantity

Milk is produced to equal demand in almost all women. If the let-down reflex is functioning adequately, insufficient milk is rarely a problem. The mother's concern may come from a well-meaning friend or relative who has casually remarked, "Mrs. X didn't have enough milk for her baby so she had to bottle-feed." Nurses and other helpers should try to impress on the new breast-feeding mother that in many societies of the world all women breast-feed their babies. And virtually *all* women in our society who really want to breast-feed can do so, too. If feeding sessions have been frequent and of adequate duration, the milk supply is probably ample. Some pediatricians suggest careful monitoring of the infant's growth by weighing every week during the first month of life. A gain of about 190 g per week is suggested. This can be reassuring to the mother and can help the clinician detect growth problems earlier.

Baby's Responses

Mothers may need to be reminded that babies do not always cry from hunger. Sometimes they may need to be "bubbled" or have diapers changed. Often they may merely require companionship and sometimes a baby seems to need to cry—for no apparent reason. If the baby is growing well and has at least six wet diapers a day, assuming he is receiving no additional water or formula, the mother should be comforted by knowing that the milk supply is adequate and that this fussy baby might be even fussier if he were being bottle-fed.

Milk Quality

Too many well-meaning "advisors" are quick to volunteer that "your milk obviously doesn't agree with him" or "he's got gas (or colic); it must be something you ate." Such comments immediately give the mother a sense of guilt. Although the protein and fat content of human milk varies slightly according to time of day, stage of lactation, and the individual woman, evidence indicates that maternal nutrient stores "subsidize" the requirements of lactation if an occasional day's dietary intake is inadequate. Therefore breast milk is seldom "too rich" or "too thin" if the maternal diet is adequate and the let-down reflex functions.

Mother's Diet and Rest

Adverse reaction to foods in the maternal diet has been known to occur. From 4 to 6 hours are required for components of metabolites of a specific food to appear in breast milk. The food producing a reaction can often be identified and omitted from the mother's diet. Most foods that could be tolerated during pregnancy will be well tolerated by the mother and the infant during lactation. If a food consistently seems to bother mother or child, it can be omitted to see if relief, real or imagined, occurs.

Adequate rest, diet, and fluids are essential, especially if the milk supply needs to be increased. Mothers do not "lose" their milk. However, sometimes a busy schedule and lack of food or rest interfere with milk production. When this happens it is wise to take a day off to "make more milk." With rest, fluids, good diet, and of course more frequent feedings, milk supply usually parallels demand within 24 to 48 hours. Growth spurts, thus increasing demand, are common at about 6 to 12 weeks of age.

Other General Anxieties

Other causes for anxiety are the softening of the breast that occurs once lactation has become established, the presence (or absence) of milk leaking, changes in infant stool patterns, and lack of sleeping through the night. All of these are normal and do not indicate lack of breast milk. Growth failure is the only true indication of inadequate nutrition in the normal breast-fed infant. When this occurs it is most frequently observed after the baby is 6 months of age. About this time some women find that their breast milk alone does not provide sufficient nutrition to maintain optimal growth. In fact, however, research has demonstrated that exclusive breast-feeding can be adequate for periods varying from 2 to 15 months and that there is no specific age at which breast-feeding becomes inadequate.

Excess Milk Flow

Sometimes the mother's concern is actually an oversupply of milk. She should be encouraged to use manual expression to slow the flow of milk before a feeding and to express to a comfort level between feedings. This expressed milk may be frozen for supplements or donated to milk banks for premature or critically ill infants. The mother should continue to offer both breasts at each feeding but decrease time to 5 to 10 minutes per side. The use of a pacifier for increasing sucking time may be desirable.

NIPPLE SORENESS

Normal Reaction vs. True Problem

Many women who breast-feed experience varying degrees of general nipple discomfort when feeding. The discomfort associated with the first few seconds of feeding and alleviated by the feeding is normal. It is caused by the stimulation of the breast tissue by oxytocin during let-down. True nipple soreness, which is accompanied by tenderness and redness of the areola, is evidence of tissue breakdown and is better prevented than treated.

Treatment

Some women, particularly those with fair skin, seem more susceptible to this problem. If nipples must be treated, they should be treated promptly rather than allowing the condition to progress to cracked and fissured nipples open to infection. In addition to the techniques already discussed for nipple conditioning and prevention of soreness, the following suggestions may be useful:

1. Check for proper tongue position below nipple and make sure the baby's grasp includes some of the areola. Express milk if necessary to allow proper grasp of nipple.

2. Feed the baby on demand. If he gets too hungry he may suck harder, causing further soreness.
3. Vary the position with each feeding, allowing the baby to suck on slightly different areas of the areola with each feeding.
4. Begin each feeding on the breast that is least tender. Allow the baby to suck until the let-down reflex has occurred, then switch to the tender side and allow the baby to empty the breast. Promptly return to the less tender side to finish the feeding.
5. Promptly terminate feedings when completed. Allowing an infant to suck on an empty breast causes increased tissue damage. From 7 to 10 minutes on each side should be sufficient if nipples are tender. Offer a pacifier if necessary.
6. Let nipples dry well before replacing brassiere flaps, allowing air to circulate on them as freely as possible. Air drying for 10 minutes after a feeding and before using any breast cream is a good procedure.
7. Avoid using soaps, alcohol, and especially petroleum-based compounds on the nipple area, as they cause further irritation. Lanolin or a commercial breast cream may be applied after the areola has dried. Tannic acid has long been recognized for its role in promoting healing. Thus some mothers have found that a used tea bag, thoroughly cooled and applied to the nipple area two or three times a day, helps to promote healing.

ENGORGEMENT

Causes

Engorged breasts are hot, heavy, and hard with milk. Many physicians and nurses see this as basically a hospital-acquired condition caused by infrequent feeding. This is at least partly true, and the consequences may be a hungry, frustrated baby and a mother suffering from pain and stress. However, in some women a general increase in circulation to the mammary tissue and edema in the tissues are thought to combine with the newly produced milk to cause mild to extreme discomfort, regardless of feeding frequency. The only component of this condition that can be remedied is the milk. There is no more effective "breast pump" than a hungry baby.

Treatment

During engorgement the baby should be put to breast at least every 3 hours. The mother should compress the areola between two fingers to make it easier for the infant to grasp (Fig. 5-13). If the milk supply greatly exceeds demand, the baby should be allowed to suck only to relieve the sensation of fullness (about 5 minutes at each breast). Some milk may be manually expressed before offering the breast to the baby if the nipple is difficult for the baby to grasp. If the baby is uncooperative or sleepy manual expression will have to be used to relieve the pressure of accumulating milk. A firmly fitting brassiere may make engorgement less painful.

Many women find relief from discomfort by the application of moist heat to the breast. This may be done with wet towels, a warm shower or bath, or steam from a sink or basin of water. For the ambulatory mother suffering from engorgement, face cloths

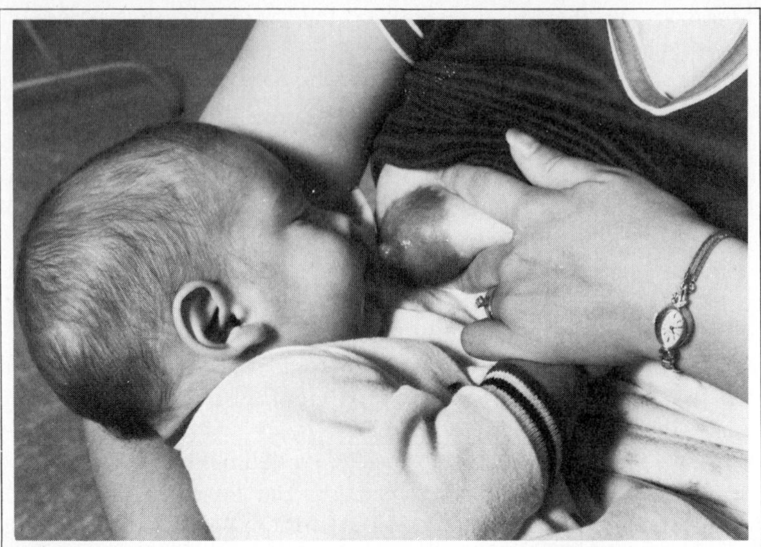

FIG. 5-13 When breast is offered to infant, areola is gently compressed between two fingers and breast supported to ensure that infant is able to grasp areola adequately.
(From Lawrence, R.: Breastfeeding: a guide for the medical profession, St. Louis, 1980, Times Mirror/Mosby College Publishing.)

wet with warm water and folded into plastic bags can be held in place by the brassiere. Since much of the discomfort is caused by edema resulting from venous stasis, moist heat to increase the circulation would seem a more beneficial prescription than ice packs. However, some women have found that ice or cold packs make them feel better, possibly because cold merely dulls the sensation of discomfort. Massage is also useful to help soften the breast and assist the baby in draining the ducts. If the mother is really uncomfortable, a mild analgesic can be recommended. Typically, engorgement occurs only on the first full day of milk production and is of short duration, usually about 24 hours.

LEAKING

A number of women experience leaking from their breasts during the first few weeks of breast-feeding. Usually it is caused by fullness in the breast or the milk letting down and is part of normal breast-feeding experience. It may occur during a nursing from the opposite breast, just before a nursing when the breasts are full, or when nursings are missed altogether. Sometimes it is caused by psychologic conditioning. For example, a woman may leak in response to hearing a baby cry, picking up her own baby to nurse, or simply thinking about breast-feeding her baby. Some mothers may be reassured by leaking, since it is a sign of a plentiful milk supply and a functioning letdown. Often the mother and baby only need time to adjust to one another, and leaking will subside as harmony develops between supply and demand.

SUPPLEMENTAL FEEDINGS

Occasional Bottle-Feeding

Rare is the mother who does not want—indeed, need—to be away from her infant for a brief period that will undoubtedly include a feeding. For this reason it is a good idea to introduce the baby to the occasional bottle at least by the end of the first month and about once a week or so thereafter. Many infants do not accept a bottle from their mothers but will take it from father or a sitter. The infant who is accustomed to breast-feeding will often swallow more air with a bottle-feeding and may need to be "bubbled" more frequently, particularly if he seems to take the milk very quickly.

Preparation of Single Feeding

Powdered formula offers advantages for use as a single feeding supplement when human milk is not available. The proper number of measures of powder can be placed in the bottle and the nipple and cap put in place. Then if the bottle is needed, about half of the required amount of cold water can be added. The bottle should be shaken thoroughly to dissolve the powder, and then the remainder of the liquid should be added as very warm water. Formula dilutions are less likely, the bottle is at serving temperature, and the cost is considerably less than ready-to-feed formula—a real advantage if the baby only takes 1 to 2 oz and the remainder has to be discarded. If the unmixed bottle is not needed, it can safely be left in the diaper bag for the next time. If refrigerated, a can of formula powder will last at least 6 months.

EXPRESSION OF MILK

Manual Technique

Manual expression of milk is a useful technique for the breast-feeding mother to learn. Although some women may find it a laborious procedure, there is often no substitute. Actually, the procedure is simple. First apply moist heat to the breast and massage for 5 to 10 minutes before expression or until a let-down reflex can be obtained. Then place the thumb on top and the forefinger under the areolar margin, gently pushing the finger and thumb back toward the chest wall to grasp behind the milk sinuses (Fig. 5-14). Squeeze gently in a "pumping" motion toward the nipple to remove the milk that has collected in the milk sinuses. Repeat the procedure, rotating the position of the grasp on the nipple occasionally so that all the sinuses are drained. Some women will find that the milk flows freely once a let-down occurs. Others will only be able to express a few drops at a time.

Breast Pump

Mothers who need to express milk for a period of a day or weeks, such as in the case of a working mother or the mother of a hospitalized infant, might find it considerably easier and more comfortable to use a breast pump. Some very good manual pumps are now on the market, and several high-quality electric breast pumps are also available. Each one simulates the nursing experience by providing alternating periods of negative and positive pressure. Many cities have rental sources of breast pumps. La Leche League maintains a rental supply of electric breast pumps in some cities. Manual breast

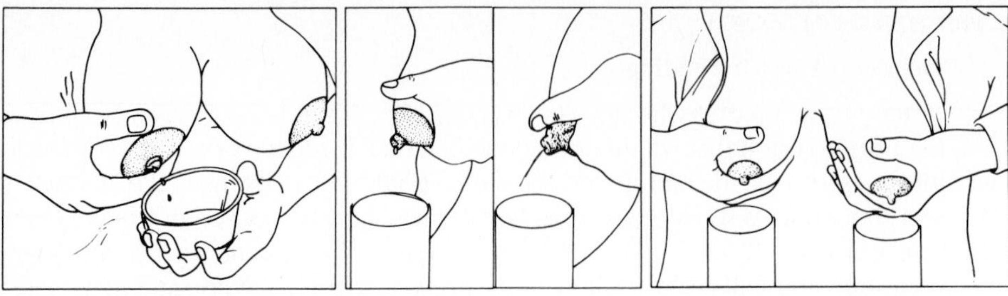

FIG. 5-14 Manual expression of breast milk. Front view, side view, and two-handed method for efficient women with good aim.

pumps frequently do not work well and can cause considerable discomfort and even nipple damage because of the tremendous uninterrupted negative pressure used to extract the milk.

STORAGE OF MILK

Safe Storage

If expressed human milk is to be saved for future feeding, care must be taken to assure that it is safe from microbes with minimal loss of its nutritional or protective characteristics. Fresh human milk is bacteriologically safe for up to, but no longer than, 6 hours after expression.[48] Freezing not only protects milk from contamination but also promotes minimal change in milk composition.[49] Membranes of milk cells are destroyed by this process and some hydrolysis of triglycerides occurs.[50] However, immunoglobulin levels, antibody titers, and nutritional properties are virtually unchanged. Heat treatment and lyophilization promote additional losses.[51,52] Fat and protein digestibility are reduced and milk cells damaged. Also, levels of many of the protective factors are substantially reduced. Recent data suggest, however, that rapid high-temperature treatment allows for retention of nutritional and immunologic qualities.[53]

Types of Containers

Several efforts have been made to determine if the type of storage container influences the quality of the milk. Paxson and Cress[54] reported that the placement of human milk into glass containers markedly reduces retrieval of the white cells even though phagocytosis is unaffected. These workers recommended that human milk be collected in plastic containers. However, Goldblum and associates[55] reported that the type of container made little difference in the number of identifiable cells after 4 hours of storage. They also found that levels of some of the protective factors declined with storage during the 4-hour period, but no one type of container proved to be superior for the storage of all of the measured immunologic factors. These investigators concluded that because of the profound loss of sIgA antibodies in polyethylene bags, the difficulty in handing the flexible bags, and the potential breakage of the Pyrex glass containers, polypropylene containers were best for future work.

DURATION OF BREAST-FEEDING

Tradition

The tradition in most parts of the world is to breast-feed for 2 to 3 years. Weaning is rather natural at this age, since the child can now feed himself and eat a full adult diet. He also has teeth and can walk and talk a little and thus express wishes and disagreements. The mother, too, may again become pregnant at this time so that her attention will need to be directed toward the new infant.

Spontaneous Termination

Many young children spontaneously give up breast-feeding at about 1 year of age or soon thereafter, especially if they are receiving adequate supplementary foods. Some mothers feel much relief, and others feel sad or rejected. Some children cling to the breast for years, and again maternal response to this behavior is mixed. There are also a few children who cling to the breast and refuse to eat solid foods. These are usually children 1 year of age who have had solids introduced too late. It is essential that these children be trained to eat solid food, and the sooner the training takes place, the easier it will be for the parent.

Individual Decision

The individual mother-child couple must determine their own ideal duration of breast-feeding. Factors to consider include:

1. Convenience of the mother
2. Needs of the child, both psychologic and physiologic
3. Availability of satisfactory alternative or supplemental foods
4. Custom in the community

Whether a mother breast-feeds her child for 2 months or 2 years, the main concern of the health-care provider is to support the mother in her decision, and to help her when necessary to avoid cutting short the period of breast-feeding against her wishes.

Special Problems

MATERNAL AND INFANT CONDITIONS

Contraindications to Lactation

Although each case must be evaluated individually, there are very few conditions that automatically preclude breast-feeding. The presence of drugs or other harmful contaminants in mother's milk may necessitate at least temporary cessation of nursing. The genetic disease *galactosemia* is one *absolute* contraindication to breast-feeding. Breast milk is a rich source of lactose, and the very survival of infants with galactosemia depends on their receiving a non-lactose-containing formula. Galactosemia is a rare disorder, occurring in approximately 1 in every 60,000 births. Another genetic disease, *phenylketonuria (PKU),* is also often mentioned as a contraindication to breast-feeding. However, breast milk has relatively low levels of phenylalanine. In fact, infants who are exclusively breast-fed may receive a phenylalanine intake near the amount recommended for treating PKU. Total or partial nursing can therefore be used through close monitoring of the infant's blood phenylalanine levels.

Negative Maternal Attitude

One factor that would definitely be against breast-feeding is a negative attitude on the part of the mother. If the mother, after having received adequate information on breast-feeding, prefers to bottle-feed her baby, she should not be encouraged to do otherwise. Rarely is lactation successful when maternal desire to breast-feed is absent. If, on the other hand, a mother begins breast-feeding and finds that she lacks the support of her family or physician and cannot continue, her decision to wean the infant to a bottle must be supported. It should be stressed again, however, that good professional support can often make the difference between success and failure.

Cesarean Birth

Mothers who have had operative deliveries usually find that they can breast-feed successfully after the effects of the anesthesia have worn off for both the mother and child. The mother can minimize the effects of pain medication on her baby by taking it 15 to 30 minutes directly before nursing. It may be possible for the mother to avoid some discomfort by requesting that the intravenous line be placed in a position that allows her maximum ability to handle her baby. Use of plenty of pillows will allow her to reduce the discomfort of pressure on her incision. If she can be comfortable in more than one position, she may be able to increase the number of nursing positions and reduce the severity of nipple soreness. Despite the few potential problems, the rate of successful breast-feeding among mothers who have just had operative deliveries is no different from that of mothers who have delivered vaginally.

Poor Let-Down Function

Some women seem to have more trouble than others in establishing a satisfactory let-down reflex. The extent to which the mother's emotional state contributes to the problem must be assessed. Anxiety and stress are known separately to decrease milk output since epinephrine inhibits oxytocin release. Anything that encourages relaxation should enhance let-down. A warm bath, moist heat to the breasts, gentle massage, and tactile stimulation, as well as soft lights and soft music, have been known to help. A moderate amount of alcohol seems to be beneficial as a relaxant for the mother and seems to enhance the let-down. Excessive amounts of alcohol and caffeine, however, have both been reported to interfere with the let-down reflex, and if this is the case, the mother who wants to smoke while nursing should wait to do so at least until the infant is sucking vigorously and the ejection is well established. Marijuana contains a psychoactive chemical (9-tetrahydrocannabinol) that acts on the hypothalamus and eventually disrupts pituitary production of prolactin as well as other hormones.

Colds and Influenza

The presence of colds or other mild viral infections such as influenza is usually no reason to discontinue lactation as long as the mother feels able to breast-feed. The infant has usually been exposed to the infection by the time the mother realizes that she is affected. There is good evidence that the infant has some immunity through maternal antibodies. If the infant is infected, the infection is often very mild. When the infant has a cold, nasal congestion will make breathing difficult during nursing. Use of a nasal aspirator to remove mucus and aid breathing may be of some help.

Clogged Milk Ducts

This condition is caused by incomplete emptying of one or more ducts. This sometimes occurs when the infant's feeding position does not allow for equal drawing on all of the milk sinuses, causing stasis. Milk or cast-off cells accumulate within a duct and form a localized plug or blockage. Milk then builds up behind the plug. Tenderness may develop in the area of the plug, and a lump may be felt at the point of blockage. Under these circumstances of simple obstruction, no fever, flulike symptoms, or systematic reactions typically occur. The remedy is: (1) more frequent feeding, especially on the affected side; (2) rest; (3) analgesics, if necessary; and (4) application of moist heat. If the mother can lie down and allow the infant to nurse on the affected breast for half an hour or longer, the improvement is often dramatic. If treatment is prompt, recovery should be nearly complete within 24 hours.

It is highly desirable that the plug be removed quickly, since plugged ducts can develop into larger blocked-off areas called a "caked breast." This may be followed by a breast infection and considerable discomfort. If the plug can be released, however, improvement can be rapid. Sometimes plugs dissolve or are reabsorbed by maternal tissues. If the plug is released and comes out with the milk, it may be brownish or greenish and thick and stringy. This is no danger for the baby, but he may temporarily reject the milk.

Mastitis

The symptoms of breast infection are similar to those of engorgement. The breast is tender, distended with milk, and may feel hot to touch. Fever may be present. Treatment consists of prompt medical attention, antibiotic therapy, bed rest, and *continued breast-feeding*. Discontinued feeding causes increased stasis and further pain. Frequently the source of the infection is an untreated infection in the infant. Recurrent breast infections may require culturing of the milk or the baby's mouth to determine which antibiotics to prescribe. Infrequently the cause of the infection may be exposure to bacteria carried by other family members. If all other treatments prove ineffective, cultures should be taken from the rest of the family to determine the source of bacteria and prescribe simultaneous treatment for all involved. In any case weaning should not be attempted until the infection has cleared up.

Abscess

When breast infections are not successfully treated, they may develop into a serious and painful condition called an abscess, in which there is localized pus and swelling of tissue. An abscess should be viewed as a serious problem requiring immediate medical attention. Diagnosis is made by culturing the secretions from the breast. Usual treatment includes antibiotics along with massage, pumping, and sometimes surgical drainage. It may be necessary to discontinue nursing on the affected side, but usually it can continue on the unaffected breast.

MATERNAL DISEASE

Chronic Disease

Heart disease, diabetes, hepatitis, nephrosis, and most other chronic medical conditions are not themselves a contraindication to breast-feeding. Usually if the condition can be managed well enough to allow successful maintenance of pregnancy, breast-feeding may be the feeding method of choice because it is less tiring for the mother.

Diabetes

Since management of the diabetic woman in pregnancy has become increasingly more successful, many diabetic mothers are now choosing to breast-feed. In fact some mothers with diabetes enjoy a postpartum remission of their diabetes, which may last through lactation and in some cases several years longer. The remission has been attributed to the hormone interactions that affect the hypothalamus and pituitary gland during pregnancy, labor, delivery, and lactation.

Since persons with diabetes are known to be prone to infection, mastitis may pose a significant threat, and vaginitis may be more common. Infection of the nipples may also occur because of *Candida albicans.* Careful anticipatory care, avoidance of fatigue, and early antibiotic management of developing problems are wise.

Thyroid Disease

When hypothyroidism is diagnosed in the mother, it is generally treated with full replacement therapy of desiccated thyroid. Under such circumstances breast-feeding is not contraindicated. If the mother is truly hypothyroid, care should be taken to rule out hypothyroidism in the infant. Diagnosis is made by evaluating blood values. Hypothyroidism is not a hazard to the nursing infant.

Unlike hypothyroidism, the diagnostic procedures and therapeutic management of the mother with hyperthyroidism present some hazards to the breast-fed infant. Treatment includes antithyroid medication, which inhibits the synthesis of thyroid hormones. Compounds in this medication may appear in breast milk and may build up in the infant's circulation. With careful monitoring and thyroid medication, nursing may proceed successfully. However, care must be taken to watch for bradycardia and other signs of hypothyroidism, including goiter.

Cancer

A mother with a diagnosis of breast cancer should not nurse her infant, in the interest of having definitive treatment immediately for herself. Not all lumps in the lactating breast are cancer, or even benign tumors. The lactating breast is lumpy by nature, and the lumps shift day by day. If a mass is located and the physician thinks it should be biopsied, it can be done under local anesthesia without weaning the infant. Usually such a lump is diagnosed as a benign mass. Immediate surgery to remove the mass may relieve tremendous anxiety without necessarily sacrificing breast-feeding.

Infectious Disease

Infectious diseases that require isolation of the mother from other adults, as well as from children, may be a contraindication to breast-feeding. Some controversy exists about the management of tuberculosis during pregnancy and lactation. Because of the hazard that tuberculosis presents to the newborn, careful family histories, including tuberculin testing and chest x-ray examinations, should be done on both the mother and the infant. If it is deemed safe for the mother to contact the infant, it is generally suspected that breast-feeding is safe, except for considerations regarding medications. Since both the mother and the infant will be taking isoniazid, care must be taken to assure that accumulation of the drug in the infant is not excessive.

FAMILY AND SOCIAL SITUATIONS

Multiple Births

It is entirely possible to nurse more than one infant and many case reports support this fact. Historical observations of wet nurses indicate that support of six babies simultaneously is within the realm of physiologic capability. The key deterrent to nursing twins or triplets is not usually the milk supply but the time. Nursing two infants at the same time is clearly more efficient. A number of tricks have been proposed to accommodate more than one infant, but as they become larger and more active, it may be a real challenge to keep them simultaneously nursing without assistance from the father or a friend. The nursing mother of more than one infant needs to conscientiously attend to her own rest and nourishment.

Working During Lactation

Many women believe that breast-feeding is not compatible with working outside the home. This is a myth, since the two can go nicely together. The reduced incidence and severity of illness in the breast-feeding infant may actually reduce the days the mother misses from work. It is desirable for the working mother to have a minimum of 4 to 6 weeks at home with her nursing infant before returning to a full-time job. This time will allow for the successful establishment of lactation and the development of a close mother-child relationship. This strong foundation will provide the mother with substantial motivation to continue breast-feeding as her work commitments increase and her time with the infant decreases. The lactating working mother will want to learn to express her milk so that she can provide it to her infant and maintain her lactation capacity on the days she has to work.

Pregnancy During Lactation

Occasionally a mother may wish to nurse an infant after she becomes pregnant again. This circumstance is physiologically possible, but the nutritional and psychologic demands on the mother are substantial. Some women may even experience uterine contractions while nursing and in some cases may need to consider weaning to avoid the possibility of spontaneous abortion. The child may become discouraged from nursing because of the changing composition and taste of the milk produced as the pregnancy proceeds. The mother's milk supply may also decrease, and this may cause her child to lose interest in nursing.

Nursing Siblings—Tandem Nursing

With sufficient sucking stimulus, most mothers can produce enough milk to successfully nurse a young infant, as well as an older child. It is important, however, to consider the emotional needs of the older sibling and the physical well-being of the mother. If the mother feels that the older child may satisfy his sucking needs and benefit emotionally from the breast-feeding experience, she may decide to continue nursing both children. However, if she feels that this undertaking is too demanding or she resents the older child's nursing, she is well advised to wean the older child as soon as possible.

If the mother decides to wean the toddler, she should go about it gradually. It may be rather difficult while she is nursing the young baby, since the older one may want to nurse when she sees the younger sibling at the breast. An obvious solution is to nurse the baby at the times when the older child is not around or is happily occupied with other things. She will need to decide on some alternative activities and snacks to take the place of breast-feeding so that the transition from nursing to total weaning will go smoothly.

RELACTATION

Reasons

Relactation is the resumption of lactation after it has been stopped some time beyond the immediate postpartum period. This process may be attempted by women who have for various reasons not nursed their infant for a while or by women who change their minds about lactation after weaning has taken place. To reactivate the lactation process requires that appropriate stimuli are provided to the breasts. The baby's sucking or manual stimulation may be accompanied by use of medications or hormones, for example, Syntocinon, synthetic oxytocin. Success generally depends on the mother's determination and the baby's willingness to suckle at the less-than-satisfying breast. The longer the interlude between initial lactation and relactation, the more likely the effort is to fail.

Motivation

A mother needs to decide if she really wishes to attempt relactation. Considerable motivation is required, and initially the effort may be very time-consuming. It should be clear to the mother that she may not be able to produce an adequate milk supply to meet all the infant's nutritional requirements. In fact such a goal may be unrealistic and undesirable. The majority of mothers who express great pleasure in their relactation experience indicate that the mother-infant relationship is of far greater short- and long-term importance than the act of the breast-feeding alone. They emphasize that breast-feeding is as much *nurturing at* the breast as it is *nutrition from* the breast. In many instances undue emphasis on a complete milk supply actually hinders the mother's ability to achieve it.

Necessary Factors

The mother who is attempting relactation needs to build up her milk supply by making sure that she receives satisfactory rest and nutrition along with frequent sucking stimulus. She may encourage the infant to suckle by simply cuddling and stroking, but in addition may apply a sweet-tasting substance to the end of the nipple. She may effectively offer the baby a supplement and avoid nipple confusion between the bottle and the breast by use of a nursing supplementer, the Lact-Aid. The Lact-Aid Nursing Trainer* is a plastic bag that can be filled with formula and affixed to the mother's clothing near the breast during a feeding. While the baby nurses at the mother's breast, he receives formula through a small tube attached to the bag at one end and taped to the mother's nipple at the other (Fig. 5-15). Gradual weaning from the Lact-Aid can be provided by putting less and less in the bag, in response to cues indicating an increase in maternal lactation, that is, excess supplement left in bag after nursing, very wet diapers, soft stools, spitting up after feedings, and increased time between feedings.

NURSING AN ADOPTED INFANT

Potential for Success

It is extremely time-consuming, and sometimes impossible, to induce lactation without having been pregnant. Even when a pregnancy has been carried out in the

*From *Lact-Aid Instruction Book,* Resources in Human Nurturing International, 3885 Forest Street, P.O. Box 6861, Denver, CO 80206.

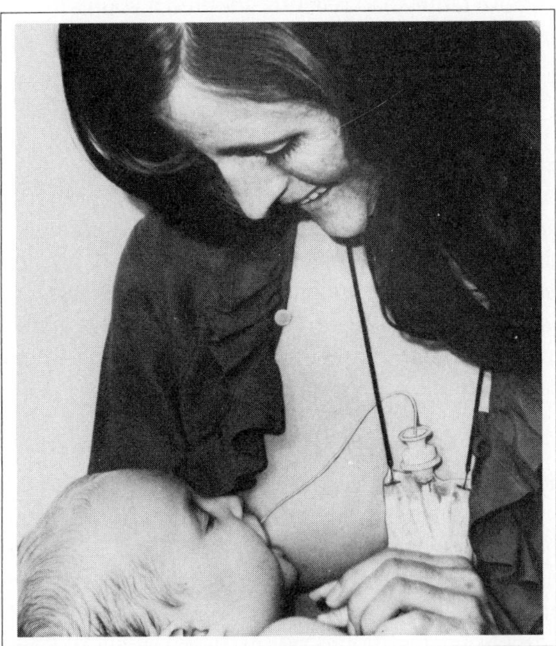

FIG. 5-15 Lact-Aid nursing trainer in use.
(Photograph compliments of Resources in Human Nurturing International, 3885 Forest St., P.O. Box 6861, Denver, CO 80206.)

past, great motivation is required to nurse an adopted infant. Chances increase if the mother has given birth or nursed another baby. If she is currently nursing another baby or has recently weaned one, her chances for success are good. A mother embarking on this nursing experience should have realistic motives and goals. She should not expect to provide all the infant's nutrition through lactation but should look forward to a satisfying emotional experience.

Process

The nipple preparation and relactation techniques described above apply also to the adoptive mother. In addition, it is useful for the mother to pump her breasts to stimulate milk production. She can gradually increase the frequency and duration of this activity until it reaches a level of about 20 minutes every 2 hours when the baby's arrival is near. The mother should realize that it may be quite a while before she sees any results from her pumping and that even a small amount of milk means success. The milk supply will increase rapidly when the baby begins suckling. If the mother is not able to obtain her baby soon after birth, however, her chances of success may decline, since the baby will have been bottle-fed and may suffer from nipple confusion.

Careful Individual Consideration

The fact that some women have succeeded in nursing their adoptive infants does not mean that all adoptive mothers can nurse or should attempt to do so. This point was well made by a physician whose family had recently adopted a young infant.[56] He points out that adoptive parents often have decided to adopt a child after a long period of reproductive failure and a trying experience with an adoptive agency. When the adopted infant finally arrives, the parents have to cope with a considerable role handicap. In view of the substantial time commitment of induced lactation and the stress and frustration that can be associated with it, one must really ask whether the advantages outweigh the disadvantages. Attempting lactation may set the mother up for another failure of physical function and loss of self-esteem, and in addition it requires much time and energy that could be devoted to more significant areas of social adjustment. *No pressure should ever be put on the adoptive mother to breast-feed.* If she wishes to try, she should have support and guidance. However, if she finds that she and her family are frustrated and exhausted, she should immediately re-evaluate her intentions and not be encouraged to continue.

TEENAGE MOTHERS

Most teenage mothers elect to keep their babies even when their home environments are neither supportive nor conducive to successful lactation. The self-image of the teenager may be poor, and she may have much doubt about her self-worth. She frequently feels uncomfortable in her new role as a mother. If the young mother expresses some interest in breast-feeding, effort should be made to determine her motives, and advantages and disadvantages should be discussed. It should be determined whether or not breast-feeding would significantly compromise her ability to continue in school or provide for the infant's other needs. Physiologically, teenagers are entirely capable of breast-feeding, although some will have less functional breast tissue than adult women. They are capable of satisfactory milk production and experience the same difficulties that other women do. When problems arise, however, they are less likely to overcome them and continue breast-feeding. They obviously require much support. Those with good support systems often breast-feed for the same amount of time as older mothers.

FAILURE TO THRIVE

Causes

Failure of some breast-fed infants to thrive has been reported for several decades and in many respects is no less puzzling today than when it was first described. A flow chart summarizing possible maternal and infant causes of the problem is provided in Fig. 5-16. In some cases there may be no history of excessive crying or dissatisfaction. The infant takes the breast well, nurses for a sufficient length of time, and sleeps well. There may be nothing to indicate abnormal nutrition until the infant shows marked signs of dehydration and even marasmus.

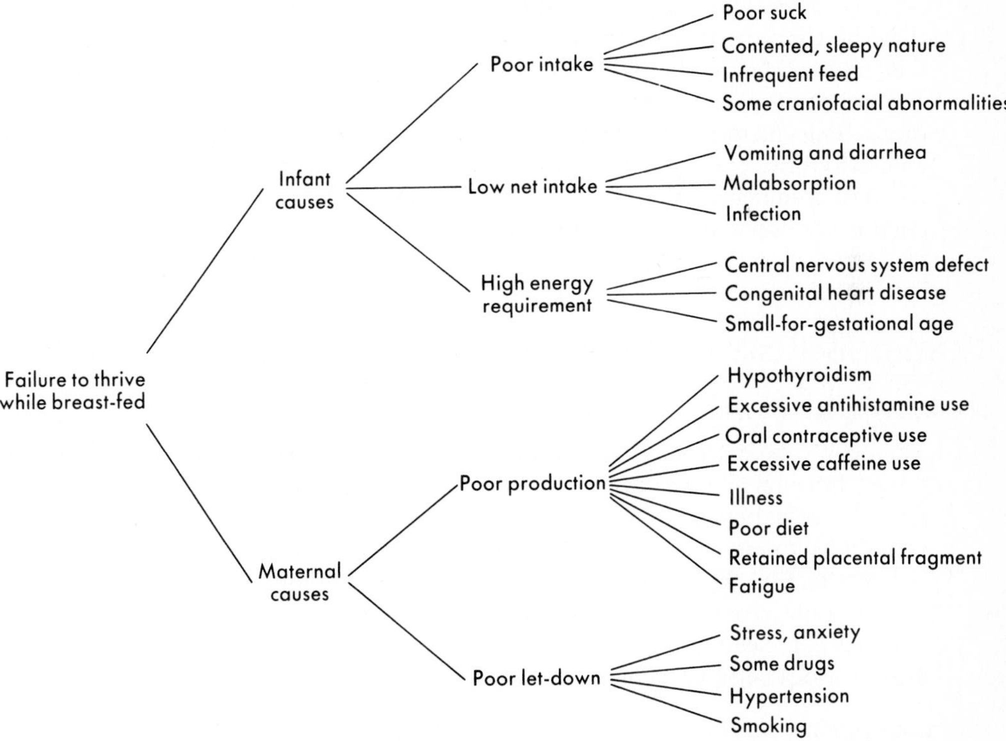

FIG. 5-16 Diagnostic flowchart for failure to thrive.

(Modified from Lawrence, R.: Breast-feeding: a guide for the medical profession, ed. 2, St. Louis, 1986, Times Mirror/Mosby College Publishing.)

Suckling Process

According to Frantz and Fleiss,[57] a major cause of failure to thrive in the totally breast-fed infant is a weak or ineffective suck. Compared to the normal suckling process, as these clinicians have repeatedly observed, the baby who is gaining weight poorly often has a rapid flutter-type chewing suckle that does not seem to have any drawing pause between the jaw motions, and swallowing occurs only every 3 to 15 suckles. On the other hand, they have noted that the babies who gain weight well also have a chew action to their jaw motions but display a slight pause in their cheeks between each suckle, and they appear to swallow with every suckle. Improvement in the quality of the suckle was often seen when an effort was made to hold the tongue down at the start of the feed and the tongue position was periodically checked. It also helped to have the mother switch breasts frequently, switching when inappropriate suckle began to develop. In some cases the Lact-Aid Nursing Trainer was found to be useful. Since minimum effort is required by infants to fill their mouths with milk, they have to create a chain reaction of suckle and swallow, suckle and swallow.

Evaluation of Growth Rate

The breast-fed infant should be evaluated regularly to determine if growth is proceeding normally. If the infant fails to thrive, even after techniques to enhance let-down and improve milk supply, and then improves when placed on a formula, breast-feeding should either be abandoned or a regular program of supplementary feeding established. The important point is to monitor growth closely enough that a life-threatening emergency and panic-weaning to bottle can be avoided. In some cases of failure to thrive at the breast, the mother should receive additional support to allay feelings of guilt and failure that will inevitably arise. Breast-feeding of a subsequent child is not necessarily contraindicated.

Common Reasons for Failure of Lactation

POOR MATERNAL ATTITUDE

Probably the chief reason for failure of breast-feeding is a poor maternal attitude toward lactation in the first place. The mother who does not sincerely want to breast-feed her infant but agrees to do so to placate her family, friends, or nurse will have a very difficult time. Fear, worry, distraction, anger, and other such emotions have a potent effect on the let-down reflex. When this reflex functions poorly, the infant receives only a portion of the milk supply because the bulk of the milk stored in the alveoli is not released. The infant cries from hunger and eventually fails to gain weight. This provides negative feedback to the mother and a vicious cycle begins.

INADEQUATE MILK SUPPLY

Failure to establish adequate milk supply by frequent feeding on demand is a great deterrent to successful lactation. Before breast-feeding is abandoned, the clinician should check to see if caloric intake has been adequate to support lactation. Are there anxieties and distractions to nursing that can be eliminated? Is the mother getting enough rest? Is she taking oral contraceptives or other medication that suppresses lactation? The problem may be inhibition of the let-down reflex rather than failure of milk production. Is the hospital routine nonsupportive? Other problems can stem from use of supplements too soon and too frequently, and from early introduction of solid foods.

LACK OF INFORMATION AND SUPPORT

Another common reason for failure of lactation is lack of information and support for the mother. Many women do not have the support of friends or relatives who have successfully breast-fed infants. These women are often poorly informed about the physiology of lactation and about the virtually fool-proof method of meeting the infant's nutritional needs. New breast-feeding mothers may have fears of the milk supply being too low in quality or quantity to support the infant's growth requirements. They may become discouraged when the infant does not feed well because he has been sedated during labor and delivery. Or they may be discouraged by nipple discomfort or engorgement, common complaints during the first few days of breast-feeding. Often a new mother feels mildly depressed around the fourth or fifth day postpartum, and any initial lactation problems will be magnified out of proportion. This is particularly true if the mother does not see these occurrences as normal. If the parents have had adequate prenatal instruction and good counseling during the hospital stay, the chances of weathering these storms are greatly increased. If the breast-feeding mother has the support of her partner and understanding professionals who can provide kind words to bolster her confidence even when things are going fine, she will feel she has a place to turn for help and advice when things go badly. Under these circumstances problems that cannot be avoided can be more easily overcome.

Summary

From many standpoints evidence supports the suitability of breast milk for the human infant. The important role of the health professional in counseling breast-feeding mothers is now recognized. Effective functioning as a breast-feeding counselor demands a thorough understanding of the process of lactation and a sincere desire to help inexperienced mothers decide for themselves about the best approaches to infant feeding in their own circumstances.

In-depth knowledge about the problems women experience with lactation needs recognition. Workable management strategies need to be devised. Because support for breast-feeding has been voiced by an array of health care disciplines and lay groups, and because breast-feeding counseling is now of high quality, lactation should remain popular in the future. Continued attention should be given, however, to early childhood exposure to lactation along with effective educational programs for both boys and girls.

Review Questions

1. Diagram the structural components of the female mammary gland and define the process of human milk synthesis and movement through the system.
2. Describe the basic physiology of lactation, referring to appropriate anatomical sites, hormonal contributions, and other significant details.
3. Outline the advantages and disadvantages of breast-feeding.
4. Define the significant characteristics of human milk that make it particularly suitable for human infants.
5. Outline a dozen concerns expressed by breast-feeeding mothers and describe appropriate approaches to counseling women about these concerns.

REFERENCES

1. Worthington-Roberts, B., Vermeersch, J., and Williams, S.R.: Nutrition in pregnancy and lactation, ed. 3, St. Louis, 1985. Times Mirror/Mosby College Publishing.
2. Shaul, D.M.B.: The composition of milk from wild animals, Int. Year Zoo Book **4**:333, 1962.
3. Chessex, P., and others: Quality of growth in premature infants fed their own mothers' milk, J. Pediatr. **102**:107, 1983.
4. Jarvenpaa, A., and others: Preterm infants fed human milk attain intrauterine weight gain, Acta Paediatr. Scand. **72**:239, 1983.
5. Gross, S.J.: Growth and biochemical response of preterm infants fed human milk or modified infant formula, New Engl. J. Med. **308**:237, 1983.
6. Lindblad, B.S., and Rahimtoola, R.J.: A pilot study of the quality of human milk in a lower socio-economic group in Karachi, Pakistan, Acta Paediatr. Scand. **63**:125, 1974.
7. Chavalittamrong, B., and others: Protein and amino acids of breast milk from Thai mothers, Am. J. Clin. Nutr. **34**:1126, 1981.
8. Packard, V.S.: Human milk and infant formula, New York, 1982. Academic Press, Inc.
9. Heitlinger, L.A., and others: Mammary amylase: a possible alternate pathway of carbohydrate digestion in infancy, Pediatr. Res. **17**:15, 1983.
10. McMillan, J.A., Landaw, S.A., and Oski, F.A.: Iron sufficiency in breast-fed infants and the availability of iron from human milk, Pediatrics **58**:686, 1976.
11. McMillan, J.A., and others: Iron absorption from human milk, simulated human milk and proprietary formulas, Pediatrics **60**:896, 1977.
12. Garry, P.J., and others: Iron absorption from human milk and formula with and without iron supplementation, Pediatr. Res. **15**:822, 1981.
13. Owen, G.M., and others: Iron nutriture of infants exclusively breast-fed the first five months, J. Pediatr. **99**:237, 1981.
14. Casey, C.E., Walravens, P.A., and Hambidge, K.M.: Availability of zinc: loading tests with human milk, cow's milk and infant formulas, Pediatrics **68**:394, 1981.
15. Hollis, B.W., Greer, F.R., and Tsang, R.C.: The effects of oral vitamin D supplementation and ultraviolet phototherapy on the antirachitic sterol content of human milk (abstract), American Society of Bone and Mineral Research Annual Meeting, 1982.
16. Greer, F.R., and others: Bone mineral content and serum 25-hydroxyvitamin D concentration in breast-fed infants with and without supplemental vitamin D, J. Pediatr. **98**:696, 1981.

17. Greer, F.R., and others: Bone mineral content and serum 25-hydroxyvitamin D concentrations in breast-fed infants with and without supplemental vitamin D: one year follow-up, J. Pediatr. **100**:919, 1982.
18. Ozsoylu, S., and Hasanoglu, A.: Vitamin D supplementation in breast-fed infants, J. Pediatr. **100**:1000, 1982.
19. Finberg, L.: Human milk feeding and vitamin D supplementation—1981, J. Pediatr. **99**:228, 1981.
20. Bachrach, S., Fisher, J., and Parks, J.S.: An outbreak of vitamin D deficiency rickets in a susceptible population, Pediatrics **64**:871, 1979.
21. Edidin, D.V., and others: Resurgence of nutritional rickets associated with breast-feeding and special dietary practices, Pediatrics **65**:232, 1980.
22. Byerly, L.O., and Kirksey, A.: Effects of different levels of vitamin C intake on the vitamin C concentration in human milk and the vitamin C intakes of breast-fed infants, Am. J. Clin. Nutr. **41**:665, 1985.
23. Felice, J.H., and Kirksey, A.: Effects of vitamin B_6 deficiency during lactation on the vitamin B_6 content of milk, liver, and muscle of rats, J. Nutr. **111**:610, 1981.
24. Borschel, M.W., and Kirksey, A.: Relationship of plasma pyridoxal phosphate levels to vitamin B_6 intakes during the first six months, Fed. Proc. **42**:1331, 1983.
25. Sandberg, D.P., Begley, J.A., and Hall, C.A.: The content, binding, and forms of vitamin B_{12} in milk, Am. J. Clin. Nutr. **34**:1717, 1981.
26. Beerens, H., Romond, C., and Neut, C.: Influence of breast-feeding on the bifid flora of the newborn intestine, Am. J. Clin. Nutr. **33**:2434, 1980.
27. Reid, B., Smith, H., and Friedman, K.: Prostaglandins in human milk, Pediatrics **66**:870, 1980.
28. Miranda, R., and others: Effect of maternal nutritional status on immunological substances in human colostrum and milk, Am. J. Clin. Nutr. **37**:632, 1983.
29. Berlin, C.M.: Pharmacologic considerations of drug use in the lactating mother, Obstet. Gynecol. **58**:175, 1981.
30. American Academy of Pediatrics, Committee on Drugs: The transfer of drugs and other chemicals into human milk, Pediatrics **72**, 1983.
31. Savage, E.P., and others: National study of chlorinated hydrocarbon insecticide residues in human milk, U.S.A., Am. J. Epidemiol. **113**:413, 1981.
32. Binkiewicz, A., Robinson, M.J., and Senior, B.: Pseudo-Cushing syndrome caused by alcohol in breast milk, J. Pediatr. **93**:965, 1978.
33. Hartmann, P.E., and others: Studies on breast-feeding and reproduction in women in Western Australia—a review, Birth Fam. J. **8**:215, 1982.
34. English, R.M., and Hitchcock, N.E.: Nutrient intakes during pregnancy, lactation, and after the cessation of lactation in a group of Australian women, Br. J. Nutr. **22**:615, 1968.
35. Butte, N.F., and others: Maternal energy balance during lactation, Fed. Proc. **42**:922, 1983.
36. Manning-Dalton, C., and Allen, L.H.: The effects of lactation on energy and protein consumption, postpartum weight change and body composition of well-nourished North American women, Nutr. Res. **3**:293, 1983.
37. Berger, L.R.: Factors influencing breast feeding, J.C.E. Pediatr., Sept. 1978, p. 13.
38. Butte, N.F., and others: Milk and mineral intake of 45 exclusively breast-fed infants, Fed. Proc. **43**:667, 1984.
39. Jakobsson, I., and Lindberg, T.: Cow's milk as a cause of infantile colic in breast-fed infants, Lancet **2**:437, 1978.

40. Evans, R.W, and others: Maternal diet and infantile colic in breast-fed infants, Lancet **2**:1340, 1981.
41. Lake, A.M., Whitington, P.F., and Hamilton, S.R.: Dietary protein-induced colitis in breast-fed infants, J. Pediatr. **101**:906, 1982.
42. Gerrard, J.W.: Allergy in breast-fed babies to ingredients in breast milk, Ann. Allergy **42**:69, 1979.
43. Auricchio, S., and others: Does breast-feeding protect against the development of clinical symptoms of celiac disease in children? J. Pediatr. Gastroenterol. Nutr. **2**:428, 1983.
44. Martinez, G.A., and Krieger, F.W.: 1984 milk feeding patterns in the United States, Pediatrics **76**:1004, 1985.
45. Martinez, G.A., and Dodd, D.A.: 1981 milk feedings in the United States during the first 12 months of life, Pediatrics **71**:166, 1983.
46. American Academy of Pediatrics, Committee on Nutrition: Nutrition and lactation, Pediatrics **68**:435, 1981.
47. American Academy of Pediatrics: The promotion of breast-feeding, Pediatrics **69**:654, 1982.
48. Pittard, W.B., Anderson, D.M., Cerutti, E.R., and Boxerbaum, D.: Bacteriostatic qualities of human milk, J. Pediatr. **107**:240, 1985.
49. Friend, B.A., and others: The effect of processing and storage on key enzymes, B vitamins, and lipids of mature human milk, I. Evaluation of fresh samples and effects of freezing and frozen storage, Pediatr. Res. **17**:61, 1983.
50. Bitman, J., and others: Lipolysis of triglycerides of human milk during storage at low temperature: a note of caution, J. Pediatr. Gastroenterol. Nutr. **2**:521, 1983.
51. Bjorksten, B., and others: Collecting and banking human milk: to heat or not to heat? Br. Med. J. **281**:765, 1980.
52. Goldsmith, S.J., and others: IgA, IgG, IgM and lactoferrin contents of human milk during early lactation and the effect of processing and storage, J. Food Protection **46**:4, 1983.
53. Goldblum, R.M., Dill, C.W., Albrecht, T.B., and others: Rapid high-temperature treatment of human milk, J. Pediatr. **104**:380, 1984.
54. Paxson, C.L., and Cress, C.C.: Survival of human milk leukocytes, J. Pediatr. **94**:61, 1979.
55. Goldblum, R.M., and others: Human milk banking, I. Effects of container upon immunologic factors in mature milk, Nutr. Res. **1**:449, 1981.
56. Carey, W.B.: Am. J. Dis. Child. **135**:973, 1981.
57. Frantz, K.B., and Fleiss, P.M.: Ineffective suckling as a frequent cause of failure to thrive in the totally breast-fed infant. In Freier, S., and Eidelman, A.I., eds.: Human milk: its biological and social value, Amsterdam, 1980, Excerpta Medica.

FURTHER READING

Brewster, D.P.: You can breast-feed your baby . . . even in special situations, Emmaus, Pa., 1979, Rodale Press, Inc.

Helsing, E., and King, F.S.: Breast-feeding in practice: a manual for health workers, Oxford, 1982, Oxford University Press.

La Leche League International: The womanly art of breast-feeding, Franklin Park, Ill., 1981, The League.

These three manuals provide easily understood discussions of lactation problems and their management, especially useful to parents.

Lawrence, R.A.: Breast-feeding: a guide for the medical profession, St. Louis, 1986, Times Mirror/ Mosby College Publishing.

This manual provides a thorough review of the process of lactation, the composition of human milk, and counseling recommendations for breast-feeding women, especially aimed at physicians and other health care professionals.

Neville, M.C., and Neifert, M.R., eds.: Lactation: physiology, nutrition, and breast-feeding, New York, 1983, Plenum Press.

This book provides a complete review of research related to lactation, human milk, and the breast-feeding experience.

Report of the Task Force on the Assessment of the Scientific Evidence Relating to Infant-feeding Practice and Infant Health: Pediatrics 4(Suppl.), October, 1984.

This task force report gives a comprehensive overview of infant-feeding practices around the world and their relationship to infant health.

United States Department of Health and Human Services: Report of the Surgeon General's workshop on breast-feeding and human lactation, Washington, D.C., 1984, U.S. Government Printing Office.

This report provides a summary of the recommendations of the expert committee that developed the policy of the U.S. Surgeon General's office about breast-feeding.

United States Department of Health and Human Serivces: Follow-up report of the Surgeon General's workshop on breast-feeding and human lactation, Washington, D.C., 1986, U.S. Government Printing Office.

This follow-up report defines the impact of the Surgeon General's recommendations (1984) regarding breast-feeding.

CASE STUDY

A young mother and her 3-month-old infant appear in the clinic for routine well-baby care. The infant appears to be healthy but small. The anthropometric measurements reveal that body weight falls on the 5th percentile and height plots on the 40th percentile. The mother reports that she is breast-feeding her baby, that things are going well although she is very tired, and that the baby is well behaved and rarely cries.

1. Define appropriate questions for the mother.
2. Outline a strategy to determine if the infant is receiving sufficient nutritional support through breast milk.
3. Propose an acceptable monitoring protocol

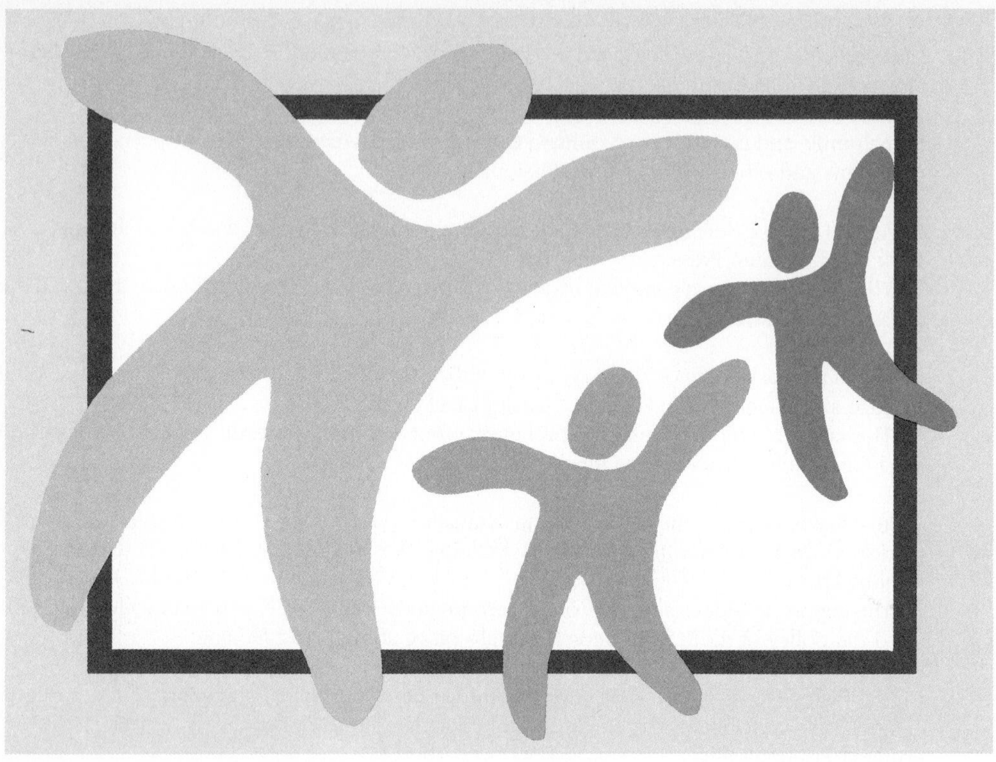

Basic Concepts

1. Early physical growth and maturation in the first year of life lays the foundation for continued development through the growth years.
2. Individual energy and nutrient needs reflect rapid growth demands for fuel, building materials, and basal metabolic rate.
3. An appropriate milk source, breast milk and alternate formulas, with gradual solid food additions, supply both nutritional and developmental needs.
4. Maturing oral structures and function determine developing infant eating skills and appropriate textures of food.
5. Infant feeding behavior follows a defined developmental sequence.

Chapter Six

Nutrition During Infancy

Peggy Pipes

The first year after birth is one of dramatic change for normal human infants. The torso grows longer and subcutaneous fat accumulates. Infants progress from being newborns with no head control to being babies who pull themselves up to a standing position and begin to take steps. They change from securing their nourishment with a reflexive suck to picking up finger foods with a precise pincer grasp. They develop voluntary and independent movements of the tongue, lip, and jaw and begin rotary chewing. At one year they are beginning self-feeding and can drink from a cup if help is provided.

In this chapter we will see that the importance of an adequate energy and nutrient intake consumed in a loving and supportive environment really can't be overstated. Milk and other foods supply the materials necessary for rapid linear growth and weight gain. Foods also support developmental progress. Adding appropriate textures and variety of food when infants are developmentally ready provides the stimulus for learning new skills. And feeding infants in a loving and nurturing environment helps them develop a sense of security and trust.

Human milk, or alternate formula if needed, is the baby's source of nutrients and energy for the first four to six months. Then added semi-solid foods progressing to "table foods" in the latter part of the first year provide important growth nutrients and support oral and fine motor development. Infants fed on demand to meet energy needs soon establish their own schedule.

Growth and Maturation

From birth to one year of age, normal human infants triple their weight and increase their length by 50%. They progress from sucking a nipple reflexively to obtain food to beginning voluntary self-feeding in a sitting position. They change from a diet solely of milk to one that includes many finger and table foods, as well as beverages, that they will consume as adults. They bond with their parents and acquire a sense of trust, and each develops an ego identity as a unique person. Growth and maturation can be compromised or accelerated by undernutrition or overnutrition. Also, the stage of maturation determines the developmental readiness to progress in food and textures of food, for example, to receive spoon foods and finger foods. Throughout this important first year of life, infant feeding and nutrition influence both physical and psychosocial growth and development.

PHYSICAL GROWTH

Weight

Birth weight is determined by the mother's prepregnancy weight and her weight gain during pregnancy. After parturition, genetics, environment, and nutrition determine rates of gains in weight and height. Immediately after birth there is a weight loss due to a loss of fluid and some catabolism of tissue. This loss averages 6% of body weight, but occasionally exceeds 10%. Birth weight is usually regained by the tenth day. Thereafter, weight gain during infancy proceeds at a rapid but decelerating rate. Average weight gains for the first 4 months are 20-25 g per day, and during the last 8 months, 15 g per day. By 4 months of age most infants weigh twice their birth weights, and by 12 months they usually weigh three times what they weighed at birth. Males increase in weight to twice their birth weights earlier than do females, and smaller newborns increase in weight to twice their birth weights sooner than do heavier infants.

Length

Infants usually increase their lengths by 50% the first year, the average length increase being 25-30 cm (10-12 in). But a period of "catch-up" or "lag-down" growth may occur. The majority of infants who are born small but are genetically determined to be longer shift percentiles on growth grids during the first 3 to 6 months. However, many infants born at or below the tenth percentile who are determined to be of average height may not achieve a new channel until a year of age. Larger infants whose genotypes are for smaller size tend to grow at their fetal rates for several months before the lag-down in growth becomes evident. Often a new percentile rating is not apparent until the child is 13 months of age.[1] Figures 6-1 and 6-2 depict catch-up and lag-down growth in the first year.

Racial differences have been noted in rates of growth. American black males and females are smaller than caucasians at birth. But they grow more rapidly during the first 2 years.[2]

GROWTH CHARTS

It is important that one concerned with infants' nutrient and energy intake be aware of how their growth is progressing. Height and weight data plotted on growth grids show how growth is proceeding. Measurements must be taken accurately as described in Chapter 3, then weight and height values recorded on growth grids so that growth velocity as well as acceleration or deceleration can be monitored.

The most commonly used growth grids in North America are those prepared by an expert committee of the National Center for Health Statistics (NCHS).[3] Data collected

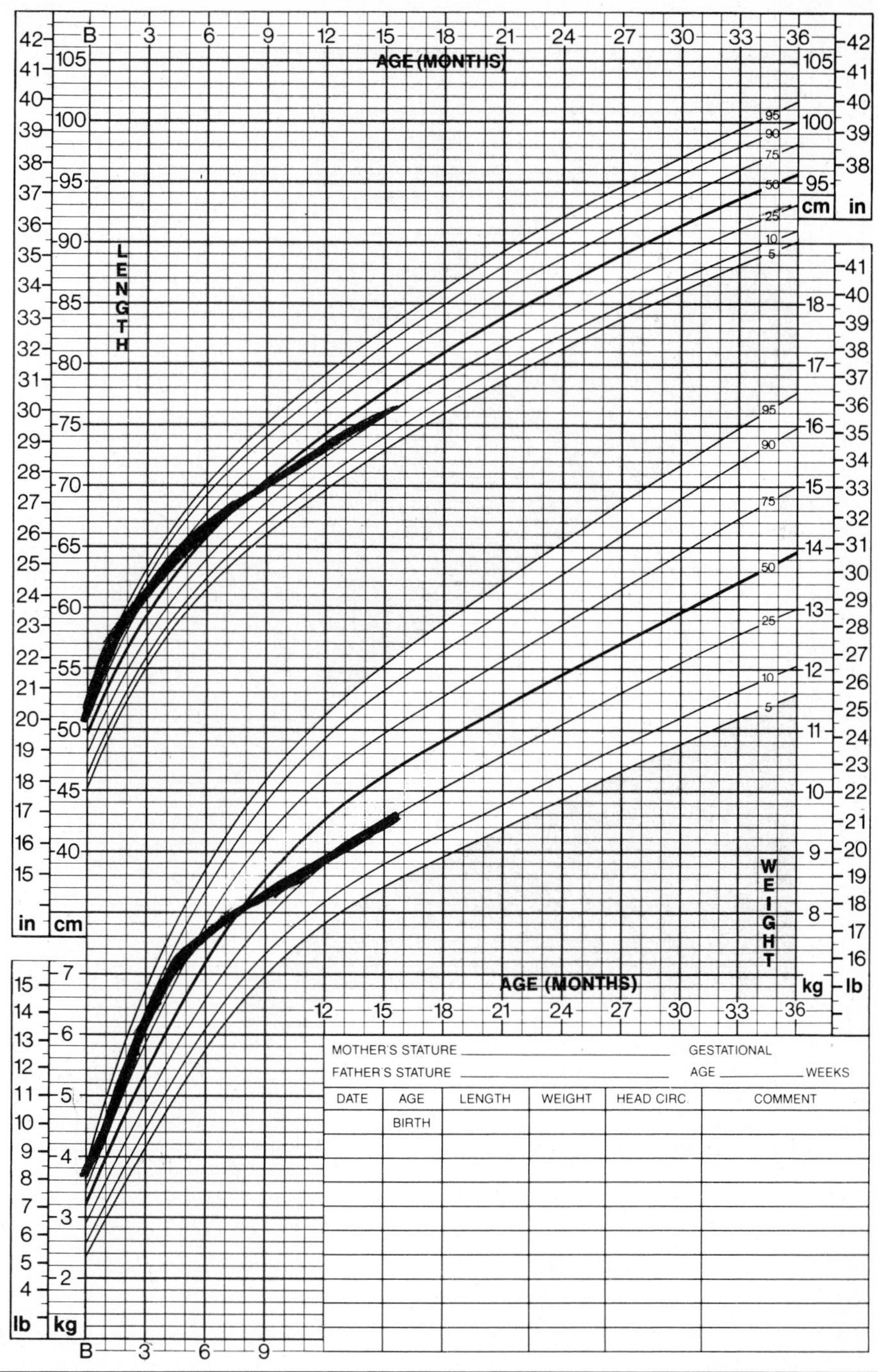

FIG. 6-1 Growth grid of a large infant who "lagged down" to her genetic potential. (Courtesy Ross Laboratories)

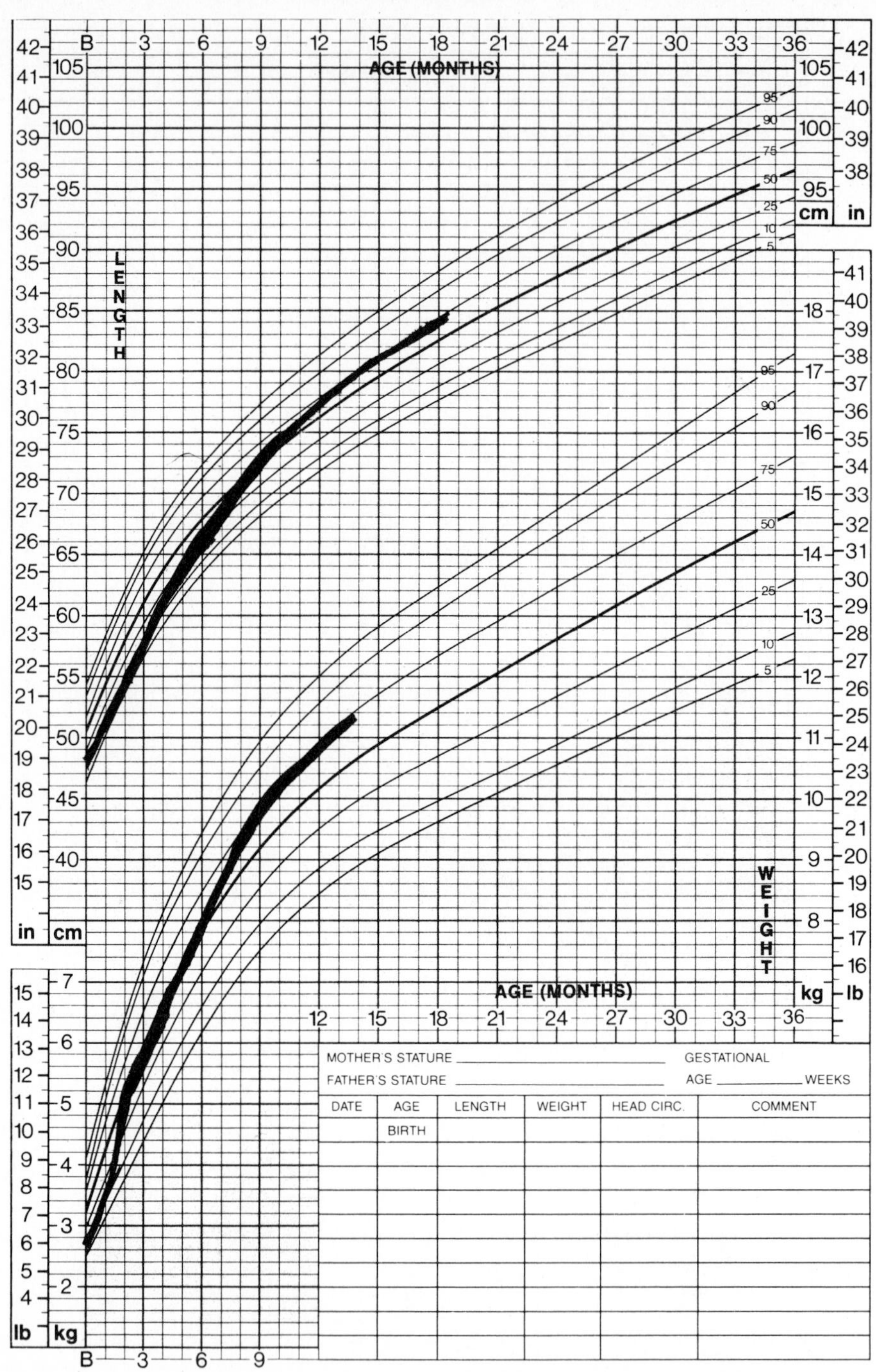

FIG. 6-2 Growth grid of a small infant who "caught up" to his genetic potential. (Courtesy Ross Laboratories)

by the Fels Research Institute from large numbers of a nationally representative sample of children were used to determine standards for children from birth to 36 months of age. The grids are prepared so that age values lie along the axis and height or weight values are plotted along the abscissa. Measurements at one age rank the baby's height or weight in relation to 100 other infants of the same age. Weight-height percentiles rank the baby's weight in relation to 100 other babies of the same length. Then sequential measurements plotted on the growth grid indicate if the baby is maintaining, reducing, or increasing the percentile rating as growth proceeds.

CHANGES IN BODY COMPOSITION

Changes during growth occur not only in height and weight but also in the components of the tissue (see Chapter 2). Increases in height and weight and skeletal maturation are accompanied by changes in body composition—water, lean body mass, and fat.

Body Water

Total body water as a percentage of body weight decreases throughout infancy from approximately 70% at birth to 60% at 1 year of age. Reduction of body water is almost entirely extracellular. Extracellular water decreases from about 42% of body weight at birth to 32% at 1 year of age. This change results from decreases in the water content of adipose tissue, increases in adipose tissue, and relative increases in lean body mass.[4]

Lean Body Mass

The fat-free mass of the body matures, the percentage of protein increasing as the percentage of water decreases. Fomon[4] estimates that the protein content of the fat-free lean body mass gained increases from 12.5% at 1 month to 17% at 1 year in males and to 16.7% at 1 year in females.

Body Fat

The fat content of the body develops slowly during fetal life. Fat accounts for 0.5% of body weight at the fifth month of fetal growth and 16% at term. After birth, fat accumulates rapidly until approximately 9 months of age. Between 2 and 6 months of age the increase in adipose tissue is more than twice as great as the increase in the volume of muscle.[5] Sex-related differences appear in infancy, the female depositing a greater percentage of weight as fat than the male.

CHANGES IN BODY PROPORTIONS

Increases in height and weight are accompanied by dramatic changes in body proportions. The head proportion decreases as the torso and leg proportion increases (Fig. 6-3). At birth, the head accounts for approximately one-fourth of the total body weight. When growth has ceased, it accounts for one-eighth of the total body length. Between birth and adulthood, leg length increases from approximately three-eighths of the newborn's birth length to one-half of the adult's total body height.

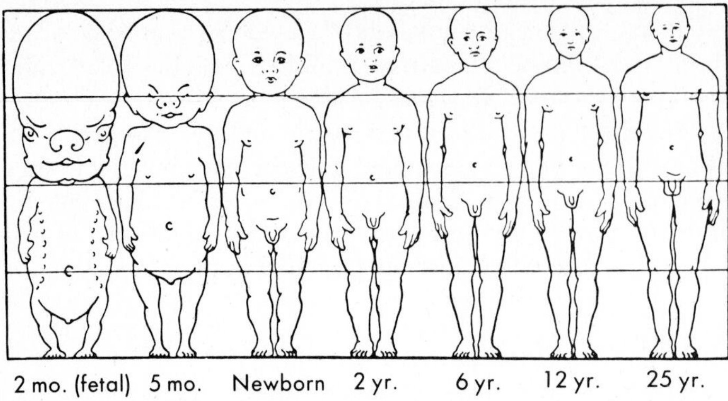

FIG. 6-3 Changes in body proportions from second fetal month to adulthood.
(From: Robbins, W.J., and others: Growth, New Haven, Conn., 1928, Yale University Press.)

PSYCHOSOCIAL DEVELOPMENT

Healthy psychosocial development in the first year involves the development of trust. In early infancy babies do not tolerate delay of gratification. However, if their needs are quickly met in the early months they accept delayed gratification later. In terms of feeding this means that in the first 2-3 months infants need to be fed as soon as possible when hunger is noted. As they grow older they can be expected to be more patient as preparation is made for feeding. Tactile stimulation is important in building trust and bonding. Infants need to be held and cuddled while feeding.

DIGESTION AND ABSORPTION

The digestive capacity of the infant matures and increases during the first year of life. The developing stomach and intestine provide an increasing ability to handle various nutrients.

Stomach Actions

The stomach capacity at birth, 10 to 12 ml, increases to 200 ml by 12 months. The gastric pH is slightly alkaline at birth but within 24 hours acid secretion reaches a peak comparable to that of a 3-year-old child. It then declines to a low level, remaining lower than that of the adult for the first few months.[6] The emptying rate of the stomach depends on the amount and composition of the food consumed.

Intestinal Actions

The early intestinal secretions of the infant provide varying enzymatic capacities to handle nutrients:

1. **Proteins.** The newborn's concentrations of trypsin are near adult levels. Concentrations of chymotrypsin and carboxypeptidase in the duodenum are only 10% to 60% of the adult levels. Babies can digest adequate protein even though the quantity is limited. Newborns can completely digest about 1.95 g per kg per day of protein, 4-month-old babies about 3.75 g per kg per day.[6]

2. **Fats.** Pancreatic lipase activity is low in the newborn, especially in the premature infant. The bile acid pool, although present, is reduced. When compared to the adult on the basis of body surface area, the newborn, although able to synthesize bile, has a bile acid pool one-half that of the adult.[7] This limited capacity prevents complete hydrolysis of lipids, resulting in inefficient lipid digestion. Lingual lipase and gastric lipase may be important for the baby's fat digestion.[6] The fatty acid composition of dietary fat influences how much of it will be digested and absorbed by the infant. Triglycerides with saturated fatty acids are not as well utilized as those with unsaturated fatty acids. Also, the position a fatty acid occupies on the fat's glycerol molecule base affects absorption. Stearic acid is poorly absorbed in any position. Free palmitic acid hydrolized from positions 1 and 3 is poorly absorbed, whereas palmitic acid occupying position 2 on the glycerol molecule remains with the glycerol base as a monoglyceride that appears to be well absorbed.[8] Fatty acids in human milk are better absorbed than those in cow's milk. Newborns absorb approximately 85% to 90% of the fat provided by human milk. Many infants absorb less than 70% of cow's milk fat.[9] Plant oils are more efficiently absorbed than animal fats. Mixtures of vegetable oils in commercially prepared infant formulas are well absorbed.
3. **Carbohydrates.** Sugars are well utilized. Maltase, isomaltase, and sucrase activity reach adult levels by 28 to 32 weeks gestation. Lactase, present in low levels at 28 weeks gestation, increases near term and reaches adult levels at birth.[10] Salivary and pancreatic amylase are low during the first months after birth. Salivary amylase concentrations rise to adult values between the ages of 6 months and 1 year.[11] Pancreatic amylase concentrations increase from birth through the preschool years. Mammary amylase may be important for starch digestion in breastfed infants. Most infants can consume limited quantities of starches. However, because of the low concentrations of amylase in intestinal secretions in early infancy it seems prudent to delay the introduction of cereals and other starches until 4 to 6 months of age.

RENAL FUNCTION

The newborn has a functionally immature kidney. The ratio of glomerular surface area to tubular volume in an infant's kidney is high, compared with the kidney of an adult.[12] The glomerular filtration rate is low. The concentrating capacity of some neonates has been reported to be as limited as 700 mOsm/L, and for others it is as great as that of older children and adults, 1200 to 1400 mOsm/L.[13,14] Human milk has a solute load of 75 mOsm/L, whole cow's milk 308 mOsm/L, and commercially prepared infant formulas 260-270 mOsm/L. Water imbalance becomes a concern in normal infants only in cases of restricted fluid intake, vomiting, and diarrhea, and in hot weather.

Nutrient Needs of Infants

Individual differences of infants in nutrient reserves, body composition, growth rates, and activity patterns make defining actual nutrient requirements impossible.

Estimates have been made from intakes of infants growing normally and from the nutrient content of human milk. Nitrogen balance studies have been conducted to establish amino acid requirements. Fat and calcium absorption have been examined. The Recommended Dietary Allowances (RDA) are planned to provide a margin of safety to allow for maximum protection. Because of the declining growth rates during the latter part of the first year, recommended intakes have been set for two 6-month periods, from birth to 6 months and from 6 months to 1 year.[14]

ENERGY

The energy requirement in infancy is determined primarily by body size, physical activity, and rates of growth. Since large variations in these variables are seen among infants at any age and in any one infant from month to month, ranges of energy needs are large. Total energy needs (kcal/day) rise during the first year but energy needs per unit of body size decline in response to changes in rates of growth. The recommended intake (Table 6-1) falls from 115 kcal/kg in the first four months to 105 kcal/kg at 1 year.

It has been estimated that approximately 50% of the energy expenditure is due to the basal metabolic rate. Energy expended for growth declines from approximately 32.8% of intake during the first 4 months to 7.4% of intake from 4 to 12 months.[9] The contribution of physical activity to total energy expenditure is quite variable but can be expected to increase with age as motor skills develop. Some are quiet and cuddly while others spend a considerable amount of time crying, kicking, or just exploring with motor skills they have acquired.

PROTEIN AND AMINO ACIDS

Protein Needs

Infants require protein for synthesis of new body tissue during growth, increases in the protein content of the body, as well as synthesis of enzymes, hormones, and other physiologically important compounds. Increases in body protein are estimated to average about 3.5 g/day for the first 4 months, and 3.1 g/day for the next 8 months.[4] The body content of protein increases from about 11.0% to 14.6% over the first year. The recommended intake is 2.2 g/kg for the first 6 months and 2.0 g/kg from 6-12 months.[9]

Amino Acid Needs

Nine amino acids are dietary essentials in infancy. Amino acid requirements have been estimated by Holt and Snyderman[17] from studies in which pure amino acids

TABLE 6-1 Recommended Energy Intakes for Infants

Age	Energy Needs (kcal)	Ranges
0.0-0.5	kg × 115	(95-145)
0.5-1.0	kg × 105	(80-135)

were supplied in proportions of amino acids in human milk. The requirement of an amino acid was defined as the least amount required to maintain satisfactory nitrogen retention and weight gain when nitrogen levels and other amino acids were held constant. Fomon and Filer[18] and Fomon and associates[20] have estimated amino acid requirements from intakes of infants between the ages of 8 and 112 days who were fed whole protein in cow's-milk formulas and soy formulas. Satisfactory linear growth and weight gain, nitrogen balance, and serum concentrations of albumin equivalent to those of normal breast-fed infants were used as criteria of adequacy.

Requirement Standards

The FAO/WHO expert committee has suggested that a composite of the lower estimates of the data from the studies of Holt and Snyderman[17] and from Fomon and Filer[17] would provide estimates of the upper range of amino acid requirements of infants aged 0 to 6 months.[19] These estimates are presented in Table 6-2. In addition, tyrosine and cystine may be essential amino acids for the premature and low-birth-weight infant.

Fomon and associates[20] have suggested that during infancy amino acid and protein requirements expressed per unit of kilocalories consumed, reflecting both size and rate of growth, would be more meaningful than expressions of requirements on the basis of body weight alone. They estimate the protein requirement to be 1.6 g/100 kcal for children 1 to 4 months of age, and 1.4 g/100 kcal for children 8 to 12 months of age.

TABLE 6-2 Estimated Amino Acid Requirements of Infants

Amino Acid	Estimated Requirements: Holt and Snyderman[17] (mg/kg/day)*	Estimated Requirements: Fomon and Filer[18] (mg/kg/day)†	Composite of Lower Values (mg/kg/day)‡
Histidine	34	28	28
Isoleucine	119	70	70
Leucine	229	161	161
Lysine	103	161	103
Methionine plus cystine	45 plus cys	58§	58
Phenylalanine plus tyrosine	90 plus tyr	125§	125
Threonine	87	116	87
Tryptophan	22	17	17
Valine	105	93	93

From Energy and Protein Requirements, Report of a Joint FAO/WHO Ad Hoc Committee, World Health Organization Technical Report Series No. 522, FAO Nutr. Meet. Rep. No. 52, Geneva, 1973, World Health Organization.

*Requirements estimated when amino acids were fed or incorporated in basal formulas. The values represent estimates of maximal individual requirements to achieve normal growth.

†Calculated intakes of amino acids when formulas were fed in amounts sufficient to maintain good growth in all the infants studied; the amino acids were not varied independently.

‡Based on a safe level of 2 gm protein/kg/day, the average of suggested levels for the period of ages 0 to 6 months.

§The values for cystine and tyrosine were estimated on the basis of the methionine:cystine and phenylalanine:tyrosine ratios in human milk.

The American Academy of Pediatrics[21] has set minimum protein standards for infant formula of 1.8 g/100 kcal with a protein efficiency ratio equal to that of casein.

FAT AND ESSENTIAL FATTY ACID

Fat Needs

Fat, the most calorically concentrated energy nutrient, supplies between 40% and 50% of the energy consumed in infancy. The energy provided by fat spares protein for tissue synthesis. Its caloric concentration is an asset during periods of rapid growth when energy demands are great. Fat provides 45% to 50% of the energy content of commercial formula and 55% of the energy content of human milk. Commercial infant semisolid foods other than egg yolks are relatively low in fat.

Essential Fatty Acid

Polyunsaturated *linoleic acid* has been proved conclusively to be essential. One of the earliest manifestations of this fatty acid deficiency recognized in animals was an increased basal metabolic rate. Infants deficient in linoleic acid have an eczema-like dermatitis. Also, infants who are fed formulas low in this essential fatty acid consume greater numbers of kilocalories than do those who receive adequate amounts of linoleic acid to maintain normal growth. Caloric utilization has been reported to vary with intakes of linoleic acid up to 4% and 5% of the total kilocalories.[22] Minimal requirements for linoleic acid are considered to be approximately 1% of the total kilocalories consumed, and an optimal intake is thought to be 4% to 5% of the total kilocalories.[23] Approximately 5% of the total kilocalories in human milk and 1% of the kilocalories in cow's milk are provided by linoleic acid. Commercially available infant formulas contain blends of vegetable oils and contribute greater amounts of linoleic acid.

The Committee on Nutrition of the American Academy of Pediatrics[21] has recommended that infant formulas contain a minimum of 300 mg of 18:2 fatty acids per 100 kilocalories, or 1.7% of the energy content (total kilocalories).

WATER

Infants require more water per unit of body size than do adults. Hence they are more vulnerable to water losses and imbalances.

Water Losses

Water is lost by evaporation through the skin and respiratory tract—insensible water loss—and through perspiration when the environmental temperature is elevated, and by elimination in urine and feces. During growth additional water is necessary since water is needed as a constituent of tissue and for increases in the volume of body fluids. The amount of water required for growth, however, is very small. The body requirement for water is the sum of the above demands.

Water lost by evaporation in infancy and early childhood accounts for more than 60% of that needed to maintain homeostasis, as compared to 40% to 50% in the adult. At all ages approximately 24% of the basal heat loss is by evaporation of water through the skin and respiratory tract.[24] This amounts to 45 ml of insensible water loss per 100 kilocalories expended. Fomon[9] estimates evaporative water loss at 1 month of age to average 210 ml/day and at age 1 year, 500 ml/day. Evaporative losses increase with fever and increased environmental temperature. Increases in humidity decrease respiratory loss. Loss of water in the feces averages 10 ml/kg/day in infancy.[9]

Water Requirements

The volume of urine in general reflects fluid intake. It includes both water needed to excrete the solutes presented to the kidney for excretion and water in excess of body need. The renal water requirement is determined by the diet and the concentrating power of the kidney. Water requirements for infants are shown in Table 6-3.

Risk of Dehydration

Because of the relatively greater demand for water due to a high rate of insensible water loss and a renal concentrating power that may be less than that of the adult, the infant is vulnerable to water imbalance and dehydration. Under normal environmental conditions infants do not need additional water. But difficulties arise when formulas are improperly prepared, when infants ingest limited volumes of milk during illness, and when extrarenal losses are greater than usual, such as during episodes of vomiting and diarrhea. To ensure adequate water intakes, infant formula should not be concentrated to more than 100 kcal/100 ml (30 kcal/oz).

MINERALS AND VITAMINS

Demands for minerals and vitamins are influenced by growth rates, mineralization of bone, increases in bone length and blood volume, and by energy, protein, and fat intakes. Recommended dietary allowances (RDA) have been established for 3 major and 3 trace minerals and for 10 vitamins, as shown in Table 6-4. Ranges of safe intakes have been suggested for 9 trace minerals.[15]

Although all of these nutrients are essential, we will focus our discussion here on those that are most commonly of concern during infancy.

TABLE 6-3 Water Requirements of Infants and Children

Age	Amount of Water (ml/kg/day)
1 week	80-100
2 weeks	125-150
3 months	140-160
6 months	130-155
9 months	125-145
1 year	120-135
2 years	115-125

Adapted from: Vaughan, V.C., McKay, R.J., and Behrman, R.E. (eds.): Nelson Textbook of Pediatrics. 11th ed. Philadelphia, 1979, W. B. Saunders Co.

TABLE 6-4 Recommended Dietary Allowances for Minerals and Vitamins for Infants*

	Age (Years)	Calcium (mg)	Phosphorus (mg)	Iodine (μg)	Iron (mg)	Magnesium (mg)	Zinc (mg)
Infants	0.0-0.5	360	240	40	10	50	3
	0.5-1.0	540	360	50	15	70	5

TRACE MINERALS

Age (Years)	Copper (mg)	Manganese (mg)	Fluoride (mg)	Chromium (mg)	Selenium (mg)	Molybdenum (mg)
0-0.5	0.5-0.7	0.5-0.7	0.1-0.5	0.01-0.04	0.01-0.04	0.03-0.06
0.5-1	0.7-1.0	0.7-1.0	0.2-1.0	0.02-0.06	0.02-0.06	0.04-0.08

ELECTROLYTES

Age (Years)	Sodium (mg)	Potassium (mg)	Chloride (mg)
0-0.5	115-350	350-925	275-700
0.5-1	250-750	425-1275	400-1200

FAT-SOLUBLE VITAMINS

Age (Years)	Vitamin A RE* (μg)	Vitamin D (μg)	Vitamin E (mgα-TE)
0.0-0.5	420	10	3
0.5-1.0	400	10	4

WATER-SOLUBLE VITAMINS

Age (Years)	Thiamine (mg)	Ribo-flavin (mg)	Niacin (mg)	Vitamin B_6 (mg)	Folacin (μg)	Vitamin B_{12} (μg)	Ascorbic Acid (mg)
0.0-0.5	0.3	0.4	6	0.3	30	0.5	35
0.5-1.0	0.5	0.6	8	0.6	45	1.5	35

*From: Food and Nutrition Board, National Research Council: Recommended dietary allowances, ed. 9, Washington, D.C., 1980, National Academy of Sciences.

CALCIUM

The recommended intake of calcium is planned to meet the needs of formula-fed infants, who retain 25% to 30% of the calcium in cow's milk. Breast-fed infants retain 67% of the calcium consumed. The RDA standard is not applicable in evaluating calcium intakes of breast-fed infants, whose intake is considered to be adequate. It is recommended that the calcium-to-phosphorus ratio in infancy be 1.5:1.0, decreasing to 1.0:1.0 at 1 year of age.[15]

IRON

Prenatal Reserves

Iron is accumulated in utero in proportion to body size. Premature and low-birth-weight infants have limited reserves that are quickly depleted. Even with the advantage of full-term iron stores, the rapidly growing infant is at risk for iron deficiency, because of the increase in blood volume as the baby grows larger.

The concentration of hemoglobin at birth averages 17 to 19 g/100 ml of blood. During the first 6 to 8 weeks of life it decreases to approximately 10 to 11 g/100 ml because of a shortened life span of the fetal cell and decreased erythropoiesis. After this age there is a gradual increase in hemoglobin concentration to 13 g/100 ml at 2 years of age.

Food Sources

Forty-nine percent of the iron in human milk, 10% of the iron in cow's milk, and 3% of the iron in iron-fortified formulas is absorbed. Many investigators believe that breast-fed infants do not need additional iron for the first year.[25] However, Garry and coworkers[26] believe that after 3 months of age exclusively breast-fed infants are not receiving sufficient iron. They found that as infants adjust to their feedings they experience a reduction in percentage of iron retained. They noted that exclusively breast-fed infants, regardless of whether they had received iron supplements, had greater total body iron than infants fed formula with or without iron at 3 months of age. However, exclusively breast-fed infants who did not receive iron supplements after 3 months of age were in negative iron balance during 4 to 6 months of age and had to use their iron reserves. They think that if no additional source of iron is given to breast-fed infants after 6 months of age, they will rapidly deplete their reserves. Infant formulas are available with or without 12 mg iron/L. Iron-fortified commercial infant cereals are fortified with electrolytically reduced iron. Absorption of this iron averages 5% of their ferrous sulfate. Many have recommended mixing this cereal with a fruit juice containing vitamin C to enhance the iron absorption. All infants would benefit from receiving a food source or supplement of iron by 4 to 6 months of age.

ZINC

Body Stores

The infant is born without zinc body stores. Tissue concentrations are similar to those of adults. Therefore, infants rapidly become dependent on a dietary source.

Variations in concentrations of plasma zinc during growth reflect the continued utilization and depletion of body stores of zinc. Although there are not enough data to state a requirement, the RDA standard has been set for 3 mg during the first 6 months of life and 5 mg during the second 6 months. One study comparing hair zinc concentration of breast-fed and bottle-fed babies during the first 6 months of life found that only male bottle-fed infants experienced a significant decline in hair zinc concentration, suggesting that males had a higher requirement for zinc during the period studied.[27]

Food Sources

Breast-fed infants receive 0.7 to 5.0 mg/day of zinc, approximately 0.2 to 1.2 mg/kg.[28] Colostrum contains 20 mg/L, three to five times as much as later milk. Levels of zinc in human milk decline after 2 months of lactation and may fall below 1.0 mg/L. Infant formulas are supplemented and contain 3 to 4 mg/L. Animal studies suggest that the bioavailability of zinc is 59.2% in human milk, 43% to 53.9% in cow's milk, and 26.8% to 39.5% in infant formula.[29]

VITAMINS

Body Stores

Most vitamins cross the placenta and accumulate in the fetus in greater concentrations than in the mother. Maternal hypovitaminemia will be reflected in the fetus.[29] Vitamins A, E, and beta-carotene concentrations are lower in the newborn's blood than in the mother's blood. The concentration of water-soluble vitamins in the blood of the neonate is higher than that of the mother.

Food Sources

Full-term infants who receive milk from a well-nourished lactating mother will receive all the vitamins they need with the exception of vitamin D. Human milk contains 40 to 50 IU/L of vitamin D activity. Although human milk does provide calcium and phosphorus in a form usable by the neonate without the presence of vitamin D, the provision of other sources of vitamin D becomes increasingly important as the infant grows older.[31]

Infants who receive a commercially available formula that is properly prepared will be adequately nourished with vitamins. Homogenized milk is fortified with vitamin D but has little vitamin C.

NUTRIENT SUPPLEMENTS

Vitamins

Vitamin K is synthesized by intestinal flora, but it takes several days or weeks to establish the flora in the newborn's sterile gut. Therefore, a prophylactic intramuscular dose of 0.5 to 1.0 mg of vitamin K, or an oral dose of 1.0 to 2.1 mg, is usually given to infants at birth.[32] After receiving the dose, infants are able to synthesize vitamin K from the bacteria in their gut and hemorrhagic disease of the newborn is no longer a risk.

Breast-fed infants should receive vitamin D by 2 months of age. Older infants who receive homogenized milk should be given a food source or supplement of vitamin C.

Minerals

Cow's milk contains 0.03 to 0.1 μg/L of fluoride; human milk contains less than 0.05 μg/L.[33] Infant formulas are not prepared by the manufacturer with fluoridated water. Unless the infant receives a formula prepared at home with fluoridated water, supplements are appropriate. The recommended intakes of fluoride are shown in Table 6-5.

The need for supplemental iron depends on the composition of the diet consumed. Solely breast-fed infants should receive a supplement by 4 to 6 months of age. Those who receive iron-fortified cereals will probably need supplements. Formula-fed infants should receive iron-fortified formula and if so will need no supplemental iron.

Milk for Infants

HUMAN MILK AND FORMULAS

The advantages of human milk for feeding human infants are numerous and breast-feeding is encouraged by most health care professionals. Many mothers breast-feed their infants for a few months and then offer them a formula. Most normal full-term infants who are not breast-fed receive a cow's-milk-base formula. Infants who do not tolerate cow's milk may receive a soy or hydrolyzed casein formula.

Differences in human and cow's milk have been discussed in the previous chapter. From such comparisons it soon becomes apparent that if cow's milk is offered to infants it must be modified. Products prepared for infant feeding do indeed modify cow's milk. In fact, most attempt to simulate human milk.

AAP STANDARDS

The Committee on Nutrition of the American Academy of Pediatrics (AAP), concerned about the composition of proprietary infant formulas, issued a policy statement

TABLE 6-5 Supplemental Fluorine Dosage Schedule (mg/day*)

	Concentration of Fluoride in Drinking Water (ppm)		
Age	**<0.3**	**0.3-0.7**	**>0.7**
2 weeks to 2 years	0.25	0	0
2 to 3 years	0.50	0.25	0
3 to 16 years	1.00	0.50	0

From Committee on Nutrition: Pediatrics 63:150, 1979. Copyright American Academy of Pediatrics 1979.

*2.2 mg of sodium fluoride contains 1 mg of fluoride.

on standards for these products.[21] These standards are based on the composition of human milk from a healthy mother. The minimum amount for each nutrient is close to that of human milk and thus is the preferable quantity. The maximum amount is given for formulas intended for low-birth-weight or sick infants who take less formula and thus need the higher nutrient content (Table 6-6). Nutrients provided by commonly used formula preparations are given in Table 6-7.

MODIFIED COW'S MILK FORMULAS

Commercially manufactured formulas prepared from nonfat cow's milk are readily available and are generously used for feeding in infancy. The protein and mineral content is decreased to reduce the solute load. The curd tension is reduced by homogenization and heat treatment to produce an easily digested protein. Two manufacturers combine whey with nonfat milk to produce a product with a whey-to-casein ratio similar to that in human milk. Combinations of vegetable oils, a high percentage of which are absorbed by infants, are added, and carbohydrate is added to increase the caloric concentration to approximately that of human milk and cow's milk. Vitamins and minerals are added. Formulas are marketed both with and without ferrous sulfate in amounts that provide 12 mg of iron/qt.

HYPOALLERGENIC FORMULAS

Soy Formulas

The most commonly used products for infants who have conditions that contraindicate the use of cow's milk are the soy milks. The most frequently used formulas are constructed of protein isolated from soy meal fortified with methionine, corn syrup or sucrose, and soy or other vegetable oils to which vitamins and minerals have been added. The trypsin inhibitor in raw soybean meal is inactivitated during heat processing. The goitrogenic effect of soy is diminished by heating and the addition of iodine.

Casein Hydrolysate Formulas

Other formulas are marketed for infants who do not tolerate either soy or cow's milk. Nutramigen, prepared from a casein hydrolysate and corn oil, and Progestimil, which contains a casein hydrolysate and medium-chain triglycerides, are examples. Both formulas have an unpleasant odor and taste and are rarely accepted by infants if not introduced before 8 to 9 months of age. The composition of non-cow's-milk-base formulas is given in Table 6-8.

SUBSTITUTE AND IMITATION MILKS

Feeding infants formulas made from recipes that have not been proved to support adequate nutrition should be strongly discouraged. Malnutrition has been observed in infants fed a barley water, corn syrup, and whole milk formula suggested in a magazine for mothers.[34] Kwashiorkor has been reported in infants fed a nondairy creamer as a substitute for milk.[35]

Substitute or imitation milks should not be offered to infants. Substitute milk is defined by the Food and Drug Administration as a nutritional equivalent to whole or

TABLE 6-6 Nutrient Levels of Infant Formulas (per 100 kcal)

Nutrient	CON 1976 Recommendations	
	Minimum	**Maximum**
Protein (gm)	1.8	4.5
Fat		
(gm)	3.3	6.0
(% cal)	30.0	54.0
Essential fatty acids (linoleate)		
(% cal)	3.0	—
(mg)	300.0	—
Vitamins		
A (IU)	250.0 (75 μg)*	750.0 (225 μg)*
D (IU)	40.0	100.0
K (μg)	4.0	—
E (IU)	0.3 (with 0.7 IU/gm linoleic acid)	—
C (ascorbic acid) (mg)	8.0	—
B_1 (thiamine) (μg)	40.0	—
B_2 (riboflavin) (μg)	60.0	—
B_6 (pyridoxine) (μg)	35.0 (with 15 μg/gm of protein in formula)	—
B_{12} (μg)	0.15	—
Niacin		
(μg)	250.0	—
(μg equiv)	—	—
Folic acid (μg)	4.0	—
Pantothenic acid (μg)	300.0	—
Biotin (μg)	1.5	—
Choline (mg)	7.0	—
Inositol (mg)	4.0	—
Minerals		
Calcium (mg)	50.0+	—
Phosphorus (mg)	25.0+	—
Magnesium (mg)	6.0	—
Iron (mg)	0.15	—
Iodine (μg)	5.0	—
Zinc (mg)	0.5	—
Copper (μg)	60.0	—
Manganese (μg)	5.0	—
Sodium (mg)	20.0 (6 mEq)‡	60.0 (17 mEq)‡
Potassium (mg)	80.0 (14 mEq)‡	200.0 (34 mEq)‡
Chloride (mg)	55.0 (11mEq)‡	150.0 (29 mEq)‡

From Committee on Nutrition, American Academy of Pediatrics: Pediatrics **57**(2):278, 1976. Copyright American Academy of Pediatrics, 1976.

*Retinol equivalents.

+Calcium to phosphorus ratio must be no less than 1.1 nor more than 2.0.

‡Milliequivalent for 670 kcal/L of formula.

TABLE 6-7 Nutrient Content of Commercially Available Cow's-milk-base Formula

	Similac	Enfamil	S.M.A.
NUTRIENT SOURCE			
Protein	Casein	Reduced mineral whey, casein	Demineralized whey, casein
Fat	Soy oil, coconut oil, corn oil	Soy oil, coconut oil	Oleo; soybean, safflower, and coconut oils
Carbohydrate	Lactose	Lactose	Lactose
NUTRIENTS PER 100 ML—NORMAL DILUTION			
Energy (kcal)	68	67	67
Protein (gm)	1.5	1.5	1.5
Fat (gm)	3.6	3.8	3.6
Carbohydrate (gm)	7.2	6.9	7.2
Vitamin A (IU)	200	207	240
Vitamin D (IU)	40	42	42
Vitamin E (IU)	2	2	1
Vitamin C (mg)	5.5	5.5	5.8
Thiamine (μg)	65	53	71
Riboflavin (μg)	10	11	11
Niacin (mg) (equiv.)	.7	.8	1.0
Pyridoxine (μg)	40	42	40
Vitamin B_{12} (μg)	.15	.16	.11
Folic acid (μg)	10	10.5	5.3
Calcium (mg)	51	46	44
Phosphorus (mg)	39	31.7	33
Magnesium (mg)	4	4	5
Iron (mg)	tr.	tr.	tr.
Zinc (mg)	.5	.5	.37
Copper (μg)	60	63.4	48
Iodine (μg)	10	6.8	7

nonfat milk based on their content of only 14 or 15 nutrients. It does not include all nutrients recommended as components of infant formulas. Imitation milk simulates milk but does not meet the standard of identity for substitute milk.[36]

FORMULA PREPARATION

Types of Formula Available

Manufacturers market three basic types of formulas, each of which is prepared according to its form: (1) *liquid concentrates* prepared for feeding by mixing equal amounts of the liquid and water; (2) *ready-to-feed* formulas that require no preparation, available in an assortment of sizes (4-, 6-, and 8-oz bottles and 32-oz containers); and (3) *powdered* formulas that are prepared by mixing 1 level tablespoonful of powder for each 2 oz of water. One recommended evaporated milk formula is prepared by mixing 13 oz (one can) of evaporated milk with 2 tablespoonsful of corn syrup and 18

TABLE 6-8 Nutrient Content of Soy Formulas and Other Milk Substitutes for Infants

	Prosobee	Isomil	Nutramigen	Progestimil
NUTRIENT SOURCE				
Protein	Soy protein	Soy protein	Casein hydrolysate	Casein hydrolysate
Fat	Soy oil	Coconut oil, soy oil	Corn oil	Corn oil, medium chain triglycer-ides
Carbohydrate	Corn syrup solids	Sucrose, corn syrup sol-ids	Modified tapioca, sucrose	Corn syrup solids, modified tapio-ca starch
NUTRIENTS PER 100 ML—NORMAL DILUTION				
Energy (kcal)	67	68	67	68
Protein (g)	2.0	2.0	1.9	1.9
Fat (g)	3.1	3.6	2.7	2.8
Carbohydrate (g)	7.1	6.8	9.4	9.4
Vitamin A (IU)	22.0	20.0	22.0	22.0
Vitamin D (IU)	44.0	40.0	44.0	44.0
Vitamin E (IU)	2.0	2.0	2.0	1.6
Vitamin C (mg)	5.7	5.5	5.7	5.7
Thiamin (μg)	55.2	40.0	55.2	55.2
Riboflavin (μg)	66.2	60.0	66.2	66.2
Niacin (mg) (equivalents)	.8	.9	.8	.8
Pyridoxine (μg)	44.1	40.0	44.1	44.1
Vitamin B_{12} (μg)	.2	.3	.2	.2
Folic acid (μg)	11.0	10.0	11.0	11.0
Calcium (mg)	66.0	70.0	66.0	66.0
Phosphorus (mg)	52.0	50.0	44.0	44.0
Magnesium (mg)	7.7	5.0	7.7	7.7
Iron (mg)	1.3	1.2	1.3	1.3
Zinc (mg)	.5	.5	.5	.4
Copper (μg)	66.0	50.0	66.0	66.0
Iodine (μg)	7.0	10.0	4.9	4.9

oz of water. All of these formulas, when properly prepared and adequately supplemented, provide the nutrients important for the infant in an appropriate caloric concentration and present a solute load reasonable for the full-term infant. Errors in dilution caused by lack of understanding of the proper method of preparation, improper measurements, adding extra water to make the formula last longer, or the belief of the parents that their child should have greater amounts of nutritious food can lead to problems.

Result of Errors in Formula Preparation

Failure to gain appropriately in height and weight has been observed as a result of dilution of ready-to-eat formulas in the manner that concentrated formulas are prepared. Mothers have been known to add extra water in the belief that more dilute formula might reduce spitting up by their infants. Also, overdiluting formula or offering water as a substitute for milk or as a pacifier can lead to serious consequences. Water intoxication resulting in hyponatremia, irritability, and coma has been reported in several infants fed 8 oz of water after each feeding or water as a substitute for milk because of financial inability of parents to buy more formula.[37]

Feeding undiluted concentrated formula increases kilocalories, protein, and solutes presented to the kidneys for excretion and may predispose the young infant to hypernatremia and tetany as well as obesity. Problems of improper formula preparation have most frequently been reported with the use of powdered formula and occur most often when an increased need for water caused by a fever or infection is superimposed on consumption of an already high-solute formula. Infants fed concentrated formula during such illnesses may become thirsty, demand more to drink, or refuse to consume more liquid because of anorexia secondary to the illness. When presented with more milk concentrated in the protein and solutes, the osmolality of the blood increases and hypernatremic dehydration may result. Cases of cerebral damage and gangrene of the extremities have been reported to be the result of hypernatremic dehydration and metabolic acidosis.[38,39]

Anticipatory guidance of parents of young infants should include information on the variety of formulas available with which to feed their infants, differences in methods of preparation of each product, and the dangers of overdiluted formula and excessive water intake.

Sterilization of Formulas

Although terminal sterilization may be recommended for infant formulas, most parents do not follow this practice but prepare formulas by the clean technique, one bottle at each feeding time, and immediately feed the infant. Several researchers have found no differences in incidence of illness or infection of infants fed formulas prepared by the clean technique or by terminal sterilization regardless of socioeconomic background or housekeeping practices.[40,41] Formulas prepared by both methods result in milk that produces aerobic bacteria.

To prepare formula by the clean technique, the hands of the person preparing the formula should be washed carefully. All equipment to be used during preparation, including the cans that contain the milk, the bottles, and the nipples, must be thoroughly washed and rinsed. Once opened, cans of formula must be covered and refrigerated. The formula is prepared immediately before each feeding as described above. After the formula has been heated and the infant has been fed, any remaining milk should be discarded. Warm milk is an excellent medium for bacterial growth.

MILKS CONSUMED BY OLDER INFANTS

Homogenized Whole Cow's Milk

Homogenized cow's milk may be offered to infants after 6 months of age. Enteric blood loss as a result of intakes of more than a quart of homogenized milk per day was at one time believed to be one factor responsible for as great as 50% of the iron deficiency in infancy.[42] However, Fomon and others[43] have since found that infants fed whole cow's milk between 112 and 140 days of age had more guaiac-positive stools than did those fed a commercially prepared formula. Infants who had been fed soy protein isolates between 8 and 112 days of age had more fecal blood loss than did those fed a cow's-milk-base formula the first 112 days. However, between 140 and 196 days of age there was no difference in the number of guaiac-positive stools between infants fed whole cow's milk or a heat-treated formula. The American Academy of Pediatrics has stated that there is no convincing evidence that feeding whole cow's milk after 6 months of age is harmful if adequate semisolid foods are given and the volume of intake is limited to 1 L/day.

Neither 2% nor nonfat milk is appropriate for infants in the first year of life. They are frequently fortified with nonfat milk solids, which increases the protein and mineral content of the milk and the solutes that must be excreted by the kidneys. It can be anticipated that infants fed nonfat milk will receive an excessive percentage of their kilocalories from protein and that their intakes of kilocalories may be sufficiently reduced that normal increments of weight gain may not be achieved. Studies of male infants who were fed nonfat milk with added linoleic acid between 4 and 6 months of age revealed that these infants increased their volume of intake of both milk and infant foods. However, since energy intakes were insufficient to meet requirements for growth, fat reserves were depleted, as demonstrated by reductions in fatfold thickness.[44]

Formula for Older Infants

One manufacturer (Ross Laboratories) markets a formula for the older infant that consists of nonfat milk, corn oil, and sucrose. The kilocalorie content is reduced to 16.5 kcal/oz as compared with 20 kcal/oz in standard formulas. The formula is fortified with both iron and vitamins. Infants fed this milk and pureed foods have been noted to increase their volume of intake, so that when compared with infants consuming a standard formula supplying 20 kcal/oz, energy intakes are similar.[44]

Foods in the Infant's Diet

In spite of the fact that no nutritional or developmental advantage can be expected from the early introduction of semisolid foods, many families feed them in the first month of infant life. Some parents add semisolid foods hoping that the added foods will encourage their infants to sleep through the night, a commonly held belief that has proved to be untrue.[45] Other parents feed semisolid foods because they think that their infants are hungry or because they consider the acceptance of these foods a developmental landmark.

Many infants receive foods with texture such as baked potato or drained tuna fish by the time they can sustain a sitting posture. When they reach out and secure foods with a pincer grasp, finger foods such as zwieback and arrowroot cookies are offered.

SEMISOLID FOODS

Age of Introduction

The age of introduction of semisolid foods to infants in the United States declined between 1920, when these foods were seldom offered before 1 year of age, and the period between 1960 and 1970 when they were frequently offered in the first weeks and months of life. Concern that this early introduction of semisolid foods predisposed infants to obesity and allergic reactions caused many health-care professionals in the pediatric community to re-examine the appropriate age to introduce these foods. It is currently recommended that the feeding of semi-solid foods be delayed until the consumption of food is no longer a reflex process and the infant has fine, gross, and oral motor skills to appropriately consume them, that is, at approximately 4 to 6 months of age. Table 6-9 gives suggested guidelines for the introduction of semisolid and table foods to normal infants.

Schedule for Adding Foods

Iron-fortified infant cereals are usually the first foods added to the infant's diet. It makes little difference whether fruits or vegetables or introduced next. New foods should be added singly, no more than one new food every 3 days. The introduction of vegetables containing nitrate, for example, carrots, beets, and spinach, is usually delayed until the infant is at least 4 months of age, because the nitrate can be converted to nitrite in the stomach of the young infant. This can result in methemoglobinemia. It is generally recommended that the introduction of fruit juice be delayed until it can be consumed by cup. Ranges of nutrients in infant foods are large (Table 6-10).

Home Preparation of Infant Foods

In spite of the fact that the manufacturers of infant foods no longer add salt or sugar to most of their commercially prepared products, many parents prefer to make their own with a food grinder, blender, or strainer. The foods should be carefully selected

TABLE 6-9 Suggested Ages for the Introduction of Semisolid Foods and Table Food

	Age (months)		
Food	**4 to 6**	**6 to 8**	**9 to 12**
Iron-fortified cereals for infants	Add		
Vegetables		Add strained	Gradually delete strained foods, introduce table foods
Fruits		Add strained	Gradually delete strained foods, introduce chopped well-cooked or canned foods
Meats		Add strained or finely chopped table meats	Decrease the use of strained meats, increase the varieties of table meats
Finger foods such as arrowroot biscuits, oven-dried toast		Add those that can be secured with a palmar grasp	Increase the use of small-sized finger foods as the pincer grasp develops
Well-cooked mashed or chopped table foods, prepared without added salt or sugar			Add
Juice by cup			Add

TABLE 6-10 Ranges of Selected Nutrients per Ounce in Commercially Prepared Infant Foods

Food	Energy (kcal)	Protein (gm)	Iron (mg)	Vitamin A (IU)	Vitamin C (mg)
Dry cereal	102-114	2.0-10.2	17.0-21.0	0-20	0-1.4
Strained and junior fruits	11-23	0.0-0.2	0.0-2.0	3-206	0.2-35.3
Strained and junior vegetables	7-18	0.2-1.0	0.1-0.4	9-3348	0.6-3.6
Strained and junior meats	27-42	3.6-4.4	.3-1.5	8-10811	.3-.7
Strained egg yolks	58	2.8	0.8	355	0.4
Strained and junior meat and vegetable dinners	20-33	1.6-2.6	0.0-0.3	22-237	0.1-0.5
Strained and junior vegetables and meat dinners	9-70	0.1-1.5	0.1-0.3	4-1114	0.2-1.2
Strained and junior desserts	17-25	0.0-0.8	0.0-0.1	4-71	0.2-8.9

From Gebhardt, S.E., Cutrufelli, R., and Matthews, R.H.: Composition of food, baby foods, raw, processed, prepared, Agriculture Handbook No. 8-3, Washington, D.C., 1978, U.S. Department of Agriculture

from high-quality fresh, frozen, or canned fruits, vegetables, and meats, and prepared so that nutrients are retained. The preparation area and all utensils used should be meticulously cleaned. Salt and sugar should be used sparingly, if at all. When the food has been cooked then pureed or strained, it should be packaged in individual portions and refrigerated or frozen so that a single portion can be heated and fed without compromising the quality and bacterial content of the entire batch (Fig. 6-4). Directions for this preparation of infant foods are given on page 243. Care must be taken not to use additional seasoning, as home-prepared infant foods usually have a greater energy content than the commercial products and many have a higher salt content. One study found that home-prepared infant foods had 1005% more salt than commercially prepared foods.

TABLE FOOD

Food from the family menu is introduced at an early age in the diets of many infants. The age of introduction and type of food offered will reflect cultural practice. For example, crumbled cornbread mixed with pot liquor (the liquid from cooked vegetables) may be fed to infants in the southern states by 3 months of age, "sticky" rice may be fed to Oriental infants in the Pacific Northwest by 6 to 7 months of age, mashed beans with some of the cooking liquid are often given to Latin American infants at 2 to 4 months of age, and mashed potatoes are offered to many infants by 3 to 4 months of age.

Form and Texture

Solid foods offered to infants should be in a form easily masticated and not given in small pieces. Choking and aspiration can occur if small pieces of hot dogs, grapes, hard candy, nuts, and other foods in small, hard pieces are consumed.

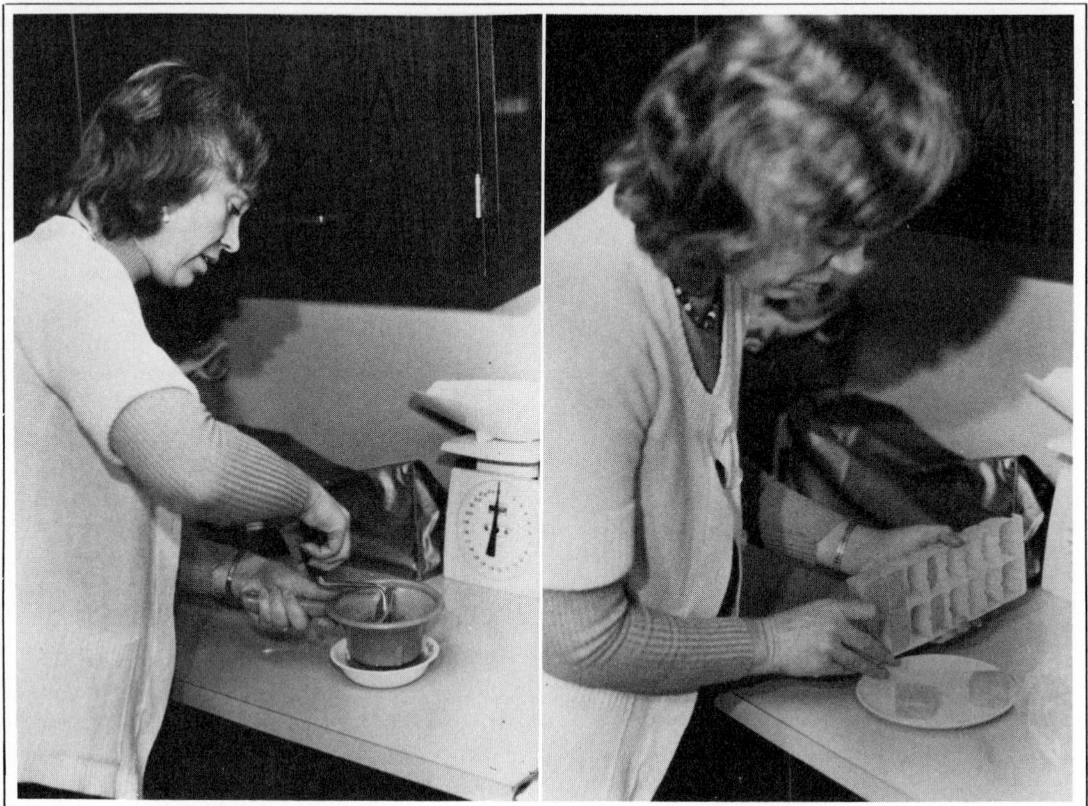

FIG. 6-4 **A,** Mother prepares food for her infant. **B,** After the food is frozen in ice-cube trays, she removes the cubes and stores them in individual portions for later use.

Honey

Sometimes honey is used as a sweetener for home-prepared infant foods and formulas, and recommended for use on pacifiers to promote sucking in hypotonic infants. However, honey has been implicated as the only food source of spores of *Clostridium botulinum* during infancy. These spores are extremely resistant to heat and are not destroyed by present methods of processing honey. Botulism in infancy is caused by ingestion of the spores, which germinate into the toxin in the lumen of the bowel. Honey should not be fed to infants less than 1 year of age.[46]

Texture Progress

Stages of development of feeding behavior indicate readiness to progress in textures of food and will be discussed in the section on development of feeding behavior. The energy and nutrient values of foods offered must also be considered. Examples of table foods often offered and their contribution to an infant's dietary intake are given in Table 6-11.

DIRECTIONS FOR HOME PREPARATION OF INFANT FOODS

1. Select fresh, high-quality fruits, vegetables, or meats.
2. Be sure all utensils, including cutting boards, grinders, knives, etc., are thoroughly clean.
3. Wash your hands before preparing the food.
4. Clean, wash, and trim the foods in as little water as possible.
5. Cook the foods until tender in as little water as possible. Avoid overcooking, which may destroy heat-sensitive nutrients.
6. Do not add salt. Add sugar sparingly. Do not add honey to foods for infants less than 1 year of age.*
7. Add enough water so that the food has a consistency that is easily pureed.
8. Strain or puree the food using an electric blender, a food mill, a baby food grinder, or a kitchen strainer.
9. Pour puree into ice cube tray and freeze.
10. When food is frozen hard, remove the cubes and store in freezer bags.
11. Unfreeze and heat in serving container the amount of food that will be consumed at a single feeding (in water bath or microwave oven).

From Pipes, P.L.: Nutrition in infancy. In Krause, M.V., and Mahan, L.K.: Food, nutrition, and diet therapy, ed. 7, Philadelphia, 1984, W.B. Saunders Co.

*Botulism spores have been reported in honey, and young infants do not have the immune capacity to resist this infection.

TABLE 6-11 Nutrient Content of Selected Table Foods Commonly Fed to Infants

Food	Portion Size	Energy (kcal)	Protein (gm)	Iron (mg)	Vitamin A (IU)	Vitamin C (mg)
Cooked cereal (farina)	¼ cup	26	0.8	Dependent on level of fortification		
Mashed potato	¼ cup	34	1.1	0.2	10	5
French fried potato	3, 1″ to 2″	29	0.4	0.2		
Spaghetti	2 tbsp	19	0.6	0.2		
Macaroni and cheese	2 tbsp	54	2.1	0.2	107	
Liverwurst	½ oz	45	2.1	0.8	925	
Hamburger	½ oz	41	3.4	0.5	5	
Eggs	1 medium	72	5.7	1.0	520	
Cottage cheese	1 tbsp	5	1.9		23.7	
Green beans	1 tbsp	3	0.15	0.2	43	1
Cooked carrots	1 tbsp	2.81			952	
Banana	½ small	40	0.5	0.35	90	5
Pudding	¼ cup	70	2.2	Trace	102	
Lollipop	1 oz hard candy	109				
Saltine crackers	1	12	0.2			
Vanilla wafer	¼″ thick, 1¾″ diameter	18	0.2			
Cheese strips	¼ oz	28	1.78		92	

From Adams, C.F.: Nutritive value in American foods in common units, Agriculture Handbook no. 456, Washington, D.C., 1975, U.S. Department of Agriculture.

Intakes of Infants

Volume of intake and energy consumption is influenced not only by the infant's requirements for maintenance, growth, and activity, but also by the parents' sensitivity to and willingness to accept cues of hunger and satiety, eagerness for the infant to feed, and skill at feeding. Infants eat differently, and mothers vary in their sensitivity to the child's cues. Thoman[47] found that primiparous mothers spent more time stimulating their infants during feeding than did multiparous mothers, yet their infants spent less time sucking during breast-feeding and consumed less from bottles at feeding than did infants of multiparous mothers. The stimulation prolonged the pauses between sucking and reduced the total consumption of food.

GROWTH RESPONSE TO FEEDING

Formula-fed infants have been reported to regain their birth weights more rapidly than breast-fed infants.[9] Thereafter, weight gains until 3 months appear similar in breast- and bottle-fed babies after which bottle-fed infants gain more rapidly.[48]

ENERGY INTAKES

Per unit of size, infants consume the greatest number of kilocalories between 14 and 28 days of age, a time referred to by many pediatricians as the hungry period.[49] After this time, although total quantity and energy intake increase, intakes per unit of size decrease. Infants consume greater amounts of food and nutrients as they grow older but less and less per unit of body size.

Wide ranges of volume of intake and energy consumption throughout the first year of life have been noted in formula-fed infants by several researchers.[50] Table 6-12 shows ranges of intake of breast- and bottle-fed infants at 1, 2, and 3 months of age in an Australian study.

TABLE 6-12 Consumption of kcal per kg Body Weight (Mean and Range) of Breast-milk Substitutes (BMS) and Breast-milk (BM) by 150 Infants Aged 1-3 Months and Fed Ad Libitum

Age (months)	BMS (kcal/kg)	BM (kcal/kg)
1	120 (78-201)	112 (74-146)
2	107 (75-168)	108 (74-145)
3	101 (76-130)	96 (70-120)

Hofvandor, Y., and others: The amount of milk consumed by 1-3 month old breast- or bottle-fed infants, Acta Paediatr. Scand. 71:953, 1982.

Feeding Behaviors

DEVELOPMENTAL READINESS

Defining developmental readiness for changes in textures of food and the acquisition of self-feeding skills is important in establishing realistic goals for normal and handicapped infants and children. Illingworth and Lister[51] have defined a "critical or sensitive" period of development in relation to eating, a time at which a specific stimulus, solid food, must be applied for the organism to learn a particular action, accepting and eating table foods. They point out that infants learn to chew at about 6 or 7 months of age; thus at this point they are developmentally ready to consume food. If solid foods are withheld until a later age, the child will have considerably more difficulty in accepting them.

In 1937 Gesell and Ilg[52] published their classic observations made during extensive studies of the feeding behavior of infants. Their observations are as valid today as they were then. Cineradiographic techniques developed since then have permitted more detailed descriptions of the actions involved in sucking, suckling, and swallowing.[53,54]

DEVELOPMENT OF ORAL STRUCTURES AND FUNCTIONS

It is important to recognize that even though the normal neonate is well prepared to suck and swallow at birth, the physical and neuromotor maturation during the first year alter both the form of the oral structures and the methods by which the infant extracts milk from a nipple. Each of these changes influences the infant's eating skills. At birth the tongue is disproportionately large in comparison with the lower jaw and essentially fills the oral cavity. The mandible is retruded relative to the maxilla, the maxilla protruding over the mandible by approximately 2 mm.[55] When the mouth is closed, the jaws do not rest on top of each other, but the tip of the tongue lies between the upper and lower jaws. There is a "fat pad" in each of the cheeks. It is thought that these pads serve as a prop for the buccinator muscle, maintaining rigidity of the cheeks during suckling.[56] The lips of the neonate are also instrumental in suckling and have characteristics appropriate for their function at this age. A mucosal fold on the free edge of the gums in the region of the eye-tooth buds of both jaws helps seal off the oral cavity as the lips close around the nipple. The mucosal fold disappears by the third or fourth month, when the lips have developed muscular control to seal the oral cavity.[56] The newborn infant sucks reflexively, the young infant beginning at 2 or 3 weeks of age suckles, and as infants grow older they learn mature sucking. Some description of these two processes, therefore, seems important.

SUCKLING

Studies by Ardran, Kemp, and Lind[53] have shown that the processes of breast and bottle suckling are similar. The nipple of the breast becomes rigid and elongated during breast-feeding so that it resembles a rubber nipple in shape, and both assume a similar position in the infant's mouth. The infant grasps the nipple in the mouth. The oral cavity is sealed off by pressure from the medial portions of the lips assisted by the mucosal folds of the jaws. The nipple is held in the infant's mouth with the tip located close to the junction of the hard and soft palates.

During the first stage of suckling, the mandible and tongue are lowered while the mouth is closed, thus creating a negative pressure. The tip of the tongue moves forward. The mandible and tongue are next raised, compressing the anterior end of the nipple. The compression is moved anteroposteriorly as the tip of the tongue withdraws, thus stroking or milking the liquid from the nipple. The retruded position of the mandible maximizes the efficiency of the stroking action.[53,54] As the tongue moves back, it comes in contact with the tensed soft palate, thus causing liquid to squirt into the lateral food channels. The location of the larynx is much higher during infancy than it is in adulthood, and the larynx is further elevated by the muscular contractions during swallowing. The epiglottis functions as a breakwater during swallowing. As the liquid is squirted back in the mouth, the epiglottis is positioned so that it parts the stream of liquid, passing it to the sides of the larynx instead of over it. Thus liquid does not pass over the laryngeal entrance during early infancy because of the relatively higher position of the larynx and the parting of the stream of liquid by the epiglottis.

SUCKING

Mature sucking is an acquired feature of the orofacial muscles. It is not a continuous process. Upon accumulation of sufficient fluid in the mouth, sucking and breathing are interrupted by a swallowing movement. The closure of the nasopharyngeal and laryngeal sphincters in response to the presence of food in the pharynx is responsible for the interruption of the nasal breathing.[57]

During swallowing the food lies in the swallow preparatory position on the groove of the tongue. The distal portion of the soft palate is raised toward the adenoidal pad in the roof of the epipharynx. The tongue is pressed upward against the nipple so that the bolus of milk follows gravity down the sloping tongue reaching the pharynx. As the bolus moves downward, the posterior wall of the pharynx comes forward to displace the soft palate toward the dorsal surface of the tongue and the larynx is elevated and arched backward. The bolus is expressed from the pharynx by peristaltic movements of the pharyngeal wall toward the back of the tongue and the larynx. The bolus spills over the pharyngeoepiglottic folds into the lateral food channels and then into the esophagus.[54]

The tonsils and lymphoid tissue play an important role as infants swallow. They help keep the airway open and the food away from the posterior pharyngeal wall as the infant is held in a reclining position, thus delaying nasopharyngeal closure until food has reached the pharynx.[56]

As the infant grows older the oral cavity enlarges so that the tongue no longer fills the mouth. The tongue grows differentially at the tip and attains motility in the larger oral cavity. The elongated tongue can be protruded to receive and pass solids between the gum pads and erupting teeth for mastication. Mature feeding is characterized by separate movements of the lip, tongue, and gum pads or teeth.[56]

SEQUENCE OF DEVELOPMENT OF FEEDING BEHAVIOR

The sequence of development of feeding behavior relates to the individual maturation of the infant.

Newborns

The "rooting reflex" caused by stroking of the perioral skin including the cheeks and lips causes an infant to turn toward the stimulus, so that the mouth comes in contact with it. Stimulus placed on the lips causes involuntary movements toward it, closure, and pouting in preparation for sucking.[58] These reflexes thus enable the infant to suck and receive nourishment. Both rooting and suckling can be elicited when the infant is hungry but are absent when the infant is satiated.[55] During feeding the neonate assumes a tonic position, the head rotated to one side and the arm on that side fisted. The infant seeks the nipple by touch and obtains milk from the nipple with a rhythmic suckle.[52] Semisolid foods, introduced by spoon at an early age into the diets of many infants, are secured in the same manner as the milk, by stroking movements of the tongue with the tongue projecting as the spoon is withdrawn. Frequently, the food is expelled from the mouth.

Age 16-24 Weeks

By 16 weeks of age the more mature sucking pattern becomes evident, with the tongue moving back and forth as opposed to the earlier up-and-down motions. Spoon feeding is easier because the infant can draw in the lower lip as the spoon is removed. The tonic neck position has faded and the infant assumes a more symmetrical position with the head at midline. The hands close on the bottle.[52] By 20 weeks of age the infant can grasp on tactile contact with a palmar squeeze. By 24 weeks of age the infant can reach for and grasp an object on sight. In almost every instance the object goes into the mouth.

Age 24-28 Weeks

Between 24 and 28 weeks of age chewing movements, an up-and-down movement of the jaws, begins. This movement, coupled with the ability to grasp and the hand-to-mouth route of grasped objects, as well as sitting posture, indicates a readiness of the infant to finger feed. Infants at this age grasp with a palmar grasp. Therefore, the shape of the food presented to the child to finger feed is important. Cookies, melba toast, crackers, and teething biscuits are frequently introduced at this stage.

Age 28-32 Weeks

Between 28 and 32 weeks of age the infant gains control of the trunk and can sit alone without support. The sitting infant has greater mobility of the shoulders and arms and is more able to reach and grasp. The grasp is more digital than the earlier palmar grasp. The infant is able to transfer items from one hand to another and learns to voluntarily release and resecure objects. The beginning of chewing patterns, up-and-down movements of the jaws, is demonstrated. The tongue shows more maturity in regard to spoon feeding than in drinking. Food is received from the spoon by pressing the lips against the spoon, drawing the head away, and drawing in the lower lip. The infant is aware of a cup and can suck from it. Milk leaks frequently from the corners of the mouth as the tongue is projected before swallowing.[52]

Age 6-12 Months

The introduction of soft mashed, but not strained, foods is appropriate at this stage of development. In fact, it is at this stage of development that Illingworth and Lister[51] believe it is critical to introduce the infant to harder-to-chew foods. Between 6 and 12 months of age the infant gradually receives greater amounts of food from the family menu and less and less of the pureed and strained items. Foods should be carefully selected and modified so that they are presented in a form that can be manipulated in the mouth without the potential of choking and aspiration, as may occur with small grains of rice or corn. Many parents mash well-cooked vegetables and canned fruits and successfully offer them to their infants. Well-cooked ground meat dishes such as ground meat in gravies or sauces appear to be easily accepted, as are liverwurst, minced chicken livers, and drained tuna fish. Custards, puddings, and ice cream soon become favorites.

By *28 weeks of age* infants are able to help themselves to their bottle in sitting postures, although they will not be able to tip the bottle adaptively as it empties until about 32 weeks of age. By the end of the first year they can completely manage bottle-feeding alone.

By *32 weeks of age* infants bring their heads forward to receive the spoon as it is presented to them. The tongue shows increased motility and allows for considerable increased manipulation of food in the mouth before swallowing. At the end of the first year, infants are able to manipulate food in the mouth with definite chewing movements.

During the *fourth quarter* of the first year, the child develops an increasingly precise pincer grasp. The bottle can be managed alone and can be resecured if it is lost. The child can drink from a cup only if help is provided. Infants at this age are increasingly conscious of what others do and often imitate the models set for them.[52] By 1 year of age the patterns of eating have changed from sucking to beginning rotary chewing movements. Children understand the concept of the container and the contained, have voluntary hand-to-mouth movements and a precise pincer grasp, and can voluntarily release and resecure objects. They are thus prepared to learn to feed themselves, a behavior they learn and refine in the second year.

This development of feeding behavior is summarized in Table 6-13, and is shown in the sequence of illustrations in Fig. 6-5.

Feeding the Infant

Presented with the breast of an adequately fed lactating mother or the nipple on a bottle of properly prepared formula, the hungry infant receives both biochemical and psychosocial nurturance.

TABLE 6-13 Sequence of Development of Feeding Behavior

Age	Reflexes	Oral, Fine, Gross Motor Development
1-3 months	Rooting and suck and swallow reflexes are present at birth Tonic neck reflex present	Head contol is poor Secures milk with suckling pattern, the tongue projecting during a swallow By the end of the third month, head control is developed
4-6 months	Rooting reflex fades Bite reflex fades Tonic neck reflex fades by 16 weeks	Changes from a suckling pattern to a mature suck with liquids Sucking strength increases Munching pattern begins Grasps with a palmar grasp Grasps, brings objects to mouth and bites them
7-9 months	Gag reflex is less strong as chewing of solids begins and normal gag is developing Choking reflex can be inhibited	Munching movements begin when solid foods are eaten Rotary chewing begins Sits alone Has power of voluntary release and resecural Holds bottle alone Develops an inferior pincer grasp
10-12 months		Reaches for a spoon Bites nipples, spoons, and crunchy foods Grasps bottle and foods and brings them to the mouth Can drink from a cup that is held Tongue is used to lick food morsels off the lower lip Finger feeds with a refined pincer grasp

Modified from Gessell, A., and Ilg. F.L.: Feeding behavior of infants, Philadelphia, 1937, J.B. Lippincott Co.

FEEDING SCHEDULE

The infant held in a semireclining position who is offered the nipple sucks and receives the major portion of nourishment in 20 minutes. Newborn infants will initially feed 6 to 8 times a day at intervals of 2 to 4 hours and will consume 2 to 3 oz at a feeding. By 2 weeks of age most infants will have increased the amount of milk consumed at a feeding and reduced the number of feedings to 6. By 2 months of age most infants are fed 5 times a day and sleep through the night. By 6 months of age most babies consume three meals and four milk feedings a day.

FOOD SELECTION

Because of the great variability in energy and nutrients provided by foods offered to infants, selection of foods and the amounts offered should be based on the infant's rate of gain in height and weight as well as on nutrient needs. The introduction and acceptance of iron-containing foods before the time homogenized milk replaces iron-fortified formula or iron supplements are discontinued is important. The infant must continue to consume foods that provide this nutrient as it is no longer available from milk

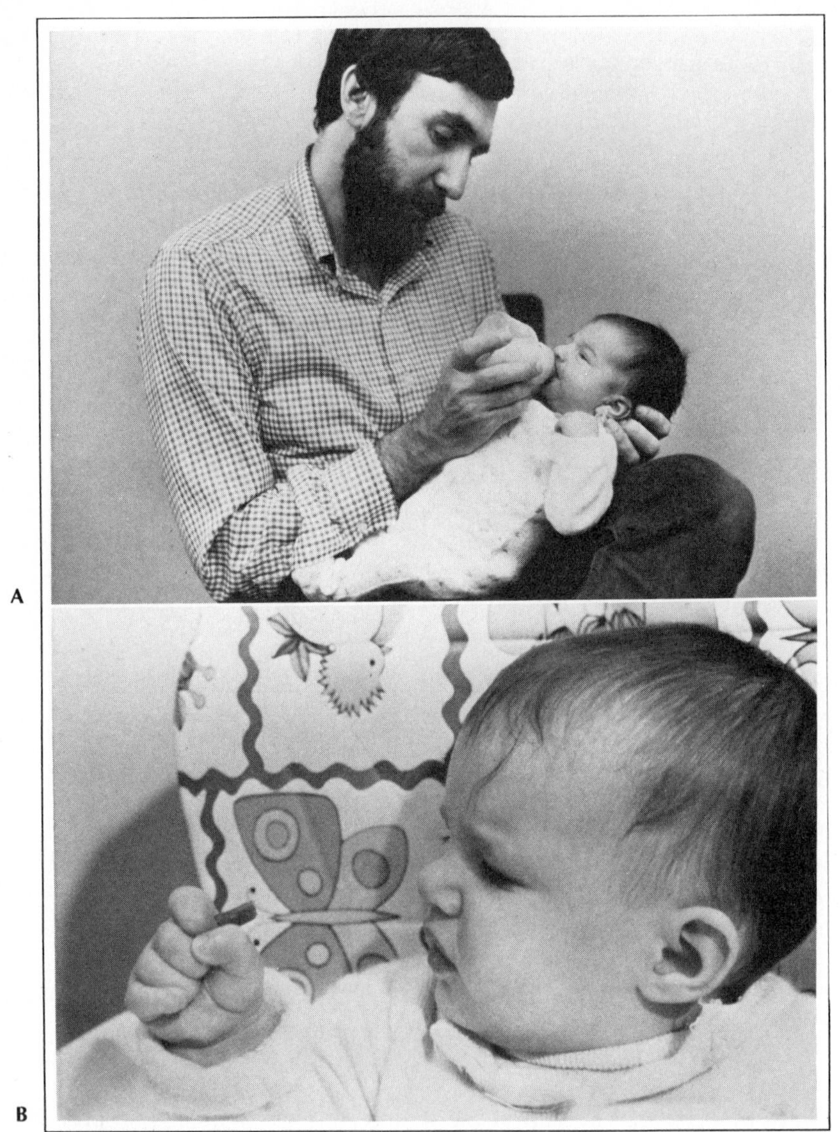

FIG. 6-5 Sequence of development of feeding behaviors. **A,** Infant sucks liquids. **B,** Five-month-old infant begins to finger feed.

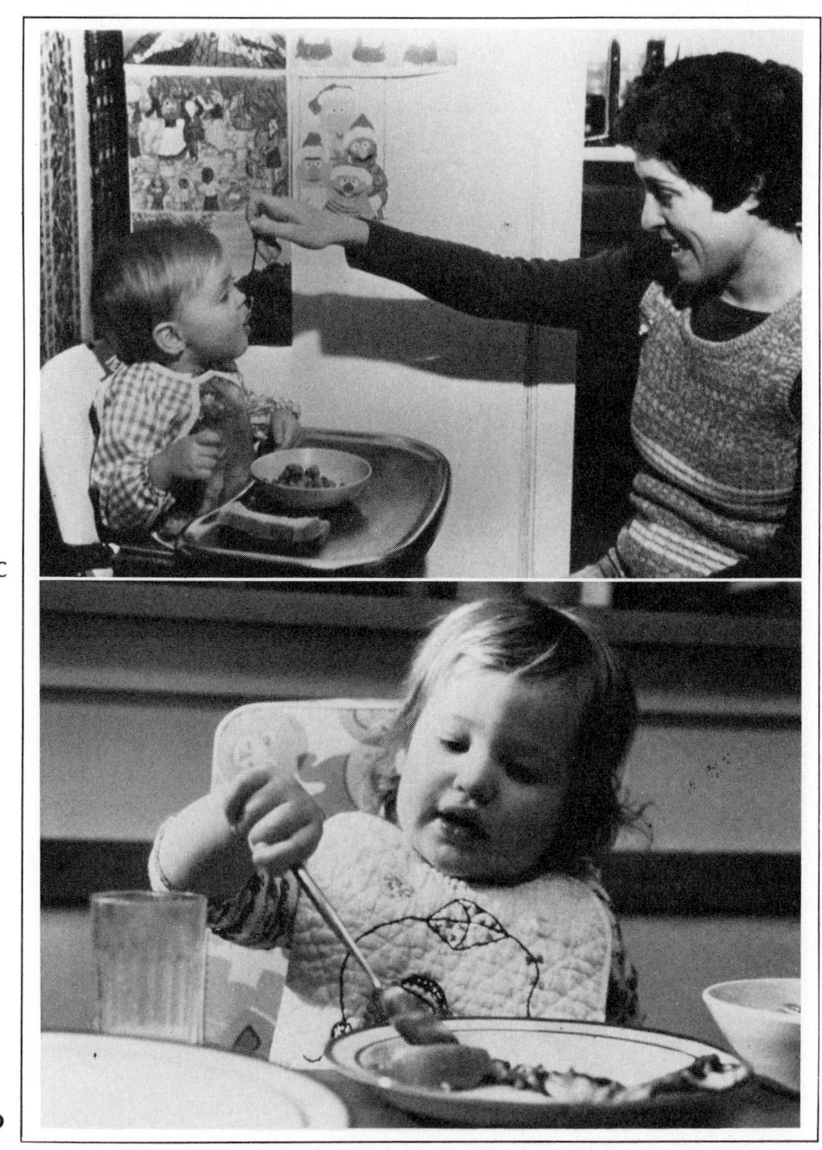

FIG. 6-5 cont'd. Sequence of development of feeding behaviors. **C,** Eight-month-old infant is fed table food. **D,** Eleven-month-old infant begins to feed herself.

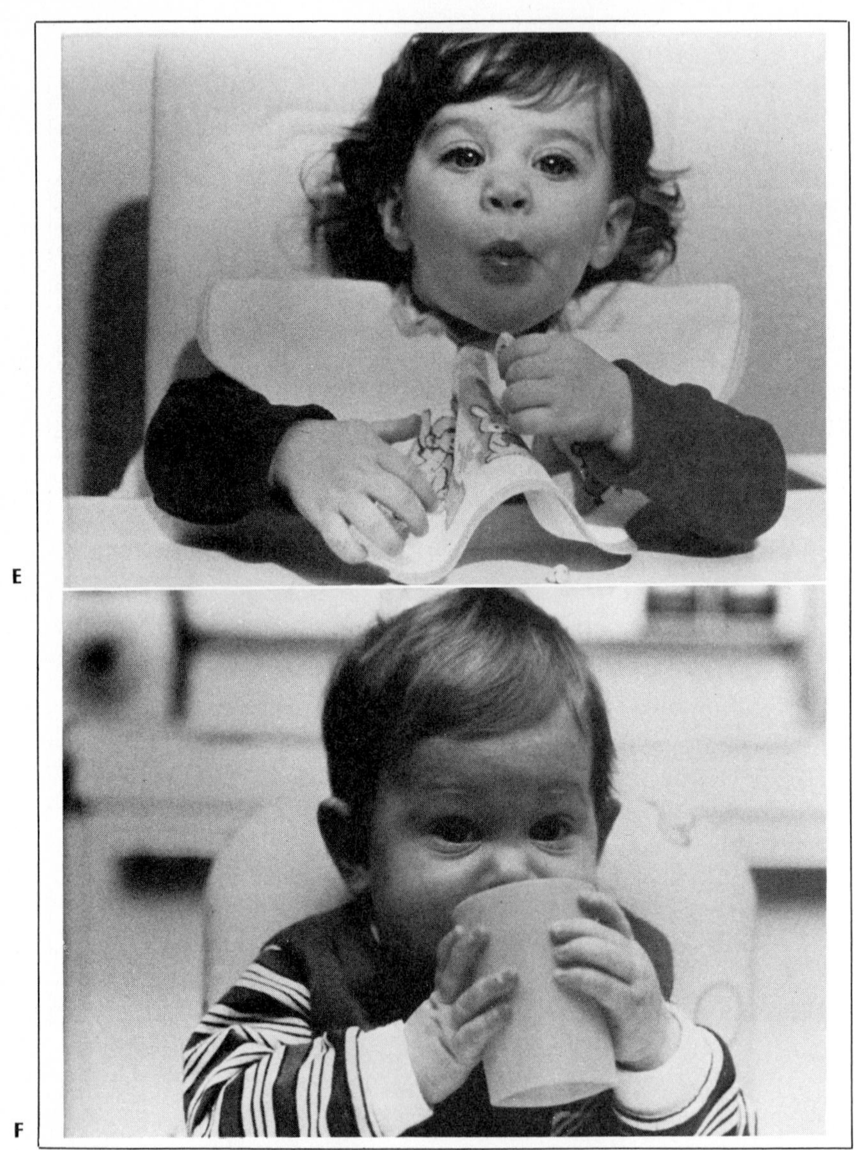

E

F

FIG. 6-5 cont'd. Sequence of development of feeding behaviors. **E,** Ten-month-old infant purses her lips. **F,** Twelve-month-old infant drinks from a cup.

or supplements. Fruit juice offers sources of vitamin C when vitamin-containing formulas are no longer consumed. It seems reasonable to encourage parents of infants whose gains in weight are more rapid than gains in length to feed the lower kilocalorie infant foods such as vegetables and dinners. Parents of infants whose increments of weight gains are small should be encouraged to feed greater amounts of the higher kilocalorie strained meats and fruits. Amounts of semisolid foods offered to infants should be adjusted to their appetites and rates of weight gain. Experiences with a variety of flavors and texture are thought to be conducive to acceptance of a variety of foods in later life.

During feeding both the mother and the infant receive satisfaction and pleasure. The infant is pleased because hunger is satiated. The mother is pleased because she has fulfilled the needs of her infant. Successful feeding provides the basis for the warm, trusting relationship that develops between infants and their mothers.

Infants swallow air as well as milk during feeding. Holding the child in an upright position and gently patting the back encourages expulsion of swallowed air and prevents distension and discomfort.

COLIC

Parents of colicky babies—those who are otherwise healthy and well fed but who cry constantly for several hours, draw their legs onto their abdomens and pass large amounts of gas—often request changes in their infants' formulas. This rarely resolves colic and frequent change in formulas should be discouraged. It has been suggested that colic in some breast-fed babies may be resolved by eliminating milk from the mother's diet.[59,60] A casein hydrolysate formula may alleviate symptoms in some but not all bottle-fed infants.[61]

SPITTING UP FOOD

Spitting up can occur in infants and usually causes concern for parents. During the early months of life some otherwise healthy infants spit up a small amount of any milk or food digested at each feeding. Although the infants do not fail to thrive, parents may seek help in resolving the situation. There is no therapy. The problem usually resolves itself by the time the infant can sustain a sitting position.

NURSING BOTTLE SYNDROME

A characteristic pattern of tooth decay in infants and young children of all the upper and sometimes the lower posterior teeth, known as nursing bottle syndrome, is often observed in children who are given sweetened liquid by bottle at bedtime or who are breast-fed frequently when they sleep with their mothers.[62] As children suck, the tongue protrudes slightly from the mouth, covering the lower front teeth. Liquids are spread over the upper teeth and the lower posterior teeth. Sucking stimulates the flow of saliva, which washes the debris from the teeth and promotes the secretion of compounds that buffer the acids in the plaque. When children are awake they swallow the liquid quickly. However, if they fall asleep, sucking stops and the salivary flow and buffering are reduced. The sweetened liquid pools around the teeth not protected by the extended tongue, and the bacterial plaque has contact with the carbohydrates during the hours of sleep.

Infant formulas, fruit juice, human milk, and cow's milk consumed when infants are falling asleep may cause this decay. To prevent this dental destruction it has been suggested that infants be held when feeding and burped and put to bed as soon as they fall asleep.

OBESITY IN INFANCY

In the past, there has been speculation that formula feeding and the early introduction of semisolid foods might be factors in excessive intakes of energy and the development of infant obesity, and that obese infants very often become obese adults. However, a number of studies have shown that neither breast-feeding nor bottle-feeding nor the age of introduction of semisolid foods are causes of obesity in infancy.[63,64] Obesity in infancy has not been found to be predictive of obesity in later life.

One study found measures of fatness at 8 years of age no greater in children who had been bottle-fed as compared to those who had been breast-fed.[65] A longitudinal study of children found that infants who were obese at 6 months and 1 year of age became progressively thinner as they grew older. Weight gain in infancy was not found to be predictive of obesity at 9 years of age.[66]

Summary

Infants can be adequately nourished consuming a variety of combinations of milks, supplements, and semisolid foods. Maturation of the oral and fine motor skills indicates appropriate stages for the introduction of semisolid and solid foods. Current recommendations include breast-feeding by an adequately nourished mother and the introduction of semisolid foods at 4 to 6 months of age, and of finger foods when the infant reaches out, grasps, and brings items to his mouth.

If the mother is unable or unwilling to breast-feed her child, a variety of properly constructed infant formulas are marketed that have been proved to support normal growth and development in infants. It is to the formula-fed baby's advantage to receive a formula with iron.

Infants should be permitted to establish their own feeding schedule and be fed to satiety. When they develop a voluntary mature sucking pattern, the introduction of semisolid foods is appropriate. When munching and rotary chewing begin, the use of soft-cooked table foods is appropriate. Infants can begin to drink from a cup with help between 9 and 12 months of age.

Review Questions

1. Why is there such a wide range of acceptable intakes of energy during infancy?
2. Under what circumstances should the infant's water intake be carefully monitored?

3. What is the difference in fat absorption of human and cow's milk?
4. What supplements should be given to a solely breast-fed 3-month-old male infant?
5. Describe the difference between sucking and suckling.
6. What developmental landmarks indicate a readiness for semisolid foods to be added to the infant's diet?
7. At what age is it reasonable to feed whole cow's milk?
8. Why is it important for a baby to go to sleep without a bottle?

REFERENCES

1. Smith, D., and others: Shifting linear growth during infancy, J. Pediatr. **89**:225, 1976.
2. Smith, D.W.: Growth and its disorders, Philadelphia, 1977, W.B. Saunders Co.
3. National Center for Health Statistics: NCHS growth charts, 1976, Monthly vital statistics report, vol. 25, no. 3, suppl. (HRA) 76-1120, Rockville, Md., 1976, Health Resources Administration.
4. Fomon, S.F., and others: Body composition of reference children from birth to 10 years, Am. J. Clin. Nutr. **55**:1169, 1982.
5. Widdowson, E. M., and Spray, C. M.: Chemical development in utero, Arch. Dis. Child. **62**:205, 1951.
6. Lebenthal, E., Lee, P.C., and Heitlinger, L.A.: Impact of development of the gastrointestinal tract on infant feeding, J. Pediatr. **102**:1, 1983.
7. Watkins, J.B.: Bile acid metabolism and fat absorption in newborn infants, Pediatr. Clin. North. Am. **2**:501, 1974.
8. Filer, L.J., Mattson, F.H., and Fomon, S.J.: Triglyceride configuration and fat absorption by the human infant, J. Nutr. **99**:293, 1969.
9. Fomon, S.J.: Infant nutrition, ed. 2, Philadelphia, 1974, W.B. Saunders Co.
10. Bayless, T.M., and Christopher, N.L.: Disaccharidase deficiency, Am. J. Clin. Nutr. **22**:181, 1969.
11. Rossiter, M.A., and others: Amylase content of mixed saliva in children, Acta Paediatr. Scand. **63**:389, 1974.
12. Nash, M.A., and Edelman, C.M.: The developing kidney, Nephron **11**:71, 1973.
13. Edelman, C.M., Barrett, H.L., and Troupkon, V.: Renal concentrating mechanisms in newborn infants. Effects of dietary protein and water content, role of urea and responsiveness to antidiuretic hormone, J. Clin. Invest. **39**:1062, 1960.
14. Polack, E., and others: The osmotic concentrating ability in healthy infants and children, Arch. Dis. Child. **40**:291, 1965.
15. Food and Nutrition Board, National Research Council, National Academy of Sciences: Recommended Dietary Allowances, ed. 9, Washington, D.C., 1980, Academy Press.
16. Fomon, S.J., and others: Recommendations for feeding normal infants, Pediatrics **63**:52, 1979.
17. Holt, L.E., Jr., and Snyderman, S.E.: The amino acid requirements of infants, J. Am. Nurs. Assoc. **175**:100, 1961.
18. Fomon, S.J., and Filer, L.J.: Amino acid requirements for normal growth. In Nyhan, W.L.: Amino acid metabolism and genetic variation, New York, 1967, McGraw-Hill Book Co.
19. Report of a Joint FAO/WHO Ad Hoc Expert Committee: Energy and protein requirements, World Health Organization Technical Series No. 522, FAO Nutr. Meet. Ser. No. 52, Geneva, 1973, World Health Organization.

20. Fomon, S.J., and others: Requirements for protein and essential amino acids in early infancy, Acta Paediatr. Scand. **62**:33, 1973.
21. Committee on Nutrition, American Academy of Pediatrics: Commentary on breast-feeding and infant formulas, Pediatrics **57**:279, 1976.
22. Wesson, L. J., and Burr, G. O.: The metabolic rate and respiratory quotients of rats on fat-deficient diets, J. Biol. Chem. **91**:525, 1931.
23. Holman, R. J., Caster, W. O., and Weise, H. F.: The essential fatty acid requirement of infants and the assessment of their dietary intake of linoleate by serum fatty acid analysis, Am. J. Clin. Nutr. **14**:70, 1964.
24. Hey, E.N., and Katz, G.: Evaporative water loss in the newborn baby, J. Physiol. **200**:605, 1969.
25. McMillan, M.A., Landau, S.A., and Oski, F.A.: Iron sufficiency in breast milk and the availability of iron from human milk, Pediatrics **58**:686, 1976.
26. Garry, P.J., and others: Iron absorption from human milk and formula with and without iron supplementation, Pediatr. Res. **15**:822, 1981.
27. MacDonald, L.D., Gibson, R.S., and Miles, J.E.: Changes in hair zinc and copper concentrations of breast-fed and bottle-fed infants during the first six months, Acta Paediatr. Scand. **71**:758, 1982.
28. Cavell, P.A., and Widdowson, E.M.: Intakes and excretion of iron, copper, and zinc in the neonatal period, Arch. Dis. Child. **39**:496, 1964.
29. Johnson, P.E., and Evans, G.W.: Relative zinc availability in human breast milk, infant formulas, and cow's milk, Am. J. Clin. Nutr. **31**:416, 1978.
30. Baker, H., and others: Vitamin profile of 174 mothers and newborns at parturition, Am. J. Clin. Nutr. **28**:59, 1975.
31. Reeve, L.E., Chesney, R.W., and DeLuca, H.F.: Vitamin D of human milk: identification of biologically active forms, Am. J. Clin. Nutr. **36**:122, 1982.
32. Committee on Nutrition, American Academy of Pediatrics: Vitamin and mineral supplemental needs in normal children in the United States, Pediatrics **66**:1015, 1980.
33. Dirks, O.B., and others: Total and free ionic fluoride in human and cow's milk as determined by chromatography and fluoride electrode, Caries Res. **8**:181, 1974.
34. Fabius, R.J., and others: Malnutrition associated with a formula of barley water, corn syrup, and whole milk, Am. J. Dis. Child. **135**:615, 1981.
35. Sinatra, F.R., and Merritt, R.J.: Iatrogenic kwashiorkor in infants, Am. J. Dis. Child. **135**:21, 1981.
36. Committee on Nutrition, American Academy of Pediatrics: Imitation and substitute milks, Pediatrics **73**:876, 1984.
37. Partridge, J.C., and others: Water intoxication secondary to feeding mismanagement, Am. J. Dis. Child. **135**:38, 1981.
38. Comay, S.C., and Karabus, C.D.: Peripheral gangrene in hypernatraemic dehydration of infancy, Arch. Dis. Child. **50**:616, 1975.
39. Macaulay, D., and Watson, M.: Hypernatremia in infants as a cause of brain damage, Arch. Dis. Child. **42**:485, 1967.
40. Hargrove, C.B., Temple, A.R., and Chinn, P.: Formula preparation and infant illness, Clin. Pediatr. **13**:1057, 1974.
41. Kendall, N., Vaughn, V.C., and Kusakeroglu, A.A.: A study of preparation of infant formula, Am. J. Dis. Child. **122**:215, 1971.
42. Woodruff, C.W., Wright, S.W., and Wright, R.P.: The role of fresh cow's milk in iron deficiency. II. Comparison of fresh cow's milk with a prepared formula, Am. J. Dis. Child. **124**:26, 1972.

43. Fomon, S.J., and others: Cow milk feeding in infancy: gastrointestinal blood loss and iron nutritional status, J. Pediatr. **98**:540, 1981.
44. Fomon, S.J., and others: Influence of formula concentration on caloric intake and growth of normal infants, Acta Paediatr. Scand. **64**:172, 1975.
45. Beal, V.A.: Termination of night feeding in infancy, J. Pediatr. **75**:690, 1969.
46. Arnon, S.S., and others: Honey and other environmental risk factors for infant botulism, Pediatrics **94**:331, 1979.
47. Thoman, E.B.: Development of synchrony in mother-infant interaction in feeding and other situations, Fed. Proc. **34**:1587, 1975.
48. Hitchcock, Gracey, M., and Gilmour, A.I.: The growth of breast-fed and artificially fed infants from birth to twelve months, Acta Paediatr. Scand. **74**:240, 1985.
49. Fomon, S.J., and others: Food consumption and growth of normal infants fed milk-based formulas, Acta Paediatr. Scand. **223**(Suppl.), 1971.
50. Hofvander, Y., and others: The amount of milk consumed by 1-3 month old breast- or bottle-fed infants, Acta Paediatr. Scand. **71**:953, 1982.
51. Illingworth, R.S., and Lister, J.: The critical or sensitive period with special reference to certain feeding problems in infants and children, J. Pediatr. **65**:839, 1964.
52. Gesell, A., and Ilg, F.L.: Feeding behavior of infants, Philadelphia, 1937, J.B. Lippincott Co.
53. Ardran, G.M., Kemp, F.H., and Lind, J.: A cineradiographic study of breast feeding, Br. J. Radiol. **31**:156, 1958.
54. Ardran, G.M., Kemp, F.H., and Lind, J.: A cineradiographic study of bottle feeding, Br. J. Radiol. **31**:11, 1958.
55. Subtelny, J.D.: Examination of current philosophies associated with swallowing behavior, Am. J. Orthod. **51**:161, 1965.
56. Peiper, A.: Cerebral function in infancy and childhood, New York, 1963, Consultant's Bureau.
57. Gwynne-Evans, E.: Organization of the oro-facial muscles in relation to breathing and feeding, Br. Dent. J. **91**:135, 1952.
58. Ingram, T.T.S.: Clinical significance of the infantile feeding reflexes, Dev. Med. Child. Neurol. 4:159, 1962.
59. Jakobsson, I., and Lindberg, T.: Cow's milk as a cause of infantile colic in breast-fed infants, Lancet **2**:437, 1978.
60. Jakobsson, I., and Lindberg, T.: Cow's milk proteins cause infantile colic in breast-fed infants: a double-blind crossover study, Pediatrics **71**:268, 1983.
61. Lothe, L., Lindberg, T., and Jakobsson, I.: Cow's milk formula as a cause of infantile colic, Pediatrics **70**:7, 1982.
62. Finn, S.B.: Dental caries in infants, Curr. Dent. Concepts **1**:35, 1969.
63. Dubois, S., Hill, D.E., and Benson, G.N.: An examination of factors believed to be associated with obesity, Am. J. Clin. Nutr. **32**:1997, 1979.
64. Ferris, A.G., and others: The effect of diet on weight gain in infancy, Am. J. Clin. Nutr. **33**:2635, 1980.
65. Fomon, S.J., and others: Indices of fatness and serum cholesterol at eight years in relation to feeding and growth during infancy, Pediatr. Res. **18**:1233, 1984.
66. Shapiro, L.R., and others: Obesity prognosis: a longitudinal study of children from the age of 6 months to 9 years, Am. J. Public Health **74**:968, 1984.

FURTHER READING

Adair, L.S.: The infant's ability to self-regulate caloric intake: a case study, J. Am. Diet. Assoc. **84**:543, 1984.

This article presents a case study of the energy intake of one bottle-fed infant growing normally for the first year of life. The infant adjusted his energy intake when semisolid foods were added by decreasing his energy intake from milk.

American Academy of Pediatrics, Committee on Nutrition: Supplemental foods for infants, pediatric nutrition handbook, Elk Grove Village, Ill., 1985, American Academy of Pediatrics.

This paper reviews developmental landmarks for the addition of nonmilk foods to the infant's diet. The contribution of these foods to the sodium intake of the infant's diet is reviewed. The implications for food sensitivity and obesity when these foods are added to the diet is discussed.

Fomon, S. J.: Reflections on infant feeding in the 1970s and 1985, Am. J. Clin. Nutr. **46**:171, 1987.

This paper discusses changes in infant feeding practices in the past two decades. There is currently a much higher incidence of breast feeding than in the early 1970s. Sugar and salt have been deleted from commercially prepared infant foods. A line of dried instant baby foods were introduced in 1984. Iron deficiency continues to be the nutrition problem of the greatest magnitude. However, many babies receive formula without iron because of unfounded ideas that these formulas contribute to fussiness, regurgitation, constipation, or diarrhea.

Martinez, G.A., Ryan, A.S., and Malec, D.J.: Nutrient intakes of American infants and children fed cow's milk or infant formula, Am. J. Dis. Child. **139**:1010, 1985.

Data from the Ross Laboratory Survey were used to assess nutrient intake of 865 infants 6.5 to 13.4 months old according to the type of milk consumed. Infants who received whole cow's milk received intakes of sodium, potassium, and chloride that exceeded the recommended safe and adequate range. Infants who did not receive an iron-fortified milk did not receive recommended intakes of iron.

Montaldo, M.B., Benson, J.D., and Martinez, G.A.: Nutrient intakes of formula-fed infants and infants fed cow's milk, Pediatrics **75**:343, 1985.

Nutrient intakes of 7- to 12-month-old infants are reported from data collected during the HANES II Survey. Nonmilk foods added to the infant's diet were relatively low in iron and linoleic acid and high in protein, sodium, and potassium. Seventy-five percent of infants fed cow's milk had intakes of iron below the RDA.

CASE STUDY

Baby P, a 5.5-month-old female weighs 7.3 kg and is 65.3 cm long. She is currently breast-fed and receives no other foods. Her mother feels it is time to add other foods to her diet.

1. List developmental landmarks that should have been reached before foods are added.
2. What foods should be introduced to the baby first?
3. How should foods be added to identify any food allergies or intolerances?

CASE STUDY

Baby D is a 6-month-old male whose grandmother is concerned about his weight gain. While the mother feels her baby is doing well, she asks for answers to questions raised by her in-laws. His heights and weights are:

	2 weeks	2 months	4 months	6 months
Weight (kg)	5.34	7.60	9.59	10.60
Height (cm)	57.10	62.50	67.10	72.60

The baby was solely breast-fed until 4 months. At that time semisolid foods were added to his diet and the infant was given a cow's-milk-base formula. His day's intake at 6 months is:

Formula, commercially prepared, (20 kcal/oz)	32-40 oz
Rice or oatmeal cereal	8 tablespoons dry
Strained pears or applesauce	½ cup
Strained squash or carrots	½ cup

1. In what percentile do his height and weight and weight-height plot?
2. Is there reason for concern about this baby's rate of weight gain?
3. Is this diet appropriate for this infant?

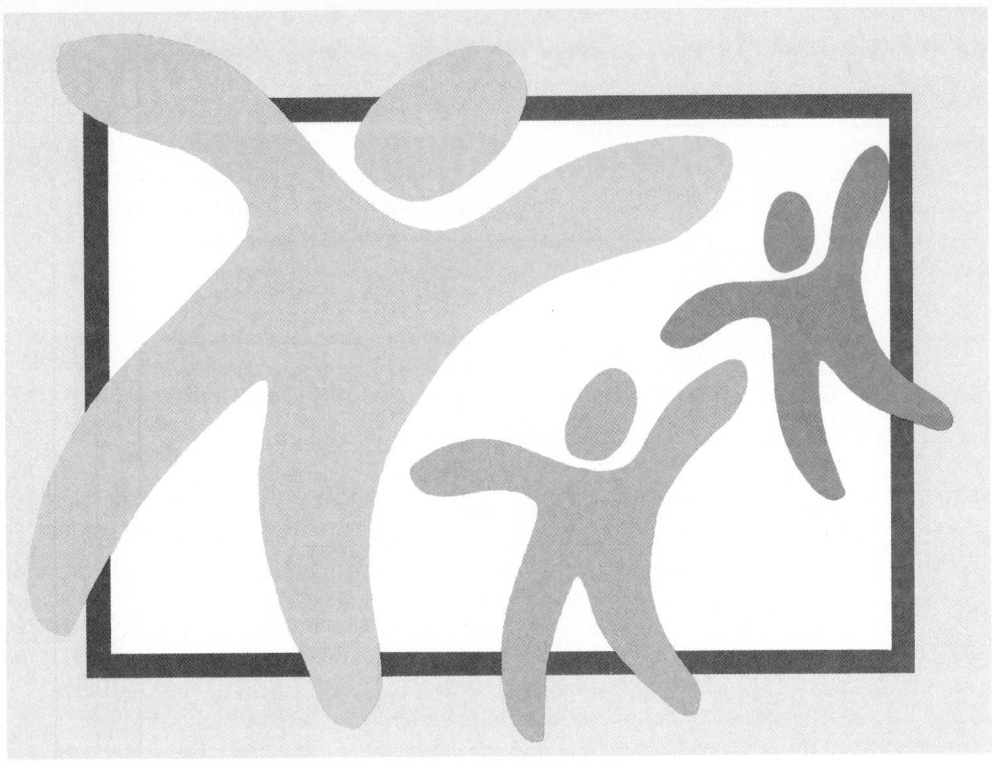

Basic Concepts

1 Nutrient requirements of children reflect varied individual needs and a generally slowed and erratic growth rate between infancy and adolescence.

2 Numerous family and community factors determine a child's food choices.

3 The young child's available food and food choices influence nutrient intake and developing food pattern.

4 Meeting physical and psychosocial needs guides considerations in feeding young children.

5 Nutrition concerns during childhood relate to growth and development needs for positive health.

Chapter Seven

Nutrition in Childhood

Peggy Pipes

After the infant's first year of rapid growth, the interval between infancy and adolescence is a period of slower growth, a time for acquisition of skills that permit independence in eating, and the development of individual food likes and dislikes. Development of gross motor skills makes increased activity possible. Preschool children learn to control body functions, to interact with others, and to behave in a socially acceptable manner. School-age children attempt to develop personal independence and establish a scale of values. Individual variations in children become more noticeable in rates of growth, activity patterns, nutrient requirements, personality development, and food intakes.

In this chapter we will see that there are wide ranges of nutrient requirements of children at any age during this period. Body size and composition, activity patterns, and rates of growth influence basic needs. The foods available to and accepted by the child are determined not only by parental food selection but also by the mealtime environment, peer pressures, advertising, and the child's food experiences. If appropriate support is provided by parents, food patterns that support normal growth and weight and good dental hygiene, and that prevent iron deficiency anemia can be established.

Physical Growth During Childhood

GROWTH RATE

The rapid rate of growth during infancy is followed by a deceleration during the preschool and school-age years. Weight gain approximates 1.8-2.7 kg (4 to 6 lbs) per year. Length increases approximately 7.6 cm (3 inches) per year between 1 year and 7-8 years of age, then 5.1 cm (2 inches) per year until the pubertal growth spurt. Between 6 years of age and the adolescent growth spurt, sex differences can be noted. At age 6 years boys are taller and heavier than girls. By age 9 years the height of the average girl is the same as that of the 9-year-old male and her weight is slightly higher.

Racial differences have been noted in rates of growth. Black American infants are smaller than white American infants at birth. They grow more rapidly during the first 2 years of life and from that age through adolescence are taller than white American boys and girls of the same age. Asian children tend to be smaller than black children and white children.[1]

BODY COMPOSITION

Muscle mass accounts for an increasingly greater percentage of body weight during the preschool years. Children become leaner as they grow older. Fatfold measurements decrease. Females, however, have more subcutaneous fat than males.

Brain growth is 75% complete by the end of the second year and 100% of adult size by 6-10 years of age. This results in a decrease in head size in relation to body size.

By 2-3 years of age, total body fluid proportion is similar to that of an adult. Rapid shifts in fluid between intracellular and extracellular compartments are less likely. The child is less vulnerable to dehydration than the infant. The extracellular fluid continues to decrease while intracellular fluid increases because of the growth of new cells. The approximate percentage of total body fluid is 59% in the toddler compared to 64% in the adult male.

Bone growth results from elongation of the legs. The school-age child with longer legs appears more graceful and slimmer.

GROWTH CHARTS

Normal differences in individual children become apparent in the percentile channel of growth followed by each child. Once the percentile ranking is established on the growth grid, children can be expected to maintain channels of growth when sequential measurements over time are recorded. It is more important to know that a child is maintaining his height and weight in relation to other children and in the weight-height percentile than it is to know that the child is tall or short.

The infant growth charts, as described in Chapter 6, are constructed to age 36 months and should be used until at least 24 months. The growth grids for children from 2 to 18 years of age were prepared from data from the national Health and Nutrition Examination Surveys (NHANES),[2] described in Chapter 3. It should be noted that length measurements for the infant grid are recumbent lengths and those for the children's grid are standing height measurements. It is not unusual for small changes to occur in length percentile ratings on growth grids when the change is made to upright measurements.

Excesses or inadequacies in energy and nutrient intakes will be reflected in patterns of growth. The child who is not eating sufficient food will drop in channel of growth grids (Fig. 7-1). If the food deprivation is severe enough and lasts long enough, rates of linear growth will be reduced or growth will cease. Intakes of energy in excess of expenditure will be noted by increases in weight percentile (Fig. 7-2).

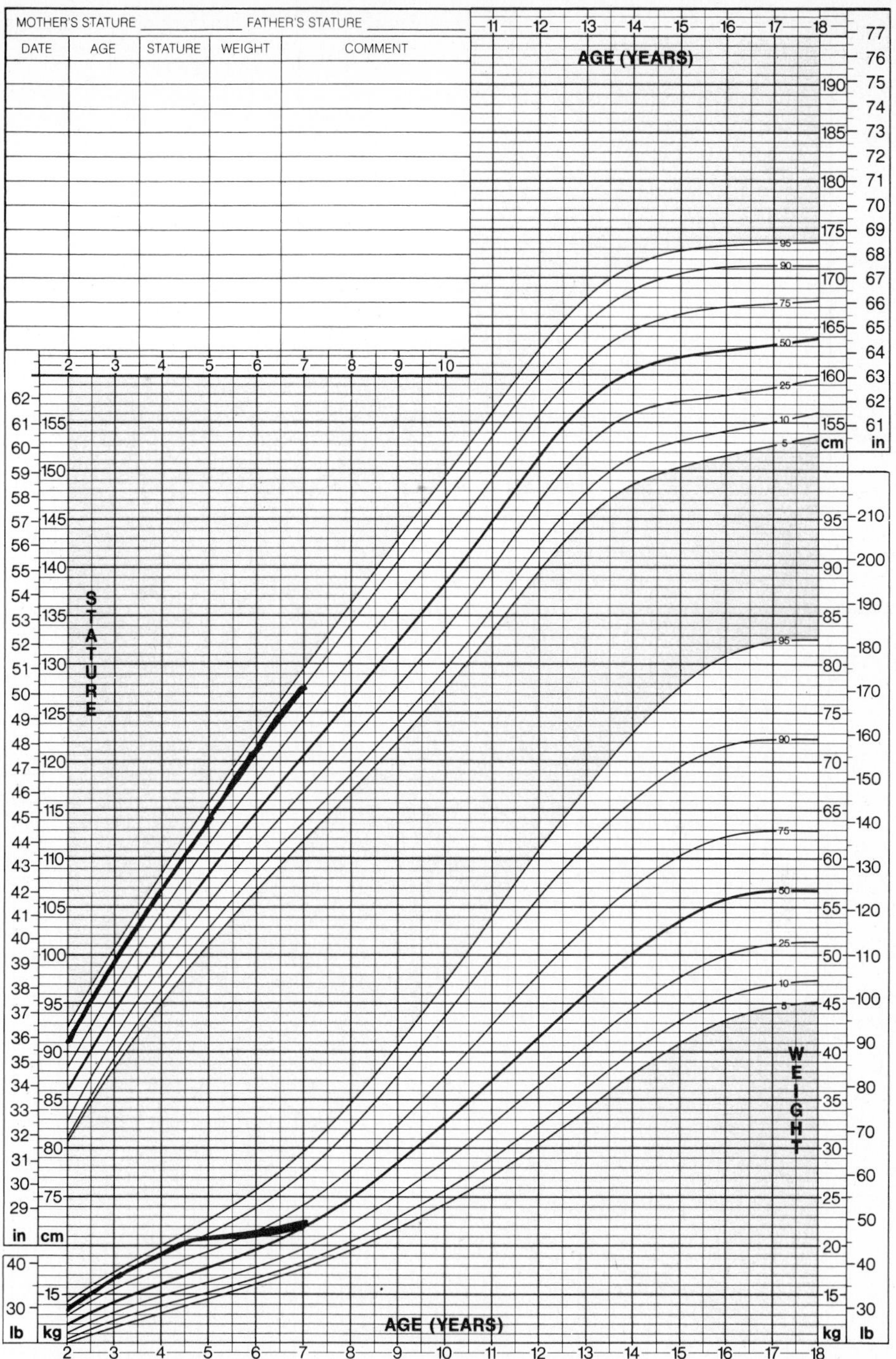

FIG. 7-1 Growth grid of a female whose weight remained in the 90th percentile over time but who became anorexic at 4½ years and did not consume enough food to support an appropriate weight gain.
(Courtesy Ross Laboratories)

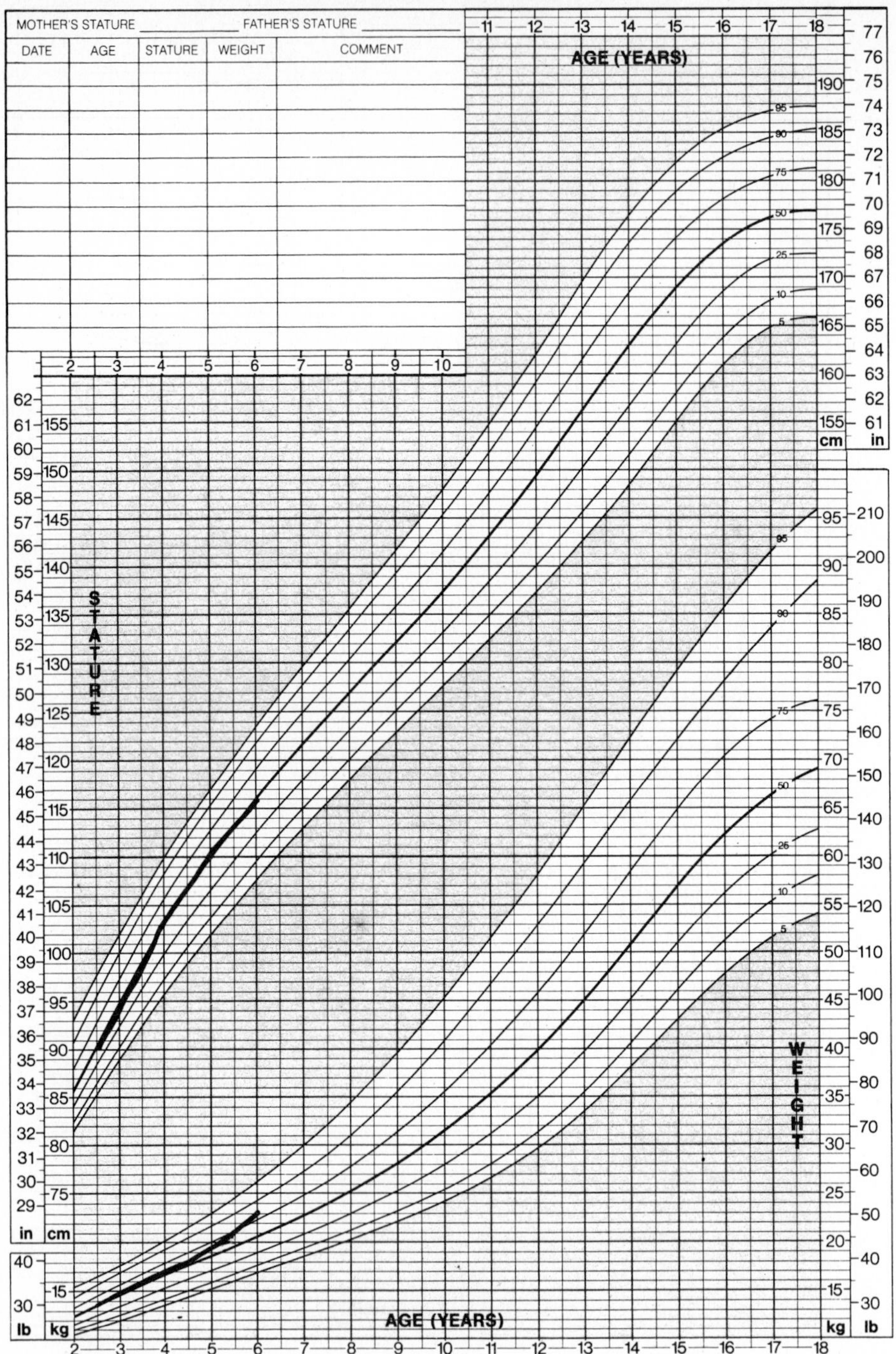

FIG. 7-2 Growth grid of a male who began eating excessive amounts of high calorie food at age 4½ years. His rate of weight gain increased.

(Courtesy Ross Laboratories)

FEEDING SKILLS

Children learn to feed themselves independently during the second year of life. The 15-month-old child will have difficulty scooping food into the spoon and bringing food to the mouth without turning the spoon upside down and spilling its contents, because of lack of wrist control.

By 16 to 17 months of age a well-defined ulnar deviation of the wrist occurs and the contents of the spoon may be transferred more steadily to the mouth. By 18 months of age the child lifts the elbow as the spoon is raised and flexes the wrist as the spoon reaches the mouth so that only moderate spilling occurs at this age, in contrast to earlier stages of self-feeding.

By 2 years of age spilling seldom occurs. Handedness is not established at 1 year of age. Children may grasp the spoon with either hand and find when they try to fill the spoon that the bowl is upside down.

A refined pincer grasp will have been developed in the first year. Finger-feeding is easy and often preferred. Foods that provide opportunities for finger-feeding should be provided at each meal (Table 7-1). Children will often place food in the spoon with their fingers and may finger-feed foods commonly spoon-fed, such as vegetables and pudding.

By 15 months of age children can manage the cup but will have difficulty in lifting and tilting a cup and in lowering it to the table surface after drinking. The cup is tilted, using the palm, and is often tilted too rapidly. By 18 to 24 months of age the cup will be tilted by coordinated movements of the fingers.

Children refine the rotary chewing movements established by 1 year of age. These chewing movements are usually well established by 2½ years of age.

TABLE 7-1 Appropriate Finger Foods for Young Children with a Refined Pincer Grasp

Appropriate Foods (no skins or peeling)	Inappropriate Foods (may cause choking or gagging)
Dry cereal: Cheerios, Kix	
Banana slices	Dried fruits: raisins, coconut, dates
Soft cut-up fruit	Small fruit with skin or peel: grapes
Mealy apple	Raw vegetables
Canned or well-cooked vegetables (green beans, broccoli, carrots)	
Cheese sticks, hard cheese (cheddar, Monterey Jack)	Processed American cheese
Large curd cottage cheese	
Small pieces tender meats (small meatballs, chicken, liver)	Hot dogs
Scrambled eggs	Nuts, including peanuts
Fish sticks (no bones)	Peanut butter
Oven-dried toast	Popcorn
Zwieback toast	Potato chips
Arrowroot biscuits	Corn chips
Graham crackers	Tortilla chips

Nutrient Needs of Children

Recommendations for energy intakes for children have been derived from intakes of normal, healthy children growing satisfactorily. Those for nutrient intakes are based on only a few balance studies, mostly extrapolated from requirements for infants and adults. It is important to remember that the range of adequate intakes is quite wide among groups of children. The Recommended Dietary Allowances (RDA) provide guidelines for studying groups of children but not for evaluating diets of individual children.[3]

ENERGY

Individual Needs

Energy requirements for individual children are determined by basal metabolic rate (BMR), rate of growth, and activity. Energy needs of individual children of the same age, sex, and size vary. Reasons for these differences remain unexplained. Differences in physical activity, in the metabolic cost of minimal and excessive protein intakes at equivalent levels of energy intake, and in the efficiency with which individuals utilize energy have all been hypothesized to exert an influence. The RDA standards established by the Food and Nutrition Board of the National Research Council are given in Table 7-2.[3] These allowances give a wide range of recommended energy intakes in each age group.

Physical Activity

The contribution of physical activity to total energy expenditure is quite variable among children and in individual children from day to day. At all ages activity patterns among children show wide ranges both in the time spent in the various activities and in the intensity of the activities. Some children may engage in sedentary activities such as looking at books or watching television, whereas their peers may be engaged in physical activities that demand running, jumping, and general body movements. Spady[4] estimated the energy expenditure for physical activity of fourth- and fifth-grade school children, for example, to be 31.2% and 25.3% of total energy expenditure for males and females, respectively.

TABLE 7-2 Recommended Energy Intakes for Children of Various Ages

	Age	Weight (kg)	Height (cm)	Energy Needs (kcal)	Ranges
Children	1-3	13	90	1300	(900-1800)
	4-6	20	112	1700	(1300-2300)
	7-10	28	132	2400	(1650-3300)

From Food and Nutrition Board, National Research Council: Recommended dietary allowances, rev. ed. 9, Washington, D.C., 1980, National Academy of Sciences.

Actual Caloric Intakes

Studies indicate that children are consuming less energy than recommended, with children 6 to 11 years of age consuming more than 20% less than the suggested intake.[5] Spady found that although the total energy expenditure of fourth and fifth grade boys approximated the recommended allowances, girls expended only 80% of the recommended allowances.[4] Farris and associates[6] noted that between 1973 and 1982 the energy intakes of 10-year-old children had declined.

The most appropriate evaluation of adequacy of a child's energy intake is based on observation of rates of growth as depicted on growth grids and on measurements of body fat.

Catch-up Growth

During a period of catch-up growth, the requirements for energy and nutrients will be greatly increased. Daily intakes of 150-250 kcal/kg of body weight have been recommended for children of preschool age. An intake of 200 kcal/kg/day should produce a weight gain of 20 g/day.[7]

PROTEIN

Basis of Need

Protein needs of children include those for maintenance of tissue, changes in body composition, and synthesis of new tissue. During growth, the protein content of the body increases from 14.6% at 1 year of age to 18-19%, which are adult values, by 4 years of age. Estimates of protein needs for growth range from 1 to 4 g/kg of tissue gained. As the rate of growth falls, maintenance requirements gradually represent an increasing proportion of the total protein requirement.

Recommended Intakes

The recommended protein intake, calculated on the maintenance requirements of the adult, growth rates, and body composition, gradually decrease from 1.8 g/kg at 1 year of age to 0.8 g/kg at 18 years of age (Table 7-3).[3] This intake approximates 6.7-7.1% of the total kilocalories, less than most children consume. Protein provided 13-15% of the energy intake in the average child's diet.

Evaluation of a child's protein intake must be based on adequacy of growth rate, quality of protein in the foods eaten, combinations of foods that provide complemen-

***TABLE* 7-3** Recommended Daily Intakes of Protein for Children

	Age (years)	Protein (gm/kg)
Children	1-3	1.8
	4-6	1.5
	7-10	1.2

From Food and Nutrition Board; National Research Council: Recommended daily dietary allowances, ed. 9, Washington, D.C., 1980, National Academy of Sciences.

tary amino acids consumed together, and adequacy of those nutrients, vitamins and minerals, and energy that are necessary for protein synthesis to proceed.

Inadequate protein intakes are rarely noted in North America. Some children have such limited energy intakes that part of the protein consumed must be used for body fuel. Children who consume vegan diets have been reported to be shorter and leaner than the average child.

MINERALS AND VITAMINS

Minerals and vitamins are necessary for normal growth and development. Inadequate intakes will be reflected in slow growth rates, inadequate mineralization of bones, insufficient iron stores, and anemia. The RDAs are shown in Tables 7-4 and 7-5.

Calcium

Attempts to establish recommended intakes of calcium have caused considerable controversy for many years. Populations that have adapted to intakes of 200-400 mg/day without adverse effects have been identified. Absorption of calcium fluctuates from 30% to 60% of intake. Lactose increases absorption. Binders such as phytic and oxalic

TABLE 7-4 Recommended Daily Dietary Allowances for Minerals

	Age (years)	Calcium (mg)	Phosphorus (mg)	Iodine (μg)	Iron (mg)	Magnesium (mg)	Zinc (mg)
Children	1-3	800	800	70	15	150	10
	4-6	800	800	90	10	200	10

TABLE 7-5 Recommended Daily Dietary Allowances of Vitamins

	Children (yr)		
	1-3	4-6	7-10
Fat-Soluble			
Vitamin A RE (μg)	400	500	700
Vitamin D (μg)	10	10	10
Vitamin E (mgα-TE)	5	6	7
Water-Soluble			
Thiamine (mg)	0.7	0.9	1.2
Riboflavin (mg)	0.8	1.0	1.4
Niacin (mg)	9	11	16
Vitamin B_6 (mg)	0.9	1.3	1.6
Folacin (μg)	100	200	300
Vitamin B_{12} (μg)	2.0	2.5	3.0
Ascorbic acid (mg)	45	45	45

From Food and Nutrition Board, National Research Council: Recommended dietary allowances, rev. ed. 9, Washington, D.C., 1980, National Academy of Sciences.

acid reduce absorption. The level of dietary protein affects the urinary excretion of calcium. As levels of protein intake increase, levels of urinary calcium increase.

Osteomalacia, which improves rapidly with calcium supplements, has been identified in three black children, a 4-year-old girl and 6- and 13-year-old boys, in South Africa.[8] Recommendations for children are set at 800 mg/day since growing children may need two to four times as much calcium per unit of body weight as adults require.

Milk and other dairy products are the primary sources of calcium. Thus children who consume limited amounts of these products risk a deficient calcium intake.

Zinc

The trace mineral zinc is essential for normal protein synthesis and growth. Variations in plasma zinc concentrations during growth reflect the continual use and depletion of body stores of zinc. The steepest decline occurs at 10-11 years of age in the female and at 12-13 years of age in the male, when growth is most rapid.[9] Zinc intakes of children 1-3 years of age have been estimated to average 5 mg/day; those of children 3-5 years of age average 5-7 mg/day.[10]

Many preschool and school-age children from low- and middle-income families may be ingesting inadequate amounts of zinc. Studies in Denver of children in the Head Start Program who were 3.5-6 years of age and whose heights were less than the third percentile revealed that 40% had low concentrations of hair zinc and 69% had low plasma and hair zinc concentrations.[11] Supplements of zinc sulfate that provided 0.2 mg zinc/kg body weight given to 5 school children with hypogeusia and low hair zinc levels resulted in normalization of taste perception and substantial increases in hair zinc content.[12]

Iron

Iron deficiency is the most common nutritional deficiency in North America. It occurs most frequently in children 12 to 36 months of age, in adolescent males, and in females in their childbearing years. It may result from inadequate iron intake, impaired absorption, a large hemorrhage, or repeated small blood losses.

The RDA standards of the National Research Council assume 10% iron absorption and are planned to meet variations of need in individuals.[3] Iron requirements of individual children vary with rates of growth and increasing blood volumes, iron stores, variations in menstrual losses of iron in adolescent females, and the timing of the growth spurt of adolescents. Larger, more rapidly growing children have the greatest requirements for iron because they are increasing their blood volumes more rapidly.

Prevention of Anemia

Many younger preschoolers do not have the oral motor strength to masticate meat and prefer nonheme sources of iron. The consumption of foods containing vitamin C along with the foods containing nonheme iron can help increase the amount of the iron absorbed. Also, directing parents to use more foods containing heme iron that are easier to chew, such as ground beef, can increase iron intake. For children whose iron intake is limited, a supplemental maintenance dose of iron (10-15 mg/day) may be indicated. Children with diagnosed iron-deficiency anemia will receive therapeutic doses of iron, 3 mg/kg/day, for 3 months.

Vitamins

The function of vitamins in metabolic processes means that their requirements are determined by intakes of energy, protein, and saturated fats. Exact needs are difficult to define. The RDA standard for most vitamins and for some trace minerals (Table 7-6) is interpolated from infant and adult allowances or calculated on the basis of energy and protein allowances.

VITAMIN SUPPLEMENTATION

The importance of appropriate vitamin supplementation of breast-fed infants is discussed in Chapter 6. After infancy, however, the percentage of toddlers who are given vitamin supplements declines. But over half of the preschool and school-age children receive multivitamin-mineral preparations.

Cook and Payne[13] found that use of vitamin supplements significantly increased the percentage of second-grade and sixth-grade children who meet 67% of the RDA compared with nonsupplemented children. Thus they consider vitamin supplementation advisable. However, Breskin[14] noted no significant differences in biochemical indices with the exception of red blood cell folate of children who used supplements compared with those who did not, even though mean intakes of vitamin B_6 of the nonsupplemented group were 30% below the RDA. Many of the nonsupplemented children ingested less than two-thirds of the RDA for folate. All blood values were in the range of accepted standards.

Table 7-6 Estimated Safe and Adequate Daily Dietary Intakes of Selected Trace Minerals and Electrolytes

	Age (years)	Copper (mg)	Manganese (mg)	Fluoride (mg)	Chromium (mg)	Selenium (mg)	Molybdenum (mg)
Children	1-3	1.0-1.5	1.0-1.5	0.5-1.5	0.02-0.08	0.02-0.08	0.05-0.1
and	4-6	1.5-2.0	1.5-2.0	1.0-2.5	0.03-0.12	0.03-0.12	0.06-0.15
adolescents	7-10	2.0-2.5	2.0-3.0	1.5-2.5	0.05-0.2	0.05-0.2	0.1-0.3
	11+	2.0-3.0	2.5-5.0	1.5-2.5	0.05-0.2	0.05-0.2	0.15-0.5
		2.0-3.0	2.5-5.0	1.5-4.0	0.05-0.2	0.05-0.2	0.15-0.5

	Age (years)	Sodium (mg)	Potassium (mg)	Chloride (mg)
Electrolytes				
Children	1-3	325-975	550-1650	500-1500
and	4-6	450-1350	775-2325	700-2100
adolescents	7-10	600-1800	1000-3000	925-2775
	11+	900-2700	1525-4575	1400-4200
		1100-3300	1875-5625	1700-5100

From National Research Council: Food and Nutrition Board, Recommended dietary allowances, rev. ed. 9, Washington, D.C., 1980. National Academy of Sciences.

Dietary Evaluation for Supplementation

Vitamin supplementation of diets of children should be recommended only after careful evaluation of the child's food intake. Diets of children who restrict their intake of milk because of real or imagined allergies, lactose intolerance, or for psychosocial reasons should be monitored for riboflavin and vitamin D. Diets of infants and children receiving goat's milk should be carefully monitored for food sources of folacin. Diets of children who consume limited amounts of fruits and vegetables should be checked for sources of vitamins A and C.

Children at Risk

The Committee on Nutrition of the American Academy of Pediatrics has defined four groups of children at particular nutritional risk and for whom vitamin supplementation may be appropriate:[15]

1. Children from deprived families, especially those who suffer from parental neglect or abuse
2. Children who have anorexia, poor and capricious appetites, poor eating habits, and who are on regimens to manage obesity
3. Pregnant teenagers
4. Children who consume vegan diets

Any vitamin supplements, especially those that are colored and sugar coated, should be stored in places inaccessible to young children.

Patterns of Nutrient Intake

INDIVIDUAL DIFFERENCES

Both longitudinal and cross-sectional studies of nutrient and energy intakes of children have shown large differences in intakes between individual children of the same age and sex. Some children consume two to three times as much energy as others.[16] After a rapid rise in intake of all nutrients during the first 9 months of life, reductions can be expected in the intakes of some nutrients as increases occur in intakes of others. Several researchers have noted sex differences in intakes of energy and nutrients. In all studies males consumed greater quantities of food, thus greater amounts of nutrients and energy.

THE PRESCHOOL YEARS

During the preschool years there is a decrease in intake of calcium, phosphorus, riboflavin, iron, and vitamin A because of discontinued use of iron-fortified infant cereals in the diets of children, a reduction in milk intakes, and a disinterest in vegetables. During this period children increase their intake of carbohydrate and fat. Protein intakes may plateau or increase only slightly.[16] Between 3 and 8 years of age there is a slow, steady, and relatively consistent increase in intake of all nutrients. Since intakes of vitamins A and C are unrelated to energy intakes, greater ranges of intakes of these nutrients have been noted. Black preschoolers in California have been noted to have higher intakes of sodium than do whites because of their frequent intake of undiluted commercially prepared soups. Between ages 2 and 4, they were also found to have greater energy intakes than whites.[17]

THE SCHOOL-AGE YEARS

By school age most children have established a particular pattern of nutrient intake relative to their peers.[16] Although wide ranges of intake of food, and thus of energy and nutrients, continue to be observed, those who consume the greatest amount of food consistently do so, whereas those consuming smaller amounts of food maintain lesser intakes of food relative to their peers. Differences in intake between males and females increase gradually to 12 years of age and then become marked. Boys consume greater quantities of food, thus energy and nutrients, than do girls.

Normal Food Behaviors

As growth and development proceed, children have predictable food behaviors that some parents consider "problems." If caretakers understand that these behaviors are normal, the behaviors usually will be only transient. If, however, parents become anxious and try to force children to eat, control becomes an issue and true problems can result. Knowledge of these behaviors can, therefore, prevent difficulties in feeding children.

FOOD JAGS AND RITUALS

Few children pass through the preschool years without creating concern about their food intake.[18] Between 9 and 18 months of age children display a disinterest in food that lasts from a few months to a few years. Food jags are also common. Likes and dislikes may change from day to day and week to week. For example, a child may demand only boiled eggs for snacks for a week and completely reject them for the next 6 months. Rituals become a part of food preparation and service. Some children, for example, accept sandwiches only when they are cut in half, and when parents quarter the sandwich the children may throw tantrums. Others demand that food have a particular arrangement on the plate or that dishes be placed only in certain locations on the table.

APPETITES

During this period appetites are usually erratic and unpredictable. The child may eat hungrily at one meal and completely refuse the next. The evening meal is generally the least well received and is of the most concern to the majority of parents. It is possible that children who have consumed two meals and several snacks have already met their needs for energy and nutrients before dinner time.

FOOD PREFERENCES

Parents report that preschool children enjoy meat, cereal grains, baked products, fruit, and sweets. They frequently ask for dairy products, cereal, and snack items such as cookies, crackers, fruit juice, and dry beverage mixes.[19] Food preferences during the preschool years seem to be for the carbohydrate-rich foods that are easier to masticate. Cereals, breads, and crackers are selected often in preference to meat and other protein-rich foods. The use of dry fortified cereals as a primary source of many nutrients is increasing.[17] Yogurt and cheese appear to be increasing in popularity among young children.

SCHOOL-AGE CHILDREN

Although school-age children usually increase the amount they eat and the varieties of food they accept, many continue to reject vegetables, mixed dishes, and liver. The range of food they voluntarily accept may be small. Sugar contributes 24% to 25% of the total kilocalories in the diets of many school-age children.[20] Milk is the primary contributor. Sweetened beverages, fruits, fruit juice, cakes, cookies, and other dessert items are also significant contributors.

Food dislikes of older children consistently include cooked vegetables, mixed dishes, and liver. Children accept raw vegetables more readily than cooked ones but often take only a limited amount. Sweetness and familiarity are significant factors that influence food preferences in all children.

A common difficulty for parents is finding a time when school-age children are willing to sit down and eat a meal. They frequently are so involved with other activities that it is difficult to get them to take time to eat. Often they satisfy their initial hunger and rush back to their activities and television programs, returning later for a snack.

FREQUENCY OF EATING

Huenemann[21] has pointed out that we are raising a generation of nibblers. Nearly 60% of children 3 to 5 years of age eat more than three times a day.[22] They consume food on an average of five to seven times a day, although ranges of three to fourteen times a day have been noted.[21] Crawford, Hankin, and Huenemann[17] found that by 6 years of age 50% of children ate five times a day. Eppright and others[23] noted that the frequency of food intakes was unrelated to nutrient intakes except when children consumed food less than four or more than six times a day. Children in this study who consumed food less than four times a day consumed fewer kilocalories and less calcium, protein, ascorbic acid, and iron than the average intakes of other children their age. Those who consumed food more than six times a day consumed more energy, calcium, and ascorbic acid than average intakes of children their age. Farris and others[6] found that snacks contributed 33% of the daily energy, 20% of the protein, 33% of the fat, and 40% of the carbohydrate consumed each day by 10-year-old children.

Factors that Influence Food Choices

The adequacy of children's food and nutrient intakes depends not only on the food available to them but also on the food environment and the models set for them by siblings, peers, parents and other important adults. Advertising and television are known to have a strong influence on children's requests for food. Working mothers may use convenience foods and fast food restaurants to feed their families, giving the food industry an impact on the development of food preferences in children.

PARENTAL INFLUENCES

Nutrition Knowledge

The nutrition knowledge of parents and other caregivers appears to be an important factor in children's food choices. The degree to which knowledge of nutrition is incorporated into family meal planning seems to be related to positive "attitude" toward self, problem-solving skills, and family organization in spite of a professed concern by all mothers interviewed about the total diet offered to young children and the importance of mealtime with children.[24] The ordinal position of the preschool child in the family appears to influence choices of specific foods regardless of equivalent knowledge of nutrition between groups of mothers.[25] When a preschool child is the youngest child in the family, the mothers appear to be less susceptible to the child's requests for new products. Mothers are willing, however, to accommodate that preference when the preschool child is the oldest child in the family.

Models

The models set for children by their families and other persons close to them exert a strong influence on their developing food patterns. Mother's and father's food preferences exert a definite influence. Food habits of siblings exert an even greater influence on food acceptance of the young child. Day-care teachers exert an influence equal to that of parents. They report that they know little about nutrition but think it is important.

Parent-Child Interactions

Children's interactions with their parents influence their acceptance of foods and the food patterns they develop. If parents accept casually the food jags and transient food dislikes preschoolers develop, these passing food behaviors are soon forgotten. However, parents who find these behaviors difficult to accept and give much attention to them by trying to bribe or encourage the child to eat, discussing the children's dislikes in front of them, or providing a preferred food when they refuse to eat may pattern that behavior into a permanent food habit.

The parent-child interaction also has an important influence on amount of food consumed. There appear to be differences between the interactions of thinner children and their mothers and fatter children and their mothers both in food and non-food situations. Thinner children and their mothers talk more with each other and eat less food more slowly than fatter children and their mothers.[26] Preferences for foods are enhanced when foods are offered as a reward or with brief positive social interactions with adults.[27]

INFLUENCE OF TELEVISION ON CHILDREN

Food Attitudes and Requests

In addition to the many family, cultural, and psychosocial influences on children's food habits, mass media have an impact on children's attitudes toward food and their requests for particular products. Of all the forms of mass media, television has the greatest impact on children because it reaches many children before they are capable of verbal communication and because it engages much of their time. Children spend more time in front of a television set than they do in any other activity than sleeping. Children from low-income families watch more television than do children from moderate- to high-income families.[28] It has been estimated that the preschool child watches television for 26.3 hours per week, and 6- to 11-year-old children watch an average of 24 hours per week.[29]

Lifestyle

Extensive television viewing can be detrimental to growth and development by encouraging sedentary and passive activities, thus promoting a lifestyle that may lead to obesity. In fact an association between obesity and time spent watching television has been documented in 6- to 11-year-old children and in adolescents.[30] Television viewing by children is also correlated with between-meal snacking. Advertisers attempt to use children to influence their parents' purchasing behavior. They present frequent cues for food and drink that often encourage consumption of a wide variety of sugared products. Television programs, as well as advertising, present models of behavior children may imitate. One study of prime-time television noted 5.31 food-related behaviors of characters per program. The behaviors that involved more nutritious food were almost equal in number to those that involved nonnutritious food.[31]

Television Advertising

It is estimated that the average child watches 3 hours of television advertising per week, or 19,000 to 22,000 commercials per year.[29] Kindergarten children often are unable to separate commercials from the program and frequently explain them as part of the program.[32] Children 5-10 years of age watch commercials more closely than do children 11-12 years of age.[33] Older children are more conscious of the concept of commercials, the purpose of selling, and the concept of sponsorship and are less likely to accept advertisers' claims without question. They perceive that television commercials are designed to sell products rather than to entertain or educate. Children in the second grade have been found to have a concrete distrust of commercials based on experience with advertised products. Children in the sixth grade have been found to have global distrust of all commercials.[32]

Food manufacturers and fast-food establishments use the greatest percentage of advertising time on television. A classic study of children's programs on Saturday and Sunday in Boston revealed that 68.5% of the advertisements were for food.[34] Of these ads, 25% were for cereal. 25% were for candy and sweets, and 8% were for snacks and other food. Quick meals and eating places were the subject of 10% of the ads. Only a few commercials were broadcast for milk, bread, or fruit. Ads for sugared cereals outnumbered those for unsugared cereals by a ratio of 3 to 1.

Certain attributes of food are promoted by television advertising as being superior to others. The main characteristics presented positively are "sweetness," "chocolatey," and "richness."[35] Many food manufacturers, in other words, de-emphasize the physiologic need for nutrients and encourage selection on the basis of sweet flavor. Exposure to such messages may distort a child's natural curiosity toward other characteristics of food such as the fresh crispness of apples or celery.

Parental Response

Children are influenced by television commercials and attempt to influence their parents' buying practices. Commercials for food have the strongest influence and mothers are more likely to yield to requests for food than for other products. They have a greater tendency to respond to requests from older children but certainly do not ignore those of younger children.[36] Highly child-centered mothers are less likely to buy children's favorite cereals than are mothers who are not as child-centered. Crawford, Hankin, and Huenemann[17] reported that two-thirds of the mothers interviewed stated that food choices were influenced by television commercials by the time the child was 4 years of age.

Feeding Children

If children are to consume an adequate diet appropriate food must be presented in a manner and an environment that supports developmental progress and the forming of sound food habits. Preschool children can be more puzzling in their response to food than school-age children. Older children may be more interested in other activities than meals and become increasingly more influenced by peers than parents. Knowledgeable parents, recognizing this, set limits on acceptable behavior yet support their children as they strive to achieve developmental landmarks and their own food patterns.

THE PRESCHOOL CHILD

In spite of the reduction of appetite and erratic consumption of food, preschool children do enjoy well-prepared and attractively served food. If simply prepared foods are presented in a relaxed setting, children will consume an appropriate nutrient intake. Meals and snacks should be timed to foster appetite. Intervals necessary between meals and snacks may vary from one child to another. Rarely can the clock be depended on to indicate appropriate intervals and times when it may be important for a child to eat. However, indiscriminate snacking dulls the appetite and such patterns should be discouraged.

Foods for Young Children

Children accept simple unmixed dishes more willingly than casseroles, and prefer most of their food at room temperature, neither hot nor cold. Food preparation is important. Children recognize poorly prepared food and are likely to refuse it. Most children eat most easily those foods with which they are familiar. Small portions of new foods can be introduced with familiar and popular foods. Even if the child only looks at the new food or just feels or smells it at first, this is a part of learning about it and accepting it.

Dry foods are especially hard for preschool children to eat. In planning a menu always balance a dry food with one or two moist foods. For example, it is wise to put a slice of meat loaf, relatively dry, with mashed potatoes and peas in a little cream sauce. Also, combinations of sharp, rather acid-flavored foods with mild-flavored foods are popular with young children. And they are pleased to find colorful foods such as red tomatoes, green peppers, and carrot sticks included in their meals.

Ease of Manipulation

Foods manipulated easily by the unskilled and seemingly clumsy hands of a young child are very important. Many small pieces of foods such as cooked peas or beans are difficult for a child to spoon up. Foods can be prepared so that a child can pick them up with his fingers. Hard-cooked eggs may be served in quarters, cooked meat can be cut in small strips, and cooked green beans can be served as finger foods. Children like oranges that have been cut in wedges, skin and all, much better than peeled and diced oranges. Mixed-up salads, when there are layers of food to be eaten, are much more difficult to eat than simple pieces of raw vegetables with no salad dressing. Serve cottage cheese or similar foods separate from the lettuce leaf on the child's plate. Creamed foods served on tough toast are difficult for children to manage.

Relatively small pieces of food that can be handled with the child's eating tools are best for preschool children. The problem of handling silverware and conveying food to the mouth at this early age is a greater task than many adults realize. Pieces of carrots that slide across the plate and are too small to remain on the fork are frustrating. On the other hand, cubes of beets so large that they must be cut into smaller pieces before they can be eaten exhaust the patience of a 2- or 3-year-old child. Most foods for these children should be served in bite-size pieces. When the child is 4 years of age and older, the skills to cut up some foods may have been developed. If, however, difficulty in managing food is noticed, small pieces should be served, with occasional encouragement to cup up some easier-to-manage foods. Canned pears and other soft fruits, for example, are usually easy to cut into bite-size pieces.

In general, the aim is to support the young child's early efforts at self-feeding and many creative adaptations can be helpful. Tomatoes or stringy spinach, for example, are a trial for anyone to eat. Much can be done with food shears in the kitchen to make these foods easier to eat. Finger foods such as pieces of lettuce or toast can be used in meals where some of the foods are difficult to handle. Small sandwiches—that is, a large one cut into four small squares—are popular with young children.

Food Characteristics

Three general food characteristics affecting taste, acceptance, and self-feeding skills development are important considerations in early feeding of young children. These aspects are texture, flavor, and portion sizes:

1. **Texture.** It is wise to serve one soft food, for easy eating, one crisp food, to allow easy chewing and enjoyment of the sounds in the mouth, and one chewy food, to use emerging chewing skills without having too much to chew, in each meal for young children. Pieces of meat seem to be hard for a young child to eat, which explains why children often prefer hamburgers to frankfurters. Most children's meat can be served as ground meat. Cook ground meat only long enough for the color to change to brown, not allowing it to become dry and crusted, hard for a child to eat. Some children may prefer moderately rare meat, which is even more moist, but care must be taken that it is cooked sufficiently to be safe.

2. **Flavor.** In general, young children reject strong flavors. Many children, however, do seem to like pickles and some spicy sauces, which may seem to contradict this. In general, it has been found that children like food only mildly salted. Pepper and other sharp spices and acids such as vinegar should also be used sparingly on children's food.
3. **Portion sizes.** Children are easily discouraged by large portions of food. Offer less than the child usually eats and permit seconds, rather than discouraging him with portions that are too large. Appropriate portion sizes are shown in Table 7-7.

Parent-Child Interaction

The environment and parent-child interaction when food is offered are important. The food should be presented without comment and the child permitted to consume a desired amount without any conversation focused on what or how much is being eaten. Portions served should be scaled to the child's appetite. When the meal is over, food should be removed and the child permitted to leave the table.

Physical Setting

Perhaps no arrangements for eating are more important than those that afford physical comfort to a child. Children should always feel secure, seated on sturdy, well-balanced chairs with their feet supported. They should be able to reach their food on the plate easily without straining their muscles. This position also enables them to eat without danger of spills. Dishes and utensils as well as table arrangements can foster success in eating. Give children sturdy utensils, as nearly unbreakable as possible, so that spills and breaking utensils will not give a sense of failure. Also, it is important not to laugh at the child, because if parents laugh at a child's mistakes the child may gain an undue feeing of being the center of attention.

Utensils

A young child's early eating experiences can be enhanced by selection of utensils that aid the eating process and meet developmental needs. Choose spoons and forks suitable for young hands. The spoon, the first eating implement a child uses, should have a round shallow bowl and a blunt tip that allows the child to shove food from the plate. A handle that is blunt, short, and easily held in the child's palm is desirable. Remember that at this age a child uses the hand as a mass of muscles. Only after 5 or 6 years of age is control of the finer muscles of the fingers accomplished. Forks with short, blunt tines are best adapted to the child's palm. Glasses that sit firmly on the table and are small enough for small hands to encircle are best for 2- to 4-year-old children. Small, delicate handles on cups are difficult for small hands to maneuver.

The shape and weight of the dishes is also very important. The young child delights in pouring his or her own milk. Interesting squat little pitchers with broad handles from which the child can easily pour milk are recommended. Parents can be encouraged to experiment with the dishes and other utensils for their children and to look for those that satisfy children's needs.

TABLE 7-7 A Feeding Guide for Children

This is a guide to a basic diet. Fats, desserts and sauces will contribute additional kilocalories to meet the needs of the growing child.

FOOD	1 year old		2-3 years old		4-6 years old		7-Puberty		Comments
	Portion Sizes	No. of Servings	Portion Sizes	No. of Servings	Portion Sizes	No. of Servings	Portion Sizes	No. of Servings	
Milk	½ cup	4-5	¼-¾ cup	4-5	½-¾ cup	3-4	1 cup	3	The following may be substituted for one-half cup of liquid milk: ½-¾ oz cheese ¼-½ cup yogurt 2½ tbsp non-fat dry milk powder
Meat and Meat Equivalents	¼-1 oz 2-4 tbsp	1	1-2 oz	2	1-2 oz	2	2-3 oz	3	The following may be substituted for one ounce of meat, fish, poultry: 4-5 tbsp cooked legumes 1 egg 2 tbsp peanut butter
Fruit & Vegetable		4-5		4-5		4-5		4-5	Include one green leafy or yellow vegetable, e.g., spinach, broccoli, carrots, winter squash
Vegetables:									
cooked	1-2 tbsp		2-3 tbsp		3-4 tbsp		½ cup		
raw	1-2 tbsp		few pieces		few pieces		½ cup		
Fruit:									
canned	2-4 tbsp		2-4 tbsp		4-6 tbsp		½ cup		Include one vitamin C-rich fruit or juice per day
raw	2-4 tbsp (chopped)		½-1 small		½-1 small				
juice	2-4 oz		3-4 oz		4 oz		4 oz		
Grains and grain products	½ slice	3	¼-1 slice	3	1 slice	4	1 slice	6	The following may be substituted for one slice of bread: ½ cup cooked cereal ½ cup spaghetti or other pasta ½ cup rice 5 saltines Whole grain products provide additional bulk to the diet.

Adapted from Lowenberg, M.E.: The Development of food patterns in young children, in Pipes, P.: Nutrition in infancy and childhood, ed. 3, St. Louis, 1985, Times Mirror/Mosby College Publishing.

Parental Concerns

Occasionally anxious or concerned parents need help with food sources of nutrients usually supplied by food the child refuses to eat or in establishing limits to the preschooler's food intakes and eating behavior. Of the commonly expressed concerns, limited intakes of milk, refusal of meat and vegetables, eating too many sweets, and limited intakes of food appear to cause the most problems.

1. **Milk.** It is important to recognize that 1 oz of milk supplies 36 mg of calcium, and many children receive 6 to 8 oz of milk on dry cereal daily. Although they consume only 1 to 2 oz of milk at a time, their calcium intakes may be acceptable when they consume milk with meals and snacks. When abundant amounts of fruit juice or sweetened beverages are available, children may simply prefer to drink them instead of milk. Other dairy products can be offered when milk is rejected. Cheese and yogurt are usually accepted. Powdered milk can be used in recipes for soups, vegetables, and mixed dishes.
2. **Meat.** Parents' perceptions of children's dislike of meat may need to be clarified, or an easier-to-chew form used. If, in fact, preschoolers do consistently refuse all food sources of heme iron, their daily intake of iron should be carefully monitored.
3. **Vegetables.** When vegetables are consistently refused, wars between parents and children should not be permitted to erupt. Small portions of 1 or 2 teaspoonfuls should continue to be served without comment and should be discarded if the child does not eat them. Preschool behavior modification programs that included token rewards when children consumed vegetables served at mealtime have been found to increase children's acceptance and intake of them.[37]
4. **Sweets.** Parents concerned about children's excessive intakes of sweets may need help in setting limits on amounts of sweet foods they make available to their children. It may be important also to help them convey their concern and the need to set limits on the availability of these foods to other family members, day-care operators, and teachers.
5. **Food intake.** If children's food intakes are so limited that their intakes of energy and nutrients are compromised, parents may need help in establishing guidelines so that the children develop appetites. They should provide food often enough so that children do not get so hungry that they lose their appetite, yet not so often that they are always satiated. Intervals of 3 to 4 hours are often successful. Very small portions of foods should be offered, and second portions permitted when the children consume the foods already served. Attention should always be focused on children when they eat, never when food is refused.

THE SCHOOL-AGE CHILD

Physical and Social Development

The school-age period is one of few apparent feeding problems. A natural increase in appetite is responsible for normal increases in food intake. Because they spend their days at school, children adjust to a more ordered routine. As they explore the environment of school and peers, children will be influenced by these experiences (Fig.

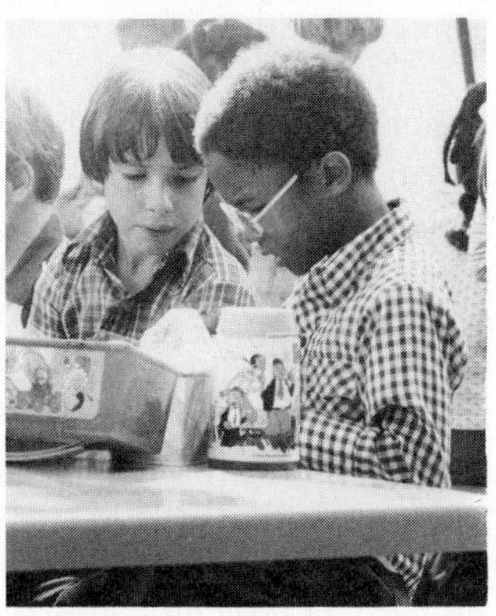

FIG. 7-3 Food habits are part of both physical and psychosocial development.

7-3). Often the credibility of parents is questioned in the face of advice from teachers, peers, or peers' parents. The school-age child has more access to money, to grocery stores, and therefore to foods with questionable nutrient values. Many school-age children have some responsibility for preparing their own breakfasts or sack lunches. Most arrive home from school looking for a snack.

Meal Patterns

Breakfast is an important meal. Even so, estimates of children who do not eat breakfast range from 8% to 29%.[38] Children will have to rise earlier to eat an unhurried and balanced meal and may have to prepare it themselves. Early morning school activities may make preplanning necessary. Some may find a glass of milk and fruit juice important before early sports activities. Studies have shown that when breakfast is consumed, children have a better attitude and school record as compared with when it is omitted.[39] Pollitt, Leibel, and Greenfield[40] found that the effect of skipping breakfast on problem-solving in 9- to 11-year-old well-nourished children was an adverse effect on accuracy of response in problem-solving but a beneficial effect on immediate memory in short-term accuracy. The effect was attributed to a heightened arousal level, which in turn had a qualitative effect on cognitive function.

Actually most children do eat breakfasts that contribute at least one-fourth of the RDA standard.[38] A larger percentage of children in the lower grades eat breakfast than those in the middle and upper grades. Reasons for skipping breakfast have been reported to be "not hungry," "no time," "on a diet," "no one to prepare food," "do not like food served for breakfast," and "foods are not available."[38] Morgan, Zabik, and Leville[41] found that children who consumed ready-to-eat cereals 3 or 4 times a week skipped breakfast less frequently than did children who ate non-ready-to-eat hot cereal. Many school-age children participate in the School Breakfast and Lunch Program administered by the Department of Agriculture, which provides cash reimbursement and supplemental foods to feeding programs that comply with federal regulations. Low-income children may receive reduced prices or free meals.

Children who do not participate in the school lunch program generally bring a packed lunch from home. Studies have indicated that, compared with the school lunch, these meals provide significantly fewer nutrients but supply energy. Little variety is seen in the lunches since favorite foods tend to be packed and repacked and lack of refrigeration limits the kinds of foods that can be carried.

The emotional environment at the dinner table may influence nutrient intake. The evening meal is not the place for family battles or punitive action toward children. If eating is to be successful and enjoyable it must occur in a setting that is comfortable and free from stress and unreasonable demands. Lund and Burke[41] found that mealtime criticism about non-food-related activities reduced the level of food consumption and adversely affected intakes of vitamins A and C in 9- to 11-year-old children.

Prevention of Nutrition and Health Problems

Nutrition concerns during childhood include iron-deficiency anemia, overweight and obesity, and dental caries. In addition some persons are worried about children's intakes of specific foods and food constituents such as artificial flavors, colors and sugar and their possible effect on behavior. Also, it is important to recognize that many risk factors for cardiovascular disease can be modified by changes in dietary patterns. Identification of children at risk and modifying fat and salt intakes as well as other contributing factors are important health promotion actions.

The prevention of iron-deficiency anemia has been discussed earlier in this chapter. Any discussion on childhood nutrition should include attention to these other concerns as well.

WEIGHT MANAGEMENT

An excessive rate of weight gain and deposition of fat occurs when energy intake exceeds energy expenditure. Over time this situation can lead to obesity. By monitoring rates of growth and deposition of adipose tissue, children can be identified who are accumulating more fat than would be anticipated, and measures to increase activity and decrease excessive caloric intakes can be taken.

Family Attitudes

Adolescents make their own decisions about what and when they eat. Counseling must be directed to the teenagers themselves. But parents control the food available to younger children, create the environment that influences their acceptance of food, and can influence energy expenditure by the opportunities they create for physical activity for their children. It may be important to explore first with parents their reasons for encouraging their children to consume amounts of food that result in rapid weight gain. Some parents may not recognize that their expectations for the quantity of food they encourage their children to consume are excessive and that the "chubby" child is not necessarily a healthy child.

Parents may need help in developing appropriate parenting skills. They may need to learn how to respond to hunger and other needs of their infants and how to interact with their children. They may need help in identifying ways to help their children develop initiative and to cultivate friends and outlets in the community.[42]

Physical Activity

The activity pattern of both the child and the family should be explored. It may be important to help parents find ways of increasing their child's level of activity. Parents who live in apartments often reinforce sedentary activities to reduce the noise level and complaints from neighbors. Those who live in one-family dwellings may have limited space for children's activities. City park departments, preschools, and schools frequently have programs that offer opportunities for increasing children's activities.

Appropriate Energy Intake

It is important to remember that at any age the range of appropriate energy intakes is large. Overweight children and children with familial trends to obesity may need fewer kilocalories than do their peers. Griffith and Payne[43] found that normal-weight 4- to 5-year-old children of obese parents expended 1174 kcal/day as compared with 1508 kcal/day expended by children of the same size and age of normal-weight parents. It was interesting that the children of normal-weight parents expended twice as much energy in physical activity as did those of obese parents. Families of children with a familial tendency to obesity may need help in identifying the kinds and amounts of food that provide an energy intake that will support normal growth and weight gain.

Nutrition Counseling

Programs of nutrition counseling should be family-oriented and based on normal nutrition, emphasizing foods that provide a balance of nutrients as well as appropriate kilocalorie intakes. Families will need to realize that efforts are directed at reduction in rates of weight gain and are not intended to effect weight loss. They must recognize that the food available and the models set for their child will determine the child's response to efforts to control weight gain. Family meals may need to be modified to include fewer fried foods, less gravy, and fewer rich desserts. Parents and siblings may have to modify their own eating practices to set appropriate examples. Teachers, babysitters, and day-care workers should be alerted to and included in programs designed to control weight. Food experiences at school may need to be modified to exclude corn dripping with butter and chocolate cupcakes so frequently provided for special occasions. Low-calorie snacks such as raw fruits and vegetables can be provided instead of cookies, candy, and hot dogs.

DENTAL CARIES

Dental caries, one of the most common nutrition-related diseases, affects children of all ages and family income levels. As in the development of other tissues, nutrition plays an important role during childhood in the development of sound teeth and the surrounding structures that hold them and in the later susceptibility of the teeth to caries. Once the tooth has erupted, the composition of the diet, the presence of acid-producing bacteria, and the buffering capacity of the saliva interact and result in control or development of dental caries. Calcified dental tissues, unlike the long bones, which are subject to constant remodeling and repair, do not have the ability to repair themselves. Tooth destruction by decay is permanent.

Etiology

Dental plaque, a prerequisite for dental caries, has been described as a sticky, gelatinous mixture that contains water, salivary protein, desquamated cells, and bacteria.[44] The plaque bacteria, using energy derived from the catabolism of dietary carbohydrate, synthesize several toxic substances including enzymes that have the potential to degrade the enamel and dentin and are precursors of acidic fermentation products. *Streptococcus mutans* appears to be the primary plaque bacteria. The acids and enzymes it produces cause demineralization of the hydroxyapatite of the enamel followed by proteolytic degradation and demineralization of the enamel and dentin. It has been proposed that when the acidic environment falls below pH 5.5, cariogenic bacteria invade the tooth and caries results. The saliva, the pH of which is 6.5 to 7.0, acts as a buffer and provides mechanical cleansing of the teeth.

Sugar

It has been well documented from animal studies and studies of humans in institutions and as outpatients when intakes of sugar could be controlled that sucrose is the most cariogenic carbohydrate and that the incidence of caries can be reduced when the intakes of sugar are reduced.[44,45] Glucose is thought to be the next most cariogenic sugar, and maltose, lactose, and fructose have been found to have equal effect. Starch can also cause the production of large amounts of plaque acid because this carbohydrate, once attacked by salivary amylase, is broken down into sugar and attacked by plaque bacteria.

Frequency of Eating

The presence of sucrose, or even the total amount of sucrose in the diet, may not be the determining factor in the incidence of dental caries. An often quoted study in an institution for the mentally handicapped in Sweden showed that the more important factors were the frequency with which the sugar is consumed and the adhesiveness of the food to the teeth.[45] The researchers who conducted this 5-year study showed that the consumption of sticky candy between meals produced a high increase in the incidence of dental caries, whereas the increase in incidence of caries from the addition of sugar-sweetened water at mealtime was small. When sucrose was fed in chocolate or bread, an intermediate increase in the incidence of caries was noted. Other studies have not supported these findings. Many researchers have found no difference between meal eating habits of caries-free and caries-prone individuals.

Snacking at bedtime is especially effective in increasing dental caries. Reduction of the flow of saliva, which occurs during sleep, reduces the natural cleansing mechanism and permits greater fermentation of cariogenic material. The ingestion of foods that alter the buffering capacity of the saliva, for example, milk and fats, which form a protective oily film on the tooth surface, may offer some protection for the teeth.[46]

Control

The less frequently sucrose-containing foods are consumed and the less ability the foods have to adhere to the teeth, the more positive will be the outlook for the control of dental caries.

1. **Fluoride.** That fluoride can reduce the incidence of dental caries has been definitely proved. It suppresses sugar metabolism by bacteria, makes enamel more resistant to acid, and stimulates remineralization of the teeth. A fluoridated water supply is important in the prevention of dental caries. Other approaches to ensuring adequate fluoride intake that are under investigation include sodium fluoride capsules that can be chewed and swallowed, the use of an aerosol that causes fluoride-containing organisms to adhere to the teeth and enhances fluoride uptake by the plaque and enamel, and the use of a small device attached to the teeth that releases fluoride at a predetermined rate for at least 6 months.[47]
2. **Diet: foods and frequency.** Dietary control continues to be a most important and effective approach to the control of dental caries. The frequency of eating breads, rolls, and cereals has not been associated with an increase in dental caries, whereas the frequency of eating candy and chewing gum has been shown to increase the number and incidence of dental caries.[48] Cookies, cakes, pies, and candies have been shown to cause large decreases in the pH of the plaque. It is interesting that the researchers found that the more acid carbonated beverages depress pH less than apple and orange juice.[49] A study of 147 junior high school students' snacking patterns in relation to caries production showed chocolate candy to be the most carious snack food selected. Children who consumed fruit drinks, cookies, or apples at bedtime and between meals had a significant caries increment during the year studied. No carious lesions developed in 47 children who had higher intakes of fruit juice and oranges and lesser use of sugar-sweetened chewing gum than the other children. As the amount of a child's spending money increased, the frequency of snacking increased.[50]
3. **Plaque control.** Researchers have studied the cariogenicity of foods in rats by noting the caries experience after food comes in contact with the teeth for designated periods and in humans by noting changes in the plaque pH before and immediately after a food is eaten. The box (p. 286) shows foods that cause the plaque pH to fall below 5.5 and are considered to be cariogenic. Certain foods do not cause the plaque pH between the teeth to fall to levels at which demineralization will occur. These foods have a relatively high protein content with basic amino acids, a moderate fat content, a strong buffering capacity, a high mineral content including calcium and phosphorus, and a pH greater than 6.0. They also stimulate saliva flow. Meats, nuts, and cheese have been found to be noncariogenic. In fact, they have a beneficial effect when consumed with other foods. Cheddar cheese has been observed to block caries formation caused by sweet snacks when sweets and cheese have been eaten alternately.[51]

A PARTIAL LIST OF FOODS THAT CAUSE THE pH OF HUMAN INTERPROXIMAL PLAQUE TO FALL BELOW 5.5

Apples, dried	Gelatin, flavored dessert
Apples, fresh	Grapes
Apple drink	Milk, whole
Apricots, dried	Milk, 2%
Bananas	Milk, chocolate
Beans, baked	Oatmeal, instant cooked
Beans, green, canned	Oats, rolled
Bread, white	Oranges
Bread, whole wheat	Orange juice
Caramel	Pasta
Carrots, cooked	Peanut butter
Cereals, nonpresweetened	Peas, canned
Cereals, presweetened	Potato, amylose
Chocolate, milk	Potato, boiled
Cola, beverage	Potato chips
Cookies, vanilla sugar	Raisins
Corn flakes	Rice, instant cooked
Corn starch	Sponge cake, cream-filled
Crackers, soda	Tomato, fresh
Cream cheese	Wheat flakes
Doughnuts, plain	

From Schachtele, C.F.: Nutr. News **42**:13, 1982. Courtesy Nutrition News, National Dairy Council.

4. **Nutrition education.** Children should be taught to select foods that provide the essential nutrients and to limit their consumption of cariogenic foods. It is important that they learn to include noncariogenic protective foods in their snacking patterns, especially when sucrose-containing foods are included in the menu. The important between-meal snacks can be carefully planned to contribute nutrients without creating an oral environment conducive to tooth decay. Sweet foods such as dessert items should be consumed as infrequently as possible within the framework of acceptability to the child and to the family.

FOOD AND BEHAVIOR

There has been considerable speculation that certain additives and food constituents such as sugar and caffeine may play a part in the etiology of hyperactivity in childhood. This condition is characterized by inattention, excess motor activity, impulsiveness, and poor tolerance for frustration, with onset before 7 years of age. It affects 5% to 10% of school-age children.

Additives

In recent years the hypothesis that artificial flavors and colors and naturally occurring salicylates cause hyperactivity in as many as 50% of children so affected has been popular. Many persons have felt that a diet that eliminates these constituents is indicated. But research has not supported this hypothesis. A very small percentage of children, however, have been identified to be "responders" to the additives.

Open clinical trials have indicated behavioral improvements in as many as 50% of hyperactive children. They have also reported that the diet improved behavior in nonhyperactive children, suggesting that behavioral changes may be due to changes in the parent-child interactions and family dynamics.[52]

Double-blind studies suggest that food additives do not play a major role in the etiology of hyperactivity in the majority of cases. Interestingly two different researchers found an order effect. In one study parents noted a slight effect if the additive-free diet had been given first, and in another study teachers noted the same effect when it was given first.[53] Studies that have challenged hyperactive children on an additive-free diet with a food containing additives or a placebo have indicated that one in 25 hyperactive children who respond to the additive-free diet show behavioral response when challenged with the constituents.[52]

Sugar

Sugar has also been hypothesized to play a role in the etiology of behavioral difficulties in children. Most of the reports that have indicted sugar have been based on clinical assessment; few have been based on controlled studies. A retrospective review of glucose tolerance curves of hyperactive children found 75% of the 261 hyperkinetic children had abnormal glucose tolerance curves following a 5-hour glucose tolerance test. Other studies have not found abnormal glucose tolerance curves.[54]

Several double-blind challenge studies have not found sugar to contribute to hyperactivity even in children whose mothers felt they were responders. However, speculation that sugar is an offender in the etiologies of the disorder continues on the basis of observations of behavior and food intake. An association was suggested between destructive aggressive behavior and sugar intake of hyperkinetic but not normal 4- to 7-year-old children on the basis of 7-day food diaries kept by the mothers and videotaped observations of behavior by trained observers.[55] Another study noted an inverse relationship in the percentage of sugar in the children's diets suggested by a 1-day dietary recall and standardized measures of intelligence and school achievement.[56] It should be noted that none of the above studies has shown a cause-and-effect relation between sugar intake and hyperkinetic behavior.

One hyperkinetic 5-year-old male and his mother were both found to become frustrated, hyperactive, and difficult to control after a double-blind challenge with sugar in lemonade.[57] However, not one of the 50 other hyperkinetic children tested in the same way responded to a sugar challenge. Definitive evidence that sugar causes behavioral problems in children has not been found.[58,59] However, there may be some children who are sensitive to sugar and further investigation using double-blind crossover design is appropriate.

PREVENTION OF ATHEROSCLEROSIS

Risk Factors

Major risk factors associated with cardiovascular disease include obesity, especially through its relation to hypertension; a strong family history of heart disease; a sedentary lifestyle; and elevated blood lipids, especially low density lipoprotein (LDL) cholesterol. These risk factors are independent and continuous variables. Modifications of dietary patterns and lifestyle of children who are at risk are important approaches to the prevention of this disease process, which is responsible for over half the mortality in the United States and other Western countries.

Studies of adults have shown a significant relation between elevated serum cholesterol, blood pressure, and the extent of atherosclerotic lesions. The extent of the raised lesion is associated with total fat, saturated fat, cholesterol, and animal protein intakes. Autopsies of young adults have also found a relationship between antemortem serum total cholesterol levels and percent involvement of the aortic fatty streak. Children with cholesterol levels between 140 and 170 mg/dl have 25% total surface involvement with fatty streaks. Those with cholesterol levels above 200 mg/dl have 50% involvement. An even stronger relationship exists between low density lipoprotein (LDL) cholesterol levels and fatty streaks. A less clear relationship exists between blood pressure in childhood and atherosclerosis. Children do show an increase in left ventricular posterior wall thickness with increasing blood pressure.[60]

Tracking will be noted in children with both high blood pressure and elevated serum lipid levels. That is, they usually maintain the same relative ranking with their peers over time. A family history of hypertension and hyperlipidemia suggests vulnerability to the development of either one of these disorders or both of them. Cholesterol levels in the first year have been found to be the most predictive factors studied of subsequent cholesterol levels. Of the children at the 90th and 10th percentiles in the first year, 45% persisted at their respective levels in the second year. Children of parents with high serum cholesterol levels are 2.57 times more likely to have serum cholesterol levels greater than the 95th percentile.[60]

Children at Risk

Children at greatest risk include: (1) those from families with a history of myocardial infarction, sudden coronary death in cardiovascular accident before age 50 in men and 60 in women; (2) those from families with hypertension or extremely abnormal lipid and lipoprotein levels; and (3) children with high levels of risk factors but who have no family history of premature cardiovascular disease.[61]

The child with risk factors is probably from a family at risk, all of whom could profit from dietary modification. A diet low in cholesterol, saturated fat, and total fat is indicated, as well as the avoidance of foods high in sodium. Obesity and overweight should be discouraged in all children. For children not at risk the Committee on Nutrition of the American Academy of Pediatrics recommends a varied diet with selections from all major food groups.[62]

GROUP FEEDING

Increasing numbers of mothers of young children are working outside the home. Many children of these women receive care and meals in family day-care homes or child-care programs. Children whose mothers work full time are often in a child care facility for 9 to 10 hours 5 days a week and receive both meals and snacks in this setting.[63] Kindergartens and preschools also offer snacks and meals along with food experiences that are often included as a part of the learning activities.

Family day-care homes and day-care centers are licensed by state agencies that mandate the meal pattern and types of snacks to be provided for the children, as well as the percentage of the recommended daily allowances that must be included in the menus. In general, a child in day care 8 hours should receive at least one-third the RDA from food and snacks, a child in day care more than 8 hours, one-half to two-thirds the RDA. Assistance is available to nonprofit, licensed day-care programs from the United States Department of Agriculture. This assistance includes reimbursement for meals in addition to donated foods.

Breakfast should be provided for children who receive none at home. Snacks should be planned to complement the daily food intakes. Small portions of food should be served, and children should be permitted second servings of those foods they enjoy. Disliked or unfamiliar foods may be offered by the teaspoonful, and the child's acceptance or rejection received without comment. Children who eat slowly will need to be served first and permitted to complete their meals without being rushed to other activities. Teachers and caretakers should eat with the children without imposing their attitudes about food.

A new setting provides an opportunity for children to have exposure to many new foods. Day-care centers, kindergartens, and preschools can provide an important educational setting for both children and their parents. Children learn to prepare food, how food grows, how it smells, and what nutrients it contains. Parents learn through participation, observation, and conversation with the staff. An organized approach to feeding children must include parents, teachers, and others who offer food to children. Teachers and day-care workers can provide important information to parents about how children successfully consume food, the nutrients children need, and the foods that provide these nutrients. Parents offer important information to the centers about their children's food acceptance and needs. Each needs to be reinforced positively by the other for their efforts to provide food for the children to be successful.

A study of 48 day-care and Head Start programs found that all participating children consumed appropriate intakes of nutrients. Total daily energy intakes were similar for all children regardless of whether one meal and one snack or two meals and two snacks were provided. In fact, when children consumed one meal and and one snack, 82% of their energy intake was provided, but when two meals and two snacks were provided, 84% of the energy intake was consumed in this setting.[64]

For older children, school lunch and nutrition education programs provide not only important nutrients but also an opportunity for them to learn to make responsible food choices. Schools may have both breakfast and lunch programs. Since its inception in 1946, the school lunch program has been administered by the U.S. Department of Agriculture, which provides both cash reimbursement and supplemental foods to feeding programs that comply with federal regulations. These regulations require that school lunches and breakfasts be sold at reduced prices or given free to children of families that cannot afford to buy them. The lunch menus must be planned to meet the guidelines established for the National School Lunch Program. Table 7-8 shows the minimal quantities of food required for the various age groups in a school lunch.

To provide variety and to encourage participation and consumption, schools are

TABLE 7-8 School Lunch Pattern—Approximate per Lunch Minimums

Components		Minimum Quantities				Recommended Quantities for Group V: 12 Years and Older; 7-12†
		Group 1: Age 1-2; Preschool	**Group II: Age 3-4; Preschool**	**Group III: Age 5-8; K-3**	**Group IV: Age 9 and Older; 4-12**	
Milk	Unflavored, fluid lowfat, skim or buttermilk must be offered*	¾ cup (6 fl oz)	¾ cup (6 fl oz)	½ pint (8 fl oz)	½ pint (8 fl oz)	½ pint (8 fl oz)
Meat or meat alternate (quantity of the edible portion as served)	Lean meat, poultry, or fish	1 oz	1½ oz	1½ oz	2 oz	3 oz
	Cheese	1 oz	1½ oz	1½ oz	2 oz	3 oz
	Large egg	½	¾	¾	1	1½
	Cooked dry beans or peas	¼ cup	⅜ cup	⅜ cup	½ cup	¾ cup
	Peanut butter or an equivalent quantity of any combination of any of above	2 tbsp	3 tbsp	3 tbsp	4 tbsp	6 tbsp
Vegetable or fruit	2 or more servings of vegetable or fruit or both	½ cup	½ cup	½ cup	¾ cup	¾ cup
Bread or bread alternate (servings per week)	Must be enriched or whole-grain—at least ½ serving ‡ for group I or one serving ‡ for groups II-V must be served daily	5	8	8	8	10

From Food and Nutrition Service, Department of Agriculture: National School Lunch Program Regulations, Nov. 16, 1982, Federal Register.

*If a school serves another form of milk (whole or flavored), it must offer its children unflavored fluid lowfat milk, skim milk, or buttermilk as a beverage choice.

†The *minimum* portion sizes for these children are the portion sizes for group IV.

‡Serving 1 slice of bread; or ½ cup of cooked rice, macaroni, noodles, other pasta products, other cereal product such as bulgur and corn grits; or as stated in the *Food Buying Guide* for biscuits, rolls, muffins, and similar products.

encouraged to provide a selection of foods. Senior high students can decline up to two items. Students below the senior high level may decline up to two or only one item at the discretion of the local school food authority. Breakfast must include liquid milk, fruit or vegetable juice, and bread or cereal. Schools are encouraged to keep fat, sugar, and salt at moderate levels.

Foods sold in competition with school lunch in snack bars or vending machines must provide at least 5% of the recommended dietary allowances for one or more of the following nutrients: protein, vitamin A, ascorbic acid, niacin, riboflavin, thiamin, calcium, and iron. This regulation eliminates the sale of soda water, water ices, chewing gum, and some candies until after the last lunch period. It should also encourage the offering of more fruits, vegetables, and fruit and vegetable juices in places that compete with school lunch.

Although elementary school children are making more decisions regarding food selection, supervision and supportive guidance may be necessary at lunchtime. Children may give priority to activities other than eating and rush through their meals. Some may refuse to eat the food on the menu. Children who need therapeutic diets will need guidance in the foods they should and should not eat.

Summary

Children between 1 year of age and the onset of puberty grow at a steady rate. They acquire new skills, learn much about their environment, and test the limits of behavior the environment will accept. All of these factors influence the food they accept and the frequency with which they eat. As they grow older, children's food intakes become more influenced by peers, activities, and stimuli in their environment.

Prevention of nutrition problems is important during childhood. Of particular concern is the prevention of iron-deficiency anemia, obesity, and dental caries.

Review Questions

1. Why do energy needs of children vary so widely at any age?
2. What independent feeding skills would you expect a normal 18-month-old child to have?
3. What factors influence food acceptance by children?
4. List food and feeding behavior concerns of most importance to mothers of preschool children.
5. List snack foods appropriate for children that are supportive of a program to prevent excessive weight gain and dental caries.

REFERENCES

1. Smith, D.W.: Growth and its disorders, Philadelphia, 1977, W.B. Saunders Co.
2. National Center for Health Statistics: NCHS growth charts, 1976, Monthly Vital Statistics Report, vol. 25, no. 3, suppl. (HRA) 76-1120, Rockville, Md., 1976, Health Resources Administration.

3. Food and Nutrition Board, National Research Council: Recommended dietary allowances, ed. 9, Washington, D.C., 1980, National Academy of Sciences.
4. Spady, D.W.: Total daily energy expenditure of healthy, free-ranging school children, Am. J. Clin. Nutr. **33**:766, 1980.
5. Food and nutrient intakes of individuals in 1 day in the United States, 1977, USDA Nationwide Food Consumption Survey, 1977-1978, Preliminary report number 2, Washington, D.C., 1980, Science and Education Administration.
6. Farris, R.P., and others: Macronutrient intake of 10-year-old children, 1973 to 1982, J. Am. Diet. Assoc. **86**:765, 1986.
7. Ashworth, A., and Millward, D.J.: Catch-up growth in children, Nutr. Rev. **44**:157, 1986.
8. Marie, P.J., and others: Histological osteomalacia due to dietary calcium deficiency in children, New. Engl. J. Med. **307**:584, 1982.
9. Butrimonitz, G.P., and Purdy, W.C.: Zinc nutrition and growth in children, Am. J. Clin. Nutr. **31**:1409, 1978.
10. Schlage, C., and Wortberg, B.: Zinc in the diet of healthy preschool and school children, Acta Paediatr. Scand. **61**:421, 1972.
11. Hambidge, K.M., and others: Zinc nutrition of preschool children in the Denver Head Start Programs, Am. J. Clin. Nutr. **29**:734, 1976.
12. Hambidge, K.M., and others: Low levels of zinc in hair, anorexia and poor growth and hypogeusia in children, Pediatr. Res. **6**:868, 1972.
13. Cook, C.C., and Payne, I.R.: Effect of supplements on the nutrient intake of children, J. Am. Diet. Assoc. **74**:130, 1979.
14. Breskin, M.W., and others: Water-soluble vitamins: intakes and indices in children, J. Am. Diet. Assoc. **85**:49, 1985.
15. Committee on Nutrition, American Academy of Pediatrics: Vitamin and mineral supplement needs of normal children in the United States, Pediatrics **66**:1015, 1980.
16. Beal, V.A.: Dietary intake of individuals followed through infancy and childhood, Am. J. Public Health **51**:1107, 1961.
17. Crawford, P.B., Hankins, J.H., and Huenemann, R.L.: Environmental factors associated with preschool obesity, J. Am. Diet. Assoc. **77**:589, 1978.
18. Beal, V.A.: On the acceptance of solid foods and other food patterns of infants and children, Pediatrics **20**:448, 1957.
19. Lamkin, G., Hielscher, M.L., and Janes, H.B.: Food purchasing practices of young families, J. Home Econ. **62**:598, 1970.
20. Morgan, K.J., and Zabik, M.E.: Amount and food sources of total sugar intake by children ages 5 to 12 years, Am. J. Clin. Nutr. **34**:404, 1981.
21. Henneman, R.L.: Environment factors associated with preschool obesity, J. Am. Diet. Assoc. **64**:489, 1974.
22. Lucas, B.L.: Nutrition in childhood. In Krause, M.V., and Mahan, L.K.: Food, Nutrition and Diet Therapy, ed. 7, Philadelphia, 1984, W.B. Saunders Co.
23. Eppright, E.S., and others: The North Central Regional Study of diets of preschool children. III. Frequency of eating, J. Home Econ. **62**:407, 1970.
24. Swanson-Rudd, J., and others: Nutrition orientations of working mothers in the North Central Region, J. Nutr. Educ. **14**:132, 1982.
25. Phillips, D.E., Bass, M.A., and Yetley, E.: Use of food and nutrition knowledge by mothers of preschool children, J. Nutr. Educ. **10**:73, 1980.
26. Birch, L.L., and others: Mother-child interaction patterns and the degree of fatness in children, J. Nutr. Educ. **12**:17, 1981.
27. Birch, L.L., Zimmerman, S.I., and Hind, H.: The influence of social-affective context on the formation of children's food preferences, J. Nutr. Educ. **13**:115, 1981.

28. Somers, A.R.: Violence, television, and the health of American youth, New Engl. J. Med. **294**:811, 1976.
29. Choate, R.: Statement presented before the House Subcommittee on Communications of the Committee on Interstate and Foreign Commerce, U.S. House of Representatives, Washington, D.C., 1975, U.S. Government Printing Office.
30. Dietz, W.H., and Gortmaker, S.L.: Do we fatten our children at the television set? Obesity and television viewing in children and adolescents, Pediatrics **75**:807, 1985.
31. Way, W.L.: Food-related behaviors on prime-time television, J. Nutr. Educ. **15**:105, 1983.
32. Blatt, J., Spencer, L., and Ward, S.: A cognitive developmental study of children's reactions to television advertising. In Rubinstein, E.A., Comstock, G.A., and Murray, J.P., eds.: Television and social behavior, vol. 4, Television in day-to-day life: patterns of use, Washington, D.C., 1972, U.S. Government Printing Office.
33. Ward, S., Levinson, D., and Wackman, D.: Children's attention to television commercials. In Rubinstein, E.A., Comstock, G.A., and Murray, J.P., eds.: Television and social behavior, vol. 4, Television in day-to-day life: patterns of use, Washington, D.C., 1972, U.S. Government Printing Office.
34. Television, 1976, North Brook, Ill., 1976, A.C. Neilson Co.
35. Gussow, J.: Counternutritional messages of TV ads aimed at children, J. Nutr. Educ. **4**:48, 1972.
36. Wackman, D.B., and Ward, S.: Children's information processing of television commercial messages, manuscript based on a symposium at the American Psychological Association Convention, Montreal, 1973. (Cited in Sheikh)
37. Harril, I., Smith, C., and Gangever, J.A.: Food acceptance and nutrient intake of preschool children. J. Nutr. Educ. **4**:103, 1972.
38. Morgan, K.J., Zabik, M.Z., and Leville, G.A.: The role of breakfast in nutrient intake of 5- to 12-year-old children, Am. J. Clin. Nutr. **34**:1418, 1981.
39. Tuttle, W.W., and others: Effect on school boys of omitting breakfast, J. Am. Diet. Assoc. **30**:674, 1974.
40. Pollitt, E.L., Leibel, R.L., and Greenfield, D.: Brief fasting stress and cognition in children, Am. J. Clin. Nutr **34**:1526, 1981.
41. Lund, L.A., and Burk, M.C.: A multidisciplinary analysis of children's food consumption behavior. Technical Bulletin No. 265, St. Paul, 1969, University of Minnesota, Agricultural Experimental Station.
42. Hertzler, A.A.: Obesity: impact of the family, J. Am. Diet. Assoc. **79**:525, 1981.
43. Griffith, M., and Payne, P.R.: Energy expenditure in small children of obese and nonobese parents, Nature **260**:698, 1976.
44. Nizel, A.E.: Nutrition in Preventive Dentistry: Science and Practice, ed. 2, Philadelphia, 1983, W.B. Saunders Co.
45. Gustafson, B.E., and others: The Vipeholm dental caries study: the effect of different levels of carbohydrate intake on dental caries in 436 individuals observed for five years, Acta Odontol. Scand. **11**:232, 1954.
46. Weiss, M.E., and Bibby, B.G.: Effects of milk on enamel solubility, Arch. Oral Biol. **11**:49, 1966.
47. Mirth, D.B., and Bowen, W.H.: Chemotherapy antimicrobials and methods of delivery in microbial aspects of dental caries. In Stiles, H.M., and others, eds.: Microbial aspects of dental caries, Washington, D.C., 1976, Information Retrieval.
48. Bagramian, R.A., and others: Diet patterns and dental caries in third-grade U.S. children, Community Dent. Oral Epidemiol. **2**:208, 1974.
49. Edgar, W.M., and others: Acid production in plaque after eating snacks: modifying factors in food, J. Am. Dent. Assoc. **90**:418, 1975.

50. Clancy, K.L., and others: Snack food intakes of adolescents and caries developments, J. Dent. Res. **56**:568, 1977.
51. Schachtele, C.F.: Changing perspectives on the role of diet in dental caries formation, Nutr. News **42**:13, 1982.
52. Levitsky, D.A., and Strump, B.A.: Nutrition and the behavior of children. In Walker, W.A., and Watkins, W.F., eds.: Nutrition in Pediatrics, Boston, 1985, Little, Brown & Co.
53. Connors, C.K., Gaysette, C.N., Southwick, D.A., and others: Food additives and hyperkinesis: a controlled double-blind experiment, Pediatrics **58**:154, 1976.
54. Langseth, L., and Dowd, J.: Glucose tolerance and hyperkinesis, Food and Cosmetics Toxicology **16**:129, 1978.
55. Printz, R.J., Roberts, W.A., and Hartman, E.: Dietary correlates of hyperactive behavior in children, J. Consult. Clin. Psychol. **48**:760, 1980.
56. Lester, M.B., Thatcher, R.W, and Monroe-Lord, L.: Refined carbohydrate intake, hair cadmium levels, and cognitive function in children, Nutrition and Behavior **1**:3, 1982.
57. Gross, M.D.: Effect of sugar on hyperkinetic children, Pediatrics **74**:876, 1984.
58. Ferguson, H.B., Stoddard, C., and Simeon, J.G.: Double-blind challenge studies of behavioral and cognitive effects of sucrose-aspartame ingestion of normal children, Nutr. Rev. **44**:(Suppl.) May 1986.
59. Rapoport, J.L.: Diet and hyperactivity, Nutr. Rev. **158**:(Suppl.) May 1986.
60. Berenson, G.S, and others: Serum high-density lipoprotein and its relationship to cardiovascular disease risk factor variables in children—the Bogalusa Heart Study, Lipids **14**:91, 1979.
61. Cresanta, J.L., Hyg, M.S., Burke, G.L, and others: Prevention of atherosclerosis, Pediatr. Clin. N. Am. **33**:835, 1986.
62. Committee on Nutrition, American Academy of Pediatrics: Prudent life styles for children: dietary fats and cholesterol, Pediatrics **78**:521, 1986.
63. Office of Human Development Services, U.S. Department of Health and Human Services: Family day care in the United States, executive summary, National Day Care Home Study DHHS, pub. no. (OHD5) 80-30287, 1981.
64. Williams, S., Henneman, R.L., and Fox, H.: Contribution of food service programs in preschool centers to children's nutritional needs, J. Am. Diet. Assoc. **71**:610, 1977.

FURTHER READING

Dwyer, J.: Promoting good nutrition for today and the year 2000, Pediatr. Clin. N. Am. **33**:799, 1986.

This timely article describes changes in nutrition problems of children from undernutrition and deficiencies to those of dietary imbalances and excessive intakes. The author, an excellent nutrition clinician and educator, outlines prevention of these problems by promoting good health for children, especially within the family, as the optimal approach.

Farthing, M.A., and Phillips, M.G.: Position of the American Dietetic Association: Nutrition standards in day-care programs for children, J. Am. Diet. Assoc. **87**:502, 1987.

This ADA position paper outlines specific recommendations for nutritional adequacy and quality of food served in day-care centers, as well as nutrition education for families, children, and day-care personnel.

Sandler, R.S., Slemenda, C.W., and La Porte, R.E.: Postmenopausal bone density and milk consumption in childhood and adolescence, Am. J. Clin. Nutr. **42**:270, 1985.

This study of postmenopausal women describes a correlation between older adult bone density and childhood milk intakes. No relationship was found between current adult milk intakes and bone density.

CASE STUDY

A 3-year-old boy's mother is concerned about his nutrient intake because he "doesn't like to drink milk and refuses vegetables."

1. How does his food behavior compare with that of other preschool children?
2. What nutrients should be assessed in the food that he does eat?
3. What nonfood parameters should be evaluated?

CASE STUDY

A 7-year-old girl's weight-for-height plots above the 95th percentile. Her rate of weight gain has increased in the past year, crossing from the 50th to the 90th percentile.

1. What factors that influence her food intake and energy expenditure should be assessed?
2. What is a reasonable goal to correct her overweight status?

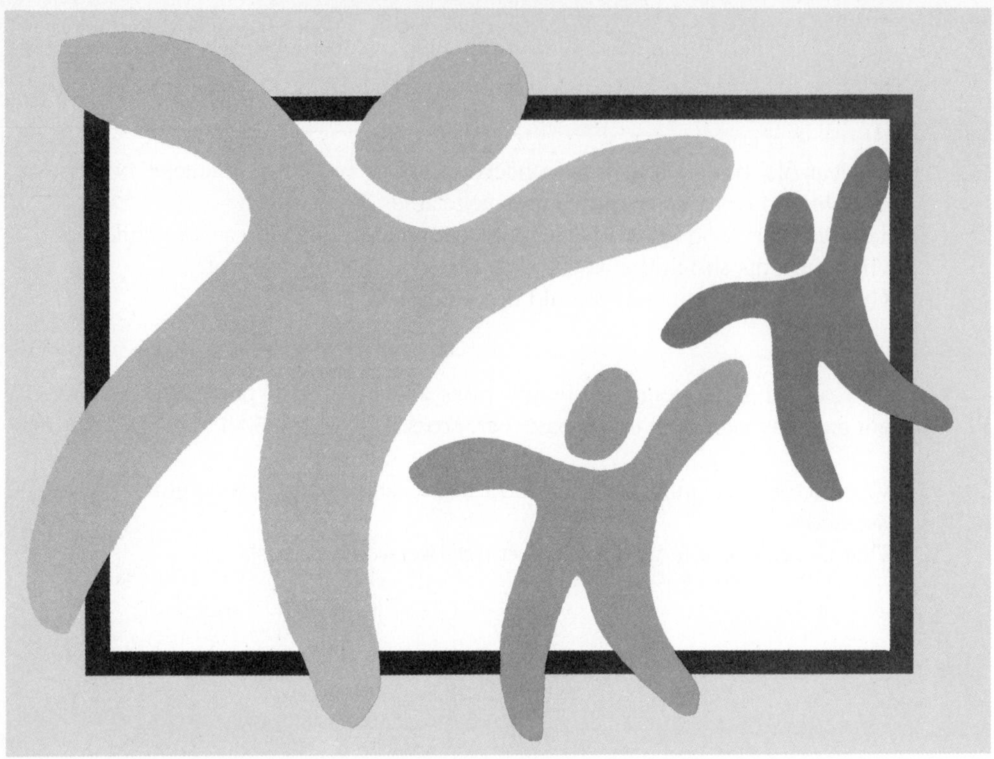

Basic Concepts

1. Adolescent growth and development involve both rapid physical growth and dramatic psychosocial development along with sexual maturation.
2. Normal adolescent growth and development require increased nutritional support.
3. Adolescent physical activities and health problems involve specific nutritional needs.
4. Individual needs guide approaches to adolescent nutrition assessment, counseling, and management issues.

Chapter Eight

Nutrition in Adolescence

Jane M. Rees and L. Kathleen Mahan

Adolescence is a phase of the life cycle that has long been puzzling to individuals and their parents as well as to health professionals. An awareness of the characteristics and needs of this special group, however, contributes to a greater understanding of teenagers in general as well as of those who have special nutritional needs. Knowledge from other disciplines in the physical and social sciences must be integrated to provide a comprehensive basis for understanding nutritional issues. The unique characteristics of adolescent growth and development, both physical and psychologic, are relevant not only to theoretical discussions of the specific topics but also to clinical protocols, in which results from controlled studies are synthesized to derive solutions to long-term problems arising in uncontrolled real-life situations.

In this chapter we will see that typical eating habits of adolescents are affected by many factors involving environment, lifestyle, and normal development. We shall also understand why counseling techniques useful in helping adolescents improve their nutritional practices must include the most sophisticated ones available from the social sciences today. In specific situations such as eating disorders, fitness activities and competitive sports, chronic disease, and pregnancy, specifically planned nutritional support for growth and development is required. Current research is beginning to shed light on the theories and myths that surround nutritional influence on adolescent behavior. While many questions related to adolescent nutrition remain unanswered, a body of sound practical knowledge exists to guide adolescents in maintaining positive nutrition and health.

Adolescent Growth and Development

PHYSIOLOGIC GROWTH

Puberty

The process of physically developing from a child to an adult is called *puberty*. Puberty, referring to maturation of the total body, is initiated by poorly understood physiologic factors. During late childhood slow growth begins to accelerate with pubescence until the rate is as rapid as that of early infancy. Fig. 8-1 shows that linear growth in cm/yr during the teen years compares with that for the second year of life. The person will gain about 20% of adult height and 50% of adult weight during pubertal growth.[1] Most of the body organs will double in size.

Initiation of Puberty

What causes the upsurge in hormonal activity that initiates pubertal development? Current radioimmunoassay techniques allow the measurement of hormonal concentrations that previously were below the sensitivity limits of earlier assays. This advance allows the hormonal changes to be measured as they occur chronologically. However, even with the development of these refined laboratory techniques, the exact factor or combination of factors that triggers these changes is still unknown.[1] Many theories have been suggested. One popular theory proposes that there is a "gonadostat," an area in the brain that is extremely sensitive to the sex steroids estrogen, testosterone,

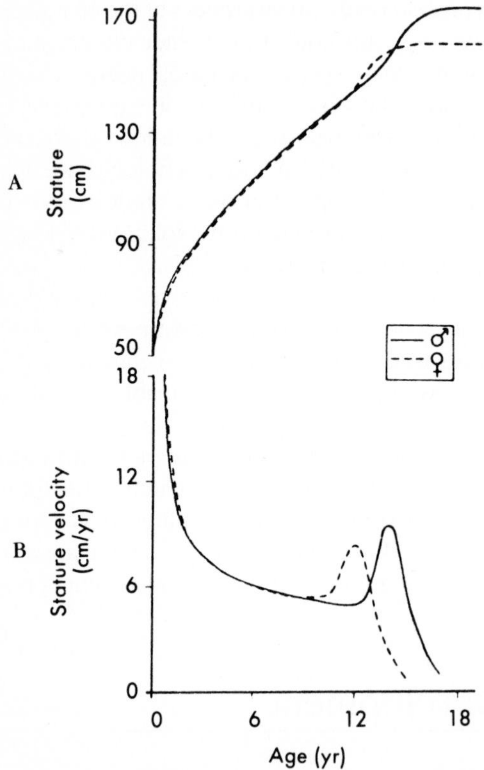

FIG. 8-1 A, Growth in stature of typical boy *(solid line)* and girl *(interrupted line)*. B, Growth velocities at different ages of typical boy *(solid line)* and girl *(interrupted line)*.
(From Marshall, W.A.: Clin. Endocrinol. Metab. 4:4, 1975.)

and progesterone. It governs the release of these hormones by a feedback mechanism that allows increased production with the onset of puberty.

Others relate pubertal onset to a change in body composition. They have observed in North American and most European females an association between menarche and the attainment of a critical body weight. They theorize that the achievement of the critical body weight of 47.8 kg (105 lb) causes a change in metabolic rate that triggers menarche and initiates the adolescent growth spurt in girls. Another way of stating this relationship is that the attainment of a minimal level of body fatness of 17% of body weight is necessary for the onset of menstruation. Other researchers acknowledge an association between change in body composition and the onset of menarche, but do not view it as a triggering factor of puberty.

Sequence and Stages of Growth

Adolescent growth is characterized by a predictable sequence of stages in sexual maturity, increased height and weight, and changes in body composition:

1. **Sexual maturity.** Throughout the approximately 5-7 years of pubertal development rapid growth continues, though a great percentage of height will be gained during the "growth spurt." Like the initiation of puberty the 18-24 month period of the peak growth velocity will occur at different ages for different individuals fitting into the sequence of overall sexual development. It occurs earlier for girls than for boys.[1] Factors known about the timing and milestones in pubertal development are summarized in Fig. 8-2.

   Data have accumulated to show that during the last century young women have gradually come to experience the menarche at younger ages, the so-called "secular trend." Improved health, including nutritional status, is thought to be responsible.
2. **Height and weight.** Following the achievement of sexual maturity, linear growth and weight acquisition continue at a much lower rate and then cease. For rare females it will continue into the late teens and for males into the 20s. Most females will gain no more than 2-3 in. (5.1-7.6 cm) after the onset of menses. The rate of weight gain following the menarche is discussed in the later section on adolescent pregnancy (pp. 362-363).
3. **Body composition.** The composition of the body changes in the process of maturation. In the prepubertal period the proportion of fat and muscle in males and females tends to be similar, with body fat about 15% and 19%, respectively, and lean body mass being about equal for both sexes. During puberty females gain proportionately more fat so that as adults the normal percentage of body fat is about 23% for females while for males it is about 12%. Males during this time gain twice as much muscle as females do. This striking difference in adolescent growth between males and females influences nutritional needs. Because the adolescent male experiences greater gain in bone and lean tissue than the female does, he requires more protein, iron, zinc, and calcium than the female for development of these tissues. Another reason for the male's larger requirements for these nutrients is his greater *rate* of growth.

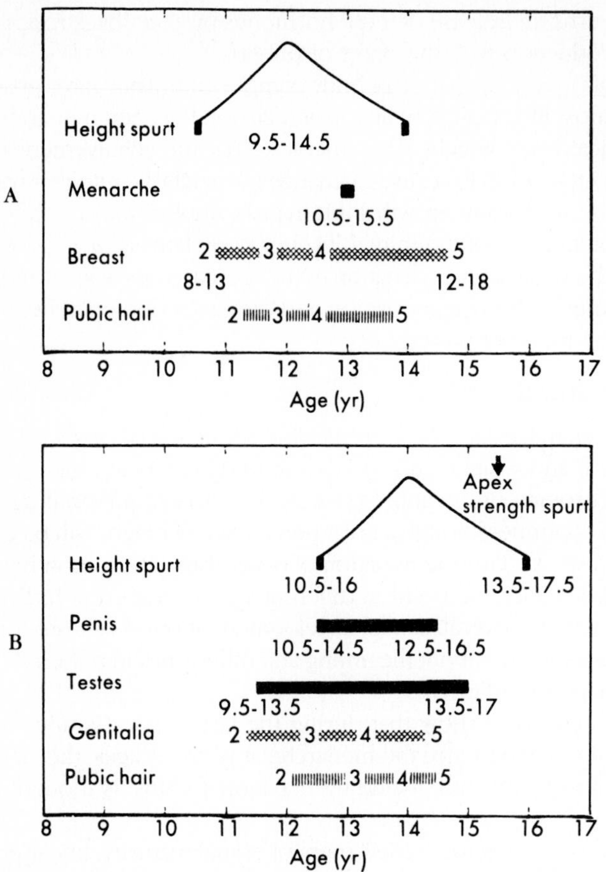

FIG. 8-2 Diagram of sequence of events at puberty in **A**, girls and **B**, boys.
(Reprinted by permission of The New England Journal of Medicine. Marshall, W.A., and Tanner, J.M.: Arch. Dis. Child. 45:13, 1970.)

Measurement of Growth

Sexual development is a measurable indicator of the process of physical maturation. The sexual maturity ratings in Table 8-1 outline the milestones of sexual maturation. Knowing the relationship between these milestones and physical growth will enable the clinician to assess the progress of growth in an adolescent at a particular time, and give some indication of the extent of future growth. Thus pubertal development can be monitored clinically by using weight and height tables and sexual maturity ratings. Excessive or less-than-normal growth can be detected by plotting height changes on the standard growth grids (see Appendix). The major cause of short stature during adolescence is genetically late initiation of puberty, though such conditions as chronic disease and skeletal and chromosomal abnormalities also account

TABLE 8-1 Stages of Sexual Maturation (Sexual Maturity Ratings)

Boys	Pubic Hair	Genitalia
Stage 1	None	No change from childhood
Stage 2	Small amount at outer edges of pubis; slight darkening	Beginning penile enlargement; testes enlarged to 5 ml volume; scrotum reddened and changed in texture
Stage 3	Covers pubis	Longer penis; testes 8-10 ml; scrotum further enlarged
Stage 4	Adult type; does not extend to thighs	Larger, wider, and longer penis; testes 12 ml; scrotal skin darker
Stage 5	Adult type; now spread to thighs	Adult penis; testes 15 ml
Girls	**Pubic Hair**	**Breasts**
Stage 1	None	No change from childhood
Stage 2	Small amount; downy on labia majora	Breast bud
Stage 3	Increased; darker and curly	Larger; no separation of nipple and areola
Stage 4	More abundant; coarse texture	Increased size; areola and nipple form secondary mound
Stage 5	Adult type; now spread to thighs	Adult distribution of breast tissue; continuous outline

Modified from Tanner, J.M.: Growth at adolescence, ed. 2, Oxford, 1962, Blackwell Scientific Publications, Ltd.

for certain children's being shorter than normal. Hormonal imbalances leading to abnormal growth are rare.[1] In the United States malnutrition as a primary cause of short stature is also rare.

Weight can be plotted on a grid similar to the one for height to determine whether or not an individual is keeping pace with peers, or exceeding them in total weight at a particular year of age. Because of the wide variation in weights seen in sample individuals in the adolescent period, some of whom were obese, the frequency distribution represented by the grids cannot be used for evaluation of weight-for-height proportion as it is used for younger children. Evaluation of weight-for-height proportion in adolescents is described here in the assessment section (pp. 311-312).

PSYCHOSOCIAL DEVELOPMENT

Span and Scope of Adolescence

Adolescence is the term applied to the period of maturation of both mind and body and therefore may be applied to humans both previous to and following puberty. Along with physical growth, the emotional, social, and intellectual development are rapid during adolescence.[2] Milestones in psychologic development are shown in Table 8-2. With the accomplishment of the developmental "tasks of adolescence" as seen in Fig. 8-3, the person is prepared for a role in adult society. The ability to use abstract thinking that the adolescent develops, as opposed to the concrete thought patterns of childhood, enables the individual to accomplish these tasks. Planning ahead and connecting facts into integrated ideas becomes possible.

TABLE 8-2 Comparison of Erikson's and Piaget's Models for Emotional and Cognitive Development

Age (yr)	Erikson (emotional)	Piaget (cognitive)
0-2	**PHASE I** Basic trust versus mistrust	**Sensorimotor Period** Learning through senses and manipulation
2-4	**PHASE II** Autonomy versus shame and doubt	**Preconceptual Period** Classification by a single feature (e.g., size); no concern for contradictions
4-8	**PHASE III** Initiative versus guilt	**Initiative Thought Period** Intuitive classification (e.g., awareness of conservation of mass concept)
8-12	**PHASE IV** Industry versus inferiority	**Concrete Operations Period** Logical thought development; learning to organize
12-20	**PHASE V** Ego identity versus role confusion	**Formal Operations Period** Comprehension of abstract concepts; formation of "ideals"
20 onward	**PHASE VI** Intimacy versus isolation	—
Middle adulthood	**PHASE VII** Generativity versus stagnation	—
Late adulthood	**PHASE VIII** Integrity versus despair	—

Implications for Nutritional Issues

Many of the tasks of adolescence relate to the nutritional health of the individual. For example, emotional maturity allows teenagers to develop their own value system. As a result they can choose foods that will enhance their health rather than making their choices by responding to less healthful characteristics of foods as they may have done in childhood. They may go through a time of experimentation while they are learning to make wise choices.

Body Image

Developing an image of the physical self that includes an adult body is an intellectual and emotional task intertwined with nutritional issues. Adolescents often feel uncomfortable with their rapidly changing bodies. At the same time, being very much affected by influences outside themselves, they want to be like their most perfect peers and the idols of their culture. Stereotypes in the mass media reinforce such images. Teenagers may wish that certain body parts were larger and that other parts were smaller. They may want to grow faster or slower. These feelings can lead them to try to change their bodies by manipulating their diets, an impulse that certain commercial

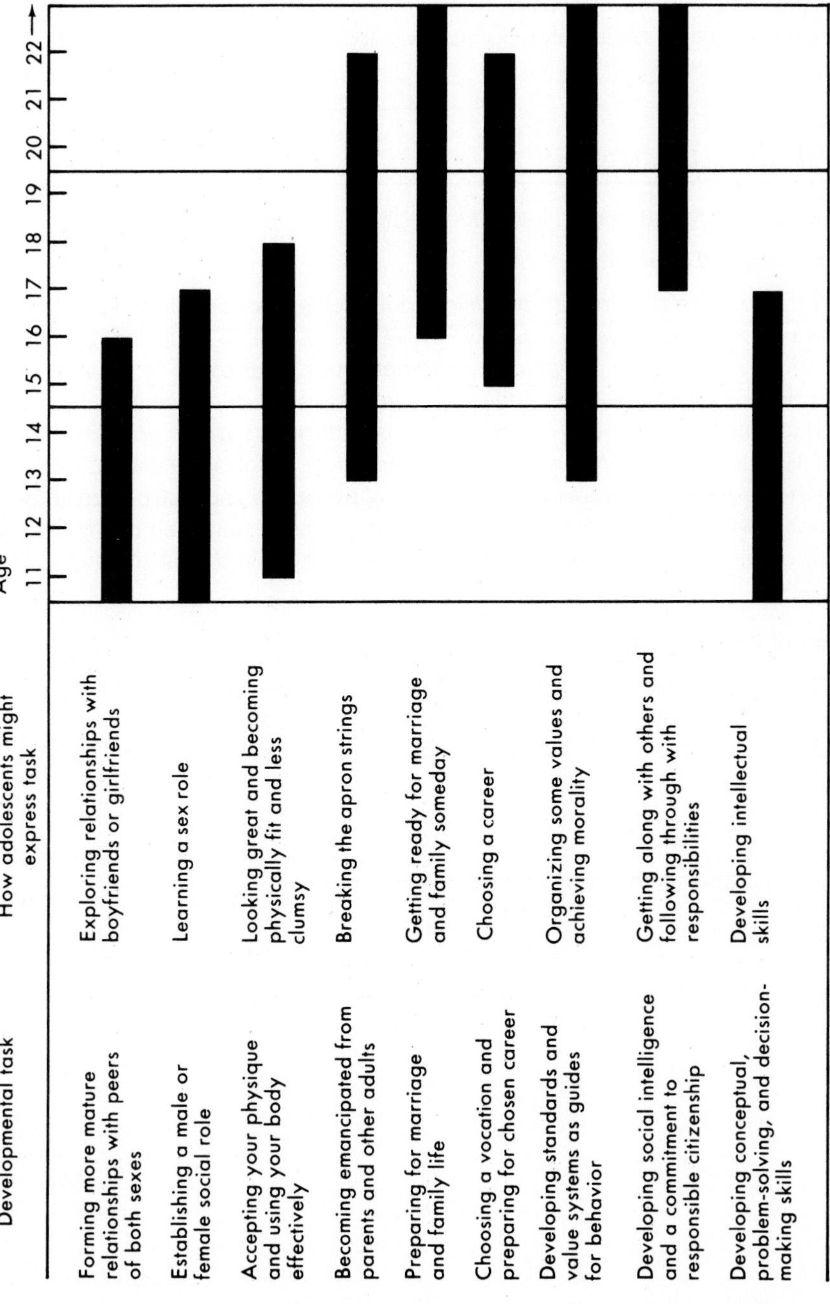

FIG. 8-3 Developmental tasks in adolescence.
(Adapted from Thornburg, H.: Contemporary adolescence: readings, ed. 2, Monterey, Cal., 1975, Brooks/Cole Publishing Co.)

interests are quick to exploit. Young women who have not developed a mature body image may unnecessarily restrict the amount of food they eat in response to weight gained in the development of secondary sex characteristics. Hoping to achieve the muscular appearance of adult males, young men are tempted to use nutritional supplements.

Nutritional Requirements

GROWTH AS A BASIS FOR NUTRITIONAL REQUIREMENTS

Limitations of the RDA Standard

Studies of the nutritional requirements of adolescents must take into account not only age but also stage of physical maturity.[3] Since studies that do so are not generally available, the research base on which recommendations are made is limited. The Recommended Dietary Allowances (RDA) are stated for three adolescent age groups, not related to stages of maturity. The highest levels of nutrients are recommended for the group assumed to be growing at the most rapid rate. Adolescents at the peak of their growth velocity will require large quantities of nutrients. They have been shown to incorporate twice the amount of calcium, iron, zinc, magnesium, and nitrogen into their bodies during the years of the growth spurt as compared to that of other years (Table 8-3).

Calculation of Needs by Height

Dividing the RDA total of a nutrient by the reference individual's height in centimeters provides a quantity of the nutrient in units/cm that can be applied to any size teenager. For example, the RDA for protein for the male 11-14 years old is 45 g/day.

TABLE 8-3 Daily Increments in Body Content due to Growth

		Average for Period 10-20 yr (mg)	At Peak of Growth Spurt (mg)
Calcium	M	210	400
	F	110	240
Iron	M	0.57	1.1
	F	0.23	0.9
Nitrogen*	M	320	610 (3.8 g protein)
	F	160	360 (2.2 g protein)
Zinc	M	0.27	0.50
	F	0.18	0.31
Magnesium	M	4.4	8.4
	F	2.3	5.0

From Forbes, G.B.: Nutritional requirements in adolescence. In Suskind, R.M., ed.: Textbook of pediatric nutrition, New York, 1981, Raven Press, Publishers.

*Maintenance needs (2 mg/basal calorie) at age 18 yr are 3500 mg and 2700 mg for males and females, respectively.

The reference height is 157 cm. Thus 0.29 g/cm would be recommended. Then the total protein need would be 39 g for the 135 cm male and 54 g for the 185 cm male. This example of variation in size during the teenage years is quite realistic, since persons experience the growth spurt at different ages. Nutrient recommendations will come closest to meeting needs when the largest quantity of nutrient/cm is suggested for those experiencing the most rapid growth, even if the age does not coincide with the age at which the highest RDA is made.

SPECIFIC NUTRIENT NEEDS

Energy

The recommended range of energy intake in the RDA for adolescents as shown in Table 8-4 reflects the different needs of teenagers. As well as growth rate, level of exercise will need to be considered in determining the needs of the individual.[4]

Protein

The protein requirement of adolescents has been studied least of all the age groups. The recommendation is that the energy value of the protein intake should make up 7% to 8% of the total energy consumed. Sex, age, nutritional status, and quality of the dietary protein must be considered in estimating the amount an individual will need. The range of total protein need will be about 39-56 g. These amounts are usually obtained in the normal diet so protein consumption should not be overly emphasized. Protein stores of adolescents should be carefully monitored and supported in situations where nutritional depletion may occur so that physical development will not be impaired.[4]

TABLE 8-4 Recommended Dietary Allowances for Energy for Children (kilocalories per day)

Age	Median*	Range†	Height per cm	Range per cm Height
CHILDREN				
7-10 yrs	2400	1650-3300	18.2	12.5-25
MALES				
11-14 yrs	2700	2000-3700	17.2	12.7-23.6
15-18 yrs	2800	2100-3900	16	12-22.2
FEMALES				
11-14 yrs	2200	1500-3000	14.0	9.6-19.1
15-18 yrs	2100	1200-3000	13.0	7.4-18.4

From Food and Nutrition Board, National Research Council: Recommended Dietary Allowances, 9th ed., Washington, D.C., 1980, National Academy of Sciences.

**Median* is the median energy intake of children of these ages followed in longitudinal growth studies.

†*Range* is the 10th and 90th percentiles of energy intake of children of these ages followed in longitudinal growth studies.

Calcium

This nutrient is important in adolescence since the requirement is based on the amount of the mineral needed for skeletal growth. Forty-five percent of the total bone growth occurs during this period. The total recommendations are the same for both sexes though accumulations are higher for males than for females because of the larger frame males will develop.[4]

Iron

Both males and females have high requirements for iron, as seen in Table 8-5. Males require more iron during adolescence because the buildup of muscle mass is accompanied by greater blood volume. Adolescent females require more than children because they will begin to lose iron monthly with the onset of menses.[3]

Zinc

This mineral is known to be essential for growth and is therefore of great importance in adolescence.[5] The retention of zinc increases especially during the growth spurt, leading to more efficient use of dietary sources of the nutrient.[4]

Other Minerals

The roles of other minerals in the nutriture of adolescents have not been extensively studied. However, magnesium, iodine, and phosphorus as well as copper, chromium, cobalt, and fluoride are important. The possibility of interactions between these nutrients cannot be overlooked. The recommendations for safe levels should be followed with moderation so that imbalances will not develop.

Vitamins

Adolescents require high amounts of thiamin, riboflavin, and niacin because of their high energy requirements. Vitamin D is especially needed for rapid skeletal growth. Recommended amounts of vitamins A, E, C, folic acid, and B_6 are the same as

TABLE 8-5 Calculated Iron Requirements for Males and Females at the 3rd, 25th, 75th, and 97th Percentile for Body Weight (from 10-16 years of age)

Percentile Rating	Calculated Iron Requirements (mg)					
	Daily Dietary Need*		Peak Daily Dietary Need*		Cumulative Need†	
	Male	Female	Male	Female	Male	Female
3rd	6.6	5.1	13.2	10.3	966	751
25th	9.3	5.2	18.6	10.4	1360	772
75th	11.0	5.5	21.9	11.0	1610	794
97th	12.9	5.7	25.8	11.9	1885	836

From McKigney, J.I., and Munro, H.N., editors: Nutrient requirements in adolescence, Cambridge, Mass., 1978, The MIT Press. Copyright © 1978 The MIT Press.

*Period of adolescent growth spurt.

†Total body iron increment represented by muscle tissue increase during 10-16 year interval.

those for adults. Often the quantity of vitamins recommended for adolescents has been interpolated from studies in adults and children.[4]

Eating Behavior

TYPICAL NUTRITIONAL PATTERNS

Surveys of nutrient intake have shown adolescents likely to be obtaining less vitamin A, thiamin, iron, and calcium than recommended. They also ingest more fat, sugar, protein, and sodium than is currently thought to be optimal.[6,7]

While concern is often expressed over the habit of eating between meals, it has been shown that teenagers obtain substantial nourishment from foods eaten outside traditional meals. The choice of foods they make is of greater importance than the time or place of eating. Emphasis should be placed on fresh vegetables and fruits as well as whole-grain products to complement the foods high in energy value and protein that they commonly choose.[8,9]

IRREGULAR MEALS

The number of meals teenagers miss and eat away from home increases from early adolescence to late adolescence, reflecting the growing need for independence and time away from home. The evening meal appears to be the most regularly eaten meal of the day. Females are found to skip the evening meal, as well as breakfast and lunch, more often than males.

Breakfast is frequently neglected and is omitted more often by teenagers and young adults under 25 years of age than by any other age group in the population.[10] A likely explanation as to why females are more apt to miss breakfast than are males is the pursuit of thinness and frequent attempts at dieting. Many teenage girls believe that they can control their weight by omitting breakfast or lunch. Young women who are dieting should be counseled that this approach is likely to accomplish just the opposite. By midmorning or lunchtime they may be so hungry that they overcompensate for the "saved kilocalories."

FACTORS INFLUENCING EATING BEHAVIOR

By the time a person reaches adolescence the influences on eating habits are numerous and the formation of those habits is extremely complex, as shown in Fig. 8-4. The growing independence of adolescents, increased participation in social life, and a generally busy schedule of activities have a decided impact on what they eat.[11] They are beginning to buy and prepare more food for themselves and they often eat rapidly and away from home.

Advertising

While the basic foundation for eating habits is found in the family, the influences on eating behavior originating outside the home in modern America are great. Teenagers are very vulnerable to the kind of advertising messages seen in Fig. 8-5. Television food commercials and the eating habits portrayed in program content have influenced

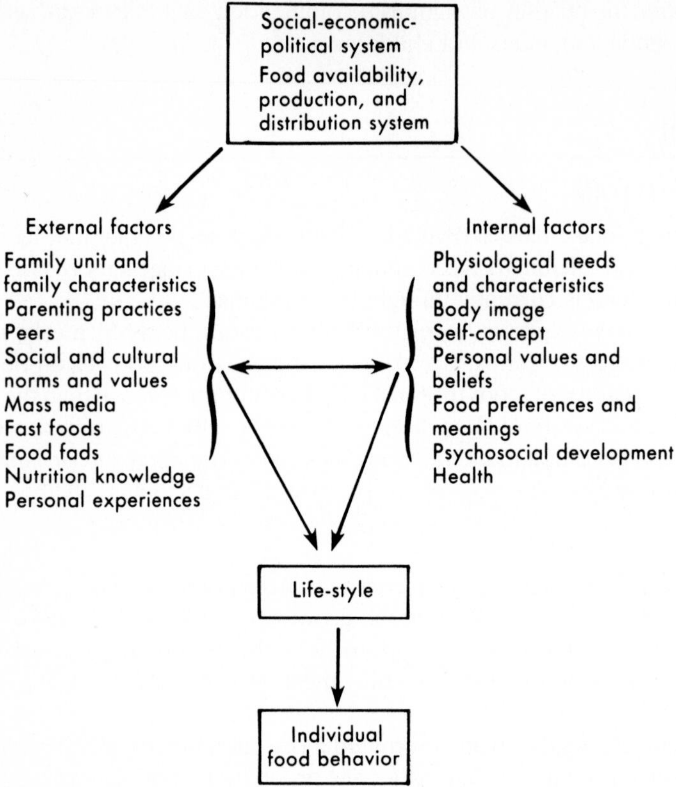

FIG. 8-4 Schematic diagram of factors influencing adolescent food behavior.

people for more than a decade by the time they become adolescents. The average teenager will have watched over a million food commercials, the majority of which are for products with a high concentration of sweetness and fat.

Ease of Obtaining Ready-to-Eat Foods

The ease of obtaining food that is ready to eat also influences the eating habits of teenagers. Through vending machines, at movies and sporting events, at fast-food outlets and convenience groceries, food is available at numerous times throughout the day. During the time of their peak growth velocity, adolescents may need to eat often and in large amounts and are able to use foods with a high concentration of energy. However, they will usually need to be more careful of amounts eaten and frequency of snacks when growth has slowed.

Nutritional Limitations of Fast Foods

The following factors appear to be the major nutritional limitations of fast-food meals:

LONDON UNIVERSITY SUPER 'CRASH-LOSS' DIET
TURNS UGLY FAT INTO HARMLESS WATER
AND FLOWS IT RIGHT OUT OF YOUR SYSTEM BY THE GALLON!
WAIST CONTROLLER
FLATTENS TUMMY INSTANTLY!
Over 153,00 sold . . .
NOW ONLY $14.99!
Lose 4-6 inches of bulging fat!
ONE-GLASS-A-DAY MEDICAL SCHOOL WONDER FORMULA-DIET . . . DOES MORE TO SLIM YOU DOWN THAN 14 MILES OF RUNNING A DAY!
LOSE WEIGHT
GRAPEFRUIT DIET PILL
90 for $2.98
500 for 9.85
Solid Black Pill
DIET Plan
SHED UGLY FAT
ONE-A-DAY DIET AID CAPSULES
Safe and Effective No Prescription Needed
30 day supply $8.95
60 day supply $16.95
90 day supply $24.95
Check One:
105 Fat Dissolving Treatments Only $17.95
210 Fat-Dissolving Treatments Only $31.50
Add $2.00 Shipping and Handling
Amount enclosed $ ____ . No C.O.D's.
IT FEELS GOOD TO BE THIN! $2 ONLY
SPECIAL TEEN DIET!
New Technique Can Suck Away Ugly Fat
"I Lost 16 lbs. in 1 Week"*
8" Off Your Waist
4" Off Your Thighs
7" Off Your Hips
Works So Fast,
You Shrink Down Your Waistline as much as
A FULL SIZE SMALLER IN JUST 24 HOURS,
4 SIZES SMALLER IN JUST 14 DAYS!
Literally turns fat to water—evaporates it by the hour—flows it right out of your system—actually burns away more fat each day than as much as 15 hours of non-stop exercise!
New Medical-School Wonder Formula Diet
BURNS AWAY AS MUCH AS 3 BULGING POUNDS AFTER EVERY SINGLE GLASSFUL!
YES! AS MUCH AS...
11 POUNDS GONE IN JUST 3 DAYS!
17 POUNDS GONE THE NEXT 7 DAYS!
23 POUNDS GONE IN JUST 2 WEEKS!
WITHOUT PILLS—DRUGS—OR BRUTAL EXERCISE!
LOSE WEIGHT & have FUN too!
NOW YOU CAN LOSE WEIGHT WITHOUT WORKING AT IT...
THANKS TO "WEIGHT AWAY"!

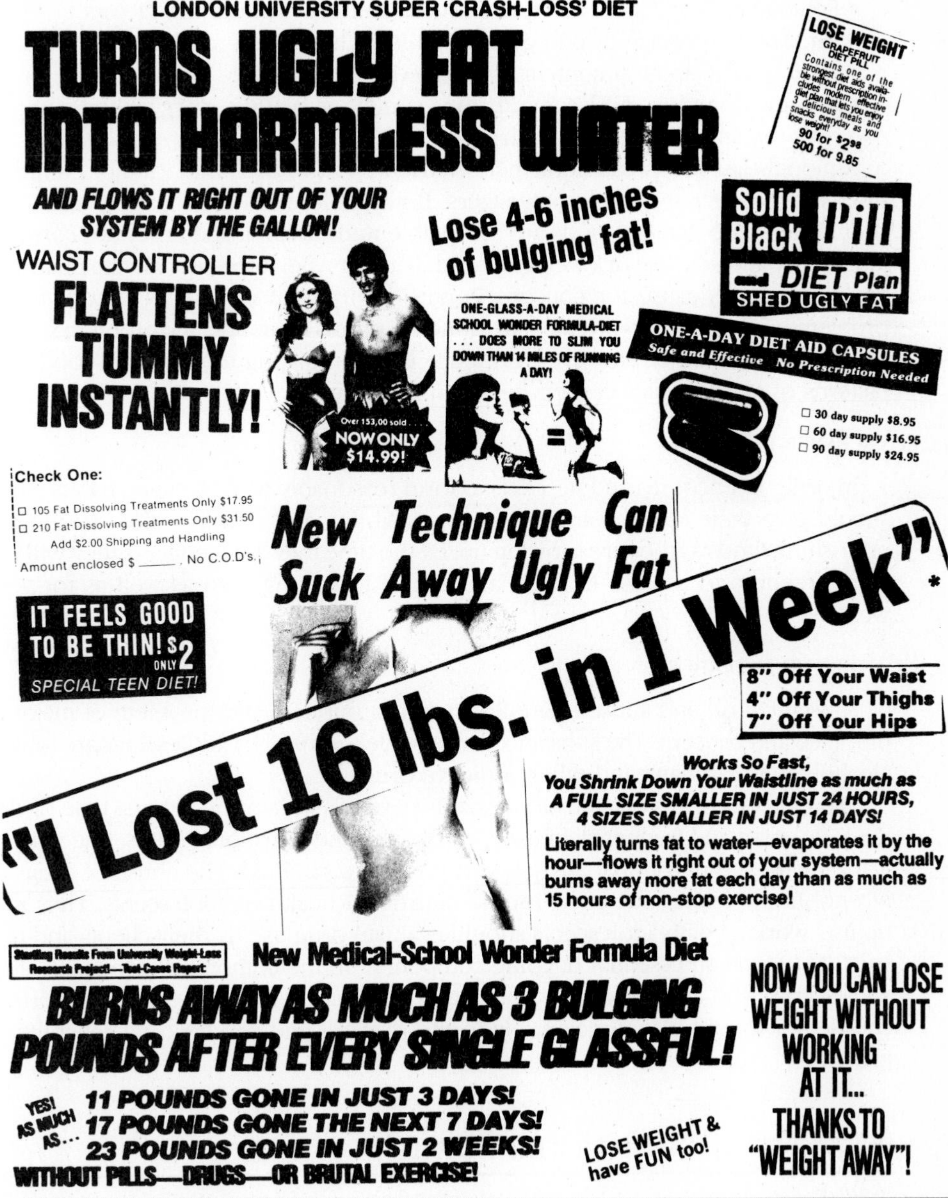

FIG. 8-5 Examples of enticements and advertisements for weight-loss products featured in popular magazines.

- **Calcium, riboflavin, vitamin A.** These essential nutrients are low unless milk or a milkshake is ordered.
- **Folic acid, fiber.** There are few fast-food sources of these key factors.
- **Fat.** The percentage of energy from fat is high in many meal combinations.
- **Sodium.** The sodium content of fast-food meals is high.
- **Energy.** Common meal combinations contain excessive energy when compared with the amounts of other nutrients provided.

Although fast foods can contribute nutrients to the diet, they cannot completely meet the nutritional needs of teenagers. Both adolescents and health professionals should be aware that fast foods are acceptable nutritionally when they are consumed judiciously and as a *part* of a well-balanced diet. But when they become the mainstay of the diet there is cause for concern. A nutrient imbalance may not *appear* to be a problem until a number of years have gone by, unless some specific problem such as a chronic disease exists. However, evidence is accumulating to show that food intake patterns of teenagers affect their health in later life.[4]

ROLE OF PARENTS

In order to encourage adolescents to form reasonably healthy eating habits parents should give their children increased responsibility and choice within the range of nourishing foods as they are growing up. By the time they are teenagers they will need some freedom to use the kitchen; this is true for young men as well as for young women.

SUBSTANCE USE AND ABUSE

Substance use and abuse in adolescence is a public health problem of major significance and concern. The substances most widely abused by adolescents are tobacco, alcohol, and marijuana and other addictive drugs.

The effect of drugs on nutritional status depends on several factors: type of drug, dose, duration and frequency of use, prior health and nutritional status, stage of physical growth, and nutritional adequacy of the diet consumed. The abuse of drugs and alcohol has a deleterious effect on the nutritional health of adolescents. Thus nutritionists working with adolescents should evaluate drug use by their clients and make such evaluation an essential ongoing component in the comprehensive team care of adolescents who are chronically abusing drugs. Nutrition intervention, support, and counseling should play a major role in the physical and psychosocial rehabilitation process.

Assessment of Nutritional Status

Teenagers are in a fluctuating state of balance between supplying their bodies with needed nutrients and using up the nutrients. At any one time, this flow is the teenager's *nutritional status.* Assessment of nutritional status is described in Chapter 3. Modification for the adolescent requires use of the sexual maturity ratings and a specific database with which to compare height, weight, and weight-height proportion.

ANTHROPOMETRIC DATA

To evaluate the relationship between the weight and height of an individual adolescent, the detailed tables of the National Health and Nutrition Examination Survey (NHANES) compiled by the National Center for Health Statistics can be used. An example is shown in Table 8-6; full tables are given in the Appendix. For each 2 cm increment in height at a particular year of age, a range of weights is given. Weight-height values for age and sex between the 25th and the 75th percentiles can be considered to be in the normal range. This range allows for the normal differences in body build of individuals.

In addition, a skinfold evaluation will yield a more precise assessment of the proportion of fat to muscle and therefore weight to height. For example, a low value for triceps skinfold measurement in an individual above the 75th percentile for weight-height indicates that the adolescent is overweight but not overfat. An assessment of midarm circumference and arm muscle area will confirm the muscular body composition. This type of evaluation is plotted in Fig. 8-6.

SEXUAL MATURITY RATING

The evaluation of sexual maturity is an essential factor in making a valid nutrition assessment of an adolescent in a normal clinical setting. By knowing the stage of sexual maturity of the adolescent it is possible to determine whether the full height has been reached or growth can still occur. Also, it is possible to determine whether the proportion of fat to muscle seen is that which the individual has developed as an adult or has obtained at one stage as a still developing adolescent. Thus if a young woman at stage 1 of sexual maturity is at the 90th percentile weight-for-height, she will continue to grow in height and has a greater potential to stay within the bounds of normal body composition than has a female of the same age, the same weight-for-height, but who has experienced menarche and is at stage 4 of sexual maturity.

TABLE 8-6 Weight in Kilograms of Girls Aged 17 Years at Last Birthday, United States, 1966-70

	Percentile						
Height (cm)	5th	10th	25th	50th	75th	90th	95th
145-149.9	38.6	38.8	40.1	45.1	45.7	51.1	51.2
150-154.9	41.6	42.3	44.6	48.9	53.5	59.2	64.1
155-159.9	44.4	45.5	48.7	53.2	57.7	61.6	76.2
160-164.9	46.8	48.0	50.2	55.4	61.5	72.3	82.3
165-169.9	47.9	50.3	55.1	59.3	65.1	69.4	71.6
170-174.9	50.6	52.9	55.5	60.2	65.7	76.1	82.7
175-179.9	54.9	56.7	60.1	61.7	75.2	75.9	83.0

Modified from National Center for Health Statistics: Height and weight of youths 12-17 years, United States. In Vital and health statistics, series 11, no. 124, Health Services and Mental Health Administration, Washington, D.C., 1973, U.S. Government Printing Office. Data from the national health survey, U.S. Department of Health, Education, and Welfare, 1973.

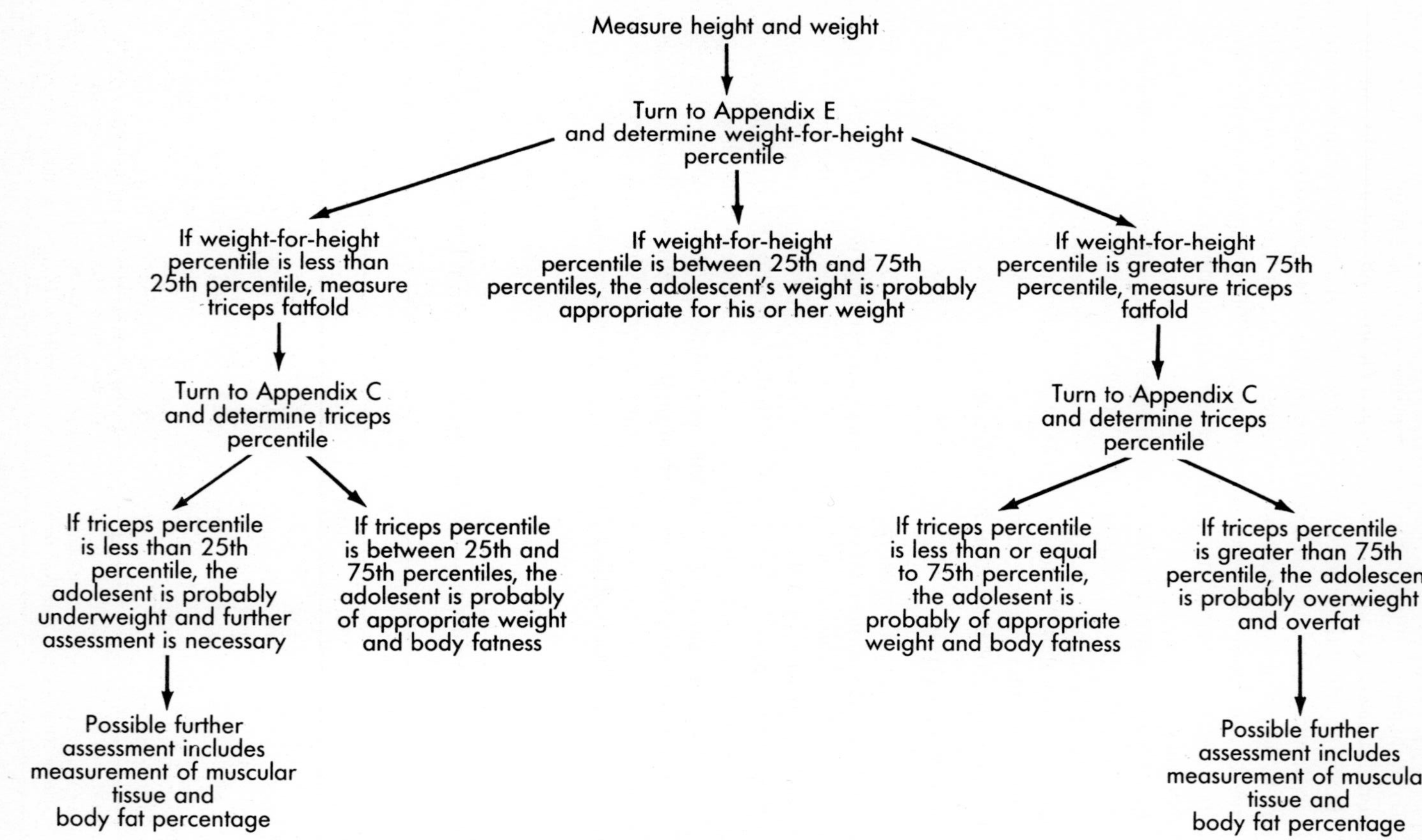

FIG. 8-6 Algorithm for evaluating an adolescent's weight.

NUTRITION ENVIRONMENT

The *nutrition environment,* the factors that influence the nutritional status, is also an important consideration. Such factors as general medical history, socioeconomic status, medications, alcohol or tobacco use, family attitudes, and peer group food practices all contribute to the adolescent's food choices. Table 8-7 summarizes the significance of each of these influences. The health professional should try to understand the effect they have on the adolescent's eating habits. *Nutrition assessment* includes study of both the nutritional status and the nutrition environment of the individual adolescent.

NUTRITIONAL CARE PLAN

Assessment of all factors in the environment that may influence nutriture is essential if appropriate action to meet needs is going to be initiated as a personal *nutritional care plan.* The extent to which the total nutrition environment is studied depends on the projected use of the nutrition assessment. For example, a great deal of detailed information reflecting nutritional status is needed for a 13-year-old male with Crohn's disease who is scheduled for a course of parenteral nutrition. Information about the nutrition environment would be less vital at this time. However, nutritional care planning for a newly diagnosed 15-year-old female with diabetes would require both nutritional status evaluation and assessment of the nutrition environment. Without both components, the care plan cannot adequately address physiologic nutritional needs and the adolescent's ability to meet them.

Nutritional Counseling for Adolescents

FACILITATING CHANGE

Attempts to help adolescents improve their nutritional status must be approached with skill, especially because of their growing independence.[11] Nutrition counselors must know adolescents' physical and psychologic development, lifestyles, and habits as well as appropriate methods of communicating with them.

Strategies for Change

Sophisticated strategies to add knowledge, alter attitudes, and change behavior must be used in any setting if the objective is to influence an adolescent's eating habits. Providing knowledge or teaching can be done in a variety of settings from the classroom to the hospital bedside.[12] Altering attitudes is much more difficult and usually demands an individualized experience. Facilitating the adoption of new behavior is even more difficult and requires a lengthy period of time. The adolescent will have to feel positive about any plan before it can succeed. In fact, much effort must be directed toward encouraging the person to want to change prior to introducing steps to bring the change about.

TABLE 8-7 Nutrition Environment Evaluation Guide

Influences	Key Issues	Significance
Likes and dislikes	Does patient dislike any particular food that is a major source of a specific nutrient (for example, milk is a major source of calcium; citrus fruits of vitamin C; meat of high-quality protein)?	Points out need to explore alternative ways to supply nutrients (for example, substitute cheese and yogurt for milk; broccoli and green peppers for citrus fruit; proper combinations of plant foods for meat)
Environment and attitudes		
Individual	Does patient express interest in his or her diet?	Gives clues to attitude toward role of nutrition in health care
	Are there any behavioral problems that influence patient's food choices?	May indicate need to work with other health team members to resolve problem that temporarily precludes nutrition intervention
	Has patient ever followed a special diet? If so, who prescribed it, what type of diet was it, and when was it prescribed? What instructions did patient receive?	Self-prescribed diet may signal inappropriate or unreliable approach toward control of health by diet; points out medical and educational considerations needed in design of care plan
	Does patient think he or she has been following the diet? Is there evidence to substantiate this?	If discrepancy exists, indicates lack of understanding of diet by patient or unwillingness or inability of patient to make dietary changes
	What difficulties if any does patient see in making dietary changes?	Focuses on issues that need consideration in design of individualized care plan
Family	Who purchases and prepares food in home (that is, partially controls patient's food supply)?	Sets scene for type of action plan suitable to patient and family
	Does patient have adequate cooking facilities and equipment or access to other resources?	May indicate need to provide basic nutrition guidelines, including personalized menu plan
	Are there any cultural, regional, or religious factors that affect patient's food choices?	Requires consideration to tailor care plan to individual needs
Peers	How often does patient eat away from home? Where and with whom does patient eat? Are there specific food intake patterns related to peer influences?	Indicates potential influences of peers on food choices; points out potential efficacy of patient- versus family-oriented care plan

TABLE 8-7 Nutrition Environment Evaluation Guide—cont'd

Influences	Key Issues	Significance
Schools	Does patient eat at school? Does patient participate in school feeding programs?	School feeding programs with their standardized composition assure minimal nutrient availability and provide reference for accuracy of reported information
	Is there anything about school schedule or cafeteria environment that may discourage appropriate nutrient intake?	"Too little time for lunch" or "no one to eat with" may necessitate consultation with other team members or school to resolve life-style problems
	Is patient in appropriate grade in school? Has patient received food and nutrition information in school courses?	Gives clues to current knowledge of nutrition and level of intellectual functioning; allows practical planning for educational aspects of care plan
Limited food funds	Is patient or family eligible for food stamps; Women, Infants, and Children program (WIC); or reduced-price or free school lunch? Do they participate in programs? Does patient or family receive other social assistance?	Indicates family has limited income and may need assistance with food buying and preparation to assure nutritionally adequate diet; points out need to consider referral to appropriate food program or nutrition education resource
Health-related concerns	Does patient have any food allergies or intolerances (as distinguished from dislikes)?	Excludes foods from diet; indicates need to plan and assure adequacy with alternative food choices
	Are there any physical conditions affecting ability to consume adequate nutrients (for example, mouth sores, swallowing problems, taste abnormalities)?	Indicates need to consider flavor, consistency, and temperature of food in care plan
	Are there any problems in digestion, absorption, or metabolism that will interfere with nutrient utilization? Will any other therapy (drugs, exercise, radiation) affect nutrient needs?	Indicates need to address these problems in diet preparation

Personalized Counseling

Besides changes in attitude the counselor must impart knowledge in an especially meaningful and individualized manner. Finally, behavior change can be approached in increments that are sufficiently realistic to ensure personal success.

Role of Parents

Parents must be appropriately involved in the counseling process. They need help in being supportive, as opposed to being intrusive, as the adolescent makes changes. Both adolescents and their parents must be helped to see the importance of focusing on the process of making change rather than solely on the desired goal of self-care. A sure understanding of both the physical and social sciences, along with a liberal injection of art, is needed in nutrition counseling for adolescents and their parents. It is indeed a challenging field.

THE HEALTH-CARE TEAM

Adolescent health care is one of the most demanding of clinical problems. As such, it is best handled as a team effort. Any one professional will generally not possess the skills to meet all the client's needs. For example, Table 8-8 lists some of the types of issues that will arise throughout the course of teenage pregnancies with a suggested list of professionals to guide clients in managing these issues. This does not mean that certain problems are the responsibility of any one profession to the exclusion of others. Each professional team member can support the messages and guidance provided by other team members. Team conferences aid in coordination of care and team efficiency in meeting identified needs and noting the client's progress in solving various problems. Nutritionists and other professionals who are in positions to influence program planning can help develop clinical teams for care of adolescents.

Eating Disorders

Although recent precise figures are not available, as many as 30% of American teenagers are said to be obese. The number with diagnosed anorexia nervosa or bulimia is growing, and many adolescents with eating disorders remain undiagnosed and untreated. Because these disorders are so common among adolescents, health professionals interested in adolescent nutrition must understand them. Eating disorders provide a good model for study of other adolescent nutrition problems and their treatment. Therefore it is valuable to study these disorders in depth.

SPECTRUM OF EATING DISORDERS IN ADOLESCENCE

Common Characteristics

Eating disorders can best be studied when the physical symptoms are viewed as a spectrum, with developmental obesity at one end and anorexia nervosa at the other (Fig. 8-7). Between are persons at normal and abnormal weights. Along the spectrum these persons hold in common basic underlying psychological problems that interfere

TABLE 8-8 Suggested Members of Health-Care Team to Guide Adolescents in Issues Arising in Pregnancy

	Discipline					
Issues	**Obstetrician**	**Adolescent Medical Specialist**	**Nurse**	**Nutritionist**	**Social Worker**	**Psychologist**
General health and planning of continuous care		X	X	X		
Complications of pregnancy	X	X	X	X		
Labor and delivery preparation	X	X	X			
School program					X	X
Economic resources			X		X	
Substance abuse (cessation and education)		X	X	X	X	X
Psychological adjustment and stress	X	X	X	X	X	X
Developmental delay			X		X	X
Infant-care education		X	X	X		
Relinquishment counseling			X		X	X
Nutritional care		X	X	X		
Education		X	X	X		
Resource coordination			X	X	X	
Family or marital conflict					X	X

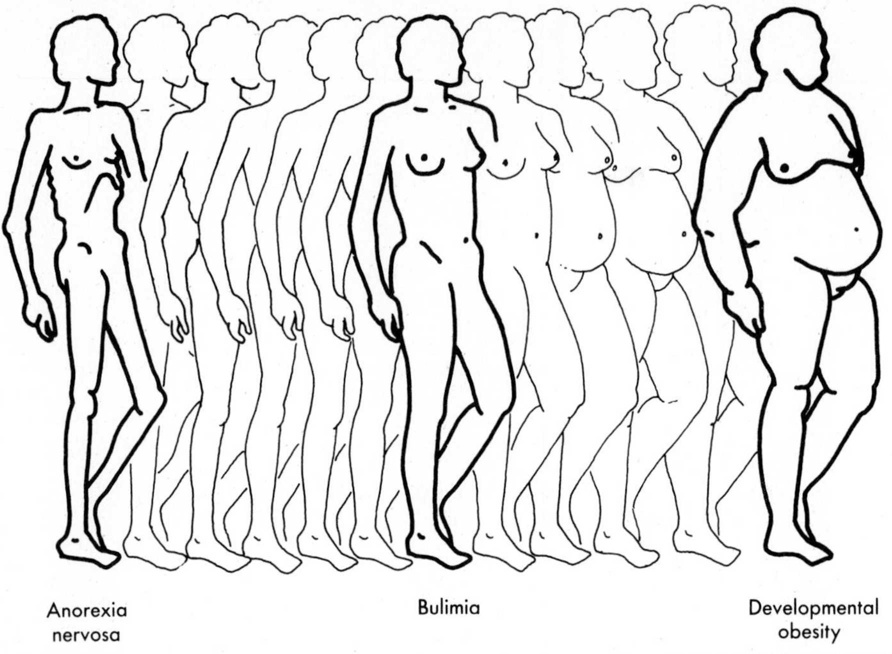

FIG. 8-7 Spectrum of eating disorders. Although physical conditions vary, underlying psychological characteristics are held in common across the spectrum.

to varying degrees with normal functioning. In developing responses to life these persons often use food inappropriately. Food-related behaviors and the resulting deviation in weight, the two most obvious aspects of these disorders, are usually the main focus of attention of the person affected, the public, and often the health professional. The underlying neurophysical and psychodevelopmental mechanisms, however, are the essential features of more fundamental study needed by clinicians who are treating the disorders.

Rapid Adolescent Growth and Body Image

Because of rapid physical growth and body-image development in adolescence, eating disorders are of special concern at this time. These changes intensify associated self-esteem problems. Anorexia nervosa, for example, is a disorder so tied to body image distortion that it is most commonly seen in adolescence, the period when a person is struggling with self-identity and most vulnerable to body image problems. Progress in adopting a normal adult body image will be interrupted for the teenager with an eating disorder. Bruch[13] and others have provided classic descriptions of distorted body images in both anorexic and obese adolescents.

Developmental Tasks

Teenagers with severe eating disorders fail in varying degrees to accomplish the development tasks of adolescence. The development problems of these persons are

DEVELOPMENTAL PROBLEMS ASSOCIATED WITH EATING DISORDERS IN ADOLESCENTS

Inability to develop and use formal operational thought processes, especially in reference to themselves
Inability to experience bodily sensations originating within themselves as "normal" and "valid"
Unrealistic perceptions of body size
Preoccupation with weight and food, reflecting dependence on social opinion and judgment
Failure to normalize eating and exercise patterns
Unrealistic expectations for themselves
Failure to develop autonomy
Difficulty in accomplishing the normal tasks of adolescence

Based on Bruch.[13]

summarized in the box above. The most striking of their problems is failure to develop autonomy.

FAMILY INTERACTION

In recent years theories about the origin of these problems have turned to the structure and interaction of the adolescent's family. Although obese teenagers are a much less homogeneous group than anorectic persons, the family patterns have much in common. Minuchin[14] has described families of persons with anorexia as being psychosomatic. They are enmeshed, rigid, and overprotective and have a low tolerance for conflict.

Anorexia Nervosa

SYMPTOMS

The term *anorexia nervosa* is actually a misnomer. The implication that affected persons have a lack of appetite has been shown to be invalid. Superficially, the motivation to be thin keeps the person with anorexia nervosa from eating. In over 100 years of description in the literature, however, a combination of symptoms has come to be recognized as characteristic of the disorder. Although certain of these symptoms may be seen in other disorders, the combination is unique in anorexia nervosa. This unique combination of symptoms has been defined by the American Psychiatric Association:[15]

- Age of onset prior to 25.
- Anorexia with accompanying weight loss of at least 25% of prior weight.
- Distorted, implacable attitude toward eating, food, or weight that overrides hunger, admonitions, reassurance, and threats: for example, (1) denial of illness with a

failure to recognize nutritional needs, (2) apparent enjoyment in losing weight with overt manifestations that food refusal is a pleasurable indulgence, (3) desired body image of extreme thinness with overt evidence that it is rewarding to the patient to achieve and maintain this state, and (4) unusual hoarding or handling of food.

- No known medical illness that could account for the anorexia and weight loss.
- No other known psychiatric disorder with particular reference to primary affective disorders, schizophrenia, obsessive-compulsive and phobic neuroses.
- At least two of the following manifestations: (1) amenorrhea, (2) lanugo, (3) bradycardia (persistent resting pulse of 60 beats per minute or less), (4) periods of overactivity, (5) episodes of bulimia, (6) vomiting (may be self-induced).

The above criteria focus more on physical symptoms at the crisis stage than on the underlying psychologic symptoms. Recognition of the psychologic symptoms, however, is of equal importance. The principal psychologic features of anorexia nervosa are "a relentless pursuit of thinness" and "a misuse of the eating function in efforts to solve or camouflage problems that otherwise would appear insolvable," that is, problems resulting from arrested normal development.[13]

INCIDENCE

The majority of persons with anorexia nervosa are adolescents, although it has been seen in other age groups. The disorder has not been commonly seen in males; 8% and 11% of anorectic teenagers were male in two groups studied. Males who develop the disorder appear to experience anorexia nervosa in essentially the same form as females. Because of the predominance of females in the population seen with anorexia nervosa, the feminine pronoun will be used in this discussion.

Anorexia nervosa occurs predominantly in affluent classes and nations and is supported by a cultural paradox in which food is abundant and used lavishly for purposes other than survival on the one hand, and slimness is highly valued on the other.[16] These cultural values are strong internal messages that have great impact on a young adolescent who has not developed autonomy. The lack of a similar value on slimness in males probably accounts for the small number of males seen with the disorder.

ETIOLOGY

Theories about the etiology of anorexia nervosa have evolved from the initial psychoanalytic idea that the disease stemmed from an inability to deal with innate sexual drives, through a period when it was ascribed to endocrine deficits, to the more recent belief that it grows out of disturbed patterns of family interaction.

Mother-Daughter Relationship

Bruch's work[13] was the first to incorporate a broader focus than simply the patient and her symptoms. An interaction pattern prevails in which the mother misperceives the needs of her child from infancy on or the child fails to express her needs clearly. In any case the child acquiesces to the mother's misguided ministrations. During the period of infancy and childhood, the daughter is so controlled by her mother that she does not develop a true sense of self as distinguished from mother.

Effect of Adolescence

As adolescence approaches, the body develops and demands for decisions and performance in many areas increase. The teenager panics at her lack of ability to cope independently. She develops rituals related to eating in an effort to be thin and "good." To gain her "independence," the teenager regresses to the period when independence ordinarily begins. In this early stage the principal manner to demonstrate growing independence open to the child is eating behavior.

Family System

Minuchin's more recent approach[14] describes how not only relationships with the mother but also interrelationships within the family system foster anorexia nervosa. If family members are enmeshed in a system that does not allow development of appropriate roles, the system can produce a variety of psychosomatic problems. The particular direction toward anorexia nervosa may be determined when the main themes of family interaction are related to food, fitness, and appearance.

Biochemical Process

The possibility that a biochemical process may be responsible for development of anorexia nervosa continues to be investigated. Although various mechanisms have been proposed, so far none has been shown to be primary or causative. These mechanisms appear to result from psychologic stress, malnutrition, and starvation. The fact that patients and their families fit such characteristic and complex patterns would raise doubt that a single primary physiologic cause exists in most cases. However, it may be found that biochemical factors contribute to development of the disorder.

PSYCHOLOGIC STATE

The physical manifestations of anorexia nervosa may be sudden, although unrecognized underlying characteristics may have been present previously. Intervention strategies must address both the psychologic and physiologic states of the patient.

Progressive Development

From the family's point of view, the anorectic teenager is usually a "model child" until she begins to develop a compulsive attitude about her weight. She has fit into the family unit and met their high expectations. She has worked extremely hard at school, being satisfied with nothing less than excellent grades.

Suddenly the whole family erupts in conflict over her eating behavior. The teenager herself has become troubled about her role in life. She is unable to sustain peer friendships and she is very anxious about relationships with males. She is confused by the need to establish more adult behavior patterns and clings to the rigid standards of childhood. She isolates herself. Life appears to be out of her control. She has conflicting feelings about living as her parents direct, is hurt by their critical comments, and begins to realize that she must assert herself. She takes a stand and will not compromise on her eating and exercise habits. She feels that she is too fat and must be slim to prove that she is a worthy person. She is increasingly preoccupied with her rituals and is angry when her family interferes. She denies her illness.[16]

Distorted Perceptions

A wide range of distorted perceptions has been noted, related specifically to body size, sex, hunger, rest, satiety, body temperature, pleasure, control, and to "feeling states" in general. The anorectic teenager has often been described as wishing to stave off adulthood. But the question remains as to whether she wishes to avoid maturation or whether maturation eludes her.

Family Problems

Although most families with anorectic teenagers would describe themselves as normal and without problems until the manifestations of anorexia nervosa, these families often have a multitude of problems. The parents may have been dominating and intrusive. They may have overlooked the *actual* (including nutritional) needs and emotions of their children, even in times when the children have been ill. By adopting a "helpless" stance, the affected children may be thoroughly manipulative and involved in their parents' conflicts. Both parents and children become locked into a system where problems go unresolved and responses are stereotyped.[14]

PHYSIOLOGIC STATE

In the initial stage of anorexia nervosa, physical symptoms are related to weight, diet, exercise, menses, and nutritional status.

Weight

In some cases the anorectic teenager is overweight when the disorder begins. The anorectic young woman is typically hypersensitive to developing breasts and hips. These young patients often recall a chance statement about their needing to lose weight by a relative or close friend, or a weight reduction plan suggested by a health professional, as the trigger for their initial weight-loss behavior.

Diet

The anorectic adolescent usually develops a personal philosophy about her diet, limiting herself by eating food only from certain categories and in certain ways. She may manipulate the fluid or sodium content of her intake. In addition, she may force herself to vomit and misuse laxatives or diuretics to rid herself of food energy and weight. Vomiting may follow episodes of gorging.

Exercise

The practice of exercise rituals is equally varied. Anorectic teenagers include excessive calisthenics and other strenuous activities in their schedules. They may limit rest and use stimulants. They are so frequently involved in junior and senior high school athletics and dancing that coaches and teachers should be educated about the disorder. Good coaches should recognize which of their students may be exercising to their detriment by compulsively training beyond reasonable endurance while losing weight at a rapid rate.

Menses

Although a young woman in a state of starvation would be expected to become amenorrheic, indications are that cessation of the menses occurs in most patients with anorexia nervosa before they have lost sufficient weight and body fat to cause an interruption of the cycle. Psychologic factors probably contribute to the problem since stressful states are known to interfere with the endocrine system regulating the menstrual cycle.

Nutritional Status

During the initial phase of an anorectic teenager's energy restriction, the body does not exhibit the effects of malnutrition to a measurable degree other than a decrease in weight. Infections are not generally seen. Deficiencies in specific nutrients have not been reported, but they may exist subclinically depending on the food habits of the individual. If weight loss continues unchecked, however, the symptoms of severe starvation may become apparent. This state indicates onset of a crisis.

INTERVENTION STRATEGIES

Initial intervention strategies include early recognition of symptoms, psychotherapy, and nutritional support.

Early Recognition of Symptoms

A recognition of the developing symptoms is the most important early intervention strategy. A protocol for assessing anorexia nervosa and other eating disorders is provided in Table 8-9. Friends, school personnel, family, and health professionals are among those who observe the growing problems and can take steps to initiate treatment.

Psychotherapy

Individual and family psychotherapy by experienced therapists will enable both the affected adolescent and her family to adopt more appropriate roles. It will also help the anorectic teenager to complete the psychologic developmental processes that have been arrested.[16,17]

Nutritional Support

Other than general monitoring of height and weight, it may not be necessary to treat the patient physically at this stage. Refocusing her attention on the primary emotional and interactional problems rather than the power struggle over food and exercise patterns will often enable the patient to abandon her compulsive striving for thinness. The patient should have access to a professional who can answer her questions about nutrition and make sure that she has the information she needs to begin to regulate her eating patterns to meet her physical needs. Information should be given in the context of the adolescent's desire to change rather than imposed as a rigid system of dietary planning by a professional. The overall disorder should not be defined as solely a nutritional problem, although nutrition counseling is an important component of therapy.

TABLE 8-9 Clinical Assessment of Eating Disorder

	Date	Date	Date	Date
MOTIVATION				
Appropriateness of weight goals				
Desire to change unhealthful habits				
Insight into problem				
EMOTIONAL/PSYCHOLOGICAL STATUS				
Depression				
Locus of control				
Body image				
Self-esteem				
Oral expression				
Coping skills				
Compulsivity				
Perfectionism				
Independence				
MENTAL FUNCTION				
Intellectual ability				
School performance				
Attitude toward school				
Ability to articulate				
FAMILY CHARACTERISTICS				
Eating disorders				
Other diseases				
Natural or other parent				
Intrusiveness				
Enmeshment				
Rigidity				
Conflict resolution				
Role of food				
Exercise patterns				
Perceptions of problem				
Attempts to intervene				
Willingness to participate in therapy				

CRISIS STAGE: PSYCHOLOGIC STATE

Overall, a lack of progress toward positive family interaction patterns during the initial therapy or continuing avoidance of intervention will often lead to physical and mental deterioration. When the crisis stage of anorexia nervosa develops, severe psychologic and physiologic symptoms appear and intervention must be directed toward the deteriorating condition.

TABLE 8-9 Clinical Assessment of Eating Disorder—cont'd

	Date	Date	Date	Date
SOCIAL RELATIONSHIPS Friends Social habits Social skills Attitude of peers				
EATING BEHAVIOR Knowledge/acknowledgement of nutritional needs Meal pattern Bizarre eating habits Personal philosophy toward eating Nutritional adequacy Control over food supply				
PHYSICAL STATUS Signs of bulimia Signs of starvation Terminal signs of starvation Thyroid status (obesity) Resting heart rate (H.R.) Exercise to reach 60% maximum (HR)				
GROWTH AND ADIPOSITY Weight/height/age percentile Triceps skinfold/age percentile Arm muscle area/age percentile Weight/height history Growth velocity Maturational stage Age				
PHYSICAL ACTIVITY Exercise patterns Hobbies/interests Personal feeling about exercise				
PLAN				

Psychologic Effects of Starvation

The anorectic teenager in crisis can cause panic in family, friends, and professionals. The family generally sees the adolescent's bizarre eating behavior as the problem and fails to understand the extent of developmental and interactional patterns. As a result, they often seek treatment that does not demand their involvement with the patient in therapy. As she becomes truly cachectic, the psychologic changes inherent in starvation, described by Keys[18] in his classic studies, become evident:

- Cognitive processes center around food. Thoughts of food intrude constantly; the major part of the waking hours are spent in contemplating it.
- Behavior around food includes toying with it and hoarding, especially during renourishment.
- Coherent creative thinking is impaired.
- Mental function is characterized by apathy, dullness, exhaustion, and depression.
- Interest in sexual function is lacking.

These effects of starvation are superimposed on the anorectic teenager's already disturbed psychologic state. The behavior pattern and weight phobia become more pronounced.

Behavior Pattern

Many patients resist what they see as intrusions by professionals. They are secretive and hide the fact that they are carrying out their rituals. Their behavior may otherwise reflect the apathy typically seen in starving people. In obsessional preoccupation they plan menus, read recipes, cook and serve food to others, cut or manipulate food before eating it, and record all that they eat. They usually have a detailed knowledge of "calorie content" but not of the energy value of foods. They may pretend to eat and then hide and dispose of the food.[16] The disturbed adolescent's fear of gaining weight becomes increasingly evident as her weight phobia intensifies.[13]

CRISIS STAGE: PHYSIOLOGIC STATE

In the crisis stage of anorexia nervosa, the physiologic state deteriorates with physical signs of starvation, endocrine abnormalities, and undeniable signs of approaching terminal starvation.

Physical Signs of Starvation

As the crisis stage develops, the individual is unable to take care of herself. The physical state of starvation is now superimposed on the other problems inherent in the disorder. These physical signs of starvation include:

- Fat-store depletion
- Muscle wasting
- Amenorrhea
- Cheilosis
- Desquamation
- Dry skin
- Hirsutism
- Thin, dry, brittle hair
- Alopecia
- Degradation of fingernails
- Acrocyanosis
- Postural hypotension
- Dehydration
- Edema

Endocrine Abnormalities

The endocrine abnormalities in anorexia nervosa are such that the body essentially reverts to a prepubertal hormonal state. As a result of hypothalamic change, the anorectic adolescent is amenorrheic, is unable to adapt to heat and cold, suffers sleep disturbances, and is unable to conserve body water. There is no interest in sex.

Terminal Starvation Signs

During the crisis, professionals must monitor the physical state of the patient and take remedial action when there are signs that starvation is approaching a terminal state. The most outstanding of these signs include:

- Fluid and electrolyte imbalance indicating inability of the body to maintain homeostasis.
- Severe cardiac abnormalities in the absence of electrolyte imbalances, indicating a wasted myocardium.
- Absence of ketone bodies in the urine, indicating a lack of fat stores for metabolic fuel.
- Concurrent infection, indicating increasing nutritional needs.

CRISIS INTERVENTION STRATEGIES

When the anorectic adolescent's condition reaches the crisis stage, hospitalization is necessary to provide comprehensive care involving nutritional therapy.

Hospitalization

For some clinicians, the decision to hospitalize an anorectic patient depends on her reaching a life-threatening physical state. However, if the goal is to renourish the individual so that she will be able to benefit from psychotherapy without semistarvation neurosis, as many authoritative therapists recommend, the anorectic patient must be hospitalized before a critical stage has been reached. The patient can be released from the hospital when she has been nutritionally rehabilitated, usually confirmed by reaching a particular weight-for-height goal (Fig. 8-8).

Comprehensive Treatment

Nutritional components of therapeutic regimens for anorexia nervosa in crisis are intertwined with the psychologic aspects of the treatment and team care is essential. Certain principles can be observed that will apply regardless of the treatment modality. Renourishment obviously will begin with a gradual increase in energy intake.

Diet Therapy

In some programs the patient will be allowed to choose anything available on the hospital menu. Other programs impose rules, make additions to what is ordered, or serve a set menu. If a diet is prescribed following the principles established for renourishing malnourished individuals, it should have adequate protein to meet basic needs with additional energy made up of complex carbohydrate and a small amount of fat.

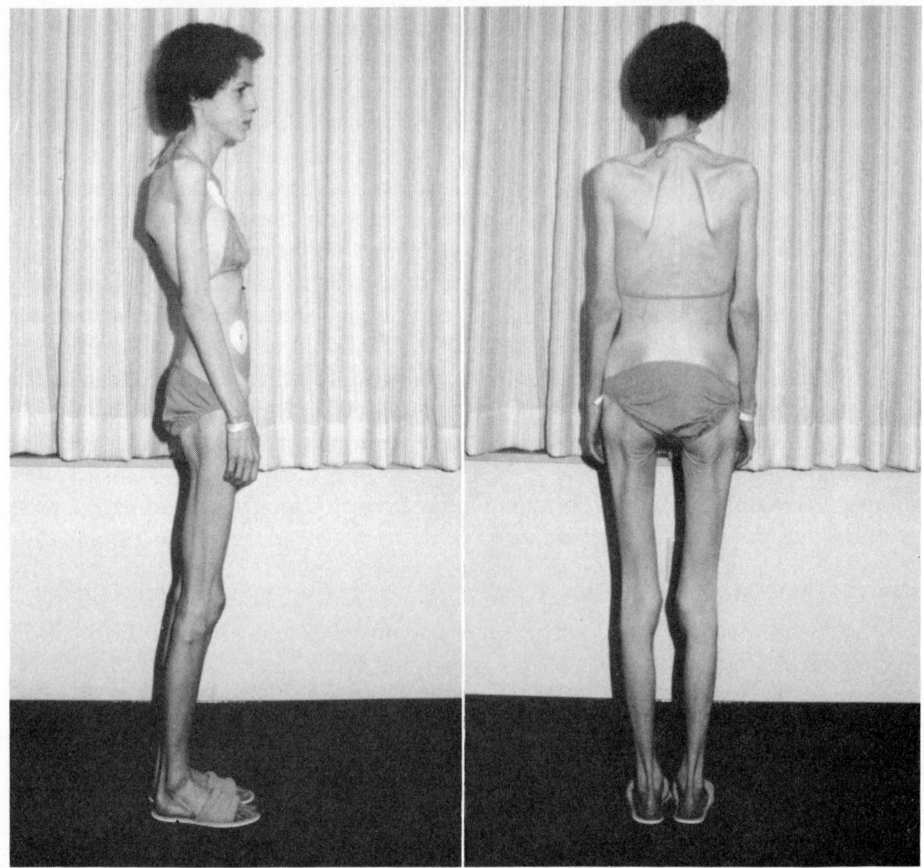

A

FIG. 8-8 A, Anorectic woman before treatment.
(Courtesy Sycamore Hospital, a division of Kettering Medical Center, Dayton, Ohio.)

Nutritional Supplements

If a patient refuses food, a nutritional supplement, which is prescribed and dispensed as a medicine, has been used. If a life-threatening state is reached at any time, with the patient refusing oral feeding, nourishment by nasogastric tube or parenteral methods may be necessary. These methods will be presented as life-saving procedures and not as punishment for refusing to eat. Nourishment by mouth is the preferred route and is possible in most cases.

Renourishment Edema and Body Image

Edema generally appears with the renourishment and can be a problem because of the anorectic patient's phobia of weight gain. The edema is seen as proof to her that she will "expand" as she feared. Some anticipatory guidance can help her accept such

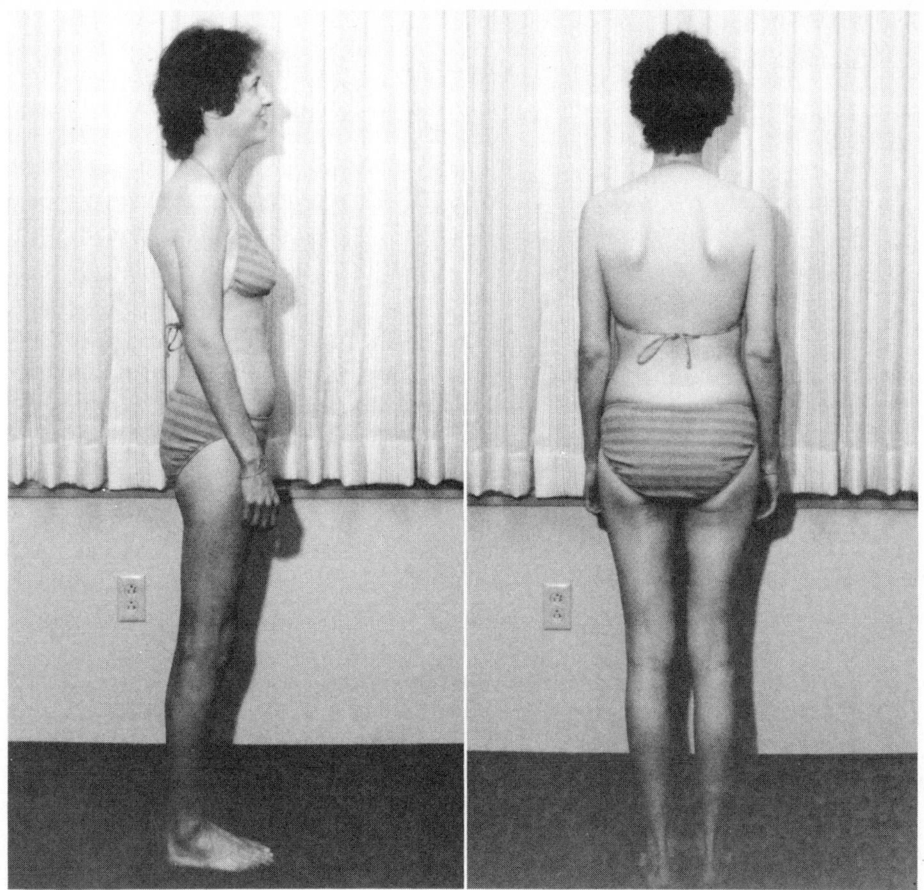

B

FIG. 8-8, cont'd. B, Same patient after *gradual* refeeding, nutritional management, and psychologic therapy.
(Courtesy Sycamore Hospital, a division of Kettering Medical Center, Dayton, Ohio.)

a development. Assurance that professionals will aid her in gaining appropriate weight, which is strengthening for her but not forming excess fat, can help desensitize the issue.

Role of the Clinical Nutritionist

The inclusion of a clinical nutritionist/dietitian on the therapeutic team gives attention to nutritional support care in a manner that does not subvert the psychotherapeutic goal of redirecting the focus of the patient's concern. The nutritionist's knowledge of energy balance as it applies to the individual is needed in determining appropriate weight goals throughout therapy and especially for termination of the hospitalization.

LONG-TERM THERAPY

Psychologic State

The anorectic teenager who has recovered from a starvation crisis by gaining a certain amount of weight to improve her physical state will still have to deal with the developmental arrest that brought her to the crisis, a process that usually requires several years. There will continue to be problems concerning vocational choices and preparation, economic stability, relationships with peers and especially with men, weight management, and body image.

Physiologic State

In the long term the anorectic young woman will often experience wide swings in weight from extreme thinness to obesity before she will be able to bring her anorexia into control. She may see herself as somewhat detached from her body and experiment with various food habits before putting food into a more normal perspective. She may keep herself sufficiently thin that she will not resume her menses. She may feel bloated and have bouts of edema, physical responses to starvation and refeeding, and carotenemia, a symptom found in anorexia.

Intervention Strategies

In the recovery period the psychotherapeutic goal will be to facilitate normal development in the anorectic teenager, to prepare her for a full adult role in society, and to enable her to function without depending on bizarre eating and exercise habits. She will need information and retraining about food and the physical aspects of life. Many of the techniques described in the section on obesity (pp. 334-346) will be useful. Issues such as the state of nourishment necessary to maintain the menstrual cycle will often resurface from time to time as development proceeds. Returning to such issues will enable her to deal more capably with them as time goes on. One well-known program incorporates training related to food experiences in cafeterias, grocery stores, cooking, and entertaining, thus helping to ready the person for managing food in her environment. The objective is to help the individual put food into a reasonable perspective rather than to overfocus on food out of ignorance. A team consisting of medical, psychologic, and nutrition specialists may provide care, or the care may be left to a single therapist who will be responsible for all aspects of therapy.

Outcome

Common features of anorexia nervosa are the strong resistance to treatment and the high incidence of relapse and partial recovery. Some of these patients will manifest varying degrees of the anorectic symptoms in adulthood. Though outcome criteria have been inconsistently used by researchers, results reported to date indicate that though weight-for-height proportion improved in about 75% of the patients, menstrual cycles were often unsatisfactorily maintained and psychosocial maladjustment was common.

Bulimia

First called *bulimarexia,* bulimia is the most recently recognized eating disorder and is characterized by gorging followed by self-induced vomiting. Although these symptoms may be a part of anorexia nervosa, they also comprise a separate syndrome. Therefore the following terminology can be used to make distinctions: (1) bulimia—gorging and vomiting without starvation; (2) bulimarexia—gorging and vomiting with voluntary starvation; and (3) gorging—binging, eating abnormally large amounts of food.

SYMPTOMS

The person suffering from bulimia generally maintains close-to-normal weight (Fig. 8-7), while gorging and vomiting on a regular basis. The bulimic teenager may have somewhat less severe distortions in body image and less restrictive weight goals than the adolescent with anorexia nervosa. She is often older at age of onset.

APA Criteria

The official diagnostic criteria established by the American Psychiatry Association (APA) includes the following behaviors:[15]

- Recurrent episodes of binge eating, rapid consumption of a large amount of food in a discrete period of time, usually less than two hours.
- At least three of the following: (1) consumption of high-caloric, easily ingested food during a binge; (2) inconspicuous eating during a binge; (3) termination of such eating episodes by abdominal pain, sleep, social interruption, or self-induced vomiting; (4) repeated attempts to lose weight by severely restrictive diets, self-induced vomiting, or use of cathartics or diuretics; (5) frequent weight fluctuations greater than ten pounds due to alternating binges and fasts.
- Awareness that the eating pattern is abnormal and fear of not being able to stop eating voluntarily.
- Depressed mood and self-deprecating thoughts following eating binges.
- The bulimic episodes are not due to anorexia nervosa or any known physical disorder.

Distinctive Behavior Pattern

The syndrome of bulimia should be differentiated from the recent behavior of many normal adolescent females who occasionally use self-induced vomiting as a means of controlling weight. A serious condition will be uncontrollable, and the psychologic features of the disorder will impair normal functioning. Bulimia sometimes develops after a serious bout with anorexia nervosa or obesity. The bulimic person is more likely to be fertile than the individual with anorexia nervosa. Therefore, certain young women will be bulimic during pregnancy.

PSYCHOLOGIC STATE

Separation anxiety is one of the important issues for the bulimic teenager. Her self-esteem is extremely low and it ties to her feelings about her body. She demonstrates excessive need for control and approval. She thinks of herself as physically unattractive, although she is well groomed and has a normally attractive physique. She develops guilt over her habits and her secret feelings of inadequacy. Superficially, she may be very responsible and keep a heavy social schedule. In reality she has few close friends and feels that no one really knows her. In contrast to the more rigid anorectic adolescent, the young woman with bulimia often demonstrates poor impulse control, abuses substances, and becomes easily enraged. By all accounts, the gorging, vomiting, and purging serve to release tension for the sufferers. However, the residual guilt feelings bring renewed tension that perpetuates an uncontrolled cycle. Social isolation is also perpetuated because of the fear that the secret will be found out.[19] If she is pregnant, the bulimic teenager may be committed to protecting the fetus but retain ideas that inhibit normal nourishment of herself, her fetus, and the child after birth.

PHYSIOLOGIC STATE

Food Behavior

The bulimic teenager periodically eats large amounts of food and then voluntarily vomits. Each person with bulimia defines what a binge is for herself. Because of distortions in thinking about food, as little as one doughnut may be thought of as a binge by one person while as much as an entire package of doughnuts may constitute a binge for another. As the duration of the habits extends, it becomes easier for her to vomit. Eventually, the vomiting is a nearly automatic response. In addition, she may take laxatives to purge herself of the energy she has ingested or use diuretics to remove body fluid.

Physical Symptoms

As a result of these behaviors, physical symptoms of the bulimic adolescent will include:

- Damage to the teeth.
- Irritation to the throat.
- Esophageal inflammation and possible tracheoesophageal fistula. (All of the above symptoms are caused by exposure of unprotected tissues to acidic vomitus.)
- Swollen salivary glands. (Caused by acidic reflux or constant stimulation.)
- Rectal bleeding. (Caused by overuse of laxatives.)

Life-threatening situations are more rare than in anorexia nervosa. They are related to fistulas or ruptures in the upper gastrointestinal tract and fluid-electrolyte imbalances. Concerns during pregnancy are the adverse biochemical environment for the mother and fetus, the mother's abnormal weight gain pattern (weight loss, lack of weight gain, inordinate gain), and the mother's unrealistic ideas about infant feeding.

INTERVENTION STRATEGIES

The techniques most frequently reported in treating bulimia are similar to those used in the long-term recovery period of the person with anorexia nervosa (p. 330). Psychotherapy, nutritional therapy, and care of any pregnancy that may occur must be included.

Psychotherapy

The emphasis of therapy is on freeing the person from guilt, facilitating gains in self-esteem, and helping her deal with anxiety. Challenging distorted goal-setting based on perfection has been tied to this emphasis. Ideally, the young woman's family or partner will be included in the therapy.

Nutritional Therapy

While she deals with the psychologic problem, the bulimic individual will still have an eating disorder and will need re-education to properly nourish herself. Physical and nutritional education can fill gaps in knowledge these teenagers have about their body functions. Over time, myths about weight management can be dispelled and more normal eating habits developed. Because of distorted feelings about food, the bulimic person may feel guilty every time she eats, despite the fact that food is necessary for life. The family often reinforces the guilt by a misguided overfocus on food, thinness, and the physical aspects of life. The bulimic teenager usually restricts her food intake to match the ideal plan she conceives for herself. Binges may thus arise from the natural need for adequate food and the desire for additional gratification.[20]

Role of Clinical Nutritionist

The clinical nutritionist on the professional team will help the young person with bulimia to see food in a more appropriate context and accept more realistic weight goals using the techniques described in the following section. Helping her understand the physiologic processes of energy balance and nutrient functions as they affect her personally is especially useful. This education, however, must be done gradually in a counseling mode, allowing time for alteration of her own rigid system of beliefs. Family and individual psychotherapy will continue concurrently, and it is necessary to deal with the underlying causes of the obsessional food behavior. Group therapy has also been used.

Pregnancy Care

The bulimic teenager who is pregnant can be helped to accept the idea that the baby she wants must be nourished. She can then be supported in learning to retain those foods that the fetus needs even if she cannot give up binging and vomiting totally. She should also be helped in learning to recognize natural hunger signals from her baby after it is born.

Obesity

At the other end of the physical spectrum of eating disorders is the very obese teenager. Unlike anorectic adolescents, persons who are abnormally heavy do not fit into a homogeneous group and may be carrying excessive weight for a variety of reasons.[21] Factors leading to obesity can be broadly divided into those that are psychologic and those that are physiologic. In any individual a combination of these factors may operate in the development and maintenance of obesity. Because of the cultural response to obesity, the adolescent whose obesity may be physiologically based will generally be subject to many of the same problems as those whose obesity is more psychologically based.

PSYCHOLOGIC FACTORS

Various psychologic factors are associated with adolescent obesity, whether it develops during earlier childhood or is related to more severe psychiatric disorders.

Developmental Obesity

Bruch[13] has described a form of obesity that primarily results from psychologic factors within the family. Thus it is termed *developmental obesity*. It is an eating disorder comparable to anorexia nervosa in that it originates in the early life of the child. The families of developmentally obese teenagers fit descriptions of the psychosomatic family. The family's attitudes and behavior thus stunt the child's psychologic development and serve as primary causes of the obesity. The obesity itself further inhibits normal development, and this in turn leads to maintenance or increase of body weight. The affected children are made to feel pressure, inappropriate responsibility, and specialness to an abnormal degree in family interactions. They become rigid, isolated, and enmeshed. They develop misperceptions about their basic physical needs and rely on coping skills based on the abuse of food. As obese teenagers, these persons may not develop their full potential as self-competent, well-functioning adults, but they are less likely to experience the complete developmental arrest that the anorectic teenager does.

Body Image

The teenager who is overweight is vulnerable to body-image disturbances. The type and extent of the disturbance depends on the length of time the person has been heavy, the amount of excessive weight carried, the person's sex, and the life situation surrounding the individual's unique development. For example, teenagers who have been heavy from childhood may react differently than those who have gained weight only during later adolescence. Like anorectic teenagers, many tie thoughts of success or failure to their weight status.

Associated Psychologic Disorders

In some teenagers, obesity may be associated with severe psychiatric disorders. In others, the overeating behavior may act as an emotionally stabilizing influence helping to maintain the person at a functioning level. Interference in such a situation without substantial support provided can cause the disintegration of the person's affect into an anxious or depressed state.

CULTURAL AND FAMILY INFLUENCES

The abundance of food and lack of necessity to expend energy in American society make it very easy for children to gain unwanted weight. In families where food intake and exercise patterns are not appropriate for dealing with this situation, an overweight state can result without other specific psychologic or physiologic origins.

BEHAVIOR PATTERNS IN OBESE TEENAGERS

The usual overweight or obese teenager is passive in interactions with others and with the environment. This response further reinforces the weight problem and leads to social isolation, lack of exercise, and disturbed patterns of eating and family interaction.

Social Isolation

The passive response pattern of the obese adolescent in contact with others creates social isolation and an increased dependence on the family for relationships, even though the family interaction patterns may be unpleasant and the parents may constantly exhibit intrusive and negative attitudes. Adolescents often react to the stigma of obesity by adopting a stereotyped lifestyle with a narrow range of activities.

Sedentary Life Style

The eating and exercise functions in the lives of obese teenagers generally become distorted. They may never feel comfortable eating in social situations. Their isolation leads them to opt out of many activities that would expend energy. They fear being seen wearing gym clothes or swim suits or doing physical activities because they feel they are the object of attention and even ridicule. Instead they usually spend an inordinate amount of time in passive pursuits such as watching television or reading. Both of these activities may be paired with eating. Commercial television, especially, fosters this behavior with frequent food-related cues.

Eating Patterns

Although many studies of teenagers after they have become obese have shown that on the average they eat no more, and sometimes less, than their normal-weight peers, they often have disturbed, unstructured patterns of eating. They may eat only in the latter part of the day, feeling nausea when eating earlier, and eat rapidly and indiscriminately.

Family Patterns

Parents in some families may be locked into power struggles with their children, attempting in vain to control what they eat. Overanxiety regarding even slight overweight may actually contribute to growing obesity. In other families overeating may be the main theme, with most interactions revolving around food.

TABLE 8-10 Physiologic Factors Observed in Obesity

Factor	Proposed Mechanism	Recent Conclusions	Therapeutic Implications
Insulin insensitivity	Obese persons are less sensitive to the action of insulin, creating the state of hyperinsulinemia.	Dietary factors and reversible changes in the metabolism of obese persons may be responsible for irregularities in body insulin levels.	Moderation of simple carbohydrate and fat intake should be encouraged. Cyclical maintenance of obesity may be interrupted by factors such as exercise, which appear to alleviate insulin sensitivity independent of weight reduction.
Thyroid dysfunction	Faulty receptor sites impair the normal function of 3,5,3′-triiodothyronine (T_3) at the cellular level.	Irregularities accompany and maintain obesity but are probably not a cause.	In most cases thyroid medication is contraindicated.
Fat cell hypertrophy	As the body gains weight, the fat cells enlarge.	The size of the fat cells can be reduced by increased energy output and decreased energy input.	Reducing fat cells to normal size is a reasonable goal.
Fat cell hyperplasia	Number of fat cells increases when sufficient weight is gained.	The heavier a body is and the longer it remains heavy, the greater the chance of an increased number of fat cells. The number of fat cells cannot be reduced with weight loss.	Preventing an increase in the number of fat cells is a reasonable goal.

Thermogenesis	Obese persons produce less heat to dissipate energy.	May be caused by specific mechanisms such as less brown fat or sodium-potassium-pump irregularity.	Increase thermogenesis in any practical way (for example, exercise).
Brown fat variability	High cytochrome content of these adipocytes causes heat production: smaller endowment leads to energy storage.	It is difficult to correlate particular amount with obese state in humans.	If operative, these mechanisms can only be overcome with extreme difficulty.
Sodium-potassium-pump irregularity	Lower number of sodium-potassium transporting units present in cells of obese persons.	Irregularity may account for decreased energy usage in metabolism of obese persons.	Reduction of body weight, if possible, may lead to a state like starvation in persons with these irregularities.
Genetic predisposition	Certain biochemical, morphologic, and histologic features are inherited.	Differences may be aggravated by decreased energy output and increased energy intake.	If obese persons have control of energy intake and output, psychologic support for living with status quo is a reasonable goal.
Physical set point	A feedback system alters intake and output of energy to maintain a particular body mass.	As above.	As above.
Lipoprotein lipase variability	Higher levels of lipoprotein lipase (LPL) in obese persons maintain obese state.	Reduced persons have higher than expected levels of LPL, favoring return to the state of obesity.	As above.

PHYSIOLOGIC FACTORS

In certain individuals physiologic factors are principally responsible for their obesity.[21] These factors are summarized in Table 8-10. Two of these underlying factors deserve note here.

Set-Point Theory

One theory that cannot be overlooked is that certain individuals may be subject to a body weight "set-point." A certain body weight may be physiologically normal for each person, and body characteristics may be tuned to keep the body at that weight.

Lower Basal Energy Needs

A decreased requirement for the amount of energy used in biochemical reactions may increase the amount of energy available in the systems of some people for storage as fat. Based on present theory, the longer the teenager has been obese and the greater the extent of the obesity, the greater the effect of these factors will be. The adolescent whose obesity was originally caused by other factors such as social, psychologic, or family influences will, as time passes, have added problems of physiologic obesity. This pattern increases the complexity of the obese state.

INTERVENTION STRATEGIES

An effective program for working with obese teenagers and their families will provide personalized care, giving attention to identifying individual needs and attitudes, setting realistic goals, developing related strategies within a comprehensive approach (see box), and evaluating outcome.

Assessment

The individual combination of psychologic and physiologic circumstances by which an individual teenager has become obese must be identified so that intervention can be directed toward specific aspects of the problem. The degree of overweight must be considered. The material in the assessment section (pp. 310-313), especially Fig. 8-6, may be used to evaluate the size of heavy adolescents. Generally they will be: (1) *overweight,* only moderately above weight-height mid-ranges for health; (2) *obese,* about 20% or more above normal weight-height ranges with higher degree of fatness; and (3) *morbidly obese,* much higher weight for height and greater amount of fat tissue, associated with multiple health problems. Among all of these persons some will suffer from hidden eating disorders such as bulimia or anorexia nervosa (recovery stage). The information needed to assess adolescent obesity (Table 8-9) may best be gathered by a team of professionals. Many of these aspects cannot be assessed immediately but will need to be explored over time. Basic initial steps assess physical status and personal attitude:

1. **Physical status.** A physical examination will disclose the stage of puberty and rule out any endocrine abnormalities or complications of the obese state. Endocrine disorders are rarely found. Most physiologic abnormalities indicated by clinical laboratory measures that are associated with obesity will respond to weight reduction.

COMPONENTS OF A COMPREHENSIVE WEIGHT MANAGEMENT PROGRAM WITH APPLICABLE TREATMENT MODALITIES

Food Management	Energy-Time Management	Psychosocial Adjustment
Food use retraining	Fitness testing and improvement programs	Supportive counseling
Nutrition education	Relaxation training	Family counseling
Behavior modification	Movement and dance therapy	Social skills training
Diet prescription	Expanded interest stimulation	Assertion training
		Psychotherapy
		Group support

2. **Personal attitude**. The most important aspect of initial evaluation is whether or not the individual is committed to making changes. The teenager's feelings must be assessed initially and at each visit. It is of no value for other persons to have goals related to weight management if the teenager is not ready to change the status quo. The question needs to be, "Are you ready to make changes?" rather than, "Do you want to lose weight?" Many teenagers will answer "yes" to the second question but remain totally passive, the implication being that the process of weight management for them is a passive one in which the professional administers treatment.

Reasons for Not Starting a Weight-Loss Program

A weight-loss program should not be instituted if: (1) the adolescent has not reached full height; (2) there is a lack of commitment; (3) it is likely to be another in a series of failures harmful to the individual's self-esteem; or (4) the individual is obviously predisposed to obesity by overwhelming physiologic factors.[22] If obese teenagers keep fit, maintain energy equilibrium, and are emotionally healthy, they will be candidates for weight loss only if they understand the physiologic aspects of obesity and are determined to test these aspects in a healthful manner. Those adolescents who are still growing in height should not be encouraged to lose weight because the level of energy restriction required to do so is inadequate to support growth.

Weight Goals

Realistic planning for weight goals should include initial goal and continuing short-term goals:

1. **Initial goal**. The initial weight goal in a *weight management* program is usually maintenance, that is, cessation of weight gain. In certain situations an even more basic change from *rapid gain* to *slow gain* is the more appropriate goal. Immature adolescents who have not completed linear growth can bring weight and, more specifically, percentage of body fat into better proportion with height by holding their weight stable or by reducing gains to a lower rate as height increases. This pattern eliminates nutritional risk to the individual from severe diet restrictions at a time of rapid growth and development. For teenagers who

have stabilized their weight and are no longer gaining in height, the next step will be a slow, steady *loss* based on re-education in the use of energy. A loss of 0.9 kg/week (2 lb/week) should not be exceeded. If this rate appears insignificant to the teenager, point out that it would add up to more than a 45 kg (100 lb) loss over 1 year.

2. **Continuing short-term goals.** These continuing short-term goals need to be based not on changes in weight but on positive changes in food-related attitudes and behaviors with appropriate rewards built in. It is especially necessary to build a program around short-term manageable goals related to behavioral change since physiologic factors may make actual weight loss a difficult, long-term achievement. The teenager should be made aware that over the long term an energy deficit will eventually lead to weight loss, however slowly.

INTERVENTION STRATEGIES: PHYSIOLOGIC FACTORS

Strategies planned to deal with the physiologic factors of obesity must be based on the laws of energy exchange and balance, address positive changes in personal food behaviors, avoid the dangers of "crash diets" and life-threatening situations, and increase physical activity and fitness.

Basic Individual Energy Balance

Whatever the reasons for a teenager's being overweight, the method for altering the situation remains the same: decreasing the body's energy intake and increasing the energy output until the appropriate deficit state is established. There is no way of knowing the exact use of energy by a particular body except by testing it over time. To lose weight an energy deficit must be achieved at the cellular level. Because this state is not measurable under normal clinical circumstances, there is no set formula that assures weight loss. It is an error to count kilocalories of food energy being eaten and assume that this amount of energy will be available within the biochemical system. Thus a deficit of 3500 kilocalories calculated at the point of intake does not necessarily lead to a loss of 1 lb of body weight. This does not imply that the second law of thermodynamics is inoperative, but simply that energy from food may be used in a variety of ways once it is in the body, as indicated previously (Table 8-10). Thus both the physiologic and the psychologic aspects of weight management are unique to the individual.

Eating Habits

Each individual teenager must be guided in learning the level of energy intake and output that produces weight gain, loss, and maintenance for that individual if the treatment is to be effective. An understanding of physiologic factors must be incorporated. The teenager must be made aware that however bleak the physiologic situation appears, the possibility of weight management has not been tested until the individual has control over energy intake and output. There is usually some potential for improvement in the diet that will help even those persons who are physiologically prone to obesity to become more fit and healthy, and to stabilize and perhaps to reduce their weight—in small amounts.

Dietary Change

Strategies for dietary change must address the issues of: (1) energy and nutrient content of the food intake; (2) circumstances of eating related to timing, place, accompanying social factors, and emotions; and (3) principles of nutrition regarding weight management.

Food Use Retraining

Specific diets have rarely achieved long-term changes in eating behavior. This result is especially true for teenagers, who tend to rebel against authoritarian techniques and hold a number of negative views about diets. Food use retraining, a series of habit changes planned jointly by the teenager and the therapist and instituted in succession over time, will be more acceptable to most adolescents and is a more realistic way to approach a complex problem.

Time Factor

Because eating habits have been developed over a number of years, it is logical that the teenager will need considerable time to make changes. A person cannot suddenly pick up a musical instrument and play it well but will need education, practice, and support to become proficient. Even so, most teenagers will not be able to learn a new food pattern or "diet" and perfect it immediately. Usually, intensive treatment will need to be continued for a year or more to accomplish major dietary changes. Breaking down the problem of food misuse into small components makes change more probable. What habit will be the initial focus, how change will be accomplished, what foods will be eaten, and what motivations and rewards will be effective are developed and clarified in counseling sessions between the therapist and the teenager.

Therapy Objective

The nutritional therapist's objective is eventually to focus on each time of day and point of environment where teenagers meet with food and to help them to *retrain themselves* in the use of food. Most teenagers will have some reasonable habits that can be supported and used as a foundation for the emerging positive patterns.

Self-Responsibility

Teenagers will need help at every stage to take responsibility for their actions. Coupled with psychologic support, the process can lead to effective change. Even those who are unsuccessful in retraining themselves during the adolescent period will have a model for the future, when they may be able to take greater control. Education regarding the physiologic factors of obesity will help teenagers avoid the harmful quick-loss plans to which they are so vulnerable.

Dangers of "Crash" Diets

A very important component of programs in weight-management education involves helping the teenager understand that rapid weight loss by either starvation or too low an energy intake is ineffective. Since the loss is in lean body mass and fluids, inevitably weight will be regained when usual eating is resumed and fat will not have been lost. The deprivation in such a regimen often leads to even greater overeating. Thus the final result of a "crash" diet is often a net gain. It is not difficult to convince those who have had the experience a few times that such practices are ineffective, but it is important to support their impressions by teaching them the physiologic reasons. Teenagers who will not be convinced that such methods and "diet aids" are unhealthy will be deterred from using them by the knowledge that they will not lose *fat.*

Morbid Obesity

There are certain life-threatening situations for very obese persons when drastic intervention will be necessary. The physical condition should be monitored to detect any rapid deterioration. The following conditions warrant hospitalization:

- Sudden changes in cardiac or respiratory function
- Inability to move, maintain balance, or travel
- Rapid weight increase because of the above factors
- Inability to fit into furniture and having to rest on floor
- Ulcerations at pressure points and friction areas

As with the anorectic teenager, a period of separation from the family may break up a pernicious cycle leading to physical deterioration. Comprehensive treatment using a modified fast as the dietary component is at present the most practical therapy. Although it is still controversial whether lean body mass can be spared, such dietary methods appear less objectionable than other radical procedures.

Physical Activity and Fitness

One of the most important concepts of weight management is that energy output must be increased. Individualized exercise programs need to be developed with the obese teenager to achieve a gradual increase in physical activity.

The fitness test shown here (see box, p. 343) is designed to be a conservative tool that can safely be used with even an extremely obese person. It can be used with or without professional help. Physically, it appears that increasing activity can be rewarding in itself, whereas denying oneself an accustomed food may seem more like punishment. Besides fitness testing and improvement, various strategies can be directed toward increasing energy output by increasing physical activity. These guidelines should be followed: (1) activities should be built into everyday life; (2) activities should be things that the person enjoys or finds useful; (3) activities should not depend on help from others or complex equipment; and (4) activities should not be stressful by causing embarrassing exposure.

INTERVENTION STRATEGIES: PSYCHOLOGIC FACTORS

Weight management for teenagers should be a total rehabilitation program. It demands a significant length of time and must be individualized. Like the physiologic component, the psychologic component of any weight management problem cannot be overlooked.[22] Activities planned to meet these needs include motivational support, psychotherapy, and counseling.

FITNESS: TESTING AND PLANNING IMPROVEMENT PROGRAMS

1. a. Have client sit quietly and relax for 3 to 5 minutes.
   b. Take pulse for 10 seconds.*
   c. Record *resting heart rate (RHR):* ____________
2. a. Find intensity of exercise required to reach *training heart rate (THR)*† immediately after exercise. THR for teens is 20 to 22 beats/10 sec.‡
   Stop with the exercise that achieves 20 to 22 beats/10 sec. This is the exercise to use initially in the improvement program.

Intensity ↑ increases	
	Run for 5 minutes
	Jog for 5 minutes
	Jog for 2 minutes—walk for 2 minutes—jog for 2 minutes
	Walk uphill or upstairs for 2 to 3 minutes
	Walk for 5 minutes at a more rapid pace
START	Walk for 5 minutes at a moderate pace

   b. Monitor pulse return toward RHR after each exercise level—it should be below 16 beats/10 sec by 5 minutes.

   ________ ________ ________ ________
   Immediate ⟶ 1 minute ⟶ 2 minutes⟶ 5 minutes⟶ . . .

3. *Improvement program:* To maintain THR for 15 minutes 4 to 5 days/wk:
   a. Work with client to design an individualized program that is comfortable for him or her.
   b. Plan 5-minute warm-up—move at level below the level that maintains THR.
   c. Exercise at intensity that maintains THR.
   d. 5-Minute cool down—back to warm-up speed—client should not sit or lie down immediately.
   e. Use a combination of exercise levels and types, if necessary.
   f. If the client is ill, he or she should begin after illness at lower intensity and return slowly to intensity achieved before illness
4. a. Retest every 3 to 4 weeks
   b. Increase intensity of exercise to maintain THR.
   c. Client can increase time spent doing the exercise by 5-minute increments, up to 30 minutes.
   d. When client has reached jogging level and maintained it for 6 to 8 weeks, increase THR to 22 to 25 beats/10 sec.
   e. Client can use any aerobic activities (for example, jogging, bicycling, skating, dancing) or combinations that the client prefers.

From Pipes, P.L.: Nutrition in infancy and childhood, St. Louis, 1981, Times Mirror/Mosby College Publishing.; developed by Scott, B., and Rees, J., Adolescent Program, University of Washington, Seattle, Wash.

*10-second time segment is easiest to measure and use.

†*Maximum heart rate (MHR)* is approximately 200 beats/min for persons under 20 years of age (Cumming, G.R., Everatt, D., and Hastman, L.: Am. J. Cardiol. 41:69, 1978). THR is 60% of MHR for persons with poor initial fitness, 75% of MHR for persons who are fit (that is, 60% of 200 = 120 beats/min = 20 beats/10 sec [20 to 22 beats/10 sec for normal variation]).

‡An adolescent of normal weight and in reasonable shape may want to start at 22 to 25 beats/10 sec.

NOTE: Contraindications for testing and initiating fitness program will be revealed by routine medical history and physical examination.

Motivation

In a short-term situation where the teenager has only a few pounds to lose, the problem is one of motivation. This support can be provided in settings such as schools and many other community settings.

Psychotherapy

With extreme developmental obesity, changes usually require extensive psychotherapeutic intervention. This includes the family when the teenager is living at home.

Counseling

For teenagers falling between these two extremes, a variable degree of supportive counseling will be needed to increase self-acceptance, to decrease stress, to facilitate development, and to enable adolescents to carry out weight-management strategies. Teenagers need help in learning to experience the body's signals related to hunger and satiety and to adopt nondestructive coping mechanisms to replace the misuse of food.

COMPREHENSIVE APPROACH

To provide a comprehensive approach to a weight-management program for teenagers, attention must be given to additional resources available. These resources include group activities applied with professional guidance, parent education and counseling, and school and community support.

Group Activities

Strategies such as camp settings, support groups, peer counseling, social skills and assertiveness training, body awareness experience, physical fitness training, and behavior modification can be used successfully with some individuals. Groups and preplanned programs will help those adolescents with mild, relatively simple problems. *Camps and other groups that provide only for short-term weight loss are detrimental and should be avoided.*

Professional Guidance

None of the group settings, however, provides a solution for all aspects of obesity. To be effective, weight management techniques must be applied within the context of ongoing supportive counseling by professionals who assess the specific problems of the individual over time and choose appropriate treatment methods. A team of professionals will be best able to carry out a comprehensive program as described here.

Parent Education and Counseling

Counseling will enable parents to support their teenagers in learning to manage weight.[22] Education about the physiologic factors involved and rational approaches to management will help dispel myths parents hold. Helping them develop a nonintrusive attitude toward their teenagers is of extreme importance. The counselor can demonstrate this by stressing the need for the teenager, not the counselor or the parent, to establish his or her own goals.

School and Community Support

Although they are rarely in the position to carry out therapy because of the complexity of the problem, teachers, school counselors, nurses, coaches, and other community leaders of adolescents have many opportunities to educate and support overweight teenagers. Curriculum materials such as those represented in Fig. 8-9 have been designed to help adolescents understand the complexity of weight management.

OUTCOME AND CONCLUSIONS

Reviews of the outcome of weight management therapies for teenagers are uniformly gloomy. In general such programs are designed as studies of *weight loss,* when informed workers in the field of adolescent health have stressed the importance of focusing on the other benefits of *weight management* programs such as increased self-esteem. Added knowledge, increased readiness to work for change, and improved practices are important outcomes of *weight management* programs for adolescents.

The spectrum of eating disorders affects adolescents physically, psychologically,

BE SIZEWISE

Don't Lose Your Balance

Nourishment	**Activities**	**Feelings**
Be good to your body—give it what it needs	Do interesting things—quiet as well as energetic	Learn to know and like yourself
Don't starve or stuff yourself	Take time to relax every day	Have realistic goals for yourself
Know what's in the food you eat	Don't let eating be your only recreation	Don't substitute food for love and companionship
	Do some strenuous activity every day	Build satisfying relationships with your family and friends
	Share active and quiet time with friends	Get help for problems you can't cope with alone

FIG. 8-9 Be sizewise—materials for clinicians, educators, and teenagers.
(© American Heart Association of Washington.)

personally, and socially. Intervention strategies must be directed toward both the nutritional and developmental aspects of these disorders to be effective. Goals must be established in relation to all aspects. Helping teenagers put food into reasonable perspective in their lives will be a principal goal of nutritional therapy. A recognition of the amount of time required for effective intervention is essential for a basic understanding of eating disorders.

Physical Fitness and Athletics

BENEFITS OF PHYSICAL FITNESS

All teenagers should be encouraged to exercise in ways best suited to their lives. The exercised body is more likely to remain healthy than one that remains sedentary, because historically the human being required great energy exchange to obtain food, protect itself, and to survive the elements. Physical activity has many benefits:[23]

- Helps maintain optimal body composition
- Increases the probability of weight loss when that is necessary
- Increases the efficiency of energy use by muscle fibers
- Increases the efficacy of hormones (insulin, lipoprotein lipase, epinephrine) in the regulation of energy metabolism
- Decreases the production of lactic acid, which interferes with energy production
- Strengthens the heart, lungs, and circulatory system
- Increases levels of HDL over LDL and decreases some triglycerides
- Raises rates of basal metabolism
- Helps control appetite

ELEMENTS OF FITNESS

Each teenager should participate in activities that maintain the elements of fitness: body composition, cardiorespiratory function, and muscular strength, endurance, and flexibility. Raising the heart rate to at least 50% but no more than 75% of maximum for 15 minutes, with 5 minutes warm-up and cool-down, at least 3 days a week, will maintain cardiorespiratory fitness. This process is incorporated in the testing and improvement protocol given here (see box, p. 343). The maximum heart rate of adolescents has been shown to be about 200. This number can be used until age 20, when the usual calculation for adults, subtracting the age from 220 to derive the maximum heart rate, can begin. Stressful exercise is unnecessary and undesirable. Continuous gradual improvement and maintenance is effective. A few well-chosen calisthenics will maintain muscular strength, flexibility, and endurance. Adolescents who participate in sports as well as those who do not should develop personal programs to assure fitness that is maintained between seasonal participation in organized programs.

NUTRITIONAL REQUIREMENTS FOR ATHLETICS

Adolescent athletes require specific nutritional support, primarily to maintain normal growth and physiologic maturation in spite of the physical stress. Energy is the basic factor in this process. The amount of additional energy needed will depend on the intensity, duration, and type of exercise being done.

Sources of Energy

Energy is best utilized if it is supplied as carbohydrate. An additional 6-7 g protein/day is sufficient in a muscle-building phase (during initial training). Thereafter 2-3 g protein/day above the daily recommended allowance will support the body maintenance in most athletes. Abnormally high levels of protein are counterproductive, leading to dehydration as the body rids itself of nitrogenous waste products. The need for carbohydrate as fuel instead of protein to build muscle is one of the most misunderstood principles among adolescent athletes.

Weight Management

Weight should be gained or lost following safe effective methods. To support normal growth successfully, weight should be maintained at an optimal level long term rather than be subjected to seasonal, or especially, weekly manipulation as is often urged by coaches of wrestling and crew during competition. The development pattern of skeletal growth and weight gain must be considered. Two problems in this area are common among teenage athletes who become too thin in trying to reduce the percentage of body fat: (1) women interrupt their menses, and (2) men stunt their linear growth. Anabolic steroids taken by men to increase weight cause stunting of growth and disturbed development of secondary sex characteristics.

Supplements

The increased dietary intake should provide sufficient amounts of nutrients, making supplements unnecessary. Supplementation of nutrients in amounts above those recommended has not resulted in benefits during competition. Of the vitamins and minerals, iron is particularly important to young athletes because "sports anemia" is associated with reduced oxygenation while the B vitamins are essential in energy production.[23]

Short-term Events

A light workout one day prior to competition combined with increased dietary carbohydrate, mainly starches, will assure a supply of liver and muscle glycogen to support the athlete during a short-term event. On the day of competition eliminate roughage, fats, and gas-forming foods from the diet to decrease discomfort and untimely need for elimination. If several short-term events are held in one day, additional carbohydrate will provide energy. Otherwise stores should be sufficient. Fluid replacement follows the same principles given below for long-term events.

Long-term Events

For events that last at least an hour, supplies of body fuel and fluids will need attention.

1. **Body fuel stores.** Modified glycogen loading before a long-term event will improve not only liver storage but also muscle reserves of glycogen. Glucose can

be taken after the event begins to spare liver glycogen stores but should not be ingested just prior to an event because it impairs lipid mobilization.

2. **Fluids and electrolytes.** Body fluid-electrolyte balance is very important during long-term events, indeed, throughout athletic training and competition.[24] Exaggerated shifts in fluids and electrolytes due to strenuous exercise are intensified by environmental temperatures and the sweat of exertion. Water must be replaced at the level of 1 pint for each pound of body weight lost in any exercise or training session. Thus fluid must be available to keep up with thirst during events and may have to be replaced at levels beyond thirst in the post-event period. Electrolytes and additional glucose can be obtained by using natural juices and fluids made with specified concentrations of glucose and electrolytes. The maximal sugar content for an efficient replacement drink is 2.0-2.5 g sugar/dl. The need for replacing fluids will vary according to loss due to the event and climate. It is unnecessary for athletes trying to keep warm on the sidelines of a soccer game in a cold northern climate to drink the electrolyte-rich fluids designed for sweat-inducing events in tropical conditions.

Overall Nutritional Goals

Maintaining appropriate weight for height is a good general guide to dietary adequacy as long as the foods eaten to attain that weight are nutrient-rich. Obtaining sufficient food may prove difficult for teenage athletes whose days may be filled from early morning to late evening with practices as well as normal activities including classes and study assignments. Parents, coaches, and school officials need to support teenagers by helping them plan specifically to obtain adequate acceptable foods at times when rigorous schedules allow them to eat.

Chronic Disorders

In a variety of chronic systemic diseases and metabolic conditions the goal of nutritional therapy is to provide nutrients for normal growth while avoiding those that increase symptoms. Monitoring and supporting protein stores, as well as height and weight, is one way to assure that physical development of adolescents is not impaired, whatever the condition.

CYSTIC FIBROSIS

Nature of the Condition

Cystic fibrosis is a chronic genetic disease whose major feature is the dysfunction of all exocrine glands. It is usually diagnosed in early childhood. With great treatment advances, sufferers of this disease are increasingly likely to survive to adolescence. Mean survival age was 3-4 years in 1950, 10.6 years in 1966, and 21 years in 1980. However, despite the increasingly optimistic prognosis, there is persistent incidence of growth failure and malnutrition. Although the main feature of the disease is usually pulmonary insufficiency, 80% to 90% of the persons have gastrointestinal involvement. Steatorrhea and malabsorption result. Fat-soluble vitamins, and fats and protein are poorly absorbed.

Nutritional Needs

To help remedy the weight loss and growth failure due to the malabsorption caused by lack of pancreatic enzymes in the intestine, these enzymes are taken orally. Dietary protein should be high and the fat usually moderate. Dividing the total day's intake into six small meals can be helpful. However, the body of each person with the disease handles food or tolerates various foods differently, and nutritional care must be planned on an individual basis.[25]

ASTHMA

Nature of the Condition

Asthma is a respiratory disorder, often a manifestation of an allergic response. Most clinical attention has been focused on the airborne allergens such as dust, mold, and pollen.[26] Whether food antigens are also likely to provoke respiratory distress is still controversial.

Nutritional Needs

The nutritionist should be open to the possibility that a food allergy may be involved. Also, there may be possible side effects on growth and bone formation from corticosteroids that may be used for medical treatment, and these effects will need nutritional attention.[25]

CROHN'S DISEASE

Nature of Condition

Crohn's disease, or granulomatous ileocolitis, was first recognized in 1932. It is a chronic disease mainly affecting young persons and is characterized by a necrotizing, ulcerating, inflammatory process. Peak frequency is between 15 and 35 years of age. The course is extremely variable, but complications tend to be frequent and severe as the person grows older. Initial symptoms are usually weight loss, diarrhea, cramps, and abdominal pain. The disease has many features of a malabsorption syndrome. It can cause alteration of gastrointestinal motility and create areas of malabsorption and obstruction of fistulas. Adolescents with this disease are subject to growth retardation or delayed sexual maturation. When malabsorption or malnutrition is a prominent feature, serum albumin may be low, macrocytic anemia may be present, and alkaline phosphatase may be elevated because of protein loss, poor absorption of folate or vitamin B_{12}, and poor absorption of calcium and vitamin D.

Nutritional Needs

To facilitate adequate nourishment and growth, a high-protein diet with vitamin B_{12}, folate, and iron supplementation is needed. The major aim of nutritional care is to maintain metabolic homeostasis and to provide adequate energy, protein, and other substrates to restore normal growth or permit catch-up growth to occur. Therapies such as food supplements, nasogastric tube feedings, and gastrostomy infusions are used. In acute attacks, total parenteral nutrition (TPN) has been advocated. It restores metabolic and nutritional homeostasis and allows the bowel to rest. When there is chronic intractability of symptoms, surgery is sometimes necessary. For the preoperative patient, parenteral nutrition decreases morbidity in those cases where there has been weight loss and extended debilitation.[25]

ULCERATIVE COLITIS

Nature of Condition

Although Crohn's disease can occur in any portion of the gastrointestinal tract, ulcerative colitis is limited to the colon and usually involves the surface and mucosal layers of the intestinal wall. Like Crohn's disease, it has no known specific cause. Its course is varied and protracted. Many investigators report that it is being seen with increasing frequency in adolescents. In this age group it is a severe disease.

Nutritional Needs

Although short stature is more often seen in Crohn's disease, 20% to 30% of prepubertal patients with ulcerative colitis also have short stature. Decreased energy intake is recognized as a major factor in this growth retardation. Combined parenteral and oral feeding that provides 130% to 140% of estimated energy needs usually will promote growth. Some authors advocate an unlimited diet based on the conviction that diet does not affect colonic symptoms and that freedom of choice is useful for overcoming anorexia and maintaining positive nitrogen balance. Others suggest restriction of roughage and spices. Folic acid deficiency is occasionally seen in patients whose diets have been restricted in fiber and leafy vegetables. Zinc deficiency may also be a factor in growth failure of children with ulcerative colitis or Crohn's disease. Thus it is wise to measure serum zinc levels in adolescents with either form of inflammatory bowel disease and use zinc supplementation if levels are low.

There is no evidence that any specific diet prevents relapse in patients with ulcerative colitis. However, persons who have diarrhea despite optimal medical management should be tested for lactose intolerance, as lactose absorption can be abnormal in up to 20% of these patients.[25]

NEOPLASTIC DISEASE

Nature of the Condition

Cancers make up the leading nonaccidental cause of death in the 10- to 21-year-old age group in the United States. The types of common tumors differ from malignancies found in adults. Leukemia, malignant lymphomas, bone tumors, and neural lesions are the ones most frequently seen in adolescents. In the past decade a significant improvement in survival has been observed in children and teenagers who are managed by aggressive use of multimodal therapies including surgery, chemotherapy, and radiotherapy. Complex interactions occur between nutrition and cancer, many of them caused by cancer therapy, and there are signs that *cachexia,* a state of severe protein and energy malnutrition, is a significant cause of mortality.

Nutritional Needs

Teenagers with cancer may be at particular risk for nutritional depletion because: (1) added energy for continued growth and development is required, (2) food preferences are strong, (3) malabsorption is often severe and sudden. Also, the immature immune system is more susceptible to the effects of malnutrition than the adult system. Nutritional problems can arise from the disease or the therapy and are best addressed immediately upon diagnosis. Thus the clinical nutritionist should be a part of the professional care team from the beginning stages of the disease. Nutrition assessment including anthropometric data levels of serum albumin and total protein, as well as a comprehensive diet history, should be the first step in the nutritional management of the teenager newly diagnosed as having cancer. This initial nutritional therapy can be followed by daily monitoring of energy intake and recommendations for continuing therapy tailored to meet the needs of each individual. Oral alimentation is the preferred route of nutritional therapy. The principal goal is prevention of weight loss.[4]

DIABETES MELLITUS

Most experts agree that a diet emphasizing regularly scheduled meals and eliminating concentrated sweets is as effective as a traditional exchange diet for controlling diabetes in adolescents. Increased fiber content appears to improve control. The diet should be limited in fat.[25]

HYPERTENSION AND HYPERLIPIDEMIA

If an adolescent is hypertensive or has a strong family history of the disease, a diet controlled in sodium and total energy is a part of long-term nutritional care. In the case of hyperlipidemia, fat and total energy intake should be controlled. All adolescents should be cautioned against a high intake of sodium, fat, and energy because of the suspected link with cardiovascular disease.[4,5]

ANEMIA

When anemia, one of the most common nutritional disorders in adolescents, is diagnosed it will need medical treatment with iron in the short term. In the long term, a diet rich in all nutrients, especially iron, in proportion to energy value is required to maintain health in all types of anemia, including sickle cell disease.[4]

INBORN ERRORS OF METABOLISM

Mandatory newborn screening laws now govern early diagnosis and care of infants with a number of these genetic disorders, and skilled professional teams including the clinical nutritionist as a key therapist have established regional metabolic centers throughout the United States. As a result, the number of children with metabolic errors who are healthy and growing normally is increasing. The basic care is nutritional, providing the necessary balance of nutrients to prevent symptoms, support normal growth and development, and thus avoid long-term harmful effects of poor control. The largest group of young persons with metabolic errors currently are those with *phenylketonuria (PKU).* It has now been well established that teenagers with PKU need to remain on their low-phenylalanine diet in order to maintain their normal mental development and a stable behavior pattern. Because of the systemic consequences, those with other metabolic errors will also need to maintain their controlled diets into adulthood.[27]

DENTAL CARIES AND PERIODONTAL DISEASE

It is becoming apparent that the cause of dental caries is a complex process involving the interaction of several factors. The minerals of the tooth enamel are in constant equilibrium with the oral environment. It is necessary therefore to consider not only the presence of fermentable carbohydrate but also such factors as food solubility, mineral composition, and the buffering capacity of the oral environment. Adolescents' propensity to snack on refined carbohydrates is conducive to tooth decay. Since 80% of the average person's total incidence of dental lesions occur in the teenage years, this is the time to encourage habits built on choosing alternatives to sugar-containing foods.

Gingivitis increases in prevalence during the teenage years, and periodontal disease often follows. Little is known about nutrition's role in periodontal disease, although deficiency in ascorbic acid has received a great deal of attention as an important cause. Vitamin A deficiency, widespread in underdeveloped countries with high incidences of periodontal disease, has also been implicated. Inadequate intake of these nutrients in the teen years can have an adverse effect on the health of the gums in later life.

ACNE

Initiated by the influence of hormones on the sebaceous glands, acne is a normal characteristic of adolescent development. It occurs in varying degrees of severity in individual teenagers, mediated by factors such as stress and phase of the menstrual cycle.[28] Almost all adolescents have acne and as many as half of all adolescent contacts with health professionals are associated with dermatologic complaints. Traditionally, dietary factors have been blamed for the appearance of acne. But studies have shown no correlation between ingestion of foods and the appearance or degree of this condition.

Education about the physiologic basis for the development of acne supports teenagers in their efforts to control it. Systemic antibiotics given orally and topical applications of benzoyl peroxide and tretinoin, as well as special cleansing agents, have been shown to be effective.

It has been suggested that pharmacologic levels of zinc and the vitamin A derivatives are useful in treating acne. Low levels of serum zinc have been found in one study among the persons suffering most, suggesting that zinc deficiency makes the condition worse. In general, while no research is available to confirm the effect, it would seem that the optimally nourished body will be best able to cope with the development of acne as with many conditions.

DEVELOPMENTAL ISSUES

For many adolescents with chronic disease the social complications of their disorder are often more debilitating than the physical effects. For these young persons it is extremely valuable to have the services of many professionals—psychologists, social workers, and nutritionists—in addition to physicians and nurses. Teenagers as a group may show poor compliance even under the best of circumstances, and the regimen has to be kept as liberal and supportive as possible. It is important to help adolescents develop the type of self-awareness and perspective illustrated in Fig. 8-10 that will enable them to become allies in the treatment of their disease.

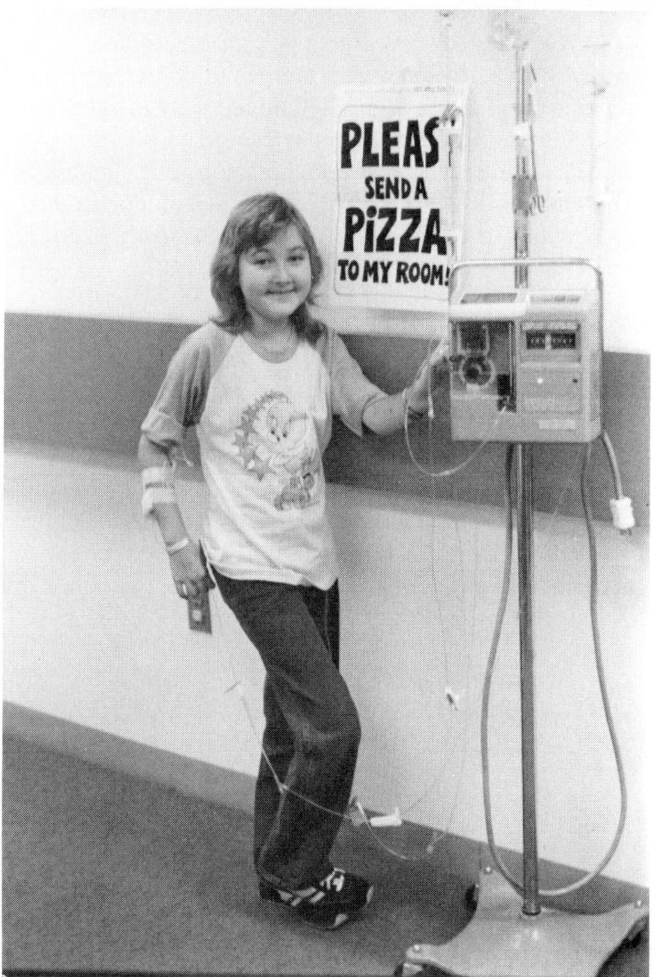

FIG. 8-10 Teenager receiving total parenteral nutrition who is asserting her independence.

Nutrition and Adolescent Behavior

POPULAR THEORIES

The popular press has given widespread attention to untested theories about the effect of nutrition on behavior, leading to the acceptance of these theories by people who do not have access to further information. Examples of these theories, some of which are discussed in the previous chapter, are that an abundance of sugar, intoxication with heavy metals, food additives, and allergic reactions are responsible for behaviors ranging from shortened attention span to learning disorders to criminal behavior. Such ideas develop as part of the effort to find environmental causes for behaviors that lead some adolescents into serious difficulties.

INFLUENCE OF NUTRIENTS ON NEUROLOGIC FUNCTION AND BEHAVIOR

Meanwhile recent research advances reveal that certain dietary factors will alter brain function or behavior by acting as dietary precursors of neurotransmitters (Fig. 8-11). At present these principles can be clinically applied only in rare neurologic disorders, with nutrients being used at pharmacologic levels. Theories that subclinical deficiences of certain nutrients influence neurologic function have centered on iron and the B vitamins, and have not led to clinically applicable intervention strategies. The types of change brought about in research studies have never been related to behaviors involved in crime.[29]

IMPLICATIONS FOR COMMUNITY RESPONSIBILITY AND POLICY

If educators and those responsible for juvenile detention facilities accept untested theories, they spend public resources in ineffective programs. To demonstrate reasonable concern about nutrition, all institutions should support the teenagers they serve by making nourishing foods available to them. Such policy will involve screening out less valuable foods that are tempting and commercially rewarding, such as those often sold in vending machines. Resulting improvements in positive nutritional status will contribute to individual physical health. But at this time such well-being cannot be counted on to prevent attention disorders or learning problems, much less criminal behavior.[29]

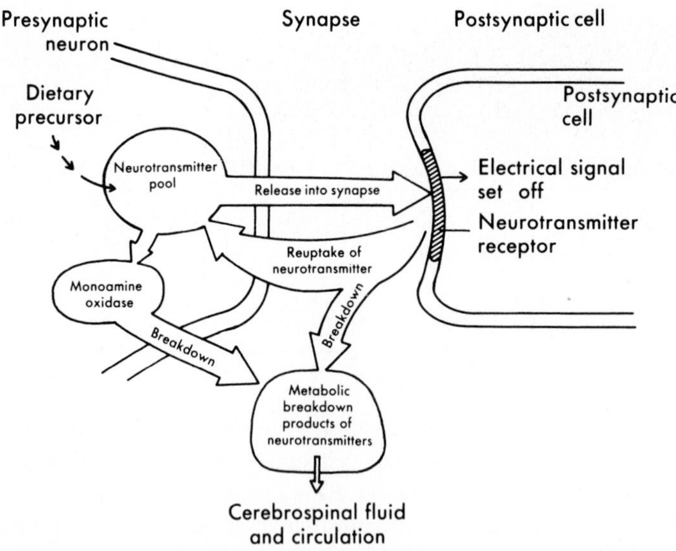

FIG. 8-11 Neurotransmitter formation and metabolism at synapse in nervous system.

Adolescent Pregnancy

DEVELOPMENTAL ISSUES

Teenage pregnancy must be studied in light of the highly dynamic nature of adolescence. Both the psychologic and the physical status of the adolescent have implications for the course of any pregnancy. The many interactions of factors in adolescent development and in reproduction have great clinical significance for all aspects of the pregnancy, including the nutritional aspect.[30] Indeed, adolescents are changing so profoundly that pregnancy for the younger, less mature teenager will be different than for the older, more mature adolescent.

Less mature teenagers will be more dependent on others and less able to act and make decisions on their own. They will be more narcissistic and less able to comprehend the needs of others. These young women will be less realistic, engage in more fantasy and wishful thinking, and have less insight into their own behaviors and motives. In general, younger teenagers will have fewer intellectual and physical skills to cope with any situation, especially a complex reproductive experience. Many of the difficulties related to pregnancy in adolescence stem from this immaturity. As development advances, a person is able to carry out reproduction and child-rearing in a more normal, less problem-fraught way. As seen in Fig. 8-12, the timeline of events in teenage pregnancy has great potential for affecting the nutritional well-being of the adolescent.

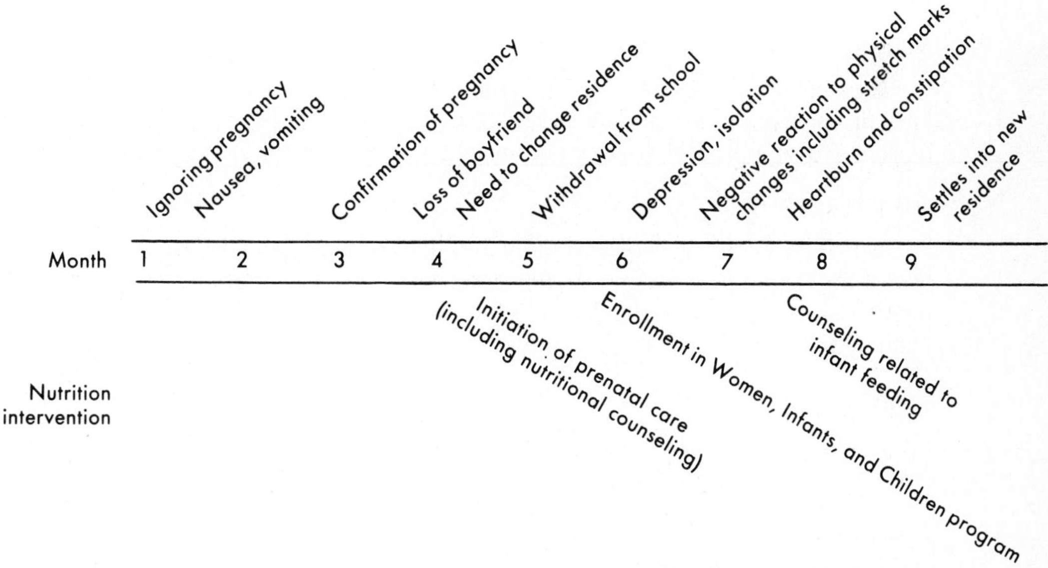

FIG. 8-12 Typical events in teen pregnancy that could affect intake or utilization of nutrients.

REPRODUCTION DURING ADOLESCENCE

The pregnant adolescent's nutritional needs are influenced by many factors. Primary influences are her growth and nutrient stores, her gynecologic age, and her preconception nutritional status.

Adolescent Growth and Nutrient Stores

The assumption that pregnant adolescents need a supply of nutrients to support their own growth along with that of the growing fetus has been questioned. Because hormone levels are high in pregnancy even the slower adolescent growth that usually follows menarche may not occur.[31] Nonetheless, whether or not actual statural growth continues for an adolescent who becomes pregnant, she will have experienced rapid growth more recently than her adult counterparts. There will have been less opportunity for storage of nutrients. Thus there may be greater physiologic risk to young women who conceive in the early years after the onset of the menses.

Gynecologic Age

The number of years between the onset of menses and conception is calculated to derive gynecologic age. Those adolescents who are more sexually mature, that is, of greater gynecologic age, share a vulnerability to physiologic stresses but appear to have no more physically based complications than do adult women. It is the young women of lower gynecologic age who carry more risk and need more nutritional support. The number of adolescents who become pregnant in the first two years following menarche will be relatively small because most of them will not be ovulating during that time though they are menstruating. Those who do become pregnant, however, are of great concern to clinicians and researchers in this area.

Nutritional Status at Conception

Pregnant adolescents who are of young gynecologic age and malnourished at the time of conception are at double risk. They appear to have the greatest need for nutrients to support a pregnancy and maintain optimal health themselves.[32]

HAZARDS TO THE MOTHER

Given the complexity of pregnancy in the adolescent period, it is logical to question how these young women fare during pregnancy. They have more complications, a higher risk of maternal mortality, and more problems in personal psychologic development and education that carry implications for economic well-being.

Complications

The variety of complications often described for the teenage mother during gestation includes:

- First and third trimester bleeding
- Anemia
- Difficult labor and delivery
- Cephalopelvic disproportion
- Pregnancy-induced hypertensive disorders including pre-eclampsia and eclampsia

Of these complications, the most common physical problem is pre-eclampsia. The disorder usually manifests itself in the third trimester by increased weight gain, fluid retention, high blood pressure, and proteinuria, and does not appear to run a different course in pregnant teenagers than in older women. Some researchers point out that it is a disease of first pregnancies. By and large, data support this observation. In addition, the harmful effects of pre-eclampsia, or the more serious state of eclampsia, may be greater in teenagers. Damage to the cardiovascular and renal systems initiated with a first pregnancy early in life and intensified by insults such as other pregnancies can increase the risk of developing renal and cardiovascular problems with increasing age.

Maternal Mortality

The serious risk of maternal mortality is also a problem. The rate is 2½ times greater for mothers under 15 years of age than for those 20 to 24 years of age.

Effect on Normal Developmental Steps

Apart from the physical sequelae, pregnancy often affects teenagers' psychological development, education, and ability to gain economic independence. Clearly these developmental steps are difficult to achieve in any case, and for many adolescents pregnancy is not a cause of failure but a coinciding event. The situations responsible for early pregnancy often remain unresolved, and many teenage mothers have additional pregnancies before the adolescent years are over.

A review of all the factors that influence the well-being of the teenage mother and implications for nutritional care are summarized in Table 8-11.

HAZARDS TO THE INFANT

Infants born to teenage mothers suffer a higher incidence of morbidity and mortality in the perinatal period than infants of older mothers experience. Problems seen more frequently include:[33]

- Prematurity
- Stillbirth
- Low birth weight, the major hazard in adolescent pregnancy
- Perinatal and infant deaths
- Physical deformities

It is difficult to compare the likelihood of these problems occurring in infants born to teenage versus older mothers, or to younger versus older teenage mothers. But it is generally agreed that the problems do occur in a considerable number of teenage pregnancies. For example, the incidence of low birth weight is far greater when the mothers are adolescents. Factors that increase risk to these infants are summarized in Table 8-11.

PATTERNS OF WEIGHT GAIN

Since the late 1960s, the suggested weight gain for pregnant women has been about 11.25 to 13.5 kg (25 to 30 lb). There is no evidence, however, that this weight gain suggested for adult women is optimal for adolescents.

TABLE 8-11 Review of Factors Affecting Well-Being of Adolescent Pregnant Women and Their Infants

Factor	Effect	Mode of Effect	Implications for Nutritional Care
IMPACT ON ADOLESCENT PREGANT WOMEN			
Economics	Economic situation is cited as single most important factor in determining outcome.	Economics determine both type and amount of medical care and health of self and ancestors.	Mobilizing food resources is of highest priority.
Prenatal care	Quantity and quality of prenatal care are universally mentioned as affecting outcome; advantages of care are evident when health complications in populations without care are compared to those with care.	There is debate as to whether incidence of pre-eclampsia can be decreased to that of adult populations; otherwise, comprehensive care appears to reduce incidence of physical complications to that of adult populations.	Care for adolescents should be comprehensive, including services of nutritionists and professionals in the psychosocial fields; teachers and others should encourage early prenatal care.
Age	Although difficult to study as sole uncontrolled variable, it is generally acknowledged that, with possible exception of eclampsia and pre-eclampsia, adolescents are not at greater physical risk for complications than older mothers; psychosocial and economic factors, however, are more likely to have an impact.	Hypothetically, physical effect may be greatest in women of low gynecological age; studies assessing impact of low gynecological age have not looked at impact on physical complications to the mother, but it was not predictive of development of pre-eclampsia in one study.	Younger adolescents need greatest attention, as they are usually without traditional supports; those of low gynecological age are possibly at greatest biological risk.
Malnutrition	Although still debated, cause-and-effect relationship is still possible.	Severe anemia is associated with high morbidity and mortality; the following nutrients have been implicated in the disease process but not conclusively shown to cause toxemia: Calcium, iron, vitamin A (because they are consistently low in diets of young women)	Effective techniques to encourage the consumption of nutrient-rich foods should be major component of prenatal counseling for adolescents.

		Thiamin Vitamin B_6 Folic acid Excess dietary sodium Greater consumption of total fats and cholesterol Generalized malnutrition When mother is malnourished, fetus draws on mother's depleted stores, resulting in decreased energy and ability to support reproduction.	
IMPACT ON INFANTS			
Maternal stress	Maternal stress is high in teen pregnancy; there is no direct evidence this causes increased problems for the fetus, but outcomes are more favorable when teens have support of others.	Stress may interfere with maintenance of satisfactory nutritional status and intrauterine environment.	Stress in pregnant teen's life must be considered in providing nutritional counseling; nutritionists and other clinicians must support pregnant teenage patients in stressful situations.
Maternal infections	The following are common infections concurrent with pregnancy: Viral infections—influenza, herpes, upper respiratory infections Protozoan infections—toxoplasmosis Sexually transmitted diseases—gonorrhea, syphilis, chlamydial infections Depending on agent, effects on fetus range from no damage to mild complications (for example, increased susceptibility to disease) to severe damage (for example, prematurity, congenital anomalies, abortion, stillbirth).	In addition to direct effect of agent, increased requirement for nutrients may create inadequacy for fetus.	Adolescents with infections during pregnancy are among priority patients for nutritional care; the goal is adequate nourishment to restore health and to meet requirements of pregnancy.

Continued.

TABLE 8-11 Review of Factors Affecting Well-Being of Adolescent Pregnant Women and Their Infants—cont'd

Factor	Effect	Mode of Effect	Implications for Nutritional Care
IMPACT ON INFANTS—cont'd			
Maternal malnutrition	Knowledge of role of specific nutritional deficiencies or excesses on development of problems in infant in human populations of developed countries is limited, although subjective evaluations suggest positive outcomes associated with well-nourished state.	Correlation is known to exist between maternal hemoglobin level and infant birth weight; it is suspected that anemia in mother augments maternal cardiac output to assure sufficient amount of inferior-quality blood is pumped to placenta to provide for fetus; with marginal malnutrition, both mother and infant will have less strength to establish bonding and feeding patterns; severe malnutrition retards cellular growth; nutritional supplementation of severely malnourished pregnant women reduces incidence of low birth weight but not necessarily anomalies; supplementation in teen population did not significantly decrease incidence of low birth weight but significantly increased mean birth weight.	Since nutrition and feeding can be controlled to assure a healthy fetal and infant environment, nutrition services are an important component of prenatal programs for adolescents; preparation for and follow-up of child-feeding practices by teen parents should be included.
Weight gain of mother	Prepregnant weight and weight gain are more important than either gynecological or chronological age in determining frequency of low-birth-weight infants born to adolescents.	Weight and height are clinically measurable evidence of nutritional status in societies with high standard of living where specific nutritional deficiencies are rare; evidence linking weight gain to infant birth weight is readily available; inadequate weight gain is associated with increased incidence of low-	Nutritional counseling for pregnant teens should place emphasis on adequate weight gain, especially for underweight patients.

		birth-weight infants and subsequent increase in neonatal morbidity and mortality; weight gain may have intergenerational effect (women small at birth are more likely to have small infants than women average or large at birth).	
Maternal age	Biological immaturity was initially suspected cause of higher fetal complications and loss found in adolescent pregnancies; when psychological stress, economics, and other variables are controlled, age not shown responsible; possible exceptions are rare teens who are pregnant at low gynecological age who have high frequency of low-birth-weight infants; two studies of this were inconclusive, as gynecological age was not sole uncontrolled variable (for example, nutritional status was not controlled); effects of young age were not overcome by improved services in years between 1978 and 1981.	It has been suggested that structurally and functionally immature uterus has less than optimal vascular system and may react unfavorably to ovarian hormones; possible biochemical evidence of nutritional risks is the competition for nutrients between immature gravida and fetus indicated by 2+ acetonuria found in 5% at age 10-14, 2% age 17-32 (fetal and neonatal death is 56% more frequent with 2+ acetonuria); psychological characteristics of "premature parents" such as unreasonable expectations for children and their parental abilities mediate unfavorable outcomes (for example, teen parents thought children would talk and be toilet trained by 6 months); failure to meet expectations contributes to infant morbidity and mortality.	Gynecological age of adolescent patients may be predictor of biological risk to infants; support for developing realistic expectations and parenting skills in younger teens affects both psychological and biological consequences for the infant and must be built into prenatal and postnatal care protocols.
Prenatal care	Specialized comprehensive prenatal care is an important factor in decreasing adverse biological effects of teen pregnancy on the newborn; nutrition services are an integral part of such care.	Comprehensive adolescent prenatal program reports 9% of infants versus 20.9% of those born to adolescents in general prenatal program weighed less than 2500 gm (5.5 lb).	Pregnant teens should be high priority among vulnerable population groups when nutrition services are scarce.

Individual Needs

Following the prenatal client's progress in weight gain has become standard clinical practice in many health-care facilities. In fact, many mothers are actively counseled to gain at the rate indicated by the curve seen in Fig. 4-9 so as to achieve a total gain in the suggested range if possible. However, variation from this pattern is normal. Each mother's optimal weight gain should be determined and sufficient nutritional support provided to help her achieve it.

Underweight Adolescents

Teenagers who were underweight at the time of conception should be encouraged to gain more weight than normal-weight or overweight teens should gain. This would allow for improvement of nutritional status, the need for which is indicated by the initial low weight-for-height proportion, and for continued nourishment during pregnancy.

Adolescent Growth Stage

Another factor supporting higher weight gain for adolescents is that the normal weight increment of the particular stage of adolescent growth and development is probably needed, in addition to the typical gestational gain. Thus, in the case of the underweight adolescent, adding both increments to the normal recommended gain yields the suggested weight gain for this teenage mother.[32] The weight gain necessary for her to reach the "critical body mass" to support a normal pregnancy might be calculated as follows:

_____ To bring weight to normal for height

_____ For the 9-month postmenarcheal interval corresponding to gynecologic age (Table 8-12)

_____ For the pregnancy 11.25 to 12.5 kg (25-30 lb)

_____ TOTAL

Research is becoming available to show that a weight gain of about 15.9 kg (35 lb) is common among adolescent mothers who bear normal-weight infants.[34]

ASSESSMENT AND MANAGEMENT OF NUTRITION

Risk Factors

In order that nutrition services can be provided efficiently and effectively, pregnant teenage clients should be screened for those risk factors most closely linked to poor outcomes. Significant factors include:

- Low gynecologic age
- Low prepregnancy weight for height, or other significant evidence of malnutrition
- Low pregnancy weight gain
- Infections during pregnancy
- Excessive pregnancy weight gain
- Excessive weight for height at conception

TABLE 8-12 Approximate Increments in Weight of Postmenarcheal Women

Postmenarcheal Year	Pounds	Kilograms
1	10.12	4.6
2	6.16	2.8
3	2.42	1.1
4 and 5	1.76	0.8

Data from Frisch, R.E.: Hum. Biol. **48**:353, 1976.

Other risk factors gathered from history:

- Unhealthy lifestyle
- Unfavorable reproductive history
- Chronic diseases

Overall assessment of nutritional status of the pregnant teenager follows more or less the general pattern for nutritional assessment of all pregnant women.

Nutrient Needs

A summary of recommended amounts of nutrients is provided in Table 8-13. It combines the allowance for pregnancy in adult women with the amounts recommend-

TABLE 8-13 Recommended Dietary Allowances for Pregnant Adolescent Females

	Age (Reference Height)			
	11-14 yr (157 cm)		15-18 yr (163 cm)	
Nutrient	Total RDA	RDA/cm	Total RDA	RDA/cm
Energy (kcal)	2500	15.9	2400	14.7
Protein (gm)	76	0.48	76	0.47
Calcium (mg)	1600	10.2	1600	9.8
Phosphorus (mg)	1600	10.2	1600	9.8
Iron (mg)	18*		18*	
Magnesium (mg)	450	2.9	450	2.7
Iodine (μg)	175	1.1	175	1.1
Zinc (mg)	20	0.13	20	0.12
Vitamin A (μg RE)	1000	6.4	1000	6.1
Vitamin D (μg)	15	0.09	15	0.09
Vitamin E (mg α-TE)	10	0.06	10	0.06
Ascorbic acid (mg)	70	0.45	80	0.49
Niacin (mg NE)	17	0.11	16	0.10
Riboflavin (mg)	1.6	0.01	1.6	0.01
Thiamin (mg)	1.5	0.01	1.5	0.01
Folacin (μg)	800	5.1	800	4.9
Vitamin B (mg)	2.4	0.02	2.6	0.02
Vitamin B_{12} (μg)	4	0.03	4	0.02

Modified from Food and Nutrition Board, National Research Council: Recommended dietary allowances, ed. 9, Washington, D.C., 1980, National Academy of Sciences.
*Supplemental iron recommended

ISSUES IN ADOLESCENT PREGNANCY THAT INFLUENCE NUTRITIONAL WELL-BEING

Acceptance of the Pregnancy

Desire to carry out successful pregnancy
Acceptance of responsibility (even if child is to be relinquished)
Clarification of identity as mother separate from her own mother
Realistic acceptance versus fantasy and idealization

Food Resources

Family meals (timing, quantity, quality, responsibility)
Self-reliance
School lunch
Fast-food outlets
Socially related eating
Food assistance (WIC program and others)
Mobilization of all resources

Body Image

Degree of acceptance of an adult body
Maturity in facing bodily changes throughout pregnancy

Living Situation

Acceptance by living partners and extended family
Role expectations of living partners
Financial support
Facilities and resources
Ethnic group (religious, cultural, and social patterns)
Emancipation versus dependency
Support system versus isolation

Relationship with the Father of Child

Presence or absence of father
Quality of relationship
Influence on decision making
Contribution to resources
Influence on mother's nutritional habits and general lifestyle
Understanding of physiological processes
Tolerance of physical changes in pregnancy and physical needs of mother and child
Influence on child feeding

ISSUES IN ADOLESCENT PREGNANCY THAT INFLUENCE NUTRITIONAL WELL-BEING—cont'd

Peer Relationships

Support from friends
Influence on nutritional knowledge and attitudes
Influence on general lifestyle

Nutritional State

Weight-for-height proportion
Maturational state
Tissue stores of nutrients
Reproductive and contraceptive history
Physical health
History of dietary patterns and nutritional status, including weight-losing schemes
Present eating habits
Complications of pregnancy (nausea and vomiting)
Substance use
Activity patterns
Need for intensive remediation

Prenatal Care

Initiation of and compliance with prenatal care
Dependability of supporting resources
Identification of risk factors

Nutritional Attitude and Knowledge

Prior attitude toward nutrition
Understanding of role of nutrition in pregnancy
Knowledge of foods as sources of nutrients and of nutrients needed by the body
Desire to obtain adequate nutrition
Ability to obtain adequate nutrition and to control food supply

Preparation for Child Feeding

Knowledge of child-feeding practices
Attitude and decisions about child feeding
Responsibility for feeding
Understanding the importance of the bonding process
Support from family and friends

ed for nonpregnant adolescents. A clinically practical way of assuring nutrient adequacy is to encourage the pregnant adolescent to gain the recommended amount of weight by consuming nutrient-rich foods. Sources of protein, calcium, iron, micronutrients, and dietary fiber are important. Contact with health professionals during prenatal care provides many important opportunities to teach adolescents about feeding themselves and their families. A clinical protocol for nutritional management of adolescent pregnancy is provided here (see box, pp. 367-368).

Economic and Psychosocial Needs

The economic instability of pregnant adolescents makes it impossible to assume that they will have an adequate food supply. The impact of lifestyle, economics, and other stressful issues on the nutritional well-being of young pregnant women is great and must be acknowledged in any program to improve their nutritional status. A summary of these issues is provided here (see box). Above all, the stage of social and emotional development will determine the mother's ability to cope with all aspects of reproduction.

Involving the Father of the Baby

When the partner of the young pregnant woman is available, he should be included in counseling sessions to build mutual nutritional support for the pregnancy. Specific outreach to the father of the baby can be beneficial. If he is employed or in school, an effort should be made to see him at least occasionally. This effort will be especially important if for some reason he is interfering with the young woman's ability to nourish herself. Sharing what is known about the father's contribution to the outcome of pregnancy helps some adolescent males become more interested in maintaining healthy living habits.

Individualized Counseling

To be effective, the clinician must work within the context of an individualized counseling relationship with the young pregnant adolescent and her partner.[30] The counselor will not "prescribe" but make practical suggestions and give support for changing of the teenager's habits, usually in small increments, throughout the pregnancy.

Benefits of Nutrition Counseling

The benefits of nutrition counseling will generally be seen more in the long term than in a particular pregnancy. Prenatal care is one of the best opportunities to teach a vulnerable group of teenagers sound nutritional information. Even if they seek care late in pregnancy and miss appointments, for most of them these contacts constitute the greatest input of health care during their adolescence.

Energy and Nutrient Intake

Helping pregnant adolescents follow the suggested weight-gain curve can ensure sufficient energy intake to support the pregnancy and the mother's own developmen-

PROTOCOL FOR MANAGEMENT OF NORMAL TEENAGE PREGNANCY

Initial Evaluation

Review social and lifestyle history
Review clinical data
- Height and weight
- Arm muscle circumference
- Physical signs of health
- Expected delivery date

Review laboratory data
- Hematocrit or hemoglobin
- Urinalysis

Begin to build relationship with the patient (and partner if available)
Assess intake patterns using dietary methodology best suited to patient and professional
Make preliminary assessment of food resources and refer to supportive agencies if necessary
Check for nausea and vomiting and suggest remedy
Assess attitude toward weight gain
Discuss supplemental vitamins and minerals
Make initial plan that sets priorities for issues
Come to agreement with patient about any initial changes and steps to take
Do initial anthropometrics—calculate allowable weight gain

Follow-up Visit

Check on referrals to other agencies.
Discuss results of evaluation and suggest any changes necessary in dietary patterns (use printed materials *as appropriate*)
Do any further investigations necessary
- Laboratory studies
  - Protoporphyrin heme or serum ferritin, Serum folate — For specific diagnosis of anemia
  - Serum albumin, Serum transferrin — For suspected undernutrition
  - Vitamin B_{12} — For vegan
- Further probing of dietary habits if necessary

Use motivating audiovisuals
Monitor weight gain and attitude of acceptance starting with patient's prepregnant weight status; discuss projected weight gain for following visit and total for gestation.
Assess and address issues affecting nutritional status in order of priority for the individual.

PROTOCOL FOR MANAGEMENT OF NORMAL TEENAGE PREGNANCY—cont'd

Subsequent Visits

Monitor and support appropriate weight gain: include discussion of fitness and encourage habitual safe exercise

Support upgrade in nutritional pattern in support of the woman and the developing infant: augment knowledge of principles of nutrition: continue to address issues affecting nutritional status.

Check for heartburn, small food-intake capacity, and elimination problems: suggest dietary interventions.

Monitor urinary ketones and protein–glucose tolerance at 28-32 wks

Final Visits

Discuss infant feeding if patient will keep infant

Help patient to understand safe methods of managing weight following delivery

tal needs. Following the guidelines demonstrates dramatically in a few months the possibility of exerting personal control over eating, as well as the effect on both weight and nutritional status, in a way the teenager can understand. There is great appeal in discussing with adolescents the effects of various events on their bodies and on the growing fetus. Learning about the physiologic needs of both her own body and her developing infant can be the teenager's impetus for upgrading the quality of her diet to keep pace with the increase in energy intake needed to support adequate weight gain. Repeated counseling sessions to review those needs may motivate the young mother to try new foods to obtain additional sources of nutrients. Attention to nutritional health in the prenatal period can become a model for taking responsibility for feeding a family. The young woman can gain experience in the use of community resources to obtain food for herself and her family.

In summary, nutrition counseling in prenatal care for teenagers can accomplish the following goals:

1. Serve as a model for exerting control over what a person eats with visible results in terms of the optimal weight-gain pattern and the quality of foods contributing to it.
2. Be an impetus for trying new foods.
3. Serve as a model for taking responsibility and using community resources to feed a family.

The nutrition counselor will be most effective when working within a clinical program designed especially for adolescents. Such programs have been shown to improve overall outcome in adolescent pregnancy.[35]

Summary

The physical and psychosocial gains in development are rapid and all-encompassing in the adolescent period of human life. The parameters of physical growth are the basis for determining nutritional needs. Eating behavior is influenced to a great extent at this time by the developing body image and by the total culture, as a result of breaking ties with the family. Thus if health professionals hope to help adolescents improve their nutritional patterns they must use appropriate tactics. They will need to sort out fact and reality in terms of the realistic role of nutrition in health and behavior. Emphasis must be placed on physical fitness as an important way to help all adolescents balance energy intake and output.

In eating disorders the overall objective is to help the individual put the eating function into proper perspective. The athlete must obtain sufficient nourishment to support a growing body subjected to stress. In chronic diseases the diet must eliminate nutrients that cause symptoms and be supplemented if necessary to allow growth to continue. If a pregnancy should occur, the adolescent will need support in nourishing herself and her developing infant during a chaotic time. While a great deal is still unknown about nutritional needs of adolescents, the growing interest in this age group should stimulate the research necessary to close gaps in our knowledge.

Review Questions

1. Define the terms *adolescence* and *puberty*. Explain how they are related.
2. Draw the growth velocity curve for males and females from birth to adulthood and describe the implications of different stages on the nutritional needs of humans.
3. Discuss the reasons for not using commonly available growth grids to assess weight-height proportion in adolescents and the alternate database that is appropriate.
4. Describe ways in which psychologic development impacts nutritional status of adolescents.
5. Discuss the commonalities and differences of specifically recognized syndromes across the spectrum of eating disorders.
6. Describe how you would set up a comprehensive weight management program for teenagers in a community where none had ever existed before.
7. It has been proposed that adolescents need to gain more weight during pregnancy than adult women do. What aspects of adolescent growth and development lead to the idea that these larger gains are beneficial?
8. What is the common goal regarding nutrition in any of the special conditions or chronic disorders an adolescent may face?

REFERENCES

1. Tanner, J.M.: Foetus into man, Cambridge, Mass., 1978, Harvard University Press.
2. Newman, B., and Newman, P.: Adolescent development, Columbus, Oh., 1986, Charles E. Merrill.

3. McKigney, J.I., and Munro, H.N., eds.: Nutrient requirements in adolescence, Cambridge, Mass., 1976, The MIT Press.
4. Gong, E., and Heald, F.T.: Diet, nutrition, and adolescence. In Shils, M., and Young, V.R., eds.: Modern nutrition in health and disease, ed. 7, Philadelphia, 1987, Lea & Febiger.
5. Thompson, P., and others: Zinc status and sexual development in adolescent girls, J. Am. Diet. Assoc. **86**:892, 1986.
6. Dwyer, J.P.: Diets for children and adolescents that meet the dietary goals, Am. J. Dis. Child. **134**:1073, 1980.
7. Penninger, J.A.T., and others: Mineral content of foods and total diets: the selected minerals in foods survey, 1982-1984, J. Am. Diet. Assoc. **86**:876, 1986.
8. Leverton, R.M.: The paradox of teenage nutrition, J. Am. Diet. Assoc. **56**:116, 1968.
9. McCoy, H., and others: Snacking patterns and nutrient density of snacks consumed by southern girls, J. Nutr. Educ. **18**:61, 1986.
10. Morgan, K.J., Zabik, M.E., and Stampley, G.L.: Breakfast consumption patterns of U.S. children and adolescents, Nutr. Res. **6**:635, 1986.
11. Story, M., and Resnick, M.D.: Adolescents' views on food and nutrition, J. Nutr. Educ. **18**:188, 1986.
12. Snetselarr, L.G.: Nutritional counseling skills: assessment, treatment, and evaluation, Rockville, Md., 1983, Aspen Publishers, Inc.
13. Bruch, H.: Eating disorders, New York, 1973, Basic Books, Inc.
14. Minuchin, S., Rosman, B.L., and Baker, L.: Psychosomatic families: anorexia nervosa in context, Cambridge, Mass., 1978, Harvard University Press.
15. Diagnostic and statistical manual of mental disorders, ed. 3, Washington, D.C., 1980, American Psychiatric Association.
16. Garfinkel, P.E., and Garner, D.M.: Anorexia nervosa: a multidimensional perspective, New York, 1982, Brunner/Mazel.
17. Crisp, A.H.: Anorexia nervosa: let me be, New York, 1980, Grune and Stratton, Inc.
18. Keys, A., and others: The biology of human starvation, Minneapolis, 1950, University of Minnesota Press.
19. Pyle, R., Mitchell, J.E., and Eckert, E.D.: Bulimia, a report of 34 cases, J. Clin. Psych. **42**(2):60, 1981.
20. Polivy, J., and Herman, C.P.: Dieting and binging: a causal analysis, Am. Psychol. **40**:193, 1985.
21. Stunkard, A.J., ed.: Obesity, Philadelphia, 1980, W.B. Saunders Co.
22. Coates, T., and Thoresen, C.: Treating obesity in children and adolescents: a review, Am. J. Public Health **68**:143, 1978.
23. McArdle, W.D., Katch, F.I., and Katch, V.L.: Exercise physiology: energy, nutrition, and human performance, ed. 2, Philadelphia, 1986, Lea & Febiger.
24. O'Neil, F.T., Hynak-Hankinson, M.T., and Gorman, J.: Research and application of current topics in sports nutrition, J. Am. Diet. Assoc. **86**:1007, 1986.
25. Krause, M.V., and Mahan, L.K.: Food, nutrition, and diet therapy, ed. 7, Philadelphia, 1984, W.B. Saunders Co.
26. Adams, L.J., and Mahan, L.K.: Nutritional care in food allergy and food intolerance. In Krause, M.V., and Mahan, L.K.: Food, nutrition, and diet therapy, ed. 7, Philadelphia, 1984, W.B. Saunders Co.
27. Trahms, C.M.: Nutritional care for children with metabolic disorder. In Krause, M.V., and Mahan, L.K.: Food, nutrition, and diet therapy, ed. 7, Philadelphia, 1984, W.B. Saunders Co.
28. Cunliffe, W.: Dermatology, acne vulgaris, Br. J. Hosp. Med. **20**:24, 1978.
29. Olson, R.E., ed.: Diet and behavior: a multidisciplinary evaluation, Nutr. Rev. **44**(suppl.): May, 1986.

30. Story, M., ed.: Nutrition in adolescent pregnancy: a selected annotated bibliography, U.S. Department of Health and Human Services, National Foundation March of Dimes, U.S. Department of Agriculture, Washington, D.C., 1987, U.S. Government Printing Office.
31. Thompson, A.M.: Pregnancy in adolescence. In McKigney, J.I., and Munro, H.N., eds.: Nutrient requirements in adolescence, Cambridge, Mass., 1976, The MIT Press.
32. Rosso, P., and Lederman, S.A.: Nutrition in the pregnant adolescent. In Winick, M., ed.: Adolescent Nutrition, New York, 1982, John Wiley & Sons, Inc.
33. Kreutner, A.K., and Hollingsworth, D.R.: Adolescent obstetrics and gynecology, Chicago, 1978, Year Book Medical Publishers, Inc.
34. Frisancho, A.R., Matos, J., Leonard, W.R., and Yaroch, L.A.: Developmental and nutritional determinants of pregnancy outcome among teenagers, Am. J. Phys. Anthropol. **66**:247, 1985.
35. Felice, M.E., and others: The young pregnant teenager: impact of comprehensive prenatal care, J. Adol. Health Care **1**:193, 1981.

FURTHER READING

McKigney, J., and Munro, H.: Nutrient requirements in adolescence, Cambridge, Mass., 1976, The MIT Press.

This in-depth series of papers provides a comprehensive discussion of the specific nutrient requirements of humans during puberty.

Thompson, P., Roseborough, R., Russek, E., and Moser, P.B.: Zinc status and sexual development in adolescent girls, J. Am. Diet. Assoc. **86**(7):892, July 1986.

This study of nutritional status is unusual in that in it the state of zinc nutrition is related to the physical developmental stage of adolescent girls.

Willard, S.G., Anding, R.H., and Winstead, D.K.: Nutritional counseling as an adjunct to psychotherapy in bulimia treatment, Psychosomatics **24**:545, 1983.

This article describes the role of nutritional therapy in the treatment of bulimia as a component of an interdisciplinary approach.

Worthington-Roberts, B.S., and Rees, J.M.: Nutritional needs of the pregnant adolescent. In Worthington-Roberts, B.S., Vermeersch, J., and Williams, S.R.: Nutrition in pregnancy and lactation, St. Louis, 1985, Times Mirror/Mosby College Publishing.

This chapter provides a comprehensive discussion of the role of specific nutrients in adolescent pregnancy and also reviews pertinent topics related to overall care of this high-risk pregnancy.

CASE STUDY

Two young women in the same class at school become pregnant. One is 16.5 years of age and her menses started when she was 14 years of age. Her weight-for-height is below the 5th percentile. The other pregnant adolescent is 15 years of age and her menses started when she was 9 years of age. Her weight for height is at the 50th percentile.

1. Describe the theoretical difference in nutritional needs of the two adolescents.
2. Which one should be given clinical priority? Why?
3. If neither young woman sought prenatal care, what might you expect as outcome for the respective infants? Why?

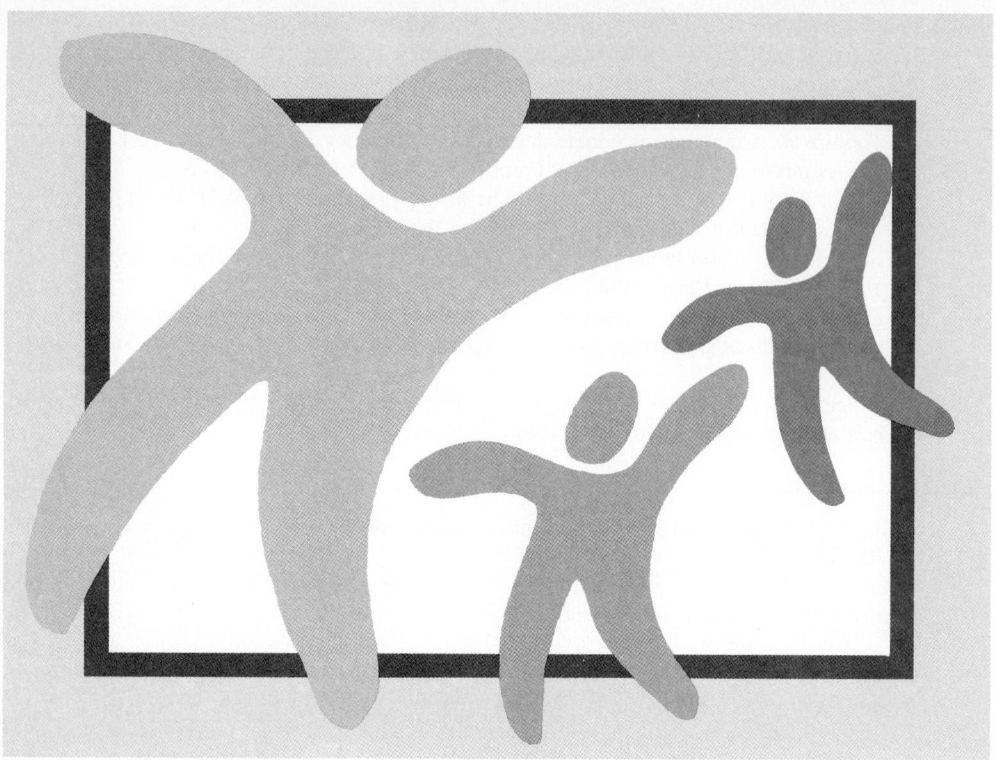

Basic Concepts

1. Although genetic factors influence adult health and longevity, personal lifestyle choices determine 50% of an adult's health status.
2. A healthy lifestyle based on health promotion and disease prevention will delay the development of chronic disease in young adults.
3. Varied personal and community health promotion programs assist individual efforts toward positive health maintenance and disease prevention.
4. Control of adult health problems requires continuing preventive care and individual therapeutic measures with optimal nutritional support.

Chapter Nine

Nutrition in the Adult

Sue Rodwell Williams and Eleanor D. Schlenker

A priority for the young adult is establishing lifelong lifestyle patterns that promote health, well-being, and fitness. Following the tumultuous teen years, when physical growth and development have reached their adult goal, nutrition education and patterns of living should focus on food and exercise behaviors that will maintain optimal physical and mental health.

Health care for adults is often directed toward particular physical problems. Rising medical costs associated with long-term treatment of chronic disorders such as heart disease and diabetes have led to our current emphasis on health promotion and disease prevention. Our goals are to help individuals identify and adopt those practices that will support good health throughout their adult years.

In this chapter we will look at some of the ways we can help meet these health goals during the adult years. If signs of chronic disease do become apparent, appropriate intervention can arrest their development and help individuals maintain the highest possible level of personal well-being. The continuing care of the chronic diseases of adulthood requires supportive therapy based on individual needs. We will see here that a fundamental part of this personal care is optimal nutritional support, with modifications in nutrients, texture, and energy levels according to particular conditions.

Adult Health, Wellness, and Lifestyle

THE CONCEPT OF WELLNESS

Health and **wellness** are words that cannot be used interchangeably. In its simplest form health is defined as absence of disease, although the world Health Organization (WHO) has expanded this definition to include complete physical, mental, and social well-being, not merely by the absence of disease or dysfunction. This WHO approach does recognize the individual as a whole person and views health as relating to both the internal and the external environments. The concept of wellness carries this process one step further. It seeks to develop the maximal potential of individuals within their own environments. This implies a balance between activities and goals: work versus leisure, personal needs versus expectations and goals of others, or lifestyle choices versus health risks. Wellness indicates a positive dynamic state as a person is motivated to seek a higher level of function.

Wellness represents a spectrum of generally high-level well-being or optimal health and of lower-level well-being or illness, as a person grows and ages along the life cycle continuum between birth and death. Various body systems or functions may differ in their level of wellness from time to time. Seldom does an individual experience the highest level of wellness in all functions at all times. As one system or function is improving, another may be deteriorating. However, often a strength in one area may compensate for a weakness or stress in another. For example, excellent physical health may help an individual cope with severe emotional stress that occurs with loss of a family member, job dissatisfaction, or disapproval of one's peer group.

APPROACHES TO HEALTH

Every day individuals are bombarded with messages that encourage actions to improve their health. However, people approach personal health decisions in many different ways and these approaches may differ at different stages in the life cycle. A healthy child may see little need for appropriate health behavior whereas an overweight man with above-normal serum lipid levels may be concerned about his risk of heart disease and consider changing his lifestyle to modify predisposing factors. In general, persons use three approaches to health care: traditional, preventive, or wellness approach.

Traditional Approach

The traditional approach to health leads to change only when the symptoms of illness or disease already exist and the individual seeks out a physician to diagnose and cure the condition. Because major chronic health problems such as heart disease or cancer develop over a period of years before overt signs becomes apparent, this approach is of little value for lifelong positive health.

Preventive Approach

The preventive approach to health focuses on identifying risk factors that increase a person's chances of developing a particular health problem and helping these persons make behavior choices that will prevent or minimize such risks. Preventive measures may include screening programs to detect the development of a problem while it is still in an asymptomatic state and thus allow early intervention. Health fairs may emphasize blood pressure screening to allow early treatment of hypertension and thus retard development of cardiovascular disease and decrease risk of stroke. The disadvantage of this approach is that it tends to be negative in style, emphasizing disease risk and "do not" rules of health care.

Wellness Approach

The wellness approach focuses on positive lifestyle choices that will enhance the achievement of a higher level of health. Individuals are encouraged to achieve a balance among all aspects of lifestyle and accept personal responsibility for choices made. On this basis persons might choose to consume more vegetables and whole-grain cereals rather than a large number of foods high in fat, salt, or sugar. The wellness approach begun early in life allows the development of full personal potential as well as retarding the onset of degenerative changes and chronic disease.

BASES OF HEALTH STATUS

Good or poor health is in large measure determined by five factors: heredity, environment, health outlook, health care, and lifestyle. The first of these factors—heredity—is beyond the individual's control. However, the remaining four factors can, at least to some extent, be modified if the person wishes to achieve a higher level of wellness.

Environment

Our environment has two dimensions: the physical environment and the social environment. The *physical environment* encompasses both the near environment and the extended surrounding area. Families living in poor housing with ineffective plumbing and no refrigerator are highly susceptible to infection and disease. Polluted air and water or food contaminated at the point of production or processing influence health status. The *social environment* can be friendly or hostile. A person may have family or friends for emotional support or be essentially alone. A person may be in a fast-paced environment with high expectations for performance or in a setting that has low expectations and few demands.

Health Outlook

Health outlook relates to personal perception of one's own health and well-being. But perception and reality may not necessarily agree. However, individuals who rate their health as excellent or good have a longer life expectancy than those who rate their health as fair or poor.[1] In fact, self-rating of health is a stronger predictor of life expectancy than actual physical status based on a medical examination. Thus individuals' thoughts and beliefs about their health may be more important than their actual health status. Positive feelings about one's health usually reflect a similar attitude toward life in general that supports positive adjustment and adaptation.

Health Care

In differing life circumstances, health care may or may not be under an individual's control. People in lower socioeconomic groups do not always have access to the same level or quality of medical care as those in higher income groups. Poor reading skills, limited education, or a language barrier may hinder an individual who is attempting to carry out instructions from a health professional about health care or treatment of disease. Health care also includes wise self-care, such as seeking medical care when symptoms so indicate, following directions when using medications, including over-the-counter drugs, practicing weight control, or exercising regularly.

Lifestyle

The term *lifestyle* refers to a person's unique pattern of living. These patterns reflect our values and beliefs. They involve what an individual may eat, how much to eat and when, whether to make time to exercise regularly, or any drugs taken. Use of time is a lifestyle choice. An individual may spend leisure time watching television and consuming large amounts of alcohol and snack foods high in sodium and fat. Another person of similar age may spend leisure time practicing tennis or walking, rather than driving, to a nearby store. A young adult may express dissatisfaction or relieve stress in harmful ways by overeating, smoking, or abusing alcohol. For another, appropriate outlets involving exercise, counseling, or relaxation techniques may be the outcome.

Young adults can significantly reduce their risk of chronic disease by adopting positive lifestyle patterns including:

- A balanced diet
- Regular exercise for fitness and weight control
- No smoking
- No or moderate use of alcohol
- Stress management

For those exhibiting early signs or symptoms of chronic disease, or those at risk because of genetic background, adoption of positive health behaviors can slow or interrupt the progress of the degenerative disease process.

Components of a Healthy Lifestyle

Health and wellness throughout adulthood are to a great extent based on lifestyle choices. When we really consider what determines health status, we find that over 50% of this influence is under one's personal control. Diet, exercise, smoking, use of alcohol, and stress management all contribute to this total. Health professionals must promote lifestyle choices that will reap positive benefits for lifelong good health.

DIET

Food Selection and Disease

Although there is general agreement that a good diet is essential to support good health and prevent degenerative changes, there has been neither systematic evaluation of such a diet nor agreement as to what it should contain. Existing research has focused on particular diseases and dietary components related to their prevention or progression. For example, nutrients evaluated on this basis have included fat in coronary heart disease, sodium in hypertension, and complex carbohydrates in diseases of the colon. Unfortunately, no studies have looked at all dietary constituents and general wellness.

Food Selections for a Healthy Diet

The two basic principles of a healthy diet to guide food selections and use are *variety* and *moderation*. Foods should be selected from all major food groups—dairy foods, protein foods, grains, and fruits and vegetables. An outline of food types and suggested servings is presented in Table 12-1. Food selections for a healthy diet would include the following types of food choices:

1. **Dairy foods.** Dairy foods are good sources of calcium, phosphorus, and riboflavin as well as protein. When selecting these foods, emphasize low-fat varieties that provide important nutrients with less energy and fat.
2. **Protein foods.** Other protein foods that are important sources of other vitamins and minerals include red meats, fish, poultry, eggs, nuts, and legumes. Limit use of red meats and eggs, which are higher in saturated fat and cholesterol, and increase use of poultry and fish, which are lower in total fat and saturated fat and higher in polyunsaturated fat.
3. **Grain foods.** These complex carbohydrates should be the primary sources of energy. They also contain plant protein. Whole grains provide good sources of fiber, thiamin, riboflavin, niacin, vitamin B_6, folic acid, iron, zinc, and other trace minerals and should constitute the majority of grain foods consumed. Refined breads and cereals, although enriched, are low in vitamin B_6, folic acid, fiber, and all trace minerals except iron.
4. **Fruits and vegetables.** This wide variety of foods provides energy and fiber as well as vitamins and minerals. These foods are receiving increased attention because vitamin A and its carotene precursors, found in dark-green and deep-yellow vegetables and fruits, as well as indole compounds, found in cruciferous vegetables such as broccoli, brussels sprouts, cabbage, and cauliflower, appear to offer some protection against certain cancers.
5. **Energy.** There is general agreement that a diet moderate in energy but supplying adequate protein and generous amounts of vitamins and minerals supports continued good health. Such a diet is high in carbohydrate, adequate in protein, and low in fat. The major source of carbohydrate should be complex carbohydrates from legumes, grains, fruits, and vegetables, with only limited amounts of added sugars, including white and brown table sugars or other sweeteners. Main dishes comprised of legumes, grains, nuts, and seeds to achieve complementary balance of the vegetable proteins, or the combination of any of these vegetable proteins with milk or cheese, are high in protein quality, high in complex carbohydrates, and low to moderate in fat.
6. **Use of processed foods.** The use of fresh foods and less processed foods is preferred. Highly processed or refined food items are lower in fiber, vitamins, and minerals—especially trace minerals—and generally have added amounts of sugar, sodium, and fat.

Fat, Saturated Fat, and Cholesterol

Since 1964 recommendations of the American Heart Association and other health agencies have led to changes in the American diet with reduced consumption of whole milk, cream, butter, eggs, and animal fats resulting in reduced intakes of total fat, saturated fat, and cholesterol. Another change occurring over this time has been a decreased mortality from coronary heart disease. Perhaps the most significant aspect of this decline is the age groups in which it has occurred. Although heart disease is still the leading cause of death among people age 65 and over, it is no longer the leading cause among those adults below age 65. Coronary mortality declined 45% among those aged 35 to 44, and 38% among those aged 45 to 54.[2]

Coronary Heart Disease Risk

Excessive intakes of fat, saturated fat, and cholesterol in children and young adults can lead to inappropriately high levels of serum cholesterol and triglycerides. Elevated serum cholesterol levels along with elevated blood pressure and cigarette smoking constitute the three major risk factors for coronary heart disease. Moreover, the risk of coronary heart disease continues to increase as serum cholesterol levels increase. Risk for adults with serum cholesterol levels above 270 mg/dl is twice that of adults with levels below 218 mg/dl.[3] Conversely, a 1% decrease in serum cholesterol level results in a 2% drop in cardiovascular risk. Diets with increasing levels of kilocalories, saturated fat, and cholesterol are associated with higher serum cholesterol levels, whereas increased intakes of polyunsaturated fats appear to lower serum cholesterol levels.

Cancer Risk

Another concern related to dietary fat is its association with cancer risk. As total fat intake increases so does the incidence of certain types of cancer, particularly breast cancer and colon cancer. Conversely, as total fat intake decreases, so does cancer risk. Of all the dietary components considered in a recent comprehensive review, fat appears to be most closely associated with cancer risk.[4] Based on available evidence it is not possible to identify the relative risk associated with different types of dietary fat.

General Dietary Recommendations

At present, recommendations concerning dietary fat intake for the adult with normal serum cholesterol levels are issues of debate. The American Heart Association recommends a diet containing no more than 30% of total kilocalories from fat, and no more than 300 mg of cholesterol daily. The Committee on Diet, Nutrition, and Cancer of the National Academy of Sciences also advocates a diet containing no more than 30% of total kilocalories from fat as a practical target, but suggests that available data might support an even greater reduction in dietary fat.[4] At this time, however, the Food and Nutrition Board of the National Academy of Sciences considers it inappropriate to make such a stringent recommendation for the general population and suggests that no more than 35% of total energy be derived from fat.[5] The typical American diet contains about 40% fat. Thus some degree of change is in order for all age groups. Suggestions for implementing such changes for healthy eating are given here (see box, p. 379).

Omega-3 Fatty Acids

Recent work suggests that omega-3 fatty acids found in cold-water fish have a serum-lipid-lowering effect even among persons with normal serum lipids.[6] In addition to lowering serum cholesterol and lipid levels, the omega-3 fatty acids also decrease serum platelet aggregation, thus lowering the risk of thrombus formation,

GUIDELINES FOR HEALTHY EATING

- *Reduce saturated fats and increase polyunsaturated fats.* Use **more** fish, poultry, lean meat, skim or low-fat milk and other dairy products low in fat. **Substitute** polyunsaturated vegetable oils and margarines for saturated ones. Use less high-fat meat, egg yolks, butter, whole milk and other dairy products high in fat. Use **less** fried foods.
- *Reduce cholesterol intake.* Use **more** skim or low-fat milk and other dairy products low in fat, lean meats, fish, and poultry. Use **less** egg yolks, butter, whole milk and other dairy products high in fat.
- *Increase complex carbohydrates and eat fewer simpler sugars.* Use **more** whole-grain breads and cereals, fruits and vegetables, and legumes. Use **less** sugar, honey, syrups, and foods high in added sugars.
- *Reduce sodium intake.* Use **less** salt in cooking and at the table. **Limit** your use of convenience foods, salty snack foods, and salty condiments.
- *Eat a variety of foods from all food groups each day.* This includes skim or low-fat milk and other dairy products low in fat; fish, poultry, legumes and lean meats; fruits and vegetables; and whole-grain breads and cereals.

and may prevent lipid molecules from entering an atherosclerotic plaque. In a retrospective study of Dutch men over a 20-year period,[6] a daily intake of 30 g of fish, about 1 ounce, resulted in a 50% decrease in risk of coronary death. Eating fish once or twice a week might be an effective deterrent to developing coronary heart disease.

Complex Carbohydrate and Fiber

Current recommendations indicate that 50% to 60% of total kilocalories should come from carbohydrates, with an emphasis on complex carbohydrates such as starch and fiber. *Fiber* is the term used to describe the indigestible carbohydrate compounds such as pectin, cellulose, and hemicellulose found in stalks, hulls, seeds, and skins of fruits, vegetables, legumes, and whole grains. Lignin, a nonpolysaccharide found in the plant cell wall, is also a dietary fiber. These various kinds of dietary fiber have several physiologic effects depending on the amount and particular type consumed. Not all types of fiber act in the same way and each type is found in particular plant foods. Therefore it is important to consume a variety of plant foods including whole grains, legumes, fruits, and vegetables to obtain all of these significant fiber components. Physiologic effects of dietary fiber serve three important functions:

1. **Water absorption.** In recent years attention has focused on the importance of fiber in the maintenance of the lower gastrointestinal tract, providing the bulk and waterbinding necessary to maintain rapid transit time and produce a large, soft stool. Lack of fiber has been implicated in the etiology of diverticular disease, colon cancer, and constipation.
2. **Binding effect.** The binding effect of certain noncellulose materials influences blood lipid levels through their capacity to adsorb or bind bile acids and cholesterol, thus preventing their reabsorption, with a subsequent lowering of serum lipids.
3. **Blood glucose control.** Studies relating dietary fiber to control of blood glucose

have demonstrated the ability of certain fibers to lower hyperglycemia.[7,8] This effect is attributed to delayed gastric emptying time, reduced intestinal transit time with subsequent reduced nutrient absorption, and slower ingestion of smaller amounts of the bulky food. Also the complex carbohydrate starch accompanying the fiber, in grains and legumes, for example, enhances this effect. Because the complex carbohydrate starch requires a longer digestive period than the simple carbohydrates, it releases glucose into the blood in a slow, sustained manner, in contrast to the rapid rise and subsequent fall in serum glucose levels occurring with the ingestion of concentrated sugars.

In addition, a diet high in complex carbohydrate foods providing a slow release of glucose is less likely to lead to obesity than a diet high in fat as a result of hormonal regulation of both appetite and energy utilization. Moreover, because of their bulk, complex carbohydrates also contribute to feelings of satiety more effectively than concentrated high-fat, high-sucrose items do. Although it is fairly easy to consume a 3-ounce chocolate bar containing about 450 kilocalories as a snack, a person is less likely to eat 3 large apples, about equal in energy value.

Some fiber components bind divalent cations and thus prevent their absorption, although the extent to which this occurs is not known. Excess dietary fiber could deplete such minerals as iron, zinc, magnesium, and chromium by binding with them and preventing their absorption. Although an appropriate diet should contain generous servings of fruits, vegetables, legumes, and whole grains (see box, p. 379), fiber supplements or unlimited use of bran is unwise.

Sodium

High intakes of sodium are associated with elevated blood pressure levels in some adults. Limiting sodium intake reduces risk among those most likely to develop hypertension in later life. A safe and reasonable intake of sodium is 1100-1300 mg per day or 3-6 g of NaCl, table salt.[5] This amount is about half the current intake in the American diet. Staying within the recommended intake level does not require limiting use of nutrient-dense foods containing natural sodium, including milk, cottage cheese, and other animal foods. It does require some substitution of other flavoring and seasonings such as spices or herbs for table salt and limited use of such salty foods as pickles, olives, sauerkraut, sardines, and snack foods. Refined cereals, canned soups, frozen dinners, and other highly processed prepared food items are high in sodium. Consumers should be encouraged to use nutrition labels to identify the sodium content of these foods.

EXERCISE

Benefits of Exercise

Regular physical exercise contributes to health and fitness in many ways. Some of these benefits include improved energy balance, body composition, cardiac efficiency, and serum lipid levels.

1. **Energy balance.** One of the most obvious health benefits of exercise may be seen in its role in energy balance and weight management. Increasing energy expenditure in exercise allows a higher energy intake in food, which helps ensure

adequate amounts of all important nutrients without inappropriate weight gain. An indirect effect of exercise is increased glucose uptake and utilization by muscle cells in the trained versus the untrained individual.

2. **Body composition.** Physical exercise strengthens muscle fibers and helps prevent age-related loss of lean body mass and increase in body fat. Exercise also prevents degenerative aging changes by strengthening of bone through stimulating bone formation and preventing bone loss. Regular physical stress on the bone provided by consistent exercise will prevent or retard the onset of osteoporosis, a common bone disorder among older women.
3. **Cardiovascular efficiency**. Regular exercise increases the individual's ability to do physical work with increased cardiovascular efficiency and decreased recovery time. Maximal oxygen consumption is increased while heart rate and blood pressure levels are decreased both during exercise and at rest. Among those persons not exercising regularly, blood pressure levels increase with age.
4. **Serum lipid levels.** Physical activity also retards degenerative changes through its effect on serum cholesterol levels. Daily exercise increases serum levels of high-density lipoproteins (HDL), which protect against coronary artery disease by removing cholesterol molecules from the blood before they can enter the arterial wall. At the same time low-density lipoproteins (LDL) that carry cholesterol to the cells and increase cardiovascular risk are significantly lowered.

Exercise and Coronary Risk

A 20-year study of nearly 17,000 male college graduates found that regular exercise throughout adulthood was associated with low coronary risk.[9] Individuals with high levels of exercise during their student years but sedentary lifestyles thereafter had high risk, whereas those who exercised little at younger years but began to exercise thereafter had low risk. This would suggest that individuals who had been sedentary can still benefit from regular exercise.

The duration and resulting energy expenditure appears to be more important than the intensity of the exercise. Maximal benefit was achieved when exercise energy expenditure from climbing stairs, walking, and sports activities equalled 2000 kilocalories per week, although significant reductions in risk still occurred within the exercise level of 500-1999 kilocalories per week. The benefit from exercise was independent of negative lifestyle factors including smoking, obesity, or family disease history. In fact, exercise reduced the risk associated with those factors as compared to individuals with sedentary habits. On this basis it was suggested that regular exercise may be most critical for those individuals who already suffer from several negative risk factors. In general, exercise appears to slow the degenerative changes associated with aging and the development of chronic disease.

Developing an Exercise Program

An individual previously sedentary, regardless of age, should undergo a physical examination before embarking on an exercise program. Also, persons should pay attention to body signals. The appearance of pain suggests that it is time to slow down or stop. Important considerations for an exercise program are:

- Safety
- Effectiveness
- Individual differences
- Cost

To prevent muscular or skeletal injury, or a cardiovascular accident, the progression in both duration and intensity must be gradual. Cardiovascular exercise requires an increase in heart rate to 60-85% of maximal rate (220 beats per minute considered maximal) that must be continued for at least 20 minutes if an improvement in fitness is to occur. However, these levels may need to be achieved over a period of time. For an individual with prior cardiovascular problems, heart rate should be carefully monitored.

People differ in their preference of individual versus group exercise. For the individual who is obese, self-conscious, or has poor athletic skills, activity such as walking, jogging, or exercising alone may be preferable to group activities or team sports. The exercise activity should be something the persons enjoy if it is to continue. Suggestions for exercise activities may be found in Table 9-1. Exercise programs have been least successful among lower-income groups. This may relate to cost of equipment or fees charged for participation.

APPROPRIATE BODY WEIGHT

Obesity and Mortality Risk

Avoidance of obesity may be the single most important factor in maintaining health and retarding the progression of chronic disease. In addition to being an independent risk factor for the development of cardiovascular disease, obesity contributes to the development of elevated blood pressure and elevated serum cholesterol levels, both of which are also independent risk factors.

Obesity can promote the development of arthritis and degenerative bone-joint disease, reducing flexibility and hindering mobility. Because physical exercise is difficult, the obese individual is more likely to be sedentary, which sustains the obesity and

TABLE 9-1 Energy Cost of Various Activities*

Activity	kcal/kg/hr
Aerobic dancing	8.9
Bicycling (moderate speed)	2.5
Bicycling (racing)	7.6
Golf	3.9
Rowing in race	16.0
Running	7.0
Skating	3.5
Skiing (cross country)	5.9
Swimming (2 mph)	7.9
Tennis	5.3
Walking (3 mph)	2.0
Walking rapidly (4 mph)	3.4

*Does not include basal metabolism.

further contributes to degenerative changes. Obesity is also a significant factor in the development of maturity-onset diabetes, as enlarged fat cells resist the action of insulin.

The influence of obesity or overweight on mortality risk has been controversial. Life insurance statistics suggest that individuals greatly above or below average weight are more likely to die at younger ages. In early reports the underweight persons had an even greater mortality risk than the overweight persons. This led to the assertion by some health professionals that being slightly overweight might actually be protective, particularly when undergoing severe illness or disease. A 26-year follow-up of the Framingham Heart Study revealed that the high mortality among the underweight men was related to cigarette smoking.[10] Eighty percent of the underweight men were cigarette smokers as compared to only 55% of the overweight men. See Chapter 2 (p. 9) for a discussion of these issues of obesity and overweight.

The age when an individual becomes obese also influences mortality from cardiovascular disease. Regardless of body weight at age 25, weight gain during the following years increases cardiovascular risk, whereas weight loss among those who are overweight reduces their risk. Men appear to be more sensitive than women to the detrimental effects of weight gain and the positive effects of weight loss. Location of body fat, in addition to body weight, also influences risk. Men with thick layers of body fat in the abdominal region have higher risk of coronary heart disease and death.

Even mild degrees of overweight can be detrimental to the maintenance of good health. For men ages 40 to 49, mortality rates are doubled in those 20% overweight as compared to those 10% overweight.[10] Moreover, a weight loss of only 10 pounds will cause a significant drop in elevated blood pressure. In general, the longest lifespans are associated with body weights below average as long as those weights are not the result of malnutrition, smoking, or drug or alcohol abuse.

Incidence of Overweight

In the United States 26% of the white population and 40% of the black population above age 24 are overweight, and the number is increasing.[11] The popularization of the slim figure, plus the recommendations of health care professionals, have led many adults to attempt to lose weight. Unfortunately, the diets chosen are frequently low in protein, vitamins, and minerals, as well as energy, and lead to nutrient depletion. Moreover, semistarvation diets do not help the dieter develop new eating patterns. Consequently, when the diet is discontinued and the usual eating pattern is resumed, the weight is regained. This can establish a cycle of weight gain, weight loss, weight gain, which may over a period of years be more detrimental to health than the initial overweight. Increasing physical exercise along with a modest decrease in energy intake, if necessary, is a more appropriate solution to lifelong weight control.

STRESS MANAGEMENT

Emotional and psychologic stress is related to both physical and mental health (see Chapter 11). Stress can result in adverse physiologic symptoms including: (1) gastrointestinal distress, for example nausea, vomiting, or diarrhea; (2) irregular sleep patterns; (3) increased muscle tension with resulting headache or backache; or (4) cardiovascular responses resulting in constriction of blood vessels and rapid pulse.

Everyone may experience one or more of these symptoms occasionally, but the danger lies in the long-term consequences resulting from continuing, unalleviated stress. Continued gastric upset and inappropriate secretion of stomach acid can lead to ulcer formation and associated stomach problems. Heart disease is significantly related to high blood pressure, which can occur over time as a stress response. Psychologic distress can have a detrimental effect on food intake resulting in patterns of overeating or binge eating leading to inappropriate weight gain, or at the other extreme bulimia or anorexia nervosa, which appear to be increasing among young adults.

Because poorly managed stress is recognized as a threat to both physical and mental health, as well as occupational safety and productivity, cognitive and behavioral approaches have been developed for stress reduction. Group and individual counseling have been directed toward improving understanding and attitude, developing constructive coping mechanisms and assertiveness, and learning positive approaches to problem-solving. Behavioral approaches include reduction in use of alcohol, caffeine, or nicotine, along with increased exercise, rest, and relaxation.

AVOIDANCE OF CIGARETTE SMOKING

Cigarette smoking is a major risk factor for many chronic conditions in both men and women. It accelerates the development of atherosclerotic lesions, leading to an estimate that 30% to 40% of all deaths from coronary heart disease can be attributed to smoking.[12] Among women who both smoke and use oral contraceptives, coronary risk is ten times greater than among those who do neither, and risk of cerebral hemorrhage is also increased. Mortality risk for both sexes increases with the number of cigarettes smoked and is higher for those who began smoking at younger ages. Even at age 30, an individual smoking two packs of cigarettes a day has a life expectancy 8 to 9 years shorter than a nonsmoker of similar age.[12]

Cigarette smoking is also the major cause of lung cancer among both sexes. Until recently prevalence of lung cancer was lower among women, reflecting their limited use of cigarettes. Presently, however, lung cancer is competing with breast cancer to become the leading cause of cancer death in women.[2]

Smokers who give up this habit experience both immediate and long-term benefits in both mortality and morbidity. Risk of cardiovascular disease decreases the first year and after several years approaches that of people who have never smoked. Risk of lung cancer also decreases as the interval of nonsmoking increases, but 15 to 20 years is required to approach that of the lifelong nonsmoker.[12] Although further deterioration of the lung is arrested, smokers with obstructed air passages cannot anticipate major improvement despite cessation of smoking.

A major concern to health professionals should be the prevalence of cigarette smoking among teenagers and young adults. Smoking is now more popular among teenage women than teenage men and nearly one-fourth of all teenage women smoke. Smoking begins at earlier ages as 15% of adolescents aged 12 to 17 now smoke, with many smoking two packs of cigarettes a day.[2]

APPROPRIATE USE OF ALCOHOL

Inappropriate use of alcohol has a negative effect on nutritional status and enhances the risk of cardiovascular disease. Alcohol has a toxic effect on the gastrointestinal tract and reduces the absorption of a variety of nutrients including vitamins B_6 and B_{12}, folic acid, and zinc. Moreover, alcohol may further contribute to malnutrition by adding kilocalories to the diet but no important vitamins, minerals, or protein. This problem relating to nutrient density is increased in some diets, especially those of young women, when alcohol kilocalories replace nonalcohol kilocalories to a level approaching one-third of the total energy intake. Although this practice may avoid weight gain, it has a significant influence on nutrient quality and may further decrease intakes of iron and calcium, nutrients already low in the diets of young adult women.

Alcohol abuse further contributes to deterioration of health through its association with elevated blood pressure and serum lipid levels. Although it was believed that liver damage resulted from malnutrition due to a lack of food intake rather than from a direct toxic effect of alcohol per se, current findings have revealed the development of liver cirrhosis in well-nourished alcohol abusers. Although the amount of alcohol consumed and the duration of consumption are of primary importance in the development of liver disease, nutrient factors do appear to modulate the degree of toxicity on liver tissue.

Growth of Health Promotion Programs

The current emphasis on wellness has led to the development of programs that provide health and nutrition education and give access to intervention activities. Schools, hospitals, and other public agencies have become involved in health promotion. In the private sector, health maintenance organizations (HMOs), businesses, and health clubs are providing health education programs for their members and employees.

HOSPITAL-BASED COMMUNITY PROGRAMS

An increasing number of hospitals are becoming involved in community health promotion. Hospital programs for the general public include community screening programs to identify those at major risk of developing chronic disease, and educational programs describing lifestyle changes to reduce risk. Others focus on weight management for those seeking a support group for long-term weight loss.

Some hospitals are marketing health promotion services to local employers including: (1) employee assistance programs offering counseling and treatment for specific problems including alcohol and drug dependency; (2) occupational health services for monitoring the safety of the work environment or treating work-related illness or injury; and (3) wellness programs emphasizing improvement of lifestyle habits.

HEALTH-MAINTENANCE ORGANIZATIONS (HMOs)

General Organization

Health-maintenance organizations (HMOs), based on a concept first developed in the early 1900s, operate currently under federal law regulating their practice enacted in the 1960s. They present the option of prepaid medical care, usually by group medical practice. Subscribers pay a set fee per individual or family and in turn are guaranteed all health services required, including visits to physicians and other health-care professionals, hospital care, and related services. HMOs negotiate fees with hospitals, pharmacies, or specialty-practice consultants.

As providers of health-care services HMOs have both advantages and disadvantages. From the consumer's point of view HMOs provide an opportunity to control one's own health-care costs as all services required will be provided for the set fee. Such a system effectively insulates an individual or family against the financial devastation that can result from a catastrophic illness or injury. Finally, HMOs have a financial incentive to encourage preventive health care. The traditional fee-for-service system rewards providers for treating illness. One disadvantage of the HMO is that in some cases individuals may not be able to choose their care provider, but rather must accept the provider under contract to the HMO. Finally, any arrangement that does not provide a fee per unit of service may result in a provider limiting services in an effort to control costs. However, this latter concern has not been a problem according to recent discussions of such units.

Health Promotion Activities

HMOs have taken a leadership role in health promotion activities, often in response to member requests. Seminars and ongoing classes are offered on such topics as diet and weight control, smoking cessation, stress management, and physical fitness. One HMO in Washington, D.C., provided extensive printed material from public sources, handouts authored in-house, lists of recommended books, and a quarterly newsletter. Over 80% of those responding to a survey of member needs considered health education to be an important component of their membership services.[13]

WORK-SITE WELLNESS PROGRAMS

Goals of Work-Site Programs

Nearly one-fourth of the nation's largest employers have health promotion programs. The incentive for establishing such programs has come, at least in part, from escalating medical care and insurance costs and efforts to identify causes of this rise. Strategies for health promotion programs for employees usually include four steps:

- Educate about common health risks
- Help identify personal health risks
- Assist in selecting lifestyle patterns to reduce health risks
- Assist in self-monitoring to reinforce lifestyle adjustments made

Evaluation

The effectiveness of work-site programs in improving employee health or reducing health costs is being evaluated. Results from many programs indicate that not only do employees lose excess weight, stop smoking, lower their blood pressure or serum cholesterol levels, or increase their physical activity, but also this reduction in risk has in some cases continued over 3-5 years. In one work-site program for treatment and monitoring of elevated blood pressure, over half of those referred for treatment and follow-up had blood pressure levels below 140/90 mm Hg after 3 years.[14] Among those referred for treatment elsewhere who had not been involved in a follow-up program only one-fifth had blood pressure readings of those levels. The success of the work-site program was attributed to the systematic monitoring and follow-up that provided employees with information about their condition and offered ongoing support.

Peer support and easy accessibility to a program at no cost contributed to the success of an employee exercise and fitness program that resulted in significant increases in maximal oxygen uptake and decreases in body weight, percent body fat, and systolic blood pressure levels.[15] These results have been sustained over 2 years. Because lifestyle habits are resistant to change, a 3-year period is considered the minimum time required to bring about lasting change. Many conditions responding to lifestyle intervention, such as heart disease and obesity, are slow to develop and will not demonstrate immediate improvement. On the other hand, stress reduction and an improvement in general well-being become evident in the short term. In one program employees with a high participation rate in fitness classes had a 42% decline in absenteeism over an 8-month period of time.[16]

Cost Effectiveness

Changing health risk factors does reduce illness and subsequent costs. According to one study, an employee who smokes costs a company $4611 per year in absenteeism, health care costs, and property damage, while a corporation smoking cessation program can be implemented at a cost of only $55 per year per person.[16] If only one-fourth of those participating in such a program actually stopped smoking, the cost benefit would be $21 saved for every $1 spent. Work-site programs appear to offer vast potential for education and intervention in all aspects of health promotion and risk.

HEALTH CLUBS

Increasing media attention to physical fitness and weight control has fostered the rapid expansion of for-profit health clubs that offer a variety of services for a comprehensive membership fee. Aerobic exercise and use of physical conditioning equipment are the most common activities, although fitness evaluations and development of personal exercise programs may also be provided. Facilities may include a swimming pool, tennis courts, or racquetball courts. Nutrition and diet counseling is often available. However, it is unfortunate that individuals providing dietary evaluations or instruction are not always professional nutritionists or dietitians.

HEALTH FAIRS

Over two million people visit health fairs each year. These health fairs are sponsored by service organizations, hospitals, home health agencies, or professional health-related associations. They take place in shopping malls, parking lots, community centers, or parks. They feature displays, posters, hand-out materials, and screening tests for common disorders. Staffed by both professional and lay volunteers, health fairs have as their major purpose health education and make an effort to attract both the general population and targeted groups.

Because health fairs are unregulated, little is known about the numbers of persons reached or screening procedures attempted. An organization that offers assistance to health-fair sponsors estimates that over 1.5 million measurements of height and weight and over 20 million blood chemistry tests are performed each year at health fairs.[17] Screening tests may be offered as an incentive to attract participants in addition to detecting health problems.

The criteria for these tests and the degree of follow-up within such screening programs concern health professionals. One program initiated telephone follow-up only when serum cholesterol levels were 360 mg/dl or above, a value considerably above that recommended.[17] False alarms for the well participants as well as false reassurance for the person at risk are at issue in situations where test conditions and the sheer numbers of tests performed contribute to error. Nevertheless, health fairs serve an important role in drawing attention to healthy lifestyle choices and emphasizing personal responsibility for one's own health.

Nutrition for Adult Growth and Development

PHYSICAL CHARACTERISTICS AND GROWTH

Faced now with an extended lifespan resulting from the advances of modern medicine and public health measures, adults are showing an increased interest in positive personal health promotion as indicated above. As they mature through the adult years, they recognize the gradual physical changes of the normal aging process.

Body Composition Changes

As the adult body reaches its overall growth in body size, its physical growth becomes that of tissue synthesis to rebuild and maintain tissue integrity, through the vigor of young and middle adulthood and declining gradually into the older adult years (see Chapter 10). The general biologic process of human growth and decline extends over the entire life cycle, with body composition changes unique to each age. These changes are described in detail in Chapter 2. During the adult years, the changes come slowly with a gradual cell loss and reduced cell metabolism, resulting in declining performance capacity of most organ systems. For example, at about age 30 the kidneys begin to lose functioning nephrons and decrease in size with accompanying decreases in renal blood flow, filtration and reabsorption capacities.[18]

Individual Differences

These gradual body changes during the adult years are not only part of the total life process, but are also highly individual in nature. They are conditioned by life experiences that have gone before and the imprint of these experiences on the genetic heritage of each unique human being. Although the biologic changes in adulthood are general, persons will display a wide variety of individual reaction and simply "grow old" at different rates.

PSYCHOSOCIAL DEVELOPMENT

Along with physical changes, psychosocial development continues in changing patterns as persons mature and grow older. The three adult stages of the human life cycle, as identified by Erikson,[19,20] complete the whole of human development.

Young Adults—Ages 20 to 40

In the young adult every person, now launched as an individual and facing adult responsibilities and fulfillments, must resolve the core psychosocial problem of *intimacy versus isolation*. If the positive adult development is achieved, the person is able to build intimate relationships leading to self-fulfillment, either in marriage or in other personal relationships. Persons who have failed to develop inner psychosocial strengths in previous years, however, may become increasingly isolated from others. These are the years of career beginnings and changes, of establishing one's own home, of parenthood, of starting young children on their way through the same life stages, and of early struggles to make one's way in the world.

Middle Adults—Ages 40 to 60

In the middle adult years, the core psychosocial problem persons face is that of *generativity versus self-absorption*. The older children may have grown and gone to make their own lives. For some middle adults these are the years of the "empty nest." For others, it is an opportunity for expanding personal growth—"it's my turn now." There is a coming to terms with what life is all about, but also a great opportunity of finding expression of stored learning in passing on life's teachings. It is a regeneration of one's life in the lives of young persons following the same way, an active nurturing transmission of culture from one generation to the next. To the degree that these inner struggles are not won, there is an increasing self-absorption, a turning-in on oneself, an immature capacity to handle stress leading to illness (p. 383), and a withering rather than a regenerating spirit of life.

Older Adults—Ages 60 to 80+

In the last stage of life, the final core psychosocial problem is resolved between *integrity versus despair*. Depending on the person's inner resources at this point, there is either a predominant sense of wholeness and completeness or a sense of bitterness, of wondering what life was all about. If the outcome of life's basic experiences and problems on the whole has been positive, the individual arrives at old age a rich person—rich in wisdom of the years. Building on each previous level, psychosocial growth will reach its individual positive human resolution. Some older adults will not have resolved these previous psychosocial conflicts, however, and will struggle still with those they have wrestled with before in younger years. They arrive at middle and later years poorly equipped to deal with the adjustments and health problems that may face them. Many others, on the other hand, will have been enriched by life's experiences in their maturing process and in turn will bring enrichment to younger lives, in relationships that are mutually rewarding.

ADULT NUTRITIONAL NEEDS

Energy

The reduced basal metabolic rate, together with reduced physical activity in most adults, combine to create less energy demand as adults grow older. Depending upon individual life situations and type of work, young adults will require more energy than older adults and will experience a gradual decline in need as age advances. Individual needs in any adult age group will vary, of course, and the RDA is expressed in ranges at each level. The average RDA standard for adult men is 2700 kilocalories for younger adults, 2400 for middle adults, and 2050 for elderly men. For women the standard average is 2000 kilocalories for young adults, 1800 for middle adults, and 1600 for elderly women. Among older adults, especially, living situations vary widely and there is need for much more information on their daily life activities and the degree of energy they may be capable of spending. Thus actual kilocalorie requirements are highly individual. Of the two major fuel sources, carbohydrate should have the greater share by far:

1. **Carbohydrate.** Although the optimal carbohydrate intake is unknown, it is usually recommended that about 55% to 58% of the total kilocalories come from carbohydrate foods, mainly complex carbohydrates in starch form, such as whole grains, legumes, potatoes and other vegetables, with the remainder in simple carbohydrate foods such as fruits, milk, and limited sweets.
2. **Fat.** Current recommendations for health promotion center on a decreased amount of total fat in the American diet, which has traditionally been relatively high in fat (p. 377). The usual recommendation is that only about 30% of the total kilocalories come from fat, with the main portion being unsaturated plant fat rather than saturated animal fat, and the fat-related substance cholesterol be lowered to about 300 mg/day. Some fat is essential in the adult diet, not only for energy but also for essential fatty acids and as a base for fat-soluble vitamins.

Protein

The traditional American diet has contained excess protein in relation to actual physiologic need, due mainly to the cultural value placed on meat as a central food, thus putting an increasing burden on the aging kidney for the resulting excess nitrogen excretion. Throughout the adult years, with physical growth achieved and need only for tissue maintenance, the protein requirement remains steady. The RDA standard for healthy adults is 0.8 g/kg body weight, making an average total for men of 56 g/day, and for women 44 g/day. Although there may be increased need during illness or convalescence, the overall mass of actively metabolizing tissue gradually decreases with age. Protein needs are influenced by: (1) the biologic value of the protein, related to such factors as the quantity and ratio of its amino acids and its digestibility; and (2) an adequate caloric value of the diet. It is estimated that 25% to 50% of the protein should come from animal food sources to assure adequate intake of essential amino acids, with the remainder from complementary plant protein foods, such as whole grains, legumes, vegetables, nuts, and seeds. Protein should supply from 12% to 15% of the day's total kilocalories.

Vitamins

There is usually no requirement for additional vitamin intake in the healthy adult. There may be gradually decreasing tissue stores with normal aging, but no difference in average allowances for the healthy adult is indicated. The problem in some individuals may stem from inadequate usual intake rather than increased need. In any event, a well-selected mixed diet from a variety of food choices usually supplies all the required vitamins in normally needed quantities. There may be increased therapeutic needs in illness or in individual special cases, but these needs should be evaluated on an individual basis.

Minerals

Usually in normal aging the standard adult requirements for minerals still apply. These same adult allowances are sufficient if provided on a regular continuing basis by a well-balanced diet. Two minerals may need emphasis: calcium and iron. For healthy adults the U.S. standard for daily calcium is 800 mg. There has been some evidence, however, that to prevent negative calcium balance, the level should be raised to about 1200 mg in women over age 50 and in men over age 60, avoiding calcium loss from bone tissue and the risk of developing osteoporosis.[21] More recent indications, however, are for greater attention to the prior adolescent years when long bones are rapidly growing to adult size and the bone calcium mass is being built up for adult years, with a recommended intake for all adolescents of 1500 mg/day to ensure this significant baseline adult mass.[22] Poor diets in adult years may also be deficient in iron, which is needed to prevent anemia. Some adults may need encouragement to ensure adequate dietary sources of iron among their daily food sources.

Use of Supplements

The question of using vitamin and mineral supplements is often raised, usually by persons having some relationship with the industry supplying them, and certainly, judging from the size of the industry, their use is widespread. However, there is little evidence that *healthy* adults eating a well-balanced diet require additional nutrient supplementation. The Food and Nutrition Board of the National Research Council has stated that it is "aware of no convincing evidence of unique health benefits accruing from consumption of a large excess of any one nutrient."[5] Professional nutritionists point out that seldom do dietary nutrient intakes in the United States fall below 70% of the recommended levels for age group populations and food provides macronutrients that supplements do not.[23] There is need for supplementation in certain instances, for example, iron, fluoride, and vitamin D for infants; iron and folic acid for pregnant women; and possibly calcium for young and middle-aged women. But there are serious concerns in the professional nutrition community about the extensive and indiscriminate use of supplements: (1) effects of resulting trace mineral imbalance; (2) the large amount of money spent on supplements, often to the detriment of adequate money for food to make up a healthy diet; (3) dangers of megadoses of nutrients used;

(4) the proliferation of "nutritional" products often with misleading health or curative claims, as well as questionable marketing schemes; and (5) frequent fads in nutrient consumption.[23] In illness or debilitated states, however, supplementation is another matter. It may well be needed in such states to help restore tissue integrity and health, but in all instances should be individually assessed and dosages of particular nutrients individually defined. As for protein supplements, for healthy adults there is no need. They are expensive and an inefficient source of available nitrogen.

NUTRIENT STANDARDS AND FOOD GUIDES FOR HEALTH PROMOTION

Changing Health Needs

For many years nutritional scientists and clinicians, together with a concerned public and various governmental agencies, have sought to help such persons as professionals or consumers to make wise food choices for promoting the health of individuals and population groups. One of the oldest such guides, commonly known as the "Basic Four Food Groups," is an example. It was developed in the post-World War II era when nutritional needs centered on dietary deficiencies of vitamins, minerals, and protein.[24] But today we live in different times and our nutrition and health problems have changed. For the most part, our diets reflect *excesses,* not deficiencies—excess fat, sugar, sodium—which contribute to our major health problems described here: heart disease, cancer, hypertension, and obesity. So other guidelines have begun to address these nutrition needs in health promotion. Three such current guides for health promotion are used here as examples of changing needs: the established nutrient standard of the recommended dietary allowances (RDA), the more recent U.S. dietary goals, and the current food exchange groups. In each case we see the broadening influence of a philosophy of positive health promotion for all ages, involving risk reduction in relation to major U.S. health problems, not limited to the concept of avoiding deficiency disease.

Recommended Dietary Allowances (RDAs)

RDAs have undergone many expansions over the years since they were first published in 1943 during World War II as a guide for planning and procuring food supplies for national defense and providing average population nutrient standards as a goal for good nutrition. Its nine revisions, one every 4 or 5 years with the most recent edition in 1980, have reflected an increasing base of scientific knowledge as well as expanding social concerns about nutrition and health.[5] Edition 10, planned for publication in 1985, was not issued due to failure of the study group to reach a consensus; this indicates the nature of our rapidly changing society and the difficult issues facing us, both scientific and social, in relating nutrition to broader standards for positive health promotion.[25-27] A newly appointed study group is now grappling with these issues in preparation of a new report for edition 10. In the meantime, edition 9 remains the standard in use.

U.S. Dietary Goals

Building upon public concerns in the 1960s and investigations of a Senate select committee studying hunger and nutrition in the U.S., these general dietary guidelines have developed from efforts to prevent or retard prevalent chronic diseases in our gradually aging population. From the first, this guide has encountered controversy, centering mainly on the broad issue of the roles of government and contemporary science in maintaining public health.[28] Reissued in 1980 by the U.S. Departments of Agriculture (USDA) and Health and Human Services (USDHHS) as the "Dietary Guidelines for Americans," these statements relate current scientific thinking to America's leading health problems. Recent review by an expert committee led to only minimal updating changes in the current 1985 edition, "Nutrition and Your Health: Dietary Guidelines for Americans" (see Fig. 12-2). These statements continue to provide a useful general guide for a concerned public.

Food Exchange Groups

This listing of food groups based on caloric and nutrient equivalences has long been a popular tool in nutrition education, especially for the management of diabetes and other obesity-related health problems. In need of revision since its previous 1976 version, this nutrition counseling tool's new 1986 edition also reflects the current guidelines relating nutrition to health promotion (see Appendix).[29] In both substance and style, the new edition combines current scientific knowledge and practical diet planning in its reorganization of material and updating of nutrition recommendations. Its companion guide for professionals is being developed on these same principles.

General Health Problems Influencing Food Intake and Use

A number of adults may suffer varying levels of discomfort and poor nutrition from numerous psychosocial and physiologic life stresses, as described in Chapter 11. Some of these problems may relate to general gastrointestinal disorders that influence food intake and its use by the body.

ORAL AND ESOPHAGEAL PROBLEMS

Oral Problems

Major dental problems leading to tooth losses may interfere with biting and chewing food properly. In middle-aged and older adults, poorly fitting dentures may also contribute to eating problems and pain, often associated with poor appetite. Also, medications may dull sensory perceptions of taste and smell, taking much of the enjoyment from eating and decreasing food intake. Other problems may stem from infections of the mouth, throat, or larynx, or from oral surgery, as well as jaw pain from problems involving the temporal mandibular joint.

Esophageal Problems

After food is taken into the mouth, masticated, and swallowed, the esophagus conducts the food mass to the stomach, aided by peristalsis and gravity. The *gastroesophageal sphincter muscle* at the entrance to the stomach forms a controlling valve. It relaxes to receive the food, then closes to hold each bolus for digestive action by enzymes in the gastric acid mix. A number of problems may interfere with this normal food passage, causing episodes of functional discomfort such as *dysphagia,* so-called indigestion, or more serious disease and complete obstruction. Nutritional care in any case is adapted to the degree of discomfort in food choices and feeding mode. Several types of esophageal conditions that interfere with eating are commonly encountered in general clinical practice, including reflux irritation, hiatal hernia, and diverticula:

1. **Reflux esophagitis.** Regurgitation of the acid gastric contents into the lower part of the esophagus creates tissue irritation. The hydrochloric acid and pepsin cause tissue erosion, with substernal symptoms of burning, cramping, pressure, or severe pain. The most common symptom is *pyrosis,* or "heartburn." Iron-deficiency anemia from chronic tissue bleeding may contribute to the general state of malnutrition.
2. **Hiatal hernia.** Normally the lower end of the esophagus enters the chest cavity at the *hiatus,* an opening in the diaphragmatic membrane, and immediately joins the upper portion of the stomach. A **hiatal hernia** occurs when a portion of the upper part of the stomach at this entry point of the esophagus protrudes through the hiatus alongside the lower portion of the esophagus (Fig. 9-1). Food may easily be captured in this upper herniated area of the stomach and, mixed with acid and pepsin, be regurgitated back into the lower portion of the esophagus. Gastritis in this area can cause bleeding and anemia. Other symptoms are similar to those of reflux esophagitis. Hiatal hernia is commonly encountered among middle-aged and older adults, frequently associated with obesity, making weight reduction a primary consideration.
3. **Diverticula.** Small outpouchings in the gastrointestinal tract called **diverticula** can also occur in the esophagus, as well as in the lower intestine. Esophageal diverticula cause general dysphagia with regurgitation of undigested or partly digested food. Difficulty in swallowing increases and eating becomes more difficult. Over time, weight loss and impaired nutrition follow.

GASTRIC PROBLEMS

Peptic Ulcer Disease

Peptic ulcers affect about 10% of the population. They are the subject of millions of dollars spent in research and cause the loss of many productive work hours as a result of illness. Often they are associated with stress. They can occur at any age, but the highest incidence is in middle adulthood, between ages 45 and 55. Gastric and duodenal ulcers, along with the complication of perforation, occur more often in men than in women, although related frequencies vary with the person's age and the type of ulcer involved.

Nutritional Care

Sound nutritional management must focus on the *person* with the ulcer. The course of the disease is conditioned by the person's unique nature and life situation, and its presence in turn affects his life. Thus two basic principles guide the current liberal approach: (1) the individual must be treated as such, with his own daily living and

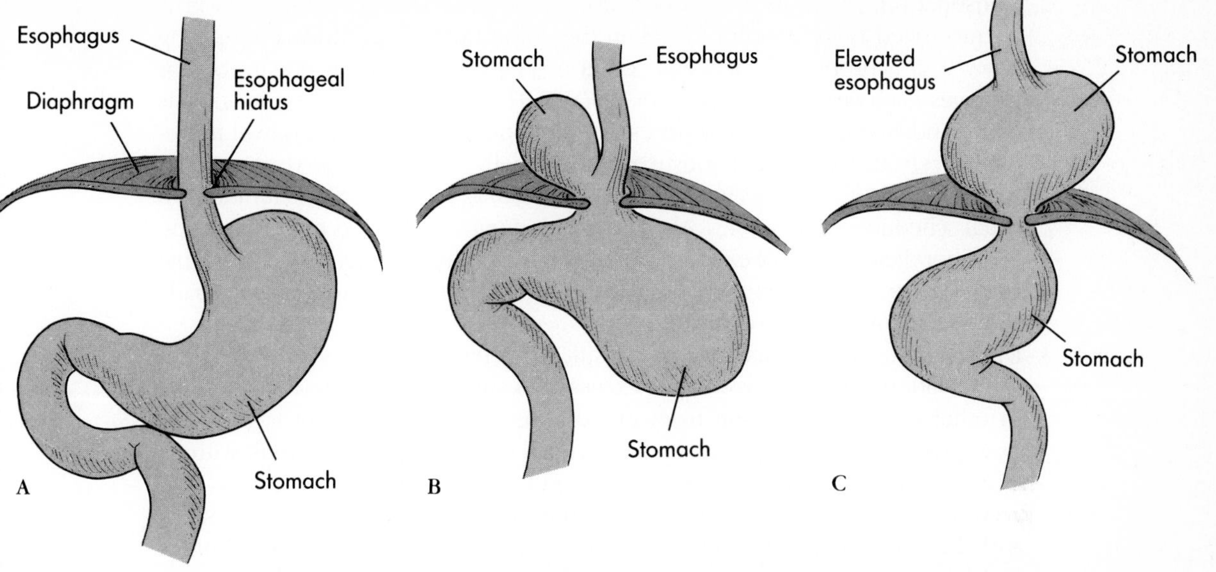

FIG. 9-1 Hiatal hernia in comparison with normal stomach placement. **A**, Normal stomach. **B**, Paraesophageal hernia (esophagus in normal position). **C**, Esophageal hiatal hernia (elevated esophagus).

working situation, attitudes, food reactions, and tolerances; and (2) the activity of the ulcer will influence dietary care. Positive individual needs and a flexible diet program guide daily food planning, and individual counseling seeks to meet personal needs and support steps toward positive health promotion.

INTESTINAL PROBLEMS

General Functional Disorders

Several common functional disorders of the intestine interfere with food use in the body and may contribute to poor nutrition in many adults. These conditions include irritable bowel syndrome, constipation, and diarrhea:

1. **Irritable bowel syndrome.** This general functional disorder may occur at any adult age and is more frequent in women. It is characterized by irritation of the mucous membrane, with symptoms varying between spastic constipation and "nervous" diarrhea. It is most often associated with stress and reflects overreactivity of the autonomic nervous system. These harried individuals develop patterns of irregular eating and bowel habits, and often resort to excessive use of laxatives, cathartics, enemas, and a variety of other medications. In general, dietary measures are designed to provide optimal nutrition and regulate bowel motility. Additional amounts of bulk foods such as fruits, vegetables, and whole grains are helpful. Supportive care must be supplied to reduce stress factors involved.

2. **Constipation.** A common disorder, usually of short duration, constipation is characterized by retention of feces in the colon beyond the normal emptying time. It is a problem Americans spend a quarter of a billion dollars on for laxatives each year but hardly ever discuss. The "regularity" of elimination is highly individual, and it is not necessary for good health to have a bowel movement every day. Extended constipation is usually a result of nervous tension, worry, and changes in diet and social setting such as vacations with alterations in usual schedules and routines. Also, it may be due to prolonged use of laxatives, low-fiber diets, or lack of exercise, all of which contribute to decreased intestinal muscle tone. General measures such as improved diet and bowel habits usually suffice to remedy the problem.
3. **Diarrhea.** Functional diarrhea may result from tension, dietary excesses with fermentation of sugars involved, or excess fiber stimulation of intestinal motility. In other cases it may result from intolerance of specific nutrient factors. For example, **lactose intolerance** is a widespread condition in which milk with its large amount of lactose cannot be digested because of lactase deficiency. The accumulated concentration of lactose in the intestine creates osmotic pressure and draws water into the gut, thus stimulating hyperactivity and resulting in abdominal cramping and diarrhea. Small amounts of milk at a time may be tolerated by some persons with lactase deficiency, or fermented products such as buttermilk and yogurt. Also, since the process of cheesemaking largely eliminates the original milk's lactose, cheese may be substituted in the diet. Often a special lactose-hydrolyzed milk treated with lactase will be tolerated.

Diverticulosis

The formation of diverticula, small tubular sacs in the intestinal wall, usually the colon, produces the condition of diverticulosis. More often it occurs in middle-aged and older adults and develops at points of weakened musculature in the bowel wall, remaining to alter its structure. The condition is usually asymptomatic unless the involved tissue becomes infected and inflamed, causing **diverticulitis.** Fecal residue causes increased irritation, increased motility brings diarrhea, and increased intraluminal pressure from luminal segmentation muscle action causes pain. If the process continues, intestinal obstruction or perforation may necessitate surgical intervention. Current clinical practice has indicated better management of diverticular disease with a high-fiber diet, although individual condition and responses will guide care.

Malabsorption Disease

Malabsorption syndromes such as **celiac disease** (sprue) or **inflammatory bowel disease** with infectious mucosal changes cause malnutrition from loss of unabsorbed nutrients released from the digestive breakdown of foods consumed. In celiac disease, the offending agent is the gliadin fraction of the plant protein gluten, found mainly in wheat, rye, and oats. Although the precise mechanism involved in the toxic effect in sensitive persons is unclear, damage to the mucosal epithelial cells and the immune system is believed to be involved. In inflammatory bowel disease, including both ulcerative colitis and Crohn's disease, the tissue changes often become chronic and can involve limited or extensive lesions that may penetrate the intestinal wall. Incidence is highest among older teenagers and young adults, with a secondary peak at ages 55 to 60. Nutritional care centers on supporting the healing process and avoiding malnutrition from deficiencies.

Health Problems of Chronic Disease

The major health problems of the United States and other developed Western societies center on the so-called diseases of civilization—heart disease and cancer—and other chronic diseases of the aging process. Additional problems stem from diabetes mellitus and its complications, mainly in relation to cardiovascular disease and renal diseases.

CORONARY HEART DISEASE AND HYPERTENSION

The Problem of Heart Disease

The major cause of death in the United States and other Western societies for the past half century has been and continues to be diseases of the heart and blood vessels. The magnitude of this health problem is indeed enormous. Every day it is estimated that 3400 American adults, more than 2 each minute, suffer a heart attack. In addition, every day approximately 1600 adults suffer strokes. Although there has been a general decline in cardiovascular mortality during the past decade, the leading cause of death in the U.S. remains coronary heart disease. It alone is responsible for some 650,000 deaths per year, with more than 150,000 of these occurring in persons less than 65 years old. In addition to its human toll, diseases of the heart and blood vessels extract a severe social and economic cost to families affected.

The Problem of Atherosclerosis

Despite enormous research efforts, the frustrating fact remains—we still do not know the precise cause of the underlying pathology of coronary heart disease, atherosclerosis. We know enough to realize that it is a multi-faceted disease process associated with the Western way of living and having multiple risk factors involved (Table 9-2). A number of these risk factors are related to nutrition and state of fitness, as discussed in opening sections of this chapter, and involve metabolism of lipids and sodium.

The Problem of Hypertension

High blood pressure presents a problem in the lives of some 60 million American adults. At least 95% of these persons have *essential* or *primary* hypertension, meaning that its cause is unknown, but with a strong genetic factor involved. Unlike many other conditions, however, hypertension develops "soundlessly" without symptoms. Yet it has become the fourth largest public health problem in America and has earned the unenviable reputation as the "silent killer" because it carries no overt signs and many persons are unaware of its presence. This is an indication of its potentially serious implications if not detected, treated, and controlled, all of which are easily accom-

TABLE 9-2 Multiple Risk Factors in Cardiovascular Disease

Personal Characteristics (no control)	Learned Behaviors (intervene and change)	Background Conditions (screen-treat)
Sex	Stress/coping	Hypertension
Age	Smoking cigarettes	Diabetes mellitus
Family history	Sedentary lifestyle	Hyperlipidemia (especially hypercholesterolemia)
	Obesity	
	Food habits	
	Excess fat	
	Excess sugar	
	Excess salt	

plished. Despite a wealth of research in past years there are few clues to its etiology, and our lack of information leaves us more confused than enlightened.

Nondrug Approaches to Hypertension Control

Since hypertension is a strong risk factor in heart disease, there is a renewed effort to screen for its presence and start control programs early, especially in young adults. A significant result of this increased public awareness and concern has been a renewed focus on nonpharmacologic approaches to control through changes in lifestyle and positive health promotion. The U.S. National Heart, Lung, and Blood Institute of the National Institutes of Health has increased its strong emphasis on nondrug therapies—diet, exercise, and behavior modification—urging that they be "pursued aggressively," not only for mild hypertension but also as an important adjunct in moderate and severe cases.[30] Experts agree that the goal of all therapy is to reduce as much as possible the quantity of drugs required. Kaplan[31] cites numerous studies to underscore the need for greater use of nondrug approaches to care through practical lifestyle changes for health—improved diet with reduced sodium, weight control, increased exercise, and stress management. Thus nutritional therapy has a fundamental role in the health care of persons with hypertension.

CANCER

Incidence

The American Cancer Society estimates that about 440,000 Americans die each year of some form of cancer. About 25% of these persons die of lung cancer, a largely preventable disease caused by the habit of cigarette smoking. In its many forms cancer has become one of the major health problems in the United States, claiming about 20% of the total deaths, close on the heels of the number one killer, heart disease, which takes about 50% of the total.

Health Promotion Approaches

Nutrition plays an important role in prevention and control of cancer. Significant nutritional relationships exist in two basic areas: (1) *prevention* in relation to environmental agents, as well as maintaining a strong body defense system; and (2) *therapy* in relation to nutritional support for medical treatment and rehabilitation.[32]

DIABETES COMPLICATIONS

Objectives of Care

The person with diabetes has three main objectives in good self-care with health-team support:

1. **To maintain optimal nutrition.** A fundamental requirement for both diabetes control and health maintenance is good nutrition for normal growth and development and a desirable lean weight.
2. **To avoid symptoms.** With sound diet, exercise, and drug therapy if needed, good health habits can keep the person relatively free from symptoms such as hyperglycemia and glycosuria, helping to avoid health problems.
3. **To prevent complications.** This basic objective recognizes the increased risk the person with diabetes carries for development of problems in tissues such as the eye (retinopathy), in nerve tissue (neuropathy), and in renal tissue (nephropathy), and in cardiovascular tissue (atherosclerosis).

Incidence

Because of these increased risks, persons with diabetes especially need to follow healthy lifestyles to maintain good control and prevent complications. Nearly 11 million Americans have diabetes, 2 million of whom use insulin. One in twenty persons has to deal with this metabolic disorder, largely through self-care, so education and support in good self-care from its onset is essential. Diabetic complications have become the fifth ranking cause of death from disease in the U.S. Among older adults with diabetes, the cause of death from diabetic complications is mainly heart attack. The underlying pathology of heart disease, *atherosclerosis,* is two to three times more common in persons with diabetes than in nondiabetic individuals. The major cause of death among younger adults with diabetes is renal failure secondary to *glomerulosclerosis.* Kidney disease affects the lives of over 8 million Americans and kills some 60,000 a year. Another 3 million or more have related infections, many of which go undetected. These kidney problems are a leading cause of lost work time and income and make up the fourth leading health problem in America today. Also, the eye complications of diabetes present a leading cause of vision problems and blindness. Good health care on a regular basis from the beginning can largely reduce risks and prevent these serious health problems from diabetes complications.

EDUCATION AND PREVENTION

In all of these health problems from chronic disease in adults, the wise approach lies in education for health promotion and prevention of risks and complications. These efforts should begin in childhood, especially in families having genetic predisposition to these health problems, and should continue throughout the life cycle with practical support of lifestyle changes for healthy living.

Summary

Adult health and wellness depend upon a healthy lifestyle through young, middle, and older adulthood. Components of a healthy lifestyle include a sound diet with attention to risk factors related to excess fat, cholesterol, and sodium, as well as excess body weight; stress management; smoking cessation; and avoidance of abuse of alcohol and drugs. To help achieve the fundamental goal of health promotion, a number of health programs have developed in response to public awareness and concern. These public and professional activities include hospital-based community programs, health maintenance organization (HMO) programs, work-site wellness programs, health clubs, and community screening programs and health fairs.

To help prevent the development of health problems, a sound nutritional base for adult health must be provided. General nutrient standards and food guides provide resources for planning such a healthy diet. A number of general gastrointestinal problems may require attention to prevent their contribution to poor nutrition. As adults grow older, chronic diseases of aging may present added health problems. These conditions include coronary heart disease, hypertension, cancer, and diabetes complications. Good nutrition plays a significant role in preventing and managing these conditions, and early education and prevention approaches are essential in health promotion.

Review Questions

1. Describe various approaches to health promotion. Which do you think has the greatest application to current health issues? Why?
2. List and describe five components of a healthy lifestyle. How is each related to high-level wellness or the prevention of chronic disease? Develop a healthy 2-day food plan for an adult of your choice, indicating daily activities that would influence meal pattern or food selection.
3. Outline a health promotion program for a particular audience. Indicate the following components of your program: (1) the intended audience; (2) the location; (3) types of publicity; (4) subject areas, topics, or activities; and (5) criteria for program evaluation.
4. Describe adult nutritional needs and factors influencing these needs. Identify and compare three nutrient or food guidelines for meeting these needs.
5. Identify five gastrointestinal problems influencing adult food intake and use. Select one of these problems and outline a day's food plan for an adult with this problem.
6. Describe five chronic disease conditions of aging that may present health problems, giving the extent of the public health problem and wise individual approaches to health management and prevention of problems.

REFERENCES

1. Mossey, J.M., and Shapiro, E.: Self-rated health: a predictor of mortality among the elderly, Am. J. Public Health 72:800, 1982.
2. Feinleib, M., and Wilson, R.W.: Trends in health in the United States, Environ. Health Perspect. 62:267, 1985.
3. Lipid Research Clinics Program: The Lipid Research Clinics coronary primary prevention

trial results. II. The relationship of reduction in incidence of coronary heart disease to cholesterol lowering, J.A.M.A. **251**:365, 1984.

4. Committee on Diet, Nutrition, and Cancer: Diet, nutrition, and cancer, Washington, D.C., 1982, National Academy of Sciences.
5. Food and Nutrition Board, National Research Council: Recommended dietary allowances, ed. 9, Washington, D.C., 1980, National Academy of Sciences.
6. Kromhout, D., Bosschieter, E.B., and Coulander, C.: The inverse relation between fish consumption and 20-year mortality from coronary heart disease, New Engl. J. Med. **312**:1205, 1985.
7. Ray, T.K., Mansell, K.M., Knight, L.C., and others: Long-term effects of dietary fiber on glucose tolerance and gastric emptying in noninsulin-dependent diabetic patients, Am. J. Clin. Nutr. **37**(3):376, 1983.
8. Simpson, H.C.R., Lousley, S., Geekie, M., and others: A high-carbohydrate leguminous-fiber diet improves all aspects of diabetic control, Lancet **1**:1, 1981.
9. Paffenbarger, R.S., and others: A natural history of athleticism and cardiovascular health, J.A.M.A. **252**:491, 1984.
10. Simopoulos, A.P., and Van Itallie, T.B.: Body weight, health, and longevity, Ann. Intern. Med. **100**:285, 1984.
11. United States Department of Health and Human Services: Health, United States, 1984, DHHS pub. no. (PHS) 85-1232, Hyattsville, Md., 1984, National Center for Health Statistics.
12. Medical Section of the American Lung Association: Cigarette smoking and health, Am. Rev. Respir. Dis. **132**:1133, 1985.
13. Foote, A., and Erfurt, J.C.: Hypertension control at the work site, New Engl. J. Med. **308**:809, 1983.
14. Blair, S.N., and others: A public health intervention model for work-site health promotion, J.A.M.A. **255**:921, 1986.
15. Reed, R.W.: Is education the key to lower health care costs? Personnel J. :40, 1984.
16. Donaldson, M.S., Nicklason, J.A., and Ott, J.E.: Needs-based health promotion program serves as HMO marketing tool, Public Health Rep. **100**:270, 1985.
17. Berwick, D.M.: Screening in health fairs, J.A.M.A. **254**:1492, 1985.
18. Epstein, M.: Aging and the kidney: clinical implications, Am. Fam. Physician **31**:123, April 1985.
19. Erikson, E.: Childhood and society, New York, 1963, W.W. Norton & Co., Inc.
20. Hall, E.: A conversation with Erik Erikson, Psychology Today **17**(6):22, 1983.
21. Review: Osteoporosis and calcium balance, Nutr. Rev. **41**(3):183, 1983.
22. Riggs, B.L., and Melton, L.J., III: Involutional osteoporosis, New Engl. J. Med. **314**:1676, June 26, 1986.
23. Guthrie, H.A.: Supplementation: a nutritionist's view, J. Nutr. Educ. **18**:130, June, 1986.
24. Ratto, T.: The four food groups revisited, Med. Self-Care **41**:43, July-August, 1987.
25. Marshall, E.: The academy kills a nutrition report, Science **230**(4724):420, October 25, 1985.
26. Hegstead, D.M.: Dietary standards—guidelines for prevention of deficiency or prescription for total health? J. Nutr. **116**:478, March 1986.
27. Food and Nutrition Board, National Research Council: Recommended dietary allowances: scientific issues and process for the future, J. Nutr. **116**:482, March 1986.
28. Miller, S.A., and Stephenson, M.G.: Scientific and public health rationale for the dietary guidelines for Americans, Am. J. Clin. Nutr. **42**:739, October 1985.
29. Franz, M.J., Holler, H., Powers, M.A., and others: Exchange lists: revised 1986, J. Am. Diet. Assoc. **87**(1):28, January 1987.

30. Dustin, H.P., Chobanian, A.V., Faulkner, B., and others: The 1984 report of the Joint National Committee on Detection, Evaluation, and Treatment of High Blood Pressure, Arch. Intern. Med. **144**:1045, May 1984.
31. Kaplan, N.M.: Nondrug treatment of hypertension, Ann. Intern. Med. **102**:359, March 1985.
32. Williams, S.R.: Nutrition and cancer. In Nutrition and diet therapy, ed. 5, St. Louis, 1985, Times Mirror/Mosby College Publishing.

FURTHER READING

Brennan, A.J.: Health and fitness boom moves into corporate America, Occup. Health Safety, July 1985, p. 38.

Corporate fitness programs, increasing in both number and scope, have had a high degree of success in reducing employee risk of chronic disease. This article describes several approaches to employee fitness programs with guidelines for planning, implementation, and evaluation.

Cancer **58**, October 15 (Supplement), 1986.

This entire supplement issue is devoted to 22 helpful articles on relationships of nutrition and cancer. Articles include such topics as debunking myths, practical guides for nutritional support, and dietary considerations for risk reduction.

Daniel-Gentry, J., Dolecek, T.A., Caggiula, A.W., and others: Increasing the use of meatless meals: a nutrition intervention substudy in the Multiple Risk Factor Intervention Trial (MRFIT), J. Am. Diet. Assoc. **86**:778, June 1986.

This article reports a nutrition education strategy for helping persons increase their use of vegetable protein and decrease their intakes of fat and cholesterol. These methods could be applied to any type of dietary modification.

Gussow, J.D., and Clancy, K.L.: Dietary guidelines for sustainability, J. Nutr. Educ. **18**:1, February 1986.

These sensitive nutritionists present an expanded basis for statements comprising the current U.S. dietary guidelines, with food choices not only based on relation to health but also influenced by knowledge of how to protect and *sustain* our precious natural resources.

Kassirer, J.P., and Harrington, J.T.: Fending off potassium pushers, New Engl. J. Med. **312**:785, March 21, 1985.

These authors present a timely article illustrating the dangers inherent in inappropriate nutrient supplementation, in this case potassium.

Lefebvre, R.C., Harden, E.A., Rakowski, W., and others: Characteristics of participants in community health promotion programs: four-year results, Am. J. Pub. Health 77(10):1342, October 1987.

This study of 25,000 participants in an ongoing community health project in heart disease prevention reports characteristics of persons making life style changes through effective programs that reached large numbers of people in the community.

Miller, R.W.: America's changing diet, FDA Consumer **19**:4, 1985.

This article provides background on factors leading to our changing diet patterns, with significant changes consumers have made in their food choices.

St. Jeor, S.T., and Winston, M.: A national educational event: The food festival designed to help consumers implement the American Heart Association dietary guidelines for healthy Americans, Nutr. Today 22(4):10, July-August 1987.

This festival, built around the theme "It's high time to lower cholesterol," provides an excellent example of how food market chains and a national health promotion association can pool their resources to increase public awareness and involve communities nationwide in health education at the point of purchase, where critical food decisions are made that affect chronic disease risks.

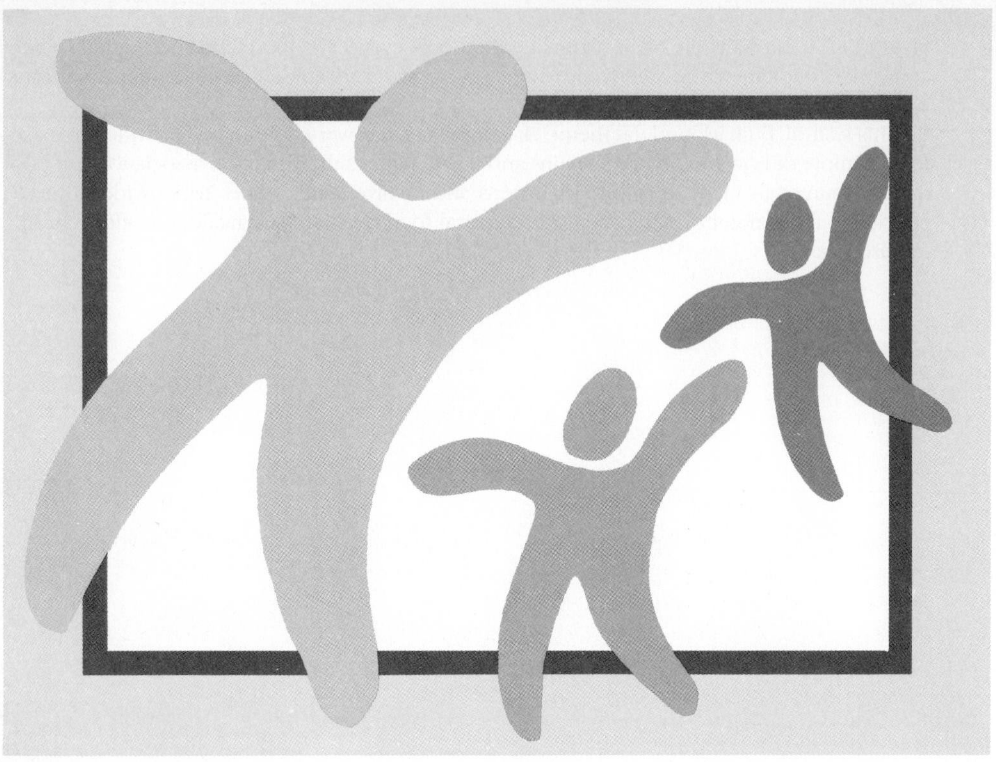

Basic Concepts

1. Persons age 60 and above, the fastest growing segment of the population, sometimes need nutrition support services to maintain independent healthy living.
2. Aging brings a gradual decline in normal physiologic functions.
3. Energy needs decrease with age but protein, vitamin, and mineral needs remain the same, making *nutrient density* important in meal planning.
4. Vitamins and minerals are the nutrients most likely to be lacking in an older person's diet and most adversely affected by multiple medications, both over-the-counter and prescription.
5. Numerous social, physiologic, and economic factors can influence food and nutrient intake in older people.

Chapter Ten

Nutrition for Aging and the Aged

Eleanor D. Schlenker

Improvements in health care, sanitation, and quality of diet have led to an increase in average lifespan and a dramatic shift in population toward older age groups. There are now more old persons in the world than at any time in history.

However, we know relatively little about the changing nutrient needs of older adults as compared to those of younger adults. For most older adults energy requirements decrease with age, but protein, vitamin, and mineral needs remain the same. And chronically ill older persons may even need nutrient increases. All of these needs, often in the face of decreased appetite, emphasize the importance of *nutrient density* in planning meals and snacks. Biologic and physiologic changes of normal aging can lead to various health problems that require dietary management.

In this chapter we will look at these changing needs of the aging population. We will explore environmental, personal, and health factors that influence them. We will see that effective nutrition intervention requires sensitive evaluation of older persons. Each is a unique individual with a complex of varying life needs affecting nutrition and nutritional care.

Demographic Aspects of Aging

POPULATION TRENDS

In the United States age 65 is frequently used as a benchmark to characterize the older population—the "retired" generation. But chronologic age is not always a measure of physical health or zest for life. Many older adults are leading active, healthy lives, and the total number of older persons in the population is growing. Actually, persons age 65 and over are increasing in number more rapidly than any other age group and now make up 11% of the total population as compared to only 4% in 1900. One in nine persons is now age 65 or over. Furthermore, this increase will continue. By the year 2020 the number of persons age 65 and over will have doubled, with the greatest rise occurring among those age 85 and older.[1]

This increase in number and proportion of older persons has implications for both the family and society. There will be fewer people of working age and greater numbers of people who will be retired. Persons age 85 and over, because of increasing disability, are more likely than those between ages 65 and 85 to require economic assistance or help with activities of daily living. Finally, older people are the largest users of health-care services and will require an ever-growing share of public and private health insurance resources.

CHANGES IN LIFE EXPECTANCY

Nature of Changes

Life expectancy is the average remaining years of life for a person of a given age. The dramatic increase in life expectancy in this century occurred primarily in infancy and childhood. For men life expectancy at birth increased from 46 to 70 years between 1900 and 1980; for women, from 46 to 78 years.[1] But despite improvements in medical care, since 1900 life expectancy at age 65 has increased by only 3 years in men and 6 years in women. Thus the growth of the older population does not reflect an increase in *maximal* lifespan, but rather the extended lifespan of those individuals who in the past died in infancy and childhood.

Influencing Factors

Gains in life expectancy have not been equal among all groups. Women can expect to live longer than men and whites longer than nonwhites. Increased smoking among women may in future years reduce their life expectancy as death rates from lung cancer continue to rise. Level of education and income are related to life expectancy and may contribute to the lower life expectancy of nonwhites.

Causes of Death

Today the three most common causes of death are heart disease, cancer, and cerebrovascular disease (stroke). All are related to degenerative changes associated with aging and the environment. In contrast, the leading cause of death in 1900 was infectious diseases, for example, pneumonia and influenza, now controlled by antibiotic drugs. A lifestyle based on a diet moderate in sucrose, fat, and sodium, with no smoking, limited or no use of alcohol, and regular exercise can delay the onset of chronic disease and lead to an improvement in health status in the expanding older population.

SOCIOECONOMIC CHARACTERISTICS OF THE OLDER POPULATION

The general public associates old age with poor health, illness, and disability. This view often leads to the assumption that the majority of older people live in institutions. In fact 95% of aged persons live within the community, either with a spouse, other family member or friend, or alone. Specific living arrangements are related to sex. About three-fourths of older men are married. In contrast, over half of older women are widows, and over one-third live alone.[1] Living situation can contribute to food problems of older people. An aged widow who lives in a rural area and cannot drive is dependent on relatives or friends for transportation to a food store.

Older women, minority groups, and those above age 84 are also more vulnerable to poor nutrition because of lower income. Usually couples have a more adequate income than single individuals. Government programs such as food stamps or congregate meals (p. 440) can help those with limited food money.

Biologic Aspects of Aging

THE AGING PROCESS

In general terms the study of aging includes all changes in body structure and function that occur throughout the lifespan as a result of growth, maturation, and senescence. In our context aging refers to the time-dependent biologic and physiologic changes that begin about age 30 and are degenerative in their effect. The pattern and sequence of the changes in normal aging are always the same although the rate at which these changes occur differs from one person to another. Both genetic and environmental factors influence this rate of aging. Individuals with long-lived parents are more likely to survive beyond age 70. Environmental factors such as irradiation or level of nutrition influence life span in experimental animals.

Cellular Level Changes

Although no one knows exactly how the aging process takes place, changes are observed first at the cellular level. Among cell types that continue to divide throughout their normal lifespan, for example, skin cells or mucosal cells lining the gastrointestinal tract, the rate of division slows as the cell nears the end of its normal lifespan and eventually stops. Cells from species having shorter lifespans will undergo fewer divisions than those from species having longer lifespans. Cells from an older donor undergo fewer divisions than those from a younger donor. Although the older person will always have some cells that are rapidly dividing, they will be fewer in number and the total cell count is reduced. Changes in nutrient absorption, observed in some but not all older persons, could relate to such changes in the mucosa.

Organ Level Changes

Highly differentiated cells including brain, kidney, and muscle that do not continue to divide throughout life undergo functional changes with time and some cells die. As a result these organ systems become less efficient as fewer cells remain to carry on body functions. The aging cell that has undergone structural or functional changes is less able to synthesize important molecules such as ones required for hormonal or neural control or for the induction of a specific enzyme. As a result, specialized organs and tissues are less able to respond to environmental stimuli and there is a breakdown in the condition of the body systems that may need to work together to carry out a physiologic function.

THEORIES OF AGING

Current theories attempting to explain the aging process point to the replication of DNA within the cell nucleus as the site of control. Two different opinions, although not mutually exclusive, have emerged:

Codon Restriction Theory

A *codon* is one of the triplet sets of bases making up the nucleotide chains of DNA and RNA, the sequence of which determines a specific genetic "code." Each specific sequence "codes" or programs for a specific amino acid, and the specific sequence of amino acids determines the polypeptide chain of a specific protein. The *codon restriction theory* proposes that aging represents a programmed series of events that is an extension of growth and maturation. It is believed that in later life particular sequences of DNA required for the synthesis of vital proteins are no longer reproduced, resulting in structural and functional changes within the organism.

Random Environmental Theory

An opposing view suggests that aging is the result of *random environmental influences* such as radiation that lead to mutations in the DNA and synthesis of abnormal proteins. Two related theories, the *error theory* and the *redundant message theory,* represent this idea. Normal aging most likely is the result of a combination of genetic and environmental events.

Physiologic Aspects of Aging

COORDINATION OF PHYSIOLOGIC FUNCTIONS

Response to Stimuli

One characteristic of physiologic aging is decreased ability to respond to changes in either the internal or external environment. The return to resting levels following a stimulus requires a longer period in older persons than it does in younger ones. The age-related decline in physiologic function occurring between ages 30 and 80 has been observed in an ongoing study of adult males at the Gerontology Research Center of the National Institute on Aging in Baltimore.[2] Functional capacity at age 30 (Fig. 10-1) is considered to equal 100% and a decline in function is rated accordingly. The degree of loss observed is influenced by the level of coordination required among one or more organ systems. Fasting blood glucose levels exhibit little change whereas resting cardiac output, requiring both neural and muscular control, declines by 30%.

Response to Added Demand

As a system becomes more complex, impairment becomes more apparent. For example, an older person may walk with comparative ease on a level surface, but climbing stairs may require heavy effort. Despite known decrements in physiologic systems most older persons function quite well on a day-to-day basis. However, when extreme demands, for example, heavy exercise or severe illness, are placed on the system, or when functional losses are excessive, problems become evident.

BRAIN AND NEURAL CONTROL

Functional Changes

Both structural and biochemical changes contribute to functional alterations in the aging brain. Although there is general agreement that neurons are lost in advanced age

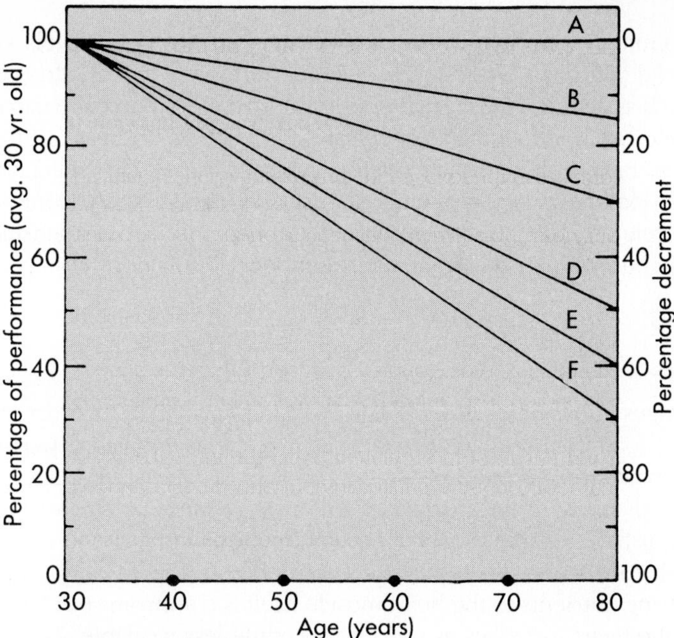

FIG. 10-1 Age-related decline in physiological function.
(From Shock, N.W.: Energy metabolism, caloric intake, and physical activity of the aging. In Carlson, L.A., ed.: Nutrition in old age, Symposia Swedish Nutrition Foundation X, Stockholm, Sweden, 1972, Almqvist & Wiksell. Used by permission.)

with estimates of losses ranging as high as 20% to 40%,[3] questions regarding changes in brain weight are still unresolved. Because brain weight is related to body size, smaller brain weights may be a secular effect (one related to outside events), and not indicative of age-related changes within the individual. Moreover, neither brain weight nor cell number appears to be related to Alzheimer-type senile dementia.

Neurotransmitters

Decreased synthesis of neurotransmitters, for example, dopamine, serotonin, or acetylcholine, required for the conduction of nerve impulses has been observed in older people. The most striking reductions in neural transmitter levels occur in the hypothalamus and cerebral cortex, which control psychomotor skills and cognitive function, activities exhibiting age-related alterations. Further work with humans should evaluate the behavioral implications of biochemical and structural changes in the aging brain.

ENDOCRINE SYSTEM

Information is limited regarding age-related changes in hormone levels or the mechanisms involved. Although blood levels of some hormones such as aldosterone decrease, others such as thyroxin (T_4) remain the same. Decreased secretion can result from either impaired hormone synthesis or release. Or reduced hormone utilization or slowed excretion may limit hormone release through homeostatic mechanisms. Current research is looking at hypothalamus-pituitary regulation of hormone secretion, storage, and release. The aged hypothalamus appears to be less sensitive to messages received and may play a role in altered endocrine function.

CARDIOVASCULAR SYSTEM

Functional Changes

Age-related changes in the heart and circulatory system involve both structure and function. The work load of the heart increases as a result of increased peripheral resistance caused by atherosclerotic deposition and loss of arterial elasticity. At the same time the effectiveness of the heart as a pump is reduced as the strength of contraction is diminished. Resting cardiac output falls measurably as the volume of blood pumped with each stroke decreases. As a result blood flow through the coronary arteries supplying nutrients to the heart muscle itself is compromised. Therefore the work load on the heart increases as nutrients become less available. As a consequence, the aged heart poorly tolerates either physiologic or emotional stress. This points to the importance of medical evaluation of older persons before they begin an exercise program.

Hypertension

Age-related changes in cardiovascular function contribute to the rise in blood pressure observed in both sexes. Hypertension is a significant medical and nutritional problem among older persons. Effective management may require weight control and sodium restriction. In a national survey,[4] about two-thirds of those above age 64 had systolic pressures above 140 mm Hg or diastolic pressures above 90 mm Hg. High blood pressure increases the risk of stroke and coronary artery disease.

RENAL SYSTEM

Functional Changes

Kidney function deteriorates with age as a result of both a loss of nephrons and a 30% decrease in blood flow, a consequence of reduced cardiac output. Total nephrons decline by 30% to 40%.[3] As the glomerular filtration rate is slowed, it takes longer to clear drugs or metabolic wastes from the blood. On that basis, excessive protein resulting in high blood urea nitrogen levels, or megadoses of the water-soluble vitamins, should be avoided. The aged kidney is less able to concentrate urine, so adequate fluid intake is essential. In the nephron tubule, nutrients including glucose, plasma proteins, and ascorbic acid are less efficiently reabsorbed while drug metabolites and H+ ions are less efficiently excreted.

Water Balance

Fluid regulation and water balance are serious needs to consider in the nutritional management of older people. An age-related increase in antidiuretic hormone (ADH or vasopressin), enlarged by drugs that induce further antidiuretic hormonal activity, can lead to water intoxication. At the other extreme, fluid restriction can result in dehydration and severely elevated serum electrolyte levels. Records of fluid intake therefore become very important in the care of an older person with limited access to water.

PULMONARY SYSTEM

Structural changes in the lung result in loss of alveolar surface area and a decrease in elasticity. Although total lung capacity does not change, the proportion of alveolar space ventilated with each breath and thus the total surface area for gas exchange decreases. Gas exchange itself is less efficient because of decreased permeability of the alveolar membranes and reduced blood flow. As a result, oxyhemoglobin saturation of arterial blood is lowered in advanced age, making oxygen transfer to the tissues more difficult. The reduced ability to effectively increase oxygen intake becomes a significant factor in exercise or physiologic stress.

Nutrition and the Lifespan

Since antiquity people have been searching for potions to preserve health and prolong life. Ponce de Leon came to the New World seeking the "fountain of youth." Francis Bacon (1591-1626) was the first author to recommend scientific evaluation of diet and longevity. He advocated a frugal diet and encouraged the study of people in various climates and living situations to determine those characteristics that influence lifespan. Unfortunately, Bacon's recommendations for study are only beginning to receive attention.

ANIMAL STUDIES

Energy Restriction

Animal studies have demonstrated that energy intake controls not only the rate of growth but also the rate of maturation and aging. Animals fed diets restricted in kilocalories, although adequate in protein, vitamins and minerals, live 40% longer than those given unlimited access to food, and chronic problems such as kidney disease appear at a later age. Diet restriction also delays biochemical alterations such as the age-related rise in serum cholesterol observed in both humans and animals.

Rate of Growth

Protein in addition to total energy influences both rate of growth and survival. In animal models, diets high in both energy and protein lead to rapid growth, large body size, and early onset and increased severity of degenerative disease. This suggestion that rapid growth and increased body weight accelerate the aging process has serious implications for current growth patterns. Children today are both taller and heavier and reach puberty at earlier ages, as compared with previous generations. Regular physical exercise is a mechanism that in animal models slows the rate of growth, lowers body weight, and increases the lifespan. This approach of regular exercise might also slow the degenerative process in humans.

HUMAN STUDIES

Little information is now available to evaluate the influence of lifelong dietary habits on health and longevity. Studies that did collect detailed nutrition information did not follow subjects at regularly scheduled intervals nor did they continue over an extended period of years. A longitudinal approach, following the same individual over time, is urgently needed to evaluate the influence of diet on physiologic and biochemical aging.

Body Weight and Mortality in the Aged

Life insurance standards, used to evaluate the body weight of individuals in relation to their peers of similar height and sex, have also been used to predict mortality risk. Since 1887 life insurance companies have compiled records on the height, weight, and subsequent mortality of their policy holders. The general conclusion drawn from these statistics is that the greater the deviation between actual body weight and standard weight (weights of policy holders who lived the longest) the greater the risk of death.

Mortality patterns, however, differ according to both sex and age. Overweight, even when extreme, carries less risk for females. Extreme underweight (25% to 35% below standard) carries greater risk for males. For both sexes underweight carries greater risk at older ages whereas overweight is more serious at younger ages. The influence of obesity on mortality seems to relate to the fact that overweight persons have a greater risk of developing diabetes, cardiovascular problems, and renal disease at younger ages.[5]

Despite the association between obesity, chronic disease, and mortality in younger age groups, the fact remains that reasonable numbers of persons have been identified who are both old and overweight. Using a weight-height index as a standard, a recent report[6] identified an equal percentage (22%) of obese men in the 25 to 34 and the 65 to 74 year age intervals. Among women the incidence actually doubled, with 21% of the younger and 40% of the older age groups identified as obese.

The disparity between life insurance data indicating a relationship between overweight and earlier death and surveys revealing significant numbers of overweight persons in older age groups has not been resolved. Overweight persons, recognizing their increased risk, may seek medical check-ups regularly and make a greater effort toward preventive health. Smoking is a factor also. A recent evaluation suggested that underweight individuals tended to be smokers, which contributed to their mortality risk, and overweight persons were less likely to smoke.[5] A major consideration in dietary management for older persons is prevention of inappropriate weight gain.

Longitudinal Studies

Longitudinal studies evaluating dietary patterns and subsequent morbidity and mortality indicate that good eating habits contribute to health and survival in middle age and beyond. Two such studies, in Michigan and in California, serve as examples.

Michigan Study

Diet quality influenced physical well-being and the length of life in a longitudinal study of 100 Michigan women over a 24-year period (1948-1972). Selected on the basis of geographical sectors to represent a socioeconomic cross-section of older women in a Midwestern city, they ranged in age from 40 to 85 years. Over a 7-year period, mortality was higher in those consuming diets containing less than 40% of the RDA for one or more nutrients. Nutrients most frequently deficient were calcium, vitamin A, and ascorbic acid.

In 1972 (24 years after the first interview) 28 of the women were located and reinterviewed by this author. Their average age was 75 years. It was apparent that survivors had reduced the quantity but not the quality of food consumed. Total energy, fat, and carbohydrate decreased by 25% although mean intakes of protein, vitamins, and minerals (with the exception of calcium) met or exceeded 67% of the RDA. Protein, fat, and carbohydrate provided 18%, 35%, and 47% of total energy, respectively.

The food pattern of the Michigan survivors could provide a model for transition from middle to advanced age. Foods high in carbohydrate and fat but providing few other nutrients were deleted from the diet. Fruits, vegetables, dairy products, and breads and cereals were used frequently. A decrease in energy intake to prevent weight gain, with continued emphasis on protein, vitamins, and minerals, is an appropriate goal.

California Study

A longitudinal study of about 7000 adults in Alameda, California,[7] examined the influence of a cluster of health practices—adequate sleep, regular meals (including breakfast), desirable body weight, not smoking, limited or no use of alcohol, and regular physical activity—on mortality. After five years it was evident that poor health practices resulted in earlier death, whereas good health habits led to longer life. Men who followed 6 or 7 health practices had a life expectancy 11 years longer than men who followed 3 or less. For women the comparable difference was 7 years. Positive gains occurred in both low- and high-income groups and in persons in poor or good health. Community education programs for health intervention should include nutrition education.

Digestion, Absorption, and Gastrointestinal Function

CHANGES IN GASTROINTESTINAL FUNCTION

Functional Disorders

Gastrointestinal discomforts including nausea, heartburn, and constipation increase in frequency with advancing age. Such symptoms can be related to poor eating and bowel habits, mental anxiety, or side effects of commonly used drugs. Gastrointestinal distress does not necessarily indicate malabsorption. Persons with no discomfort may absorb nutrients poorly whereas others with persistent distress may absorb nutrients normally.

Eating Problems

Changes in muscle innervation and reduced secretion of saliva can lead to difficulty in swallowing, particularly among frail aged persons. The result may be fear of choking and food may be refused. General dehydration or certain drugs causing dry mouth can add to this problem. Older people should eat only when seated in an upright position. Being fed in a supine position increases the risk of food aspiration and pneumonia.

Bowel Problems

At present there is little evidence to support the generally held concept of age-related degenerative changes in the stomach, small intestine, and colon. Constipation, a problem for many older people, is more likely related to low fluid intake, diets low in fiber and bulk, medications, and general lack of exercise. Constipation is more often perception than fact. Many older people have an exaggerated concern with bowel habits and the belief that a daily bowel movement is essential for good health. True constipation is characterized by: (1) fewer than two bowel movements per week, (2) persistent difficulty in passing stools, (3) bleeding with bowel movements, or (4) pain with bowel movements. Any bleeding from the rectum should be reported to a physician immediately.

Laxative Use

Individuals with normal bowel function who do not have a daily bowel movement sometimes turn to laxatives in an effort to relieve the perceived problem. After the purging effect of the laxative, normal bowel movements may not resume the following day. This reinforces the idea that the individual is constipated and leads to a vicious cycle. Use of laxatives over a prolonged period results in loss of normal bowel function. Diets generous in whole-grain breads and cereals, and fruits and vegetables, along with adequate fluid intake (1500-2000 ml daily) contribute to the formation of large, soft stools and more frequent bowel movements.

ENZYME SECRETION, DIGESTION, AND ABSORPTION

Lack of digestive enzymes does not appear to impair nutrient absorption in healthy older people. Because digestive enzymes are normally secreted at levels substantially above what is required, actual enzyme levels (though sometimes reduced) are still sufficient to adequately break down all food consumed into the forms required for absorption.

Carbohydrate Digestion and Absorption

Absorption is slowed but there is no evidence to suggest that it is incomplete in the healthy older person. The absorption of common monosaccharides is evaluated using

D-xylose as a test substance. Since this sugar is not metabolized, completeness of absorption is measured by recovery of D-xylose in the urine. Equal amounts of the test substance are recovered in younger and older subjects.

Lactose Intolerance

Reduced lactase levels have been evaluated in relation to low milk consumption among many older persons. It appears that psychologic attitudes toward milk are as important, if not more so, than physiologic factors in lactose intolerance. Malabsorption was not related to incidence of digestive symptoms as equal numbers of absorbers and malabsorbers reported symptoms following the lactose-containing drink.[8] Conversely, several malabsorbers complained of distress after both the lactose-containing and the lactose-free beverage, suggesting that a component other than lactose was causing the problem. Over half of the malabsorbers reported drinking more than one glass of milk per day, indicating that other factors in addition to lactose malabsorption influence low milk consumption in this age group.

Fat Digestion and Absorption

Both the rate and to some extent the absolute amount of fat absorbed decrease with age. Under normal conditions neutral fat (triglyceride) comprises only a minor portion of fecal fat with fatty acids the predominant form. Some older individuals, particularly those with extremely high levels of dietary fat, do have higher-than-usual fecal fat. Existing levels of pancreatic lipase are believed to be the limiting factor.

Protein Digestion and Absorption

Despite the importance of protein and amino acids little is known about the rate and degree of digestion and absorption of these nutrients as influenced by age. In older subjects both the total volume and the hydrochloric acid concentration of gastric juice, and the volume of pepsin, are decreased, but hydrochloric acid and pepsin are most affected. It is of interest, however, that individuals with lowered enzyme levels do not report any abdominal discomfort following eating.

Changes in gastric secretion result from decreases in both the number of parietal cells and the secretory capacity of remaining cells. Other changes in the mucosal lining can reduce secretion of intrinsic factor resulting in vitamin B_{12} deficiency. In light of the current controversy regarding the protein needs of older persons in general, and the apparently elevated requirements of physically impaired older persons, possible changes regarding this nutrient need to be clarified.

Vitamin and Mineral Absorption

Age-related alterations in vitamin and mineral absorption are poorly understood. For the most part these nutrients have been studied in a clinical context, considering age-related changes in nutritional status or incidence of deficiency disorders. For this reason absorption of vitamins and minerals will be discussed in a later section.

Nutrient Requirements of Older People

RECOMMENDED DIETARY ALLOWANCES

Limitations

The Recommended Dietary Allowances (RDA) as applied to older adults have many limitations. Because studies of older individuals have been few, the RDAs for persons above age 50 have for the most part been extrapolated from those developed for young adults. For the majority of nutrients, recommended intakes are the same for younger (ages 23 to 50) and older (age 51 and over) adults.[9] Energy is the only factor for which there are adjustments beyond age 51 (Table 10-1).

Older Adult Differences

This RDA pattern fails to recognize that people age 51 differ from those age 85 in body composition, physiologic function, and metabolic adaptation. Physiologic changes in digestion or absorption could increase the need for a particular nutrient. Estrogen withdrawal following menopause alters calcium absorption and metabolism. Reduced efficiency of the renal system in excreting nitrogenous or other wastes contraindicates excessive intakes of protein or water-soluble vitamins.

Disease Interaction

A second issue is the interrelation between nutritional status and degenerative disease. Chronic disorders influence requirements both as a result of the disease process and in relation to drugs prescribed in therapeutic management. Kidney disease can result in excessive loss of albumin in the urine. Diuretics prescribed in management of hypertension can lead to depletion of potassium, pyridoxine, folic acid, or zinc, depending on the particular drug. For that individual, the RDAs may not provide a realistic estimate of nutrient needs. Based on this premise Munro[10] advocates the development of recommendations for both healthy aged persons and those with chronic disease. This emphasizes the importance of evaluating each older client as an individual, considering general health, level of physical activity, and presence of chronic disease.

TABLE 10-1 Recommended Energy Intakes for Older People

	51-75 Years	76+ Years
FEMALES		
Energy (kcal)	1800	1600
Range	1400-2200	1200-2000
MALES		
Energy (kcal)	2400	2050
Range	2000-2800	1650-2450

Modified from Food and Nutrition Board, National Research Council: Recommended dietary allowances, ed. 9, Washington, D.C., 1980, National Academy of Sciences.

ENERGY NEEDS

Energy needs decrease with age as the result of changes in both basal metabolism and physical activity. Basal needs are not under the individual's control, but energy expended in physical exercise varies according to individual activity patterns. Such physical activity can play a major role in maintaining energy balance.

Basal Metabolism

Basal oxygen consumption (ml per min) is influenced by sex, age, body size, and body composition, but mainly by lean body mass. Women at all ages have lower basal needs per unit of body height and weight because of their higher proportion of body fat and lower proportion of lean body mass. Although basal oxygen consumption begins to decline about age 20, substantial changes occur beyond age 45 and each decade thereafter. This decline in oxygen consumption results from the age-related loss of lean body mass described in Chapter 2. The metabolic activity of remaining cells, however, appears to be unchanged. Decreases in basal metabolism in later life are not the result of impaired thyroid function. Basal energy needs of older persons range from 1100 to 1300 kilocalories for women and 1100 to 1400 for men. For sedentary aged persons, the total energy requirement is very close to the basal need.

Physical Activity

Physical fitness is the state in which a person's muscular, cardiovascular, and respiratory systems have the ability to respond to physical work with rapid recovery and minimal fatigue. Changes in physical fitness occur as a result of smoking, lack of exercise, and age-related deterioration. Regular exercise can lead to improved functional capacity that will enhance the individual's ability to carry on daily activities and remain independent. Regular walking improves aerobic capacity, with decreased fatigue, increases mental alertness and effectiveness, and increases bone strength. No strenuous exercise regimen should be undertaken, however, without a physical examination beforehand and professional supervision.

Energy Intake and Expenditure

An increase in body weight throughout adulthood will result if energy intake continues at the same level as both basal metabolism and physical activity decline. Diaries of food intake and physical activity of 252 healthy men ages 30-80 indicated that total energy intake declined on an average of 12.4 kilocalories a day each year.[2] Physical activity fell more rapidly than basal requirements (7.8 kilocalories as compared with 5.2 kilocalories a day per year). The steepest drop in total energy needs (physical activity plus basal needs) occurred between ages 70 and 80.

Other work suggests that the most precipitous decline in physical activity occurs in young adulthood rather than later in life.[11] Decreases in daily energy expenditure were 40 kilocalories between ages 35 and 44, 17 between ages 55 and 74, and 23 between ages 75 and 84. This pattern emphasizes the importance of developing an exercise program early in life that with modifications can be continued throughout adulthood.

The National Research Council[9] points out that diets containing less than 1800 to 2000 kilocalories may not be adequate in required nutrients unless intakes of sugar, fat, and alcohol are restricted. In a national survey of women above age 65, mean intakes of low and high income groups ranged from 1170 to 1620 kilocalories a day.[10]

Long-Term Energy Balance

Analysis of long-term energy balance suggests that individuals possess a regulatory mechanism that acts to ensure energy homeostasis. Shifts in basal metabolic rate will conserve energy when fewer kilocalories are ingested and in some individuals will dissipate unneeded kilocalories as heat when intake exceeds expenditure. This raises questions regarding the efficacy of low-energy diets to achieve weight reduction in older persons for whom a metabolic pattern has developed over a lifetime. Decreasing energy intake may be necessary to prevent weight gain. However, if energy expenditure declines due to increasing disability, a severe restriction that results in weakness and further limitation of physical activity may not accomplish the intended goal. A moderate energy intake balanced by an increase in energy expenditure within the physical capabilities of the older adult is a more effective plan.

ESSENTIAL FATTY ACIDS

Although linoleic acid deficiency in adults is virtually unknown under normal conditions, efforts to control both fat and energy intakes can result in a low intake of linoleic acid, the essential fatty acid. Including one tablespoonful of vegetable oil or equivalent in the daily diet will provide both linoleic acid and appropriate amounts of vitamin E.

PROTEINS AND AMINO ACIDS

Protein Needs of Adults

Protein metabolism continues as a dynamic process throughout adult life. Although physical growth has ceased, sufficient protein must be consumed to replace obligatory nitrogen losses through desquamated cells from the skin or gastrointestinal tract, body secretions, and metabolic end products. When nitrogen excretion exceeds intake, as might occur following surgery, in debilitating illness, or when the diet is poor, protein depletion ensues.

Even well-nourished adults appear to lose body nitrogen as a function of age. It is estimated that total body nitrogen decreases from 1320 g in the young adult to 1070 g in the aged adult.[12] Skeletal muscle contributes a major portion of the protein that is lost with lesser amounts coming from vital organs such as heart and liver. Muscle mass comprises 45% of body weight in the young adult but only 27% of body weight beyond age 70. As a result body protein turnover—protein breakdown and synthesis—shifts in location from the muscle to the visceral organs.

Changes in body nitrogen content have led to different interpretations of protein requirements of older people. First, a decrease in active metabolic tissue and protein synthesis could reduce the need for protein and amino acids. Second, an alternate point of view is that an inadequate intake of nitrogen over adulthood ultimately leads to the observed loss in body nitrogen. Evaluations of protein metabolism and nitrogen requirements have not resolved this question.

Evaluating Protein Requirements

The methods used to evaluate protein requirements in adults are the *factorial method* and *nitrogen balance study*. The factorial method involves measuring obligatory nitrogen losses on a protein-free diet and calculating the daily protein intake required to replace these losses. Nitrogen balance studies evaluate the level of dietary protein that must be fed to replace obligatory losses and achieve nitrogen balance. Unfortunately, in older subjects results obtained by the two methods do not agree.

Total obligatory nitrogen losses do not appear to differ between younger males and older males when calculated per kg of body weight. Differences between males and females related to the higher proportion of muscle and lower proportion of body fat in males. When calculated on the basis of body cell mass, obligatory nitrogen losses are higher in older than in younger individuals. This reflects the shift in protein turnover from muscle to visceral organs. Despite similar nitrogen losses per kg of body weight, protein requirements may still differ between old and young of the same sex if dietary protein is less efficiently used by the older adult.

Factorial estimates of obligatory nitrogen losses, adjusted to allow for efficiency of use and individual variability, predict a safe level of protein intake to be 0.42 g per kg body weight per day for older women and 0.55 g for older men. These values are lower than those suggested for young adults of 0.52 and 0.57 g per kg body weight per day for women and men, respectively. Older people given egg protein, however, cannot maintain nitrogen balance on the "safe" levels of intake suggested for either young or aged adults (see Fig. 10-2).

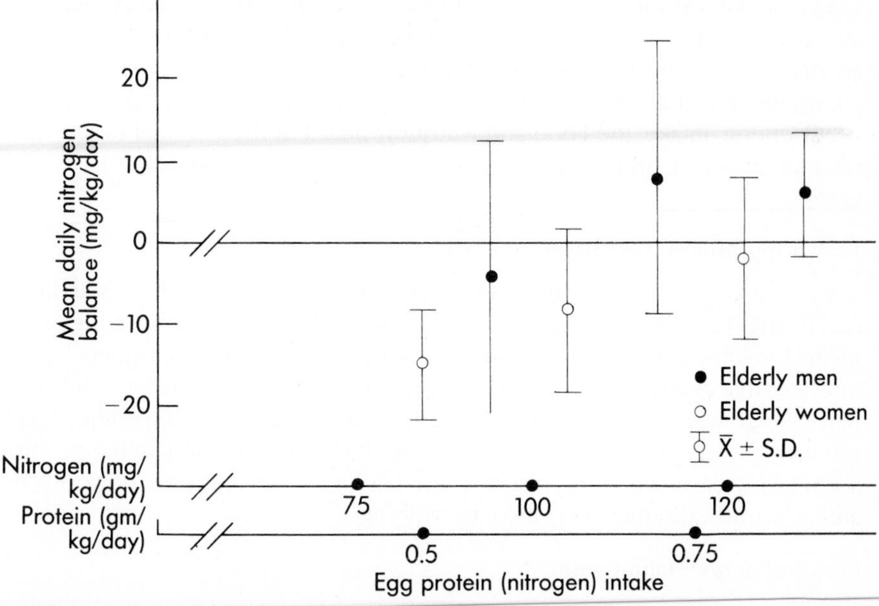

FIG. 10-2 Nitrogen balance in older people given graded levels of egg protein.
(From Uauy, R., Scrimshaw, N.S., and Young, V.R.: Human protein requirements: Nitrogen balance response to graded levels of egg protein in elderly men and women, Am. J. Clin. Nutr. **31**:779, 1978. Used by permission.)

A recent study evaluated the current RDA (0.8 g per kg body weight per day), given as egg protein, in 15 men and women ranging from 70 to 85 years of age and consuming various prescription drugs.[13] These workers concluded that the recommended level of protein, even high-quality protein, is not adequate to prevent nitrogen loss in many persons above age 70 with chronic disease.

Factors Affecting Protein Requirements

The inability of some older persons to achieve nitrogen balance on the test diets fed may relate to the type and level of protein consumed in the months preceding. On self-selected diets older people can maintain nitrogen balance on lower levels of protein than when fed a test diet. Individuals may over the years adapt to a diet actually considered inadequate by general standards. Then if they maintain reasonable health they may retain that accommodation throughout life. Thus previous diet should be considered when developing a therapeutic regimen for an older person.

Emotional and physical stress can increase protein requirements. Inflammation or infection leads to negative nitrogen balance and loss of labile body proteins, mediated in part by the stress response of the adrenal corticosteroid hormones.

Classic studies have described the protein-sparing action of carbohydrate and pointed to the need for sufficient nonprotein energy intake to promote use of the protein consumed to maintain body protein mass. When kilocalories are limited protein metabolism is compromised regardless of protein intake. The inability of some older individuals to maintain nitrogen balance on what appears to be adequate levels of protein may relate to the energy value of the diet. Although protein use is maximal at a level of 40 kilocalories per kg body weight, the recommended energy intake for those above age 50 is only 29-32 kilocalories per kg body weight. Encouraging physical activity to allow greater flexibility in energy intake should be a priority in nutrition counseling for older persons. In order to approach a sufficient intake of protein on a lower energy intake, the Food and Nutrition Board of the National Research Council recommends that protein contribute 12% to 14% of total kilocalories in older age groups.[9]

Evaluating Amino Acid Requirements

Present knowledge of amino acid requirements of aged persons is both limited and conflicting. Early studies suggested that older individuals may have higher requirements for some amino acids. But these reports have not been confirmed. Recent work indicates that essential amino acid requirements calculated on the basis of body weight may change with age, although the direction of change is not consistent. Tryptophan requirements appear to decrease with age, but threonine and valine requirements seem to increase. When estimated on the basis of body cell mass, however, essential amino acid requirements do increase with age.[12]

Protein-Energy Malnutrition

The older person with a history of debilitating disease and poor diet is likely to have low nutrient reserves and is particularly vulnerable to overt malnutrition. The nutritional impact of chronic disease and hospitalization no doubt contributes to the poor nutritional status observed in some institutionalized aged persons. But their condition may also relate to intake before as well as after admission. Poorly nourished persons may have had a disability before entering the health-care facility and consequently had inadequate meals. Protein-energy malnutrition is difficult to identify in this age group because normal assessment values specific for older persons have not been developed. Measurements such as skinfold thickness and arm circumference or serum albumin and transferrin levels, described in Chapter 3, may change as a function of age.

Protein Intake

Protein intake for most older Americans appears to be adequate but protein status is income-related. Low-income people are more likely to have low intakes. In a recent national survey about 10% of higher-income women ages 65 to 74 consumed less than two-thirds of the RDA, although 25% of lower income women consumed less than that amount.[14] At greatest risk are those consuming inadequate levels of both protein and energy. Over 50% of the low-income women had less than two-thirds of the recommended level of kilocalories. It is reasonable to assume that some of those low in one nutrient value were also low in the other. Inadequate energy intake results in less efficient use of the protein that is available. Thus, vulnerability to both infection and chronic disease increases.

FAT-SOLUBLE VITAMINS

Absorption of fat-soluble vitamins requires the secretion of pancreatic lipase and bile salts for breaking down dietary fat and "packaging" it in fat micelles for transport. Thus persons with gallbladder disease might have impaired fat absorption. Decreased intakes of fat could also interfere with this process. Because of competition for binding sites, highly concentrated supplements, particularly of vitamin A, can produce imbalances as well as general toxicity.

Vitamin A and Vitamin E

Increasing age as such does not appear to increase the requirements for these vitamins nor hinder their absorption. When deficient serum levels are detected in older individuals they usually relate to low intake and respond to dietary improvement. Liver stores of vitamin A are not lower in older adults as compared to younger ones. But questions have been raised about the ability of older persons to mobilize vitamin A from storage sites in the liver.

Recent data suggest that many older persons consume less than 67% of the RDA for vitamin A (5000 IU for men; 4000 IU for women). One-fourth of those age 65 to 74 consumed less than 2000 IU daily.[14] Blacks and Spanish Americans are particularly vulnerable to low vitamin A intakes. Dietary deficiency can be influenced by income, since dark-green and deep-yellow vegetables and fruits, high in carotene (provitamin A), tend to be expensive, especially in cold winter months. Vitamin E may be less of a problem as reasonably priced vegetable oils are a good source.

Vitamin D

Although vitamin D can be obtained from food or by exposure to sunlight, the vitamin status of many older people based on either dietary intake or serum vitamin D metabolite levels is less than optimal. Dietary sources make only a limited contribution to the requirement. In a recent study of aged persons living in the community, one-fourth had less than 50% of the RDA.[15] The seasonal variation in serum vitamin D metabolite levels in older individuals emphasizes the importance of sunlight in meeting the requirement. Indoor lighting providing ultraviolet exposure has been evaluated as an alternative to sunlight for those who are housebound, but its use is currently being reviewed because of possible harm to the eyes.

Age-related problems with vitamin D focus on: (1) its absorption, which is less efficient in some older people; and (2) its metabolic conversion to the active vitamin D hormone form. Vitamin D, whether ingested in food or synthesized in the skin from its precursor cholesterol, undergoes two hydroxylation steps in the liver and kidney, respectively, to form the active vitamin D hormone, 1,25-$(OH)_2D$, which promotes calcium absorption in the small intestine and calcium reabsorption in the nephron tubules. Some older persons have low serum levels of the active vitamin D hormone, which is produced in the kidney, despite adequate to high levels of the intermediate metabolite 25-OH-D, which is produced in the liver. This points to a metabolic problem with the second and final hydroxylation step in the kidney.

In healthy older people a daily vitamin D intake of 160 IU (4 μg) is adequate to maintain normal serum metabolite levels, even if exposure to sunlight is minimal.[16] The current RDA for all adults is 200 IU (5 μg) of cholecalciferol. In light of the danger of vitamin D toxicity and subsequent hypercalcemia, supplements containing more than 400 IU are hazardous.

WATER-SOLUBLE VITAMINS

Thiamin, Riboflavin, and Niacin

These three B vitamins are all coenzyme factors in energy metabolism. Thus their requirements are based on energy intake and decrease in men beyond age 50 in response to lowered energy needs. Poor status usually relates to low dietary intake or excessive alcohol consumption. Surveys suggest that many older persons consume less than the recommended amounts of thiamin and riboflavin.[14] However, little actual biochemical deficiency based on red blood cell enzyme activity is observed. Blacks have lower intakes of riboflavin, possibly related to lower consumption of dairy products.

Vitamin C

Older men and women differ in their metabolism of ascorbic acid as men have lower plasma levels despite intakes equal to or greater than those of women.[17] This increased requirement could relate to the higher proportion of lean body mass in males. An important factor in ascorbic acid metabolism is the total body pool of the vitamin, which is estimated to reach a maximal tissue saturation of 20 mg per kg body weight at a plasma concentration value of about 1.0 mg per dl.

Calculation of the plasma vitamin concentration per unit of ascorbic acid intake indicates that older women require 75 mg and older men 150 mg daily to maintain a body pool of 20 mg per kg. Garry and coworkers[17] concluded that the differing vitamin C requirements of older men and women should be considered when establishing the

RDA. However, to date the recommendation has not changed. In younger men smoking increases the ascorbic acid intake required to maintain the body pool from 100 to 140 mg. Thus older men who smoke would have a requirement about 40% higher than nonsmokers.

Among older people socioeconomic status relates to ascorbic acid status. Aged persons with lower incomes are more likely to have deficient serum ascorbic acid levels. Limited intakes of vitamin C–rich fruits and vegetables may contribute to this problem. Ascorbic acid is lost if cooked vegetables are held at serving temperature for long periods of time, as sometimes happens with quantity meal programs. Citrus fruits are a better source under such circumstances.

Vitamin B_6

Vitamin B_6 (pyridoxine) is a problem nutrient for some older persons. Both serum levels of the vitamin and the activity levels of red-blood-cell enzymes requiring it as a cofactor decrease with age. Reasons proposed for these observed changes include: (1) decreased intake, (2) impaired absorption, or (3) less efficient metabolic conversion to its active form. The majority of older people consume less than recommended amounts of vitamin B_6 and for nearly half, intake falls below 50% of the RDA.[15] Thus the problem is more likely caused by poor intake rather than impaired absorption, since a daily supplement equal to the RDA can reverse deficiency symptoms. Altered vitamin B_6 metabolism and storage may also be a factor because the vitamin is stored in muscle tissue, which is decreased in older age. Absorption may, however, be impaired in older persons using high levels of prescription drugs known to interfere with vitamin B_6.

Decreased use of meat, poultry, and fish because of chewing problems or less food money also influences vitamin B_6 intake. Frail aged persons with low energy intakes may not be able to meet their requirements through food only and may need a supplement. Because vitamin B_6 can be destroyed by heat processing, prepared foods can be poor sources.

Folic Acid

Recent interest in the folic-acid status of older persons has centered on the absorption of this vitamin and the enzyme required to hydrolyze folylpolyglutamates to folylmonoglutamates, the form in which the vitamin is absorbed. It appears that healthy older persons have hydrolase levels equal to younger persons. But questions still remain regarding folic-acid requirements because many older persons, particularly those in low-income groups, have less than adequate serum folate levels. On the other hand, overt deficiency is seldom observed in healthy financially advantaged older people despite intakes as low as 50% of the RDA.[18] Older persons in hospitals or other long-term health-care facilities have the highest incidence of folate deficiency.

Incidence of poor folate status is related to high use of prescription drugs known to interfere with folate metabolism, combined with relatively low food intake. Cooking practices can contribute to folate deficiency, since boiling vegetables for long periods of time destroys the vitamin. Nutrition education and counseling should stress low-cost food sources of folic acid and cooking practices that retain it.

Vitamin B_{12}

Intrinsic factor found in the gastric secretions is required for the absorption of vitamin B_{12}. Lack of intrinsic factor causes a deficiency of the vitamin and *pernicious anemia.* Eventually, degenerative changes occur in the brain and spinal cord bringing mental deterioration.

Impaired vitamin B_{12} absorption does exist in some older people. Various conditions such as gastrectomy, achlorhydria, chronic gastritis, or decreased gastric secretions reduce available intrinsic factor and subsequent vitamin B_{12} absorption. The problem is sometimes associated with general malabsorption syndromes, steatorrhea, and deficiencies of iron and folate. There may be atrophy of the intestinal mucosa, although physical findings may be similar in older people with normal absorption. Laxatives that reduce transit time interfere with vitamin B_{12} absorption.

The nutritional significance of the observed decrease in serum vitamin B_{12} levels as a function of age has not been resolved (see Fig. 10-3). Although impaired absorption may play a role, older people may also consume less meat, fish, or poultry because of low incomes or chewing problems and not compensate with increased intakes of milk or cheese. In one community group study,[15] about half of the persons above age 60 had vitamin B_{12} intakes below the RDA. The relation of food intake to biochemical status is underscored by the fact that low serum vitamin B_{12} levels are found more

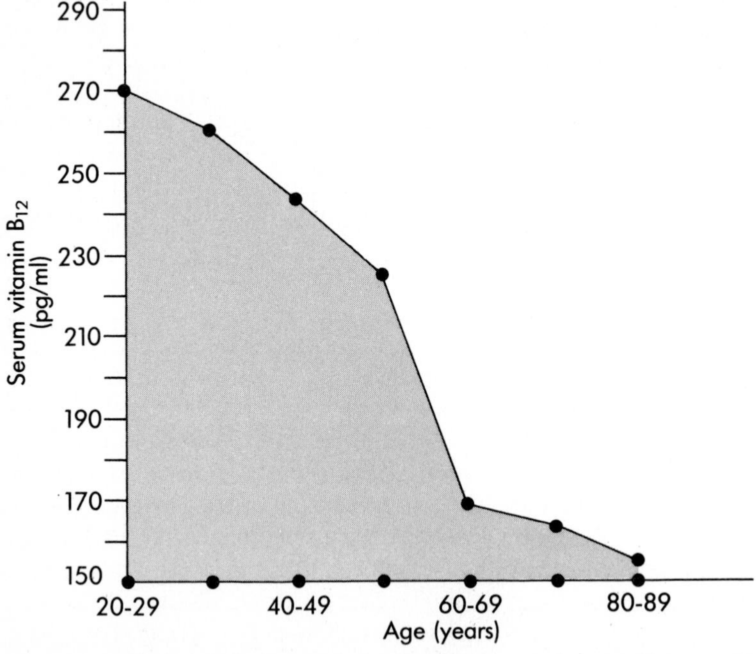

FIG. 10-3 Serum vitamin B_{12} levels according to age.
(Data from Gaffney, G.W., and others: Vitamin B_{12} serum concentrations in 528 apparently healthy human subjects of ages 12-94, J. Gerontol. 12:32, 1957.)

frequently among those persons over age 75 who live alone and have problems with food shopping and preparation. At the same time, physiologic aging and chronic disease may exert an influence, since older persons taking B_{12} supplements may continue to have low serum levels. In light of the role of vitamin B_{12} in maintaining nerve tissue and function, further evaluation of the significance of lowered serum levels is essential.

MINERALS

Iron

Absorption of iron, a complicated and inefficient process in people of all ages, is even more difficult in older people with gastrointestinal changes. When gastric secretions, including hydrochloric acid, are absent or reduced, iron absorption is limited. Components of these secretions bind to iron and enhance its absorption, and the hydrochloric acid reduces iron from its ferric form in food to its ferrous form necessary for absorption. Also, the absorbing surface "brush border"—microvilli of the small intestine mucosa—undergoes age-related morphologic changes that can modify the rate of absorption. And finally, antacids that raise gastric pH levels and certain drugs (for example, cholestyramine) that bind both inorganic iron and iron complexes can further decrease iron uptake.

Highly processed bread and cereal items are attractive to older people because they have a long shelf life, are easily chewed, and require little preparation. Naturally occurring iron, lost in the milling process, is replaced with inorganic iron salts, which are less easily absorbed. A liberal intake of fiber, to promote normal bowel function, may bind trace minerals and decrease iron absorption. However, iron absorption does not appear to be a problem for many older people who are able to maintain adequate iron status on intakes approximating the RDA.

Daily iron losses in the form of desquamated cells have been estimated to be less than 1.0 mg per day in older men and in nonmenstruating older women. But pathologic conditions such as peptic ulcers or excessive aspirin use leading to continual blood loss can significantly deplete iron reserves. In general, iron reserves in the bone marrow and liver are similar in older and younger men. Older women may have considerably higher iron storage levels than younger women, which reflects cessation of menses and monthly iron loss. At the same time, older women are vulnerable to poor iron intake based on their relatively low energy intakes. In a recent survey 10% of older men as compared to 25% of older women consumed less than two-thirds the RDA for iron.[14] Low-income older people may obtain a greater proportion of their dietary iron from fortified cereal products, necessitating the combining of foods to best advantage for maximum iron absorption.

Calcium and Phosphorus

Calcium metabolism has important implications for both nutritional and physical health. To ensure normal function of the heart and nervous system serum calcium must be maintained within very narrow limits (9 to 11 mg per dl). A decrease in serum calcium levels or increase in serum phosphate levels triggers the release of parathyroid hormone (PTH), which restores serum calcium levels by: (1) releasing calcium from the bone (resorption), (2) increasing calcium absorption in the intestine, and (3) increasing calcium reabsorption in the kidney nephrons.

Prior to menopause estrogen exerts a protective effect on bone, balancing the action of PTH in promoting bone calcium release. Following menopause and estrogen withdrawal, bone becomes increasingly sensitive to PTH and calcium mobilization accelerates. As bone resorption continues to bring about high serum calcium levels, release of PTH is reduced, resulting in lowered intestinal calcium absorption and reduced renal calcium resorption. Thus loss of body calcium is increasing while net absorption is decreasing. If this process continues, eventual loss of bone density and strength increases the susceptibility to fracture.

Recker and Heaney[19] propose that calcium balance in older women can be improved by increasing dietary calcium. Although the percentage of absorption may be low, the net amount absorbed from a larger intake will be greater. Based on their studies, postmenopausal women can approach calcium balance on intakes of 1500 mg calcium per day. This level is substantially above the current RDA for women of all ages. The NHANES data (Chapter 3) show median calcium intakes of older women to be 475 mg per day; older men had higher intakes (median levels = 597 mg).[14] Based on the recommendations of Recker and Heaney, postmenopausal women are consuming only 32% of the calcium needed.

The RDA for calcium remains controversial. The position of the Food and Nutrition Board is that: (1) persons have been shown to achieve calcium balance on intakes well below the current RDA of 800 mg, and (2) higher intakes of calcium have not been shown to prevent or reverse bone loss.[9] Individuals achieving calcium balance on fairly low intakes of calcium, however, were consuming vegetarian diets low in protein and phosphorus as compared to the typical Western diet. High-protein diets result in elevated urinary calcium levels in persons of all ages, because the catabolism and excretion of sulfate from the sulfur-containing amino acids interfere with renal tubular reabsorption of calcium. Recent data indicate that women with calcium intakes above 800 mg per day and vitamin D intakes of 400 IU per day have increased bone density at older ages, as compared to others of similar age and lower nutrient intakes.[20] This suggests that bone loss can be retarded if not prevented.

Current research also implicates low calcium intakes with elevated systolic blood pressure levels. Older women consuming less than 800 mg of calcium daily have significantly higher systolic blood pressure.[21] Since calcium intakes between 1000 and 1500 mg have not been shown to produce any harmful effects in healthy individuals, a higher recommendation, particularly for postmenopausal women, would appear to have potential in preventive health.

Chromium

The suggested daily intake of chromium is 50 to 200 μg. Healthy older persons consuming self-selected diets containing these levels of chromium appear to maintain appropriate tissue stores. Age as such does not seem to be a factor in chromium deficiency. Chromium tends to be lost in food processing and can be low in diets made up largely of highly processed items. Whole grains, meats, and cheese are good sources.

Zinc

Dietary zinc is influenced by total energy intake, total money spent for food, and food selection. Older men with an energy intake of 1800 kilocalories consume about 10.6 mg of zinc. Older women consuming about 1300 kilocalories take in only 7.2 mg of zinc, less than 50% of the RDA.[22] In the average American diet about 40% of the zinc is provided by meat, fish, and poultry, relatively expensive items in the food budget. The most common food source is beef. A diet based on dairy products and processed breads and cereals will be limited in zinc. Older people with low intakes from the meat group as a result of limited income or chewing difficulties are at risk.

Both hair and plasma zinc concentrations are used to evaluate zinc status although both have limitations. Among low income people above age 60, only 8% had hair zinc values indicating a deficiency, despite the fact that mean zinc intake was well below the RDA.[22] In a recent NHANES report[14] 39% of women age 65 and over had serum zinc levels considered to be less than adequate and levels were consistently lower in poor versus nonpoor groups. Whether the serum levels observed reflect reduced intake or a metabolic response associated with aging requires further study.

Zinc plays an important metabolic role in taste, wound healing, and immune response. These functions are sometimes altered in older people. However, zinc supplementation does not reverse such changes in older persons with adequate zinc status. Zinc status is particularly important in older individuals with decubitus ulcers or recovering from surgery.

FLUID INTAKE

Water is supplied to the body by food, liquids consumed, and water of oxidation. In younger people the thirst mechanism ensures adequate fluid intake. Diminished sensitivity to dehydration can reduce fluid intake in the older person. The disabled individual who cannot drink without help is particularly vulnerable to low fluid intake. Those subject to incontinence may consciously restrict fluid intake to avoid embarrassment. Patients given high protein supplements are subject to dehydration if fluids are limited. Because older persons are less able to concentrate urine, fluid intake becomes more critical. Unless they have cardiac or renal complications, older people should be encouraged to drink at least six to eight glasses of fluid each day.

Nutritional Disorders in the Aged

CARBOHYDRATE METABOLISM AND GLUCOSE TOLERANCE

Glucose tolerance, or the ability to metabolize a glucose load, deteriorates with age. In younger individuals abnormal glucose tolerance is associated with development of diabetes. In older individuals the difference between the pathology of disease and normal aging is less clear.

Fasting Blood Glucose

In older persons fasting blood glucose levels are not significantly higher than those in younger individuals. However, two hours following administration of glucose under standard conditions, blood glucose levels remain significantly higher in older persons.

Many factors contribute to this alteration in glucose tolerance. The age-related decrease in lean body mass and increase in body fat play a role as excessive fatness in younger people leads to impaired glucose tolerance. Increased physical activity enhances metabolic activity and glucose uptake in the skeletal muscle for fuel. Conversely, bed rest or limited exercise reduces glucose entry. Finally, potassium depletion resulting from inadequate intake or prolonged use of particular diuretics can impair glucose tolerance as potassium ions are required for glucose movement into cells.

Comparison with Diabetes

In diabetes a major factor is the deficiency of the active form of insulin required to facilitate both the entry and metabolism of glucose into the cell. This is not the case in older persons. In fact, insulin levels may even be higher in older than in younger groups. One problem is that older fat cells are less sensitive to the action of insulin and the rate of glucose entry and metabolism is slowed. Fat cells in older people are larger than those found in normal-weight younger people and have fewer insulin receptors. Older people may also secrete a different form of insulin (proinsulin) with limited effectiveness on fat and muscle cells.

Diet Effects

High-carbohydrate (especially complex carbohydrate) high-fiber diets can improve glucose tolerance in older persons. Fiber slows the rate at which glucose is released into the blood from the small intestine, thereby lowering blood glucose levels after eating. Efforts at weight control and exercise throughout adulthood may pay dividends in avoiding deterioration in glucose tolerance.

CHANGES IN BONE METABOLISM

Definitions

Loss of bone mineral and matrix, a physiologic effect of aging, has been identified in prehistoric skeletons from the year 2000 BC. Osteoporosis (porous bone) is the clinical syndrome resulting when over one-third of the bone is lost. Beginning at age 30 to 40, women lose about 10% of their bone mass per decade; men lose about 3%.[23] All people lose bone as a result of aging. But not all develop osteoporosis. Bone loss can occur in many locations including the spine, hip, or femur. Loss of bone (and bone strength) increases susceptibility to fracture and possible disability. The incidence of spontaneous fractures (resulting from little or no trauma) increases at an accelerating rate among older persons, especially women. The resulting immobility can change lifestyle. For example, an older woman may be forced to give up her home after breaking her hip.

Osteoporosis

This is the most common bone disorder among older persons. Decreased bone mass occurs with no change in the chemical ratio of mineral to protein matrix. Existing bone is normal. There is just less of it. In *osteomalacia* (adult rickets) bone density is decreased because of poor mineralization of available matrix. These conditions are illustrated in Fig. 10-4. Relative bone mass at older ages is influenced by the total bone laid down during periods of growth. Men at all ages have greater bone mass than women and are less likely to develop osteoporosis.

Factors Influencing Bone Loss

Many factors affecting bone loss have been identified:

Diet—calcium, protein, vitamin D, fluoride, calcium-phosphorus ratio, alcohol
Hormones—estrogen, parathyroid hormone
Other—age, sex, race, physical exercise, smoking

The most obvious predisposing factor is being female.

Heaney and coworkers[24] have summarized two general theories describing age-related bone loss. The first theory considers bone loss the result of a deficiency of 1,25-$(OH)_2$ D, the active metabolite form of vitamin D hormone that, in partnership with PTH, controls body calcium balance. This active metabolite regulates calcium absorption in the intestine and calcium deposit in the bone. The primary problem is reduced production of this metabolic hormone in the kidney, most likely related to estrogen withdrawal. With less calcium absorbed and supplied to the blood, serum calcium falls, resulting in secretion of PTH, mobilization of bone calcium, and eventual development of osteoporosis.

The second theory proposes that an underlying imbalance exists between bone resorption and bone formation. Bone remains a dynamic tissue throughout life with remodeling occurring at many locations at any given time. When because of age, estrogen withdrawal, or lack of physical activity, bone resorption occurs at a faster rate than bone replacement, osteoporosis will result. Both theories agree that calcium absorption is reduced and production of the active vitamin D hormone is depressed. Both theories may be correct depending on the individual and the severity of bone loss.

A

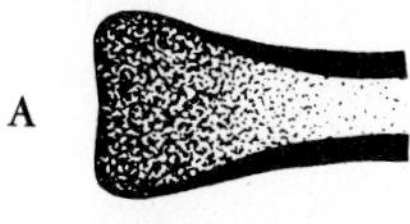

B

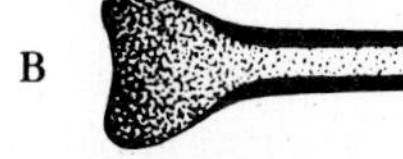

C

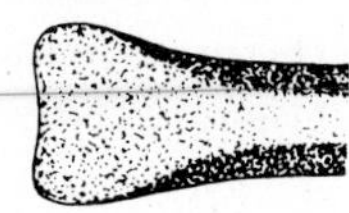

FIG. 10-4 Normal bone, osteoporosis, and osteomalacia. **A**, normal bone; **B**, osteoporosis in which there is a reduced amount of bone of normal composition; **C**, osteomalacia in which the amount of bone is normal but the composition is abnormal.

Prevention of Osteoporosis

No effective treatment now exists for replacing bone that has been lost. For this reason, prevention must be the focus, beginning with adolescent girls and young women, to reduce the risk factors involved. Smoking and excessive use of alcohol appear to accelerate bone loss. Regular physical exercise and muscle pull on the bone are necessary to maintain bone tissue. Body weight must be exerted on the bone. In fact, weightlessness, as shown by space flights, results in rapid loss of bone tissue similar to that experienced in prolonged bed rest, despite normal calcium intakes and efforts to exercise. Even general inactivity contributes to calcium loss. Older persons who exercise only infrequently have significant bone loss in contrast to those who exercise several times a week.

Calcium intakes of 1000 to 1500 mg along with 400 IU of vitamin D have been shown not only to reverse bone loss but in some cases bring about a slight increase in bone density. Some researchers dispute these findings and consider increased calcium intakes to be of no benefit in preventing bone loss unless estrogen is given simultaneously. Determining whether or not higher calcium intakes can actually replace bone previously lost requires long-term evaluation. However, retarding bone loss is in itself a worthy goal. Since malabsorption of calcium is a significant risk factor for development of osteoporosis, physiologic doses of 1,25-$(OH)_2$ D, the active vitamin D hormone, are being evaluated as a prophylactic measure. But the extreme physiologic potency of this metabolite and the need for constant monitoring of patients make this inappropriate for large-scale use at this time.

Calcium Supplements

Current publicity regarding the ability of high calcium intakes to prevent bone loss has led to mass marketing of calcium supplements. Calcium intakes up to 1500 mg appear to have no adverse effects in women with no previous history of kidney problems. Hypercalcemia has been reported in persons consuming large amounts of both calcium and alkali (sodium bicarbonate) and individuals should check with their physicians before using such combinations.[24] However, a recent report evaluating calcium carbonate supplements versus milk as a source of calcium concluded that milk provided calcium in a readily absorbable form that did not inhibit bone remodeling as did calcium carbonate, and milk also provided the vitamin D necessary.[19] Helping older persons select high-calcium foods that are reasonably low in fat and energy should be a component in all nutrition counseling.

Osteomalacia

Osteomalacia is usually the result of vitamin D deficiency. It is characterized by demineralization of the bone matrix. Among older people this can relate to: (1) low vitamin D intake coupled with nonexposure to sunlight, (2) malabsorption of ingested vitamin D, or (3) liver or renal disease that interferes with the conversion of the vitamin to its active form. The active form of vitamin D or an analogue is being used in treatment. Daily calcium supplements (1500 mg) in addition to vitamin D therapy may be required.

NUTRITIONAL ANEMIA

Anemia results from changes in either the number or characteristics of the erythrocyte. A decrease in the oxygen-carrying capacity of the blood and the consequent oxygen deficit in the tissues leads to increased heart rate, shortness of breath, and weakness. Unfortunately, such symptoms are often considered typical of older people and may go unnoticed as danger signs of a developing anemia.

Iron-Deficiency Anemia

The most common cause of anemia in older people is iron deficiency, although vitamin deficiencies may complicate the problem. Blood loss through the gastrointestinal tract is a frequent and critical cause of iron deficiency in older people. Excessive blood in the stool may go unnoticed. Extreme blood losses impart a dark red or black color to the stool, but abnormal losses are frequently not visible (occult) and require chemical analysis for detection. Conditions associated with gastrointestinal bleeding include gastric or duodenal ulcers, diverticulitis, hiatus hernia, hemorrhoids, and cancer. Long-term use of aspirin with irritation of the stomach lining can lead to significant blood loss.

Healthy older people have hemoglobin levels similar to those of young people, although several trends are apparent with age. Among men hemoglobin levels decrease with age and prevalence of anemia is higher after age 65. Women have lower hemoglobin levels throughout child-bearing years, but improve in iron status when menstruation ceases. Aged black persons, particularly women, are more likely to have hemoglobin levels below 12 g per dl. Older people in general have reduced numbers of red blood cells as compared with established standards. Mean cell hemoglobin concentration, however, is relatively unchanged, suggesting that red blood cells produced have normal hemoglobin concentration.[25]

Erythropoiesis can be less efficient in advanced age as a result of changes in the bone marrow or a lack of nutrients. Protein-energy malnutrition depresses red blood cell production. Decreased erythropoiesis will result if body iron is not released for hemoglobin synthesis as occurs in infection. This appears to be a body defense mechanism, making iron less available to the disease organism. Chronic low-grade infection as occurs with fever, inflammation, renal disease, and other chronic conditions produces an anemia characterized by reduced erythropoiesis, reduced numbers of red blood cells normal in size and hemoglobin content, and low serum iron. Uncomplicated iron-deficiency anemia will respond to iron therapy; anemia of chronic disorders is highly resistant.

Treatment of iron-deficiency anemia must be preceded by careful evaluation. Administering supplemental iron to persons who in fact have megaloblastic anemia caused by a lack of folic acid or vitamin B_{12} has serious consequences, since the B_{12} deficiency and neural damage continue. Equally unwise is the shotgun approach including iron and all necessary cofactors. A healthy nonanemic individual who is not consuming adequate iron should be helped to select iron-rich foods. If the diet cannot be improved, a supplement of the recommended allowance for iron (10 mg) is a reasonable alternative. Self-medication with iron supplements above the recommended intake is *extremely dangerous.* It can lead to hemochromatosis and liver damage or mask a pathologic condition causing gastrointestinal blood loss.

Pernicious Anemia

A megaloblastic "pernicious" anemia occurs in less than 1% of the population, with an average age at onset of 60 years. It was originally given the name "pernicious" anemia before its underlying cause was discovered to be a vitamin B_{12} absorption defect, and its persistent downward course led to death. Now it can be treated with B_{12} injections to bypass the intestinal absorption defect. A general age-related decline in serum vitamin B_{12} levels has been reviewed in relation to its possible significance as a predictor of vitamin B_{12} deficiency or onset of pernicious anemia. If vitamin B_{12} is poorly absorbed and body stores are systematically being depleted, overt deficiency is imminent. On the other hand, many people with serum levels below normal, observed over time, do not develop overt anemia. The need for a sensitive and specific method for detecting B_{12} deficiency is underscored by the report that several older patients with no abnormal blood parameters were found to have neurologic damage resulting from pernicious anemia.[26]

Increasing numbers of older people are being treated with intramuscular injections of vitamin B_{12} as a preventive measure. Those diagnosed and treated for pernicious anemia must be made aware of the need to return periodically for continued treatment to prevent subsequent deterioration.

Drug-Nutrient Relationships

DRUG USE BY AGED PERSONS

Older people are among the chief users of drugs in the United States. A 3-year follow-up[27] of over 1700 persons age 65 and over living in the community reported that 77% used at least 1 drug regularly; those under age 70 used at least 1 to 2, and those above age 84 used at least 2 to 3. Drugs most commonly used were antihypertensive agents, vitamins, cardiovascular agents, and analgesics. Drug use is even higher among older adults with severe chronic disease in long-term health-care facilities.

Aged persons are particularly vulnerable to adverse nutritional effects from drug therapy. Nutritional status may already be jeopardized by physiologic changes and less-than-optimal nutrient intake influenced by social and economic conditions. Chronic disease necessitates long-term drug therapy that can contribute to gradual depletion of nutrient reserves. Multiple drug intake compounds nutritional problems. Moreover, the effects of most drugs have been tested and validated on younger individuals who have different rates of drug absorption, metabolism, and excretion, based on differences in body composition and renal function.

NUTRITIONAL ASPECTS OF OVER-THE-COUNTER DRUGS

Analgesic and Gastrointestinal Drugs

Because over-the-counter (OTC) drugs are easily obtained and commonly used they are often perceived to be without risk. Use of these drugs may not be reported to a physician, creating the possibility of a dangerous interaction with a prescription drug. The person may have increased dosage above that recommended if the desired effect had not been achieved.

The analgesic most used by older persons with arthritis, headache, and muscle pain is aspirin (acetylsalicylic acid). Prolonged use can induce iron-deficiency anemia from irritation of the gastrointestinal mucosa and subsequent blood loss. Among the gastrointestinal drugs, laxative abuse can lead to depletion of sodium and potassium as well as chronic diarrhea. Mineral oil used as a cathartic interferes with the absorption of fat-soluble vitamins. Sodium bicarbonate and other antacids increase gastric pH, which inactivates thiamin and hinders the absorption of iron and folic acid. Aluminum-hydroxide–containing antacids that bind phosphate have been shown to cause phosphate depletion and accelerate bone loss.

Alcohol

A significant number of older people use alcoholic beverages regularly, but the number of abusers is not known. Physical and emotional upset, loneliness, and bereavement all contribute to increased use of this drug. Among 270 healthy older people in New Mexico,[15] 46% of the men and 41% of the women consumed alcohol at least once over a 3-day period; total intake decreased with age. As persons grow older, tolerance to alcohol decreases and adverse side effects increase, even in chronic alcoholics. The risk of nutritional deficiency arising from use of other drugs is markedly increased by excessive use of alcohol or when prior alcoholism has depleted nutrient stores. Moreover, alcohol interacts with some drugs and conditions to make worse any negative effects. Both alcohol and aspirin irritate the gastric mucosa and can lead to bleeding; when combined, the anticoagulant effect of aspirin can result in serious hemorrhage. High alcohol intakes decrease potassium levels, making the cardiac patient on digitalis at risk for toxicity. The person with insulin-dependent diabetes can become hypoglycemic following high alcohol intake as the alcohol interferes with gluconeogenesis.

Alcohol has both primary and secondary effects on nutritional status. It interferes with the absorption of thiamin by inhibiting the active transport mechanism required to move the vitamin across the mucosal cell and into the blood. As a result thiamin deficiency is common among alcohol abusers. Alcohol-induced damage to the intestinal mucosa results in malabsorption of both vitamin B_{12} and folate. Excessive zinc excretion is associated with alcohol abuse. Pancreatitis is common in alcoholic patients and is believed to contribute to the general malabsorption syndrome sometimes observed. Alcohol intake may in itself lead to lower intakes of food. Among moderate users of alcohol, alcohol kilocalories may be substituted at the expense of kilocalories from carbohydrate, fat, and protein, in an effort to limit total energy intake.

USE OF VITAMIN AND MINERAL SUPPLEMENTS

Many older persons regularly use vitamin and mineral supplements. However, the specific supplements chosen do not necessarily provide those dietary nutrients in shortest supply. Although calcium is frequently the nutrient lowest in intake relative to the RDA, calcium supplements have begun only recently to gain popularity.

Of concern is the excessive use of vitamin-mineral supplements by some older individuals. Among healthy aged persons in New Mexico, 95% of those taking a multivitamin preparation daily also used other vitamin or mineral products.[15] The nutrient supplemented at the highest level was vitamin E, with median supplemental intake 18 times the RDA. Supplements did, however, contribute toward meeting the recommended daily intake of vitamins B_6 and D and folic acid. For those not taking supplements, median intakes of those vitamins were less than 67% of the RDA. Some individuals, however, were routinely consuming at least five times the recommended levels of vitamins A and D, intakes that over a prolonged period are potentially toxic.

MECHANISMS OF DRUG-NUTRIENT INTERACTIONS

Modes of Metabolic Interference

Drugs may interfere with nutrients at the point of ingestion, absorption, utilization, or excretion. Food intake may decrease because of drugs that depress appetite or cause nausea and vomiting. Interference with the secretion of digestive enzymes or alterations in pH or transit time by particular drugs can prevent the digestion or conversion of nutrients into the forms required for absorption. Competition for binding sites on the mucosa may reduce nutrient uptake. Drugs may prevent the metabolic conversion of a vitamin into its active form, thereby negating its physiologic function. Some drugs form insoluble complexes with nutrients that cannot then be metabolized and are therefore eliminated. In general, vitamins and minerals are most affected.

Nutrient Depletion

Nutrient depletion is most likely to occur with a drug that inhibits nutrient absorption or with a drug taken for an extended period of time. A drug that acts as a vitamin antagonist, or affects a nutrient such as folic acid that participates in a variety of metabolic processes, will result in impaired biochemical function. Finally, nutritional effects of drugs will be more serious in individuals with pre-existing subclinical malnutrition. Those with marginal status who consume multiple drugs over periods of years are at greatest risk of nutrient depletion.

Food Selection Patterns of Older People

ENVIRONMENTAL FACTORS AND FOOD PATTERNS

Living Situation Changes

In the older person food patterns reflect lifelong attitudes and habits as influenced by the changing environment. To better understand the influence of lifestyle, health, and economic status on the food choices of older people, review the examples listed in Table 10-2. Many influencing factors have been identified that can act both singly and in combination. The older woman who has prided herself on "cooking from scratch" may have to rely on heat-and-serve items or home-delivered meals if her worsening arthritis makes it difficult to help with food preparation. Solving the food

TABLE 10-2 Factors Influencing Food Selection Patterns of Older People

Psychologic	Physiologic	Socioeconomic
Loneliness	Loss of appetite	Age
Bereavement	Loss of taste	Sex
Social isolation	Dental problems	Level of income
Food aversion	Prescribed diets	Cooking facilities
Symbolism of food	Chronic disease	Daily schedule
Mental awareness	Food intolerance	Retirement/leisure time
Feelings of self-worth	State of health	Level of education
Food faddism	Physical disability	Distance to food store
Nutrition knowledge	Degree of physical exercise	Availability of transportation
		Availability of familiar foods

problems of older people often involves seeking alternatives as living situations and resources change and things have to be done differently than before.

Adequate Diets

Living alone and having less money to spend on food results in poor nutrient intake in *some* older people, but this is not true for *all* older people. The stereotype of an old person who subsists on tea and toast is not substantiated by survey data from the United States or Great Britain. Although there are individuals who follow this pattern, it is *not typical* of this age group. The mere fact of their survival indicates their ability to select a reasonably adequate diet over a period of years.

CHANGES IN LIFELONG FOOD PATTERNS

Decreased Energy Needs and Nutrient Density

Normal aging brings about a decrease in energy requirements and the quantity of food consumed. According to NHANES data,[14] mean daily intake decreases by about 900 kilocalories in men and 350 kilocalories in women between the ages of 25 and 65. If older persons decrease their energy intakes by consuming less of all foods usually eaten, rather than selectively reducing intakes of items low in *nutrient density,* the overall quality of the diet will suffer. Among 194 older Canadians,[28] perceived health benefit was a stronger determinant of food choices than convenience, price, or prestige value. These results support the idea that nutrition education can be effective in helping older persons modify their food patterns.

Food Market Changes

Changes in agriculture, food preservation, and food processing over the past 35 years have multiplied the food forms now available to the consumer. Frozen orange juice, unheard of during the early adult years of people now over 60, is a common item. Adoption of new food items by older persons suggests that nutritious foods not used previously may be accepted if introduced in a positive way.

PSYCHOLOGIC ASPECTS OF FOOD SELECTION

Eating Alone

Throughout life eating is a social activity. The birthday party, the wedding breakfast, the family sharing at the table are all social acts. Loss of spouse or friends results in a loss of eating companions for the older individual who may now be eating alone for the first time in life. It is important, however, to differentiate between isolation and desolation. Isolates are content living alone and may have done so most of their lives. Desolates, on the other hand, live alone but are both lonely and unhappy. Emotional frustration or need for attention may be expressed in the form of food-related problems.

Retirement

Retirement results in a change in lifestyle for older single people and couples. Less money may be available for food. Since both husband and wife are now at home both may be involved in meal planning and food preparation. Among one group of retired couples not only did husbands participate in food-related decisions, but their level of participation also had nutritional implications.[29] The greater the husband's involvement in meal planning and actual food purchase, the better the diet. Women who expressed dissatisfaction with their traditional role consumed poorer diets and may have had less commitment to meal preparation. Food programs are often directed toward women, but leaders should make an effort to involve men who: (1) may be less bored with food activities and therefore more receptive, and (2) strongly influence the food decisions within a retired family.

Mental Disorders

Psychologic and mental disorders in the older person can result in confusion, irritability, acute depression, or in extreme situations dementia. Those with organic brain syndrome may forget to eat or be unable to differentiate between breakfast, lunch, and dinner. If they are unable to prepare food, meals may consist of bread and jam or prepackaged foods, thus limiting nutrient intake both in quantity and quality. Patients with Alzheimer-type senile dementia may not know how to use a knife and fork or how to lift a cup to the mouth. Disinterest in food and feeding problems can result in extremely low energy intakes.

PHYSIOLOGIC ASPECTS OF FOOD SELECTION

Sensory Loss

The majority of older persons living in the community describe their appetite as good, but anorexia is a common side effect of many prescription drugs used in treating chronic diseases. Taste and odor also influence the older person's selection and enjoyment of food. Sensitivity to all four basic tastes—sweet, sour, salty, bitter—declines with advancing age, and accelerates in heavy smokers. This results from decreases in both the number of tongue fungiform papillae and the number of taste buds per papilla. Prescription drugs can contribute to unpleasant or disordered taste. Even healthy aged persons have a diminished sense of smell, which also plays a role in altered taste perception. In practice, the tendency to use generous quantities of salt may be an effort to strengthen flavor when sensitivity has declined.

Dental Problems

Loss of teeth is often thought to alter dietary patterns among older people, particularly those who are edentulous—without any teeth. Economic problems may prevent seeking professional services for preparation or repair of dentures. In general, lack of dentures influences the enjoyment of eating more than it does actual nutrient intake. Dairy products, eggs, ground meat, and well-cooked chicken and fish can provide high-quality protein for those with chewing problems. Fruit juices and cooked vegetables are good sources of vitamins A and C and folic acid. Most fresh fruits can be eaten if ripe, peeled, and cut into small pieces.

Physical Health

Older persons limited in vision or movement find it difficult to shop for groceries or prepare meals. Moving about the kitchen requires special effort for a person who must grasp a cane or walker. Poor eyesight can preclude reading a nutrition label or package directions for use. Preparing vegetables is painful or in some cases impossible for a person whose hands are crippled with arthritis. All of these problems can result in increased use of heat-and-serve items that tend to be high in sodium and fat, and somewhat low in vitamins and trace minerals.

Special Diet

Impaired physical health, or multiple high-risk factors in a reasonably healthy older person, sometimes necessitates a specially prescribed diet limited in energy, fat, sodium, or cholesterol. Other diets may be self-prescribed such as a diet to prevent or alleviate arthritis. Many older people following a special diet obtain their food information from someone other than a clinical nutritionist-registered dietitian, nurse, or physician. These diets include low-fat, "diabetic," and various weight-loss regimens that in many cases are not appropriate for the individual.

SOCIOLOGIC ASPECTS OF FOOD SELECTION

Living Situation

Older people living in their own homes usually have adequate facilities for food storage and preparation including a working stove, oven, and refrigerator. The type and size of appliance can affect its use. With rising utility costs older people may hesitate to heat their conventional oven for one item such as a baked potato. A small electric appliance that functions as an oven is a wise investment for the person cooking for one or two. Individuals who rent a room with no kitchen facilities must eat in restaurants or elsewhere. They may heat some foods on a hotplate or use a heating coil to heat water for soup or beverages.

Access to Food Market

Lack of access to a grocery store may present additional problems. In rural areas stores may be at some distance, requiring either a car or a ride. Even in urban settings the older person may be required to ride the bus or walk to the store and carry bundles home (Fig. 10-5). During the winter months icy sidewalks may present special difficulties for the infirm. For inner-city aged persons the nearby store may be a convenience store with higher prices and poor selection, since supermarkets in such areas

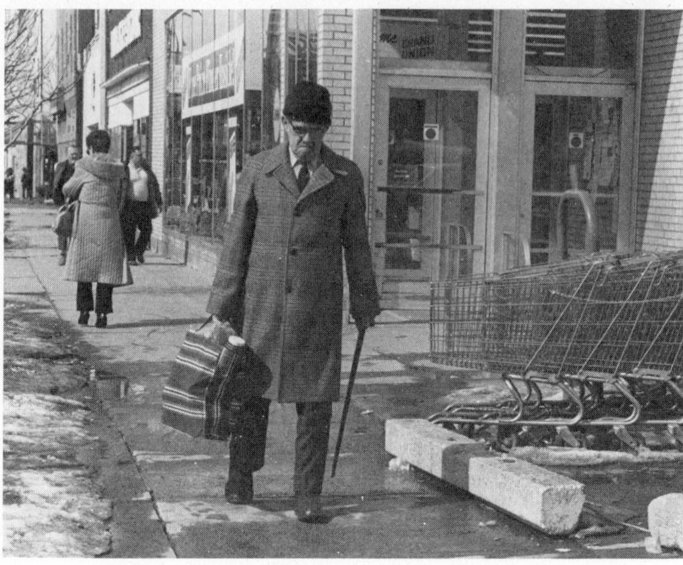

FIG. 10-5 Carrying groceries from the store is a difficult task for older people.

are closing because of poor profit margins and growth of suburban shopping malls. Shopping services would be a valuable program for a volunteer community agency to undertake.

Lifestyle

Some persons eating alone may not feel motivated to prepare adequate meals. But available evidence does not support the generalization that older individuals residing in one-person households have poorer diets than those in households of two or more. Socioeconomic status influences both social participation and nutrition in older people living alone. Those with higher incomes entertain friends in restaurants more frequently and tend to have more nutritionally adequate diets. Low-income older people have few mealtime visitors and those that do serve food items that they usually eat themselves, such as macaroni and cheese or tomato soup. Company at meals can have a positive influence on food intake, particularly among those who may not care to cook just for themselves.

Single older men tend to have poorer diets than single older women. Older men may not be accustomed to food preparation, but other factors such as education, income, or food preferences may enter in. Single men consume few fruits and vegetables and have poor intakes of vitamins A and C, although they drink generous quantities of milk, providing riboflavin and calcium.

ECONOMIC ASPECTS OF FOOD SELECTION

Food Patterns

Women and minority groups are most likely to be poor. This influences food patterns in various ways: (1) the level of income will determine how much money can be spent for food; (2) the low-income individual is less likely to own a car to simplify grocery shopping; and (3) the individual is more likely to live in either the inner city or a rural area where food is more expensive. Therefore the buying power of the money available is reduced. Older households spend a larger proportion of their total income on food but less of their food dollar goes toward food away from home. While younger people eat in restaurants, older people are more likely to eat at each other's homes, congregate meal programs, or "pot luck" socials.

Income and Ethnic Group

Both income and ethnic group influence nutrient intake and food selection. National survey data[14] revealed that energy levels—kilocalories—decreased with income in both black and white women, ages 65 to 74, although black women consumed less food regardless of income. Iron intake per 1000 kilocalories was 8.2 mg in older women in both higher and lower income groups. The nutritional vulnerability of low-income women in general and black women in particular is emphasized by the fact that median intakes in this study were about 75% the RDA for iron and vitamin A. Therefore, half of those surveyed were consuming less than these amounts.

FOOD ASSISTANCE PROGRAMS

Programs that increase food buying power can improve dietary quality. Unfortunately, eligible older persons are less likely to participate in programs such as food stamps than eligible younger persons. Older persons may be less well informed concerning available programs, may lack transportation to the appropriate office, may be in poor health generally, or may not apply because of pride.

A USDA evaluation of 854 older persons either receiving or eligible to receive food stamps indicates that men over age 64 and both sexes over age 75 benefit most.[30] Intakes of protein, calcium, magnesium, and vitamin A did not differ between participating and nonparticipating women ages 65 to 74. Those using food stamps had higher intakes of vitamin B_{12} but all met at least 100% of the RDA. Vitamin B_6 intake fell to below two-thirds the RDA among all women evaluated. Men age 75 and over who were not using food stamps has less than 67% of the RDA for energy, magnesium, and vitamin B_6, and only 71% of the RDA for vitamin A. Men of similar age who used food stamps met at least three-fourths the RDA for all nutrients except vitamin B_6.

IMPLICATIONS FOR NUTRITION EDUCATION

Food preference patterns of older people indicate that bread and ready-to-eat cereals, both enriched and whole grain, are consumed regularly as are whole and low-fat milk. Unfortunately, actual quantities consumed were not recorded so daily use of milk could reflect the small amounts used with coffee, tea, or cereal. Eggs and luncheon meats were the most common foods from the meat or protein group. Orange juice, bananas, and apples and lettuce and potatoes were the fruits and vegetables included most regularly in meal planning.[31]

Immediately apparent is the absence of a dark-green leafy vegetable as a source of both folic acid and vitamin A. Orange juice brings ascorbic acid, folate, and potassium to the diet, and bananas supply both potassium and vitamin B_6. Increased use of milk and other dairy products should be encouraged and whole grain products emphasized. Alternatives to costly luncheon meats, high in fat and sodium and low in other nutrients, should be explored. Such practical approaches as these could be used in nutrition education programs.

Nutrition Programs for Older People

COMMUNITY-BASED LONG-TERM CARE

Long-term care refers to the medical and support services, including nutrition services, required to maintain the functionally impaired older person at an optimal level of well-being. Long-term care can take place in an institutional or community setting. In a community setting nutrition support services provided by family members, neighbors, or community agencies can allow the older person to continue to live independently for an extended period of time. Such services may take the form of a ride to the grocery store with a daughter or delivery of meals by a community-sponsored home-delivered meals program. Congregate meals providing both a nutritious meal and a social outlet can help to maintain health and well-being in the relatively fit adult.

CONGREGATE MEAL PROGRAMS (Title III-C)

Basic Authorization

The Older Americans Act of 1965 as amended is the major piece of legislation providing programs for persons age 60 and over. When establishing the nutrition program in 1972, Congress directed attention toward elderly persons who might not eat adequately because they

- cannot afford to do so
- lack the skills to select and prepare nourishing meals
- have limited mobility that hinders shopping and cooking
- feel rejected and lonely and lack incentive to cook and eat alone

The congregate meal program, currently funded under Title III-C of the Older Americans Act, is designed to provide meals at little or no cost in a social setting. It operates through meal sites in community or recreation centers, municipal buildings, public housing, senior citizens centers, or churches. Important criteria in selecting a location are accessibility and familiarity to the older people in the community. Recent amendments to Title III-C have authorized funds for home-delivered meals for those unable to leave their homes.

Menu Planning

Under current guidelines a hot (or cold when appropriate) meal is served 5 days each week at noon. In rural areas meals may be served 1 to 4 days each week. Generally meal sites do not operate on weekends, which presents a serious problem for the participant whose personal food resources are limited. Nutrition programs may choose to prepare their own food or purchase food from a caterer. Meals are expected to provide one-third of the RDA for this age group.

The method most commonly used for planning menus to meet this standard is the Title III-C Meal Pattern (Table 10-3). Maximal nutrient quality of the meals can be

TABLE 10-3 Title III-C Meal Pattern Meeting Federal Guidelines

Food Type	Recommended Portion Size*
Meat or meat alternate	3 ounces of cooked edible portion
Vegetables and fruits	Two ½ cup servings
Enriched white or whole grain bread or alternate	One serving (one slice bread or equivalent)
Butter or margarine	1 teaspoon
Dessert	½ cup
Milk	½ pint (one cup)

From United States Department of Health, Education and Welfare: Guide to effective site operations: the Nutrition Program for the Elderly, Corvallis, 1973, Oregon State University.

*A vitamin C-rich fruit or vegetable is to be served each day; a vitamin A-rich fruit or vegetable is to be served at least three times per week.

maintained by the selection of foods with high *nutrient density*. Bread products prepared from enriched flour are acceptable, but whole-grain items increase intakes of fiber, vitamins, and trace minerals. Whole-grain breads and pasta might be introduced gradually to improve acceptance among those not accustomed to these items.

Because rising food prices limit the frequency of meat, fish, or poultry use, other sources of iron, zinc, and important vitamins need emphasis. One alternative is legumes, including lentils. If cheese or other dairy product is the primary protein source, iron could be provided in the form of a whole-grain bread and a dessert containing eggs or iron-rich fruit. Milk consumption may increase if there is a choice of whole, lowfat, nonfat, or buttermilk. Nonfat dried milk or grated cheese can fortify soups or sauces, increasing the calcium, protein, and riboflavin content.

Dessert should be a significant source of nutrients as well as a pleasant climax to the meal. Fruit desserts such as a baked apple or apple crisp contribute important nutrients, particularly if made with whole grains. Pudding, custard, or ice cream provides calcium as well as high-quality protein for those who do not drink milk. Moist, flavorful baked products prepared with whole grains, oatmeal, raisins, applesauce, pumpkin, carrots, or banana add iron, B-complex vitamins, vitamin A, and trace minerals. Recipes containing sugar, fat, and little else are generally avoided.

Limited funding and lack of professionally trained personnel make modified diets impractical in most locations. For persons with diabetes or those limiting energy intake, the Title III-C pattern is likely to be acceptable if portion size is controlled, skim milk is available, and fruit is offered as an alternative to a high caloric dessert. General modifications limiting sodium, sugar, and fat in food preparation benefit all participants.

Program Evaluation

Title III-C participants consume better diets on days that include a site meal. Further, they consume better diets than their nonparticipating neighbors of similar age and socioeconomic background. Calcium and vitamin A are most influenced by participation. This suggests that older people consume less milk and other dairy products, as well as dark-green and deep-yellow fruits and vegetables, at home. Participants with the best diets tended to be younger and more socially active, with higher incomes.

Kohrs and coworkers[32] evaluated the impact of Title III-C on the nutritional status of 466 rural aged persons. They reported that menus provided considerably more than one-third the RDA for all the nutrients calculated. For women the meals contained at least 80% of the RDA for protein, vitamins A and C, and riboflavin, and at least 40% of the RDA for energy, calcium, iron, and the B vitamins. It cannot be assumed, however, that all food served is consumed, including the cup of milk. Both men and women received about half of their daily intakes of protein, calcium, iron, vitamin A, and vitamin C from the Title III-C meal. Women who live alone and individuals with limited education and lower income consume a greater share of their daily nutrient intake at the meal site.

HOME-DELIVERED MEALS

General Organization

Meal delivery programs have been developed by community nonprofit organizations and health and social service agencies, such as hospitals, churches, nursing homes, and visiting nurses associations. Within community-sponsored programs, meals are usually delivered by volunteers who pay their own transportation costs. People who deliver meals for the Title III-C program are usually reimbursed for both time and mileage.

Meal delivery programs operate Monday through Friday. A hot meal is delivered at noon, sometimes accompanied by a cold meal to be eaten later. Some programs include additional cold lunches on Friday or before a holiday to provide for days when meals are not delivered. Delivery of cold lunches requires that the recipient have a refrigerator to safely store the additional food. No program provides meals on all days or for all meals of the day.

Eligibility Requirements

Older people can request meal delivery directly or be referred by a family member, physician, visiting nurse, dietitian or nutritionist, outreach worker, or social worker. Programs receiving Title III-C funding require that: (1) recipients be age 60 or over, although spouses below 60 can be served; and (2) recipients must be unable to leave their homes because of disability or other extenuating circumstances.

When meal delivery is not appropriate the client should be assisted in exploring other options. If the individual can leave home, transportation to a Title III-C meal site provides an opportunity for both food and social activity. A two-person household may be in need of home-delivered meals if one person is so burdened caring for an invalid partner that he or she has little time or incentive or energy to prepare adequate meals. Implementation of diagnostic related group (DRG) guidelines, resulting in earlier release of older patients from medical facilities for extended convalescence at home, has led to a dramatic increase in requests for home-delivered meals.

INNOVATIVE APPROACHES TO FOOD DELIVERY

One alternative to daily delivery of hot meals is weekly delivery of several frozen meals. This allows recipients to choose what they want to eat on a particular day and at what time. Supplementing one or two home-delivered meals each week with several frozen meals presents another option. Milk, fruit, and canned or freeze-dried items could accompany the frozen meals. However, recipients must have freezer space for storing meals as well as an oven for reheating.

For homebound persons able to move about within their homes, groceries can supplement either frozen or hot meals. Canned, dehydrated, and freeze-dried foods developed for use in the space program are also suitable for home delivery. Shelf-stable foods could replace either a congregate or home-delivered meals program. They are also appropriate as a supplementary food source for weekends or other nondelivery days. Analysis of the relative cost-effectiveness and cost-benefit of alternative food delivery systems, particularly in rural areas where daily delivery costs accelerate, should be a priority for community-based long-term care.

Summary

People above age 60 are increasing in number faster than any other segment of the population. Control of infectious diseases has reduced the number of early deaths. Now major causes of death are heart disease, cancer, and stroke. The aging process, with loss of cells, results in declining heart, renal, and pulmonary functions. Those functions that require the greatest degree of coordination among systems show the greatest rate of change. Both structural and functional alterations in the brain and target organs contribute to the changes observed.

For the most part the RDAs for older persons have been extrapolated from those for younger adults. Energy requirements decrease with age due to the decline in basal metabolic rate and physical activity. Protein needs may be increased among aged persons with serious chronic disease, but a wider problem may be the inefficient use of ingested protein because of inadequate energy intakes. Vitamin needs do not increase in healthy aged persons. Biochemical deficiencies more likely relate to low intake or use of prescription drugs that interfere with nutrient absorption and utilization.

Trace-mineral intake tends to be low among older persons who rely on highly processed food items or who have low energy intakes. Iron-deficiency anemia is most often due to occult blood loss. Age-related bone loss may be retarded by generous calcium intake, adequate supplies of vitamin D, and regular exercise.

Loneliness, physical disability, and poverty contribute to inadequate nutrient intakes. Individuals over age 75, older men living alone, and the homebound are most vulnerable to poor dietary intake. Government and community programs including food stamps, congregate meals, and home-delivered meals make positive contributions to the nutritional status of older persons.

Review Questions

1. What factors have led to the significant increase in life expectancy that has occurred since 1900? Why has life expectancy at age 65 not changed proportionately over this same period?
2. Describe several physiologic changes that occur with normal aging. Give a nutritional implication of each.
3. How do the RDAs for persons above age 50 differ from those for younger adults? What are the limitations of the current RDAs for older persons?
4. Serum levels of folic acid, pyridoxine, and vitamin B_{12} appear to decline with age. Does this relate to decreased dietary intake, decreased absorption, or the aging process? Explain.
5. Define osteoporosis. What physiologic, socioeconomic, and dietary factors have been related to this problem? Can osteoporosis be prevented? Explain.
6. What are some nutritional implications of common OTC drugs? By what mechanisms can prescription drugs adversely influence nutritional status?
7. How may age, sex, loneliness, physical disability, poverty, and living alone influence nutrient intake in older persons?
8. Describe several types of community-based nutrition programs that serve older people. What levels of nutrient intake are provided by each?

REFERENCES

1. United States Senate Special Committee on Aging: Aging America: trends and projections, 1985-86 ed., Washington, D.C., 1986, U.S. Government Printing Office.
2. Shock, N.W.: Energy metabolism, caloric intake and physical activity of the aging. In Carlson, L.A., ed.: Nutrition in old age, Symposia Swedish Nutrition Foundation X, Stockholm, 1972, Almqvist & Wiksell.
3. Kenney, R.A.: Physiology of aging: a synopsis, Chicago, 1982, Year Book Medical Publishers, Inc.
4. United States Department of Health and Human Services: Hypertension in adults 25-74 years of age, United States, 1971-1975, DHHS pub. no. (PHS) 81-1671, Washington, D.C., 1981, U.S. Government Printing Office.
5. Simopoulos, A.P., and Van Itallie, T.B.: Body weight, health and longevity, Ann. Intern. Med. **100**:285, 1984.
6. United States Department of Health and Human Services: Obese and overweight adults in the United States, DHHS pub. no. (PHS) 83-1680, Washington, D.C., 1983, U.S. Government Printing Office.
7. Breslow, L., and Enstrom, J.E.: Persistence of health habits and their relationship to mortality, Prev. Med. **9**:469, 1980.
8. Rorick, M.H., and Scrimshaw, N.S.: Comparative tolerance of elderly from differing ethnic backgrounds to lactose-containing and lactose-free dairy drinks: a double-blind study, J. Gerontol. **34**:191, 1979.
9. Food and Nutrition Board: Recommended Dietary Allowances, ed. 9, Washington, D.C., 1980, National Academy of Sciences.
10. Munro, H.N.: Major gaps in nutrient allowances: the status of the elderly, J. Am. Diet. Assoc. **76**:137, 1980.

11. Elahi, V.K., and others: A longitudinal study of nutritional intake in men, J. Gerontol. **38**:162, 1983.
12. Young, V.R., and others: Protein and amino acid requirements of the elderly. In Winick, M., ed.: Nutrition and aging, New York, 1976, John Wiley & Sons, Inc.
13. Gersovitz, M., and others: Human protein requirements: assessment of the adequacy of the current Recommended Dietary Allowance for dietary protein in elderly men and women, Am. J. Clin. Nutr. **35**:6, 1982.
14. United States Department of Health and Human Services: Dietary intake source data: United States, 1976-80, DHHS pub. no. (PHS) 83-1681, Washington, D.C., 1983, U.S. Government Printing Office.
15. Garry, P.J., and others: Nutritional status in a healthy elderly population: dietary and supplemental intakes, Am. J. Clin. Nutr. **36**:319, 1982.
16. Vitamin D status of the elderly: contributions of sunlight exposure and diet, Nutr. Rev. **43**:78, 1985.
17. Garry, P.J., and others: Nutritional status in a healthy elderly population: vitamin C, Am. J. Clin. Nutr. **36**:332, 1982.
18. Garry, P.J., Goodwin, J.S., and Hunt, W.C.: Folate and vitamin B_{12} status in a healthy elderly population, J. Am. Geriatr. Soc. **32**:719, 1984.
19. Recker, R.R., and Heaney, R.P.: The effect of milk supplements on calcium metabolism, bone metabolism and calcium balance, Am. J. Clin. Nutr. **41**:254, 1985.
20. Sowers, M.F.R., Wallace, R.B., and Lemke, J.H.: Correlates of mid-radius bone density among postmenopausal women: a community study, Am. J. Clin. Nutr. **41**:1045, 1985.
21. Sowers, M.F.R., Wallace, R.B., and Lemke, J.H.: The association of intakes of vitamin D and calcium with blood pressure among women, Am. J. Clin. Nutr. **42**:135, 1985.
22. Sandstead, H., and others: Zinc nutriture in the elderly in relation to taste acuity, immune response, and wound healing, Am. J. Clin. Nutr. **36**:1046, 1982.
23. Avioli, L.V.: Postmenopausal osteoporosis: prevention versus cure, Fed. Proc. **40**:2418, 1981.
24. Heaney R.P., and others: Calcium nutrition and bone health in the elderly, Am. J. Clin. Nutr. **36**:986, 1982.
25. United States Department of Health and Human Services: Hematological and nutritional biochemistry reference data for persons 6 months to 74 years of age: United States, 1976-80, DHHS pub. no. (PHS) 83-1682, Hyattsville, Md., 1982, U.S. Government Printing Office.
26. Norman, E.J.: Vitamin B_{12} deficiency in the elderly, J. Am. Geriatr. Soc. **33**(5):374, 1985.
27. Hale, W.E., Marks, R.G., and Stewart, R.B.: Drug use in a geriatric population, J. Am. Geriatr. Soc. **27**:374, 1979.
28. Krondl, M., and others: Food use and perceived food meanings of the elderly, J. Am. Diet. Assoc. **80**:523, 1982.
29. Schafer, R.B., and Keith, P.M.: Social-psychological factors in the dietary quality of married and single elderly, J. Am. Diet. Assoc. **81**:30, 1982.
30. United States Department of Agriculture: Food and nutrient intakes of individuals in 1 day, low-income households, November 1979 to March 1980. Nationwide Food Consumption Survey 1977-1978, preliminary report no. 13, Washington, D.C., 1982, U.S. Government Printing Office.
31. Fanelli, M.T., and Stevenhagen, K.J.: Characterizing consumption patterns by food frequency methods: core foods and variety of foods in diets of older Americans, J. Am. Diet. Assoc. **85**:1570, 1985.
32. Kohrs, M.B., O'Hanlon, P., and Eklund, D.: Title VII Nutrition Program for the Elderly, I. Contribution to one day's dietary intake, J. Am. Diet. Assoc. **72**:487, 1978.

FURTHER READING

Fanelli, M.T., and Stevenhagen, K.J.: Characterizing consumption patterns by food frequency methods: Core foods and variety of foods in diets of older Americans, J. Am. Diet. Assoc. **85**:1570, 1985.

This article, using national survey data, evaluates the variety of foods consumed by persons ages 55-75+ with emphasis on age-related changes in food selection and the implications for nutrient intake and nutrition education.

Garry, P.J., and others: Nutritional status in a healthy elderly population: Dietary and supplemental intakes, Am. J. Clin. Nutr. **36**:319, 1982.

This article describes the nutrient intake, including both food and supplements, of a group of healthy aged people. Reported intakes are compared with the RDA, and implications for possible vitamin and mineral deficiencies and excesses are discussed. The high level of use and the impact of vitamin and mineral supplements upon the nutrient intakes of this group are especially pertinent in light of the current advertising directed toward older people.

Harris, L.J., and others: Comparing participants' and managers' perception of services in a congregate meals program, J. Am. Diet. Assoc. **87**:190, 1987.

These authors evaluated the nutrient quality of the menus served at 14 Title III-C congregate meal sites and interviewed managers and participants regarding the quality of the meal and other services, including nutrition education. The differing perceptions expressed by managers and participants provide a broad orientation to both program and food management issues for nutrition professionals.

Hollonbeck, D., and Ohls, J.C.: Participation among the elderly in the food stamp program, Gerontologist **24**:616, 1984.

This article describes the factors that can discourage or prevent eligible older people from participating in the food stamp program and suggests approaches to be used with older clients to overcome some of these difficulties and encourage participation.

Pardini, A.: Exercise, vitality and aging, Aging, April-May, no. 344, p. 19, 1984.

The author presents an overview of the health benefits of exercise, practical suggestions on how to get started on an exercise program, and the cautions to be observed. A list of helpful publications and resources is also included.

Recker, R.R., and Heaney, R.P.: The effect of milk supplements on calcium metabolism, bone metabolism and calcium balance, Am. J. Clin. Nutr. **41**:254, 1985.

This article describes a two-year study evaluating the effectiveness of milk as a source of calcium to support bone health in postmenopausal women. The discussion comparing milk and calcium carbonate as possible sources of added calcium provides valuable information for use in nutrition counseling.

Roe, D.A.: Therapeutic effects of drug-nutrient interactions in the elderly, J. Am. Diet. Assoc. **85**:174, 1985.

This article highlights important nutrient-drug-food interactions and describes the role of the dietitian in planning meals that will minimize such interactions.

Suter, P.M., and Russell, R.M.: Vitamin requirements of the elderly, Am. J. Clin. Nutr. **45**:501, 1987.

This article provides a comprehensive review of current knowledge regarding the vitamin requirements of both healthy and chronically ill older persons. The 1980 RDAs for vitamins are evaluated in relation to the particular nutrient needs of aging individuals.

Turner, M., and Glew, G.: Home-delivered meals for the elderly, Food Technol. **36**(7):46, 1982.

The authors provide a detailed evaluation of the nutrient content of home-delivered meals as influenced by recipe development, food holding time, and length of delivery routes. This article would also apply to hospital and nursing home food service as well as food delivery to congregate meal sites.

Yung, L., Contento, I., and Gussow, J.D.: Use of health foods by the elderly, J. Nutr. Educ. **16**:127, 1984.

This survey report describes the extent and type of health-food use by older people, as well as the socioeconomic and motivational factors related to health-food decisions. These findings have important implications for nutrition education for older people.

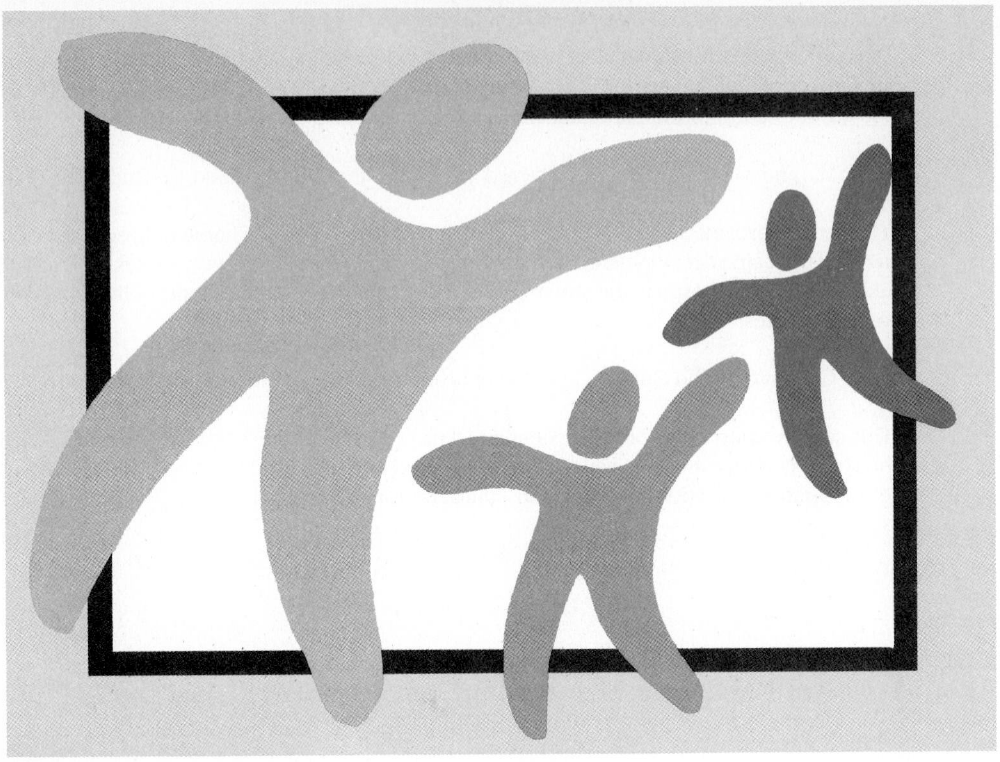

Basic Concepts

1. The common nutrition and health risk factor of stress in many forms flows from life's changes and events in a rapidly developing modern society.
2. Stress activates a series of generalized neuroendocrine responses designed to protect the body from harm, but constant modern stressors contribute to malnutrition and disease.
3. Persons and population groups more vulnerable to both physical and psychosocial stress carry higher risk of malnutrition and disease.
4. Health promotion requires stress management, which involves both personal and social approaches as well as physical and nutritional support.

Chapter Eleven

Nutrition for High-Risk Populations

Sue Rodwell Williams

Have you ever dropped a small pebble into a body of water and watched the ripple effect? It moves quickly from the point of contact across the water surface in all directions in ever widening circles. In a similar way the human body responds to various forms of life's stress, either physical or psychosocial, causing high-risk situations for malnutrition and disease. Modern society is fast paced and competitive, with its pressures and problems, and with its rapidly changing environment in a complex technologic age affecting air, water, and food. Constant life changes and events, large and small, bring varying degrees of individual stress, causing an automatic internal cascade of physiologic reactions requiring adaptation and affecting health. These adaptive reactions are triggered through the neuroendocrine system, producing the familiar "fight or flight" response. Through some 40,000 years of human development this physiologic response has readied the body to confront or escape danger.

However, today these automatic physiologic responses are not well adapted to the relatively high-pressured and unphysical modern civilization and lifestyle. Sometimes it's hard to fight or flee. Yet the body continues to respond to all stresses with the same automatically triggered set of reactions as if one's life were threatened—as indeed it often actually is, depending on one's individual capacity to manage life's stressors. These physiologic reactions are linked to reduced immune function and the emergence of many of the "diseases of civilization"—coronary heart disease, hypertension, diabetes, and cancer.

Stress and its related diseases are also bound with a composite of other lifestyle factors. These are simply different pieces of the way members of Western society live their lives and the values—or lack thereof—they place on human need. So when we talk about reducing or managing stress and the related risks of malnutrition and disease, we are really talking about rethinking the Western way of living. In this chapter, we will look at some of these issues in relation to nutrition and health. We will seek first to understand the ever present underlying physiology of stress, so that we can then apply these principles to nutritional support needs, especially in those high-risk population groups that are more vulnerable to both physiologic and psychosocial stress with resulting malnutrition and disease. Finally, we will seek ways in which life stress may be managed, to help both ourselves and our clients toward more positive nutrition and health through reduction of risk factors or more successful coping with illness.

The Role of Stress as a Risk Factor

The classic work of Canadian physician Hans Selye[1] has clearly shown the close relationship of stress, which he called "the rate of wear and tear in the human machinery which accompanies any vital activity,"[2] to the risk and incidence of disease. He also established the pattern of individual physiologic response to a given stress agent, with different reactions in different persons depending on *conditioning factors,* which can selectively inhibit or enhance one or more stress effects. These factors may be endogenous, such as genetic predisposition, age, or sex. Or they may be exogenous, such as poor diet or drug abuse. Numerous investigators have reinforced the validity of Selye's early foundation work, with applications in many areas of health and disease. Thus stress management has become a necessary consideration in nutrition assessment and nutritional-care planning based on identified human needs (p. 41) and an essential component in current health-promotion programs (p. 383).

HUMAN NEEDS: THE PROCESS OF LIFE CHANGES AND EVENTS

Both change and balance are basic concepts to the perpetuation of life. The changing human body throughout the life cycle presents dramatic evidence of the dynamic interior metabolism interfacing with the changing exterior environment. Normal physiologic stress is an integral part of this dynamic development. For example, the normal physiologic stress of pregnancy brings multiple synergistic changes and balances adapting the maternal body to sustain and support fetal growth and prepare for birth. Also, the normal stress of inserted skeletal muscles on bones helps maintain calcium balance between the bone compartment and the interfacing serum calcium. And the general stress of pain warns of injury or illness. However, it is the severe, prolonged, or uncontrolled stress, be it physical or psychosocial hunger and pain, that contributes to exhaustion of resources and illness, since the adaptability of individuals is always finite. Thus health-team members in any situation seek to provide care based on identified human needs in four basic areas: life cycle growth and development, health-disease status, stress-coping balance, and general human needs for self-fulfillment, all of which involve nutritional concerns.

Life Cycle Growth and Development Continuum

From the initiation of life at conception to its cessation at death, a steady one-way integrated continuum of physical growth and psychosocial development ensues. Each stage of human life brings unique physical characteristics and psychosocial maturation, both of which are integral aspects of every person's total life and health. Over the past 30 years Erikson's outline of human development has influenced our view of this life cycle progress.[3,4] This leading American psychoanalyst has provided much insight to our understanding of human personality and growth throughout critical periods of our development. He has identified eight stages of human growth and the basic psychosocial problem each person struggles with at each stage. Each developmental problem has a positive ego value and a conflicting negative counterpart:

1. Infant: trust versus distrust
2. Toddler: autonomy versus shame and doubt
3. Preschooler: initiative versus guilt
4. School-age child: industry versus inferiority
5. Adolescent: identity versus role confusion
6. Young adult: intimacy versus isolation
7. Adult: generativity versus stagnation
8. Older adult: ego integrity versus despair

Given favorable circumstances, the person develops positive ego strength at each life stage and thus builds positive resources to meet the next life developmental crisis. However, the struggle at any age is not forever won at that point. A residue of the negative remains, and in periods of stress some degree of regression may occur. But as the child and then the adult gains mastery at each stage of development, assisted by significant positive support, integration of self controls and strengths takes place. Various related developmental tasks surround each of these life stages and are learnings that, when accomplished, contribute to successful resolution of the core problem. These developmental tasks are integrated and associated with the normal physical maturation at each point. Various neuromuscular motor skills enable the person to accomplish related physical activities.

Health-Disease Spectrum

Throughout the life cycle, persons move back and forth across a spectrum of degrees of health and disease. Many fortunate ones remain on the positive side due to their "luck of the draw" in physical heritage and life circumstances and live relatively healthy lives free from major disease. Others experience varying degrees of disease or injury, both physical and mental, with individual responses depending on personal resources, physical and mental as well as psychosocial and economic. Thus any person's health and nutrition status and needs will always involve data from two sources: (1) objective information in quantified terms from various technologic sources, such as laboratory and X-ray tests, performance measures, nutrition analyses, physical findings, clinical and behavioral observations; and most significantly (2) subjective information gained from talking with and listening to the person and family, such as perceived pain, tolerances, feelings about health status or care, perceptions of their own problems, goals, priorities. Too often health practitioners dwell primarily with their technology of modern health care, when many roots of disease, especially in high-risk populations, lie in the area of personal stresses and needs—psychosocial, economic, and mental pressures as well as physical ones.

Stress-Coping Balance

Since stress is a fact of life, there must also be a coping balance to maintain positive health. Physiologic stress, either normal or abnormal, is met with a number of automatic physiologic responses to maintain the body in a state of dynamic equilibrium or *homeostasis.* For example, to meet the physiologic effects of stress from disease, injury, shock, or increased physical exertion, various homeostatic mechanisms automatically respond to restore the body's fluid-electrolyte and acid-base buffer balances, which are vital to sustain normal metabolism. Similarly, psychosocial stress is met with *learned* mental defense mechanisms, which may or may not be constructive in the circumstances. For example, such defense mechanisms as rationalization, compensation, suppression, repression, depression, or substitution are developed during the growing years to cope with stress, relieve tension, and preserve the inner self-concept. Often such mechanisms are the only means of making a painful situation psychologically tolerable, but some are less constructive than others.

Basic Human Needs Hierarchy

Human needs and motives, including nutrition-related ones, are highly personal. People are not the same the world over; those of differing cultures and life circumstances are not motivated by the same needs and goals. Even primary biologic drives, such as hunger and sex, are modified in their interpretation, expression, and fulfillment by many cultural, social, and personal influences. A hierarchy of human needs, such as that developed by the classic work of Maslow[5] with persons exhibiting characteristics of positive mental-health behavior, helps us to understand human strivings. He described five levels of human need that operate in turn, each building on successful achievement of the prior ones and having priority at different times depending upon related personal circumstances:

1. Basic physiological needs: hunger, thirst
2. Safety needs: physical comfort, security, protection
3. "Belongingness" needs: giving and receiving love and affection
4. Self-esteem needs: sense of self-worth, strength and self-confidence, status, recognition, capability, adequacy
5. Self-actualization needs: self-fulfillment, creative growth

Although these levels of need overlap and vary with circumstance and time, we can use them to help us understand human needs and plan nutrition and health care accordingly, both for our clients or patients and for ourselves.

THE NATURE OF STRESS

Perception of Stress

Individual responses to stress vary according to its reality and how it is perceived. Perception enables human beings to make sense out of an otherwise chaotic assortment of impressions. It enables them to live in an environment that feels relatively stable. Perception also limits understanding, however; every phenomenon that the outer world offers is understood through a social and personal lens. In every life experience one perceives a blend of three factors: (1) the external *reality,* (2) the *message* of the stimulus that is conveyed by the nervous system to the brain's integrative centers where thinking and evaluation go on, and (3) the *interpretation* that one puts on every bit of experience. A host of subjective elements, such as hunger, thirst, hatred, fear, self-interest, values, and temperament, influence response to the phenomena presented by the outer world.

Common Life Stressors

As with any force meeting a resistant force, the effect of life stresses will reflect three basic influencing factors: (1) the nature of the stress, whether it is relatively mild with minor consequences or severe with major results; (2) the duration, whether it is a fairly transient event or long term and relentless to the extent of exhausting both psychic and physiologic reserves; and (3) the nature of the personal coping resources, whether they are strong, relatively positive, effective, and constructive, or whether they are more negative, ineffective, and destructive. As indicated, these common life stressors are twofold in nature: (1) physical or physiologic stress from physical abuse, injury, disability, and disease, or normal physiologic demands of pregnancy and growth; and (2) psychologic, social, or economic stress from verbal abuse, emotional pressures, or lack of financial resources. Undoubtedly, emotional tension from multiple causes is the most common human stressor agent. It can contribute to such serious conditions as cardiac and gastrointestinal diseases, especially if the body is conditioned by malnutrition or faulty diet or poor housing, as is often the case with high-risk families in the grip of poverty.

The General Adaptive Syndrome: Physiologic Response to Stress

When any form of stress occurs, the body automatically responds to defend itself from harm. This common physiologic response to stress has been named by Selye the *general adaptive syndrome.*[2] An understanding of this automatic "cascade of physiologic events" provides a basis for planning nutritional support, both immediate and long term, for identifying needs and resources, and for rebuilding reserves.

ACTIONS OF THE NEUROENDOCRINE SYSTEM

Both parts of the nervous system, the central nervous system and the autonomic or sympathetic nervous system, are constantly involved in controlling the body's reactions to sensory stimuli and to stress. Together with hormones and other chemical messengers, the overall neuroendocrine system provides a vast network of both conscious and unconscious reactions to protect the body.

Conscious Response: The Central Nervous System

Certain processes in the body are under conscious direction. One decides to behave or act in a definite way in a given situation. In response to conscious decisions and directions, the brain and central nervous system send messages to the muscles, which in turn carry out the specific actions involved. For example, one may choose to eat some available food, take a walk, read a book, call someone on the phone, watch television, or do some other conscious act.

Unconscious Response: The Autonomic Nervous System

There are other processes, however, such as breathing and the beating of the heart, that are essential to life and must always go on. Such processes are automatically regulated. This essential control is managed by the autonomic, or sympathetic, nervous system. For many years Western science considered the autonomic functions to be beyond the reach of conscious control. However, Eastern traditions have included such phenomena in "holy men" who are able to slow their heart rate, control blood pressure and respiration, or show no evidence of pain in response to apparently painful stimuli. It has only been in recent years that Western medicine has evidenced interest in conscious control over unconscious processes and has been able to put forth theories about it with scientific credibility.

Combined Neuroendocrine Response

In response to stress the autonomic nervous system and its integrated hormones and other chemical messengers mobilize the body's reserves for protection. It is this immediate and continuing automatic physiologic response to stress that Selye called the *general adaptive syndrome.*[1,2] From his research he identified three stages of this generalized response process: (1) the *initial alarm reaction* in which the body's forces are mobilized for action; (2) the *adaptation-resistance stage* in which energy reserves are adjusted or rebuilt; and (3) the *exhaustion stage* in which resources give out if severe stress continues unabated. These stages overlap in the body's response to daily life stresses, reflecting the intensity of one's life situation. The rate of stress and its automatic physiologic response process is increased during nervous tension, physical injury, infections, muscular work, or any other strenuous activity, as a major defense mechanism that increases resistance to stressful agents.

STAGE I: THE INITIAL ALARM REACTION TO STRESS

Brain Signals

In response to a perceived threat, the brain initiates an instantaneous ripple effect throughout the body metabolism. It triggers the release of chemical messengers, **neurotransmitters**, in the cortex, which relay impulses along neuron tracks in the brain's outer edge to the hypothalamus. The hypothalamus at the head of the brain stem is the part of the brain originating in the earliest primitive era of the development of the human species. It governs the autonomic functions of the body, such as heart rate, blood pressure, peripheral temperature, breathing, digestion, blood-sugar level, hormonal balance, and many other vital activities. The hypothalamus has been called the "automatic pilot" or the "brain's brain." Upon instant receipt of the stress message, the hypothalamus triggers two responses: (1) it stimulates the release of the neurohormone **norepinephrine** from the cells of the autonomic/sympathetic nervous system to act as a chemical messenger; and (2) with continued stress it sends out another chem-

gency fuel. They also mobilize free amino acids from protein, which can thus serve not only for fuel but also as an important source of nitrogen for new protein synthesis, should the stress response require it. Two other important glucocorticoid-triggered stress responses are **glycogenolysis** and **gluconeogenesis**, which help maintain liver and muscle glycogen as a readily available fuel source. The glucocorticoids, along with epinephrine, suppress the action of insulin. Insulin is the body's key anabolic hormone, promoting storage of metabolic fuel inside cells. Suppressing this action of insulin to remove glucose from circulation sustains an elevated blood-sugar level, thus keeping metabolic fuel mobilized.

2. **Mineralocorticoids.** The main mineralocorticoid, **aldosterone**, causes the resorption of sodium by the nephron tubules and with it water, thus helping to protect the body's vital water and electrolyte balance. Aldosterone secretion by the adrenal cortex is also stimulated by the renin-angiotensin-aldosterone mechanism (p. 15) in response to threatened fluid loss. The process of inflammation, a localized protective response to injury or infection, is stimulated by the mineralocorticoids, whereas it is inhibited by the glucocorticoids.

Other hormones. In response to the stress signals, the anterior pituitary also secretes the **thyroid stimulating hormone (TSH)**, which triggers the release of T_3 and T_4—**thyroxine** from the thyroid gland to increase the basal metabolic rate (BMR) and accommodate the greatly enhanced metabolic activity induced by the body's stress responses. Two other anterior pituitary hormones, **growth hormone** and **prolactin**, both of which have generalized anabolic tissue-building effects, are mobilized to help protect tissue integrity. Growth hormone is anabolic in relation to protein, but catabolic in relation to fat and carbohydrate storage. Thus fats and carbohydrates are mobilized for emergency fuels, and free amino acids are readied for synthesis into stress-demanded hormones and only secondarily used as a source of the carbon skeleton for fuel from gluconeogenesis. The small posterior lobe of the pituitary secretes a major antidiuretic hormone, **vasopressin**, which in the face of stress guards the body's vital water supply by increasing water resorption in the kidneys' nephrons.

STAGE II: RESISTANCE AND ADAPTATION TO STRESS

Following the initial alarm reaction described above, if the particular stress has not been so potent that continued exposure overwhelms the person's coping resources, a second stage of resistance and adaptation necessarily follows. Hormonal feedback and rebuilding of reserves support this period of adjustment allowing a certain tolerance to build up.

Hormonal Feedback Mechanism

The body's normal hormonal feedback mechanism controls the output of the initiating agent and helps return the blood level of the target gland's hormone to a lower maintenance level. For example, during the alarm reaction the outpouring of thyroid hormone and adrenal cortex corticoids that manage massive immediate metabolic needs raises the blood levels of these substances, which in turn feed back to the controlling master gland, the anterior pituitary, to shut off or lower its stimulating hormones TSH and ACTH for a period of automatic adjustment to normal balance.

Rebuilding Reserves

As a result of the massive alarm reaction, normal body reserves are rapidly depleted, the blood becomes concentrated with metabolic materials, and there is marked loss of body weight. A period of restoration must eventually follow, in which the glands and other body tissue reserves are built, the blood dilution resumes normal levels, and the body weight returns toward normal.

Adaptive Homeostasis

The level of this adaptation to the initial or chronic stress will depend upon the extent of the stress and the person's coping powers. The stress reaction is generalized throughout the body as described, always resulting in this general adaptation syndrome identified by Selye,[2] no matter what type of stress is applied. Under the influence of stress, some higher-risk persons may develop gastric ulcers, cardiovascular diseases, hypertension, headache, or neurosis, depending on their physiologic and psychosocial status. When stress is superimposed on persons made vulnerable by nutritional deficiency or disorder or disease, the effect is to make a bad situation worse. Often this is the situation, for example, of high-risk populations suffering the chronic stress of poverty and malnutrition.

STAGE III: EXHAUSTION OF STRESS-COPING RESOURCES

After still more prolonged exposure to stress, the adaptation powers of the body weaken and a stage of exhaustion follows. If the stress is severe enough and applied long enough, particularly if disease compounds it, the person's adaptation energy becomes exhausted and must be restored if life is to continue.

Immunity

Persons under stress of life events, crises both large and small, experience depressed immune function and increased vulnerability to disease. Miller[7] reports results of recent studies at Ohio State University in which groups of people under stress showed measured reduction of immune response and increased episodes of infectious disease. One of the immune functions, especially that of "natural killer cells" activity, was depressed. These important cells are members of the T cell population of lymphoid cells, the **lymphocytes**, a type of white blood cell making up a major component of the body's remarkable defense system. Together with a companion B cell population of lymphoid cells, these lymphocytes are derived from precursor cells in the bone marrow (Fig. 11-1). The T cells comprise the majority of the circulating pool of small lymphocytes in blood and lymph and in certain areas of the lymph nodes and spleen. A T cell recognizes invading antigens by means of specific special receptors on its surface.[8] Upon contact with an **antigen**—a foreign intruder, a "nonself" or alien substance such as a virus—the T cells multiply and initiate specific cellular immune responses: (1) they activate the **phagocytes**, special cells of the reticuloendothelial system that have intracellular killing and degrading mechanisms for destroying invaders; and (2) they start the inflammatory process by releasing chemical mediators. Some T cells can do even more by becoming "killer" cells themselves and attacking antigens. These special double-duty T cells have been called "helper cell-independent cytotoxic T lymphocytes," abbreviated more graphically to the name **HIT cells**.[9]

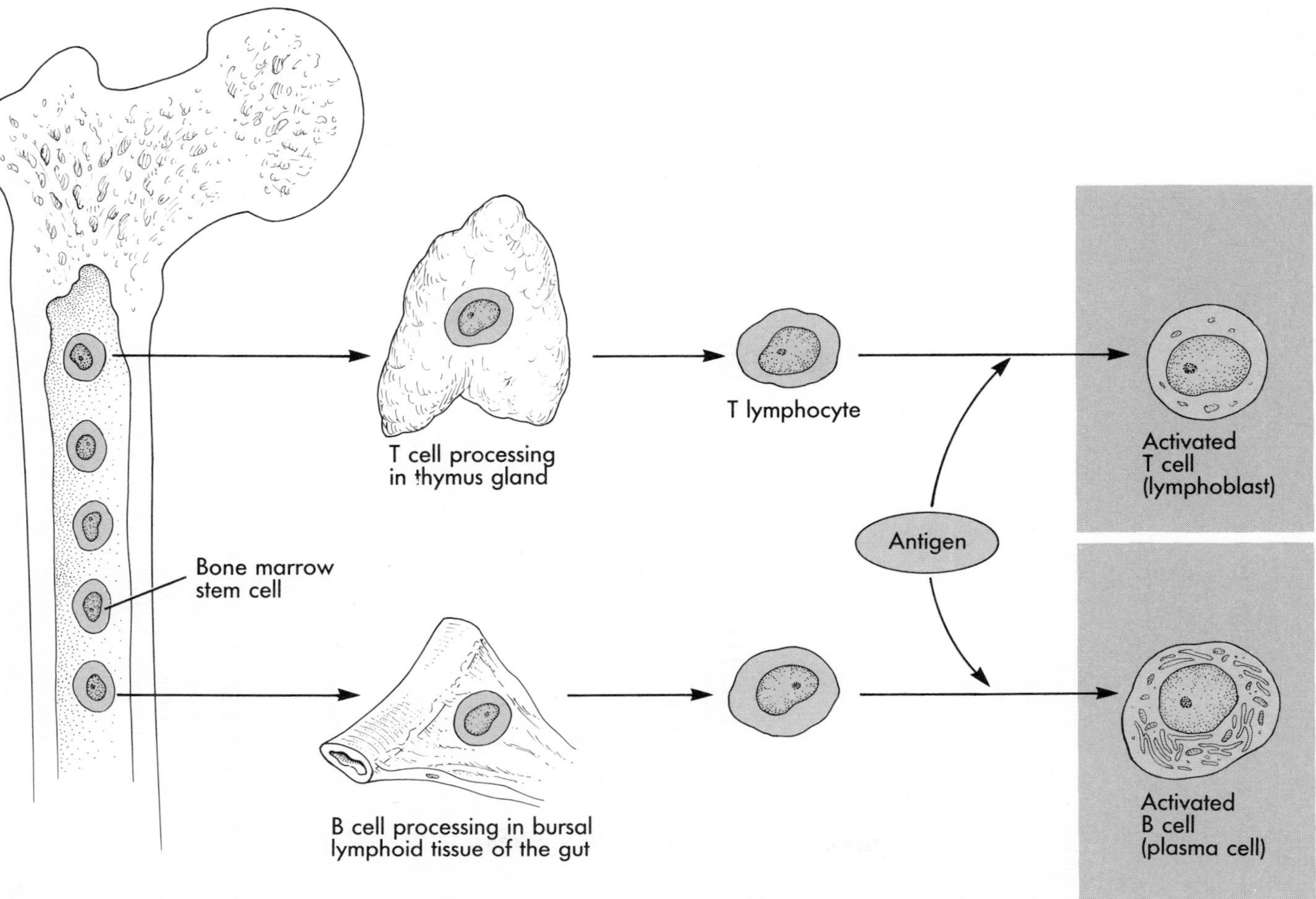

FIG. 11-1 Development of the T and B cells, lymphocyte components of the body's immune system.

Disease

The Ohio scientists[7] studying crisis-related immunity concluded that heightened and sustained distress can suppress immune function, but whether this condition leads to disease depends on individual conditioning factors such as psychologic resources, prior health and nutrition, and exposure to infectious diseases. They suggest that stress-related immunosuppression has its most significant consequences in elderly persons and others who have pre-existing deficiencies in immune function.

Death

The exhaustion stage of response to stress cannot be maintained for long periods of time as body systems begin to wear out in their ability to cope. If restoration of resources does not occur, and the stress is relentless and prolonged, finally the body's energy sources are depleted and death follows. Intervention must occur earlier to reduce stress, prevent disease, and promote health. A vital part of such intervention is nutritional support.

Life Cycle Stress: High-Risk Population Groups

GENERAL NUTRITIONAL RISKS

Throughout the life cycle, a number of general nutrition and health behaviors place persons at risk. These general nutritional risks, reviewed in preceeding life cycle chapters in various ways, include such factors as poor eating habits, bizarre diets, extreme vegetarianism, substance abuse as with alcohol and illicit drugs, various food-nutrient-drug interactions, megadoses of food supplements, nutrient imbalances, eating disorders, lack of exercise, or poor mental attitude. Each of these situations present special needs to meet numerous physiologic and psychosocial stresses involved and help provide the necessary related nutritional support.

SPECIFIC LIFE CYCLE STRESS PERIODS

At each stage of the human life cycle, specific physiologic growth and psychosocial development create nutrition-related stress for both the physical body and the person. Nutritional needs can only be met within the total life context at any particular point. Also, additional risks and health problems are imposed by the added stress of physical trauma, disease, or disability. Other risks may relate to the workplace, heavy exercise, or the rapidly changing environment. And the painful stress of over-riding poverty brings physical, psychosocial, and mental-health problems to many persons.

Here we will review some of these high-risk populations throughout the life cycle and consider approaches to nutritional care. Then we will look at some ways of managing high-risk stress as a means of more positive nutrition and health promotion in general.

Physiologic and Psychosocial Stress of Pregnancy

NORMAL PHYSIOLOGIC STRESS AND ADAPTATION

In Chapter 4 a detailed review of the multiple physiologic processes of pregnancy has been provided. For our discussion here, three concepts form a fundamental framework for understanding the *normal* physiologic stress of pregnancy and the hormonally controlled maternal responses adapting the body to meet these increased demands.

Perinatal Concept

As knowledge and understanding increase, it is evident that the whole of the mother's life experiences surrounding her pregnancy must be considered. For any woman in any culture the first pregnancy is a profound experience, a veritable "rite of passage." And any following pregnancy continues to change life situations for parents and family. Cultural and social influences have shaped values and beliefs of both parents about pregnancy. Genetic heritage and previous years of living and food habits have determined the mother's current health and nutritional status and pre-conception nutrient reserves for the present pregnancy. All of these influences are important.

Life Continuum Concept

Each child becomes a part of the ongoing family and the continuum of life. At conception the child receives a unique genetic foundation and from the food the mother eats, she gives to her unborn child the nourishment required to initiate, develop, and sustain the tremendous fetal growth. Then after the child's birth, the family carries over its nutritional beliefs and practices in its feeding and teaching of the growing child. These attitudes and values are internalized and passed on to future generations of children.

Synergism Concept

The term *synergism* is used to describe biologic systems in which the integrated interaction of two or more factors produces a total effect greater than and different from the sum of their parts. In short, a new whole is created by the unified, joint blending of the parts in which each part potentiates the action of the other. Of the many biologic and physiologic interactions in nature providing examples of synergism, pregnancy is a prime case in point. Maternal organism, fetus, and placenta all combine to create a new whole, not existing before, producing a total effect greater than and different from the sum of their parts, all for the purpose of sustaining and nurturing the pregnancy and its offspring. Physiologic parameters change, blood volume increases, cardiac output increases, respiration changes with increased ventilation rate and tidal volume. The physiologic norms of the nonpregnant woman do not apply. These normal physiologic adjustments of pregnancy cannot be viewed as the same signs would be interpreted in an abnormal state, nor can the treatment procedures for these same signs in an abnormal condition be applied to pregnancy. For example, a normal generalized edema of pregnancy is a protective response. It reflects the normal increase in total body water necessary to support the increased metabolic work of pregnancy and as such it is associated with enhanced reproductive performance.

NORMAL PREGNANCY: GENERAL RISK FACTORS

The normal physiology of pregnancy, as described in Chapter 4, places stress upon the mother to meet the demands of rapid fetal development and growth, the growth and functioning of the placenta, and the maternal tissue development and increased metabolic activity. But optimal nutrition support and good prenatal care meet these added physiologic stresses and help produce a healthy course and outcome of the pregnancy.

HIGH-RISK PREGNANCY: ADDED RISK FACTORS

A number of added risk factors, however, may contribute to a poor pregnancy outcome. In a joint report, the American College of Obstetricians and Gynecologists and the American Dietetic Association have issued a set of risk factors to identify women with special nutritional and health-care needs during pregnancy.[10] These factors are summarized in Table 11-1 and relate to nutritional status, habits, needs, and problems. The nutritional factors identified in this report are based on clinical evidence of inadequate nutrition. But a better approach suggested by King[11] provides useful criteria for predicting nutritional risk, instead of waiting for clinical signs of poor nutrition to appear. Three types of dietary patterns, she summarizes, would not support optimal maternal and fetal nutrition: (1) insufficient food intake, (2) poor food selection, and (3) poor food distribution throughout the day. These patterns, added to

TABLE 11-1 Nutritional Risk Factors in Pregnancy

Risk Factors Presented at the Onset of Pregnancy	Risk Factors Occurring During Pregnancy
Age	Low hemoglobin or hematocrit
15 years or younger	Hemoglobin less than 12.0 g
35 years or older	Hematocrit less than 35.0 mg/dl
Frequent pregnancies: three or more during a 2-year period	Inadequate weight gain
	Any weight loss
Poor obstetric history or poor fetal performance	Weight gain of less than 2 lb per month after the first trimester
Poverty	Excessive weight gain: greater than 1 kg (2.2 lb) per week after the first trimester
Bizarre or faddist food habits	
Abuse of nicotine, alcohol, or drugs	
Therapeutic diet required for a chronic disorder	
Inadequate weight	
Less than 85% of standard weight	
More than 120% of standard weight	

the list of risk factors in Table 11-1, would be much more sensitive for nutritional risk. On this basis, practitioners can plan personal care and provide for special counseling needs.

Personal Care

Women identified as having higher risks in their pregnancies need careful attention. Some of them may have low reserves due to their obsession with thinness and pattern of constantly "dieting." Others may be strict vegetarians or "vegans" and need exploration of ways to achieve high-quality complete protein intake. Others may be food faddists or follow some bizarre food pattern. Still others may be athletes and need help in planning a lighter program to avoid major risks to the fetus, such as hypoxia, disruption of fuel supply, hyperthermia, or cardiac failure, from continued strenuous exercise.[12] By working closely with each woman and her personal patterns of food intake, nutritionists can help mothers develop a reasonable personal food plan to ensure a positive intake of all the nutrient and energy increases demanded for the support of the pregnancy and its successful outcome.

Special Counseling Needs

Several special problems require sensitive and supportive counseling to reduce risks:

1. **Age and parity**. Pregnancies at either reproductive age extreme pose special problems. The adolescent pregnancy, described in detail in Chapter 8, is fraught with both psychosocial and nutrition-related risks. Imposed on a still-growing teenaged body are the additional demands of the pregnancy. *Nulligravidas* 15 years of age and younger are especially at risk, since their own growth is incomplete. Sensitive counseling provides both information and emotional support and should involve family and other significant persons. On the other hand, the older *primigravida* over 35 years of age also requires special attention. She may be at more risk for hypertension, either pre-existing or gestational, and need more monitoring of rate of weight gain and amount of sodium used. In addition, a mother with a high *parity* rate, having several pregnancies within a limited number of years, is usually drained of nutritional resources and enters each successive pregnancy at higher risk. Counseling may well include discussions of acceptable means of contraception, as well as nutritional support and information.
2. **Alcohol, cigarettes, and drugs**. These three personal habits create serious risks and are contraindicated during pregnancy. Studies indicate that intrauterine growth retardation has been the most consistently observed and dramatic effect of fetal alcohol exposure.[13] Extensive and habitual alcohol use during pregnancy leads to the well-described fetal alcohol syndrome, a specific set of alcohol-related birth defects (p. 126). Cigarette smoking during pregnancy (p. 135) poses special high-risk problems resulting in placental abnormalities and fetal damage including prematurity and low birth weight.[14] Drug use, both recreational and medicinal, also carries problems. Even self-medication with over-the-counter

drugs has numerous adverse effects. The use of "street drugs" carries special hazards, resulting not only from the drugs themselves but also from the various impurities they contain. Also, megadosing with various nutrients during pregnancy can be damaging.

3. **Socioeconomic problems.** Special counseling is essential for women living in high-risk, low-income or extreme poverty situations. Numerous studies and clinical observations indicate that lack of prenatal care, often associated with racial prejudices and fears as well as poverty, places the mother in grave difficulty. Sensitivity for personal needs can help in planning for necessary resources of food assistance, such as the Special Supplemental Food Program for Women, Infants, and Children (WIC), the results of which are shown in Fig. 11-2. (See Chapter 12.)

HIGH-RISK PREGNANCY: CLINICAL COMPLICATIONS

Any complication of the pregnancy adds still more risk. Examples of these conditions include anemia, pregnancy-induced hypertension, and pre-existing disease.

Anemia

Various forms of anemia are common risk factors in pregnancy. Anemia may be caused by nutritional deficiency of iron or folic acid or by hemorrhage:

1. **Iron-deficiency anemia.** About 10% of the women attending large prenatal clinics in the United States have hemoglobin concentrations of less than 10 g/dl and

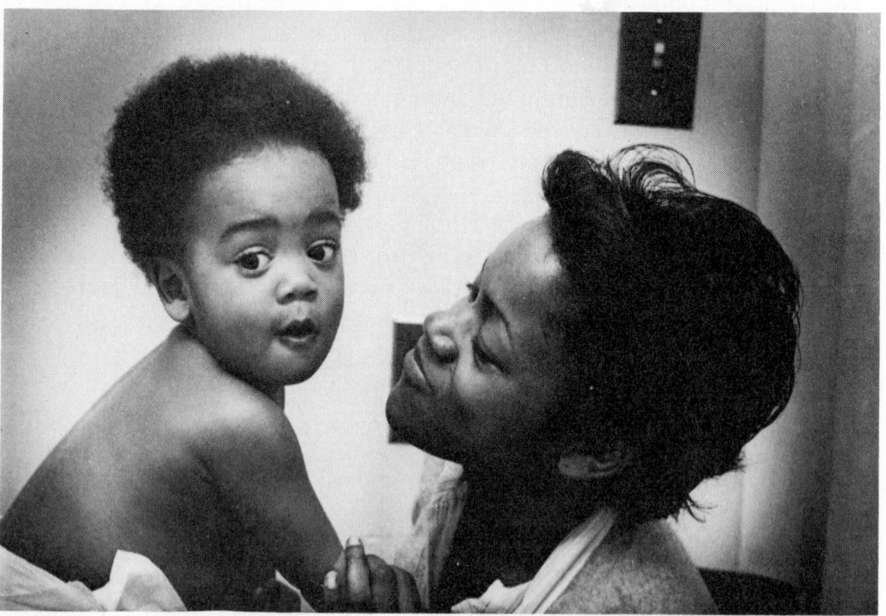

FIG. 11-2 A healthy child and mother—happy participants in the WIC Program.

hematocrit readings below 32%. Anemia is more prevalent among the poor, many of whom live on diets barely adequate for marginal existence. But it is by no means restricted to lower economic groups. The *iron cost* of a single normal pregnancy is high—500 to 800 mg. Of this amount, nearly 300 mg is used by the fetus. The remainder is used in the normal physiologic expansion of maternal red-blood-cell volume and hemoglobin mass, a requirement exceeding the available iron reserves in the average woman. In some women the iron level is borderline before pregnancy and insufficient to meet the augmented needs during pregnancy. Usually the iron requirement of the fetus, which increases during the last trimester of rapid growth, will continue to be met by transfer of iron across the placenta. It is the mother who will suffer from iron deficiency. Thus the RDA standard recommends a daily iron supplement during pregnancy of 30 to 60 mg for preventive care. Treatment of highly deficient states in high-risk women requires daily therapeutic doses of 120 to 200 mg, continued for 3 to 6 months after the anemia has been corrected, to rebuild the depleted stores. Meanwhile, ways of including more iron-rich foods in the mother's diet must be explored.

2. **Folic acid deficiency anemia.** A less common form of nutritional anemia of pregnancy results from deficiency of folic acid. An analysis of the diets of women with this *megaloblastic anemia* usually reveals that they eat few if any vegetables, especially green leafy ones, and seldom have animal protein. Symptoms include intensified nausea, vomiting, and anorexia. As the anemia progresses, the anorexia becomes marked, further compounding the nutritional deficiency. During pregnancy, both the fetus and trophoblast cells helping to form the placenta are sensitive to folic acid inhibitors and thus have increased metabolic requirements for folic acid and its derivatives. To prevent this anemia, the RDA standard recommends a preventive supplement for pregnant women of 400 μg of folic acid daily.
3. **Hemorrhagic anemia.** Anemia caused by blood loss is more likely to occur during the period after labor and delivery than during gestation. Blood loss may occur earlier, however, as a result of abortion or ruptured tubular pregnancy. Most patients undergoing these problems receive blood by transfusion, and iron therapy may be indicated for adequate replacement of hemoglobin.

Pregnancy-Induced Hypertension (PIH)

Formerly labeled *toxemia,* PIH is a risk factor related to nutrition and treated according to its symptoms:

1. **Relation to nutrition:** Clinical experience indicates that PIH is a disease of malnutrition, especially related to diets poor in protein, kilocalories, calcium, and salt,[15] and that the malnutrition affects the liver and its metabolic activities. Certainly, as many practitioners have observed, PIH is classically associated with poverty. It has been encountered most often in women subsisting on inadequate diets and having little or no prenatal care. Much of the PIH problem could be prevented by good prenatal care, which inherently includes attention to sound

nutrition. It is this sound nutritional status, which a woman brings to her pregnancy and *maintains* throughout, that provides her with optimal resources for adapting to the physiologic stress of gestation. Her fitness during pregnancy is a direct function of her past nutrition and her optimal nutrition during pregnancy.

2. **Clinical symptoms.** PIH is generally defined according to its manifestations, which usually occur in the third trimester toward term. Among its symptoms are hypertension, abnormal and excessive edema, albuminuria, and in severe cases, convulsions or coma—*eclampsia.*
3. **Treatment.** Specific treatment varies according to the patient's symptoms and needs. In any case, optimal nutrition is a fundamental aspect of therapy. Adequate dietary protein is essential. Correction of plasma protein deficits stimulates normal operation of the capillary fluid shift mechanism and restores circulation of tissue fluid, inducing subsequent correction of the *hypovolemia.* In addition, adequate salt and sources of vitamins and minerals are needed for correction and maintenance of metabolic balances.

Pre-existing Disease

Pre-existing clinical conditions complicate pregnancy and increase risks. They are managed according to the general principles of care related to pregnancy and to the particular disease involved. Examples of these pre-existing conditions include hypertension, diabetes mellitus, and phenylketonuria:

1. **Hypertension.** Preventive screening and monitoring of blood pressure are essential. The hypertensive disease process begins long before any signs and symptoms appear and later symptoms are inconsistent.[16] Risk factors for hypertension before and during pregnancy are given in Table 11-2. Nutritional care will center on prevention of weight extremes, either underweight or obesity, and correction of any dietary deficiencies by maintaining optimal nutrition. Sodium intake can be moderate but should never be unduly restricted, because of its relation to fluid and electrolyte balances during pregnancies.

TABLE 11-2 Risk Factors in Pregnancy-Induced Hypertension

Before Pregnancy	During Pregnancy
Nulligravida	Primigravida
Diabetes mellitus	Large fetus
Pre-existing condition (hypertension, renal or vascular disease)	Glomerulonephritis
Family history of hypertension or vascular disease	**Fetal hydrops**
Diagnosis of pregnancy-induced hypertension in a previous pregnancy	**Hydramnios**
Dietary deficiencies	Multiple gestation
Age extremes	**Hydatidiform mole**
20 years or younger	
35 years or older	

2. **Diabetes mellitus.** The management of diabetes in pregnancy presents special problems. Thus routine screening is necessary to detect gestational diabetes, and team management is required for control of pre-existing insulin-dependent diabetes mellitus (IDDM).[17]

   Screening. Most prenatal clinics do routine screening for diabetes and provide careful follow-up for every patient who shows glycosuria. Risk factors detected in initial history include: (1) family history of diabetes, (2) previous unexplained stillbirths, (3) large babies weighing 4 kg (9 lb) or more, (4) recurrent miscarriage, (5) births of babies with multiple congenital anomalies, and (6) excessive obesity.

   Gestational diabetes. During pregnancy glycosuria is not uncommon because of the increased circulating blood volume and its load of metabolites. But only 20% to 30% of women showing glycosuria or somewhat abnormal glucose tolerance subsequently develop diabetes. Nonetheless, identification of women with this condition and their close follow-up observation are important because of the higher risk of fetal damage during this period. Most of these women revert to normal glucose tolerance after delivery.

   Pre-existing IDDM. Because of the course of diabetes during pregnancy, as well as the altered course of pregnancy in the presence of diabetes, a team of specialists is necessary for sound management and prevention of problems to reduce risk of fetal death and increase the probability of a successful outcome. Close personalized nutritional care by the team nutritionist is mandatory throughout. The insulin requirement increases during the pregnancy and drops dramatically upon delivery.
3. **Maternal phenylketonuria (PKU).** Mandatory screening of all newborns for the genetic disease PKU and low-phenylalanine diet have supported normal growth in PKU children. Now a generation of young women with childhood PKU are having children of their own. Maternal PKU presents potential fetal hazards associated with increased abortions and stillbirths, congenital anomalies often causing death, and intrauterine and postnatal growth and development retardation in surviving infants.[18] A planned pregnancy, with careful management of the mother's diet *before* conception and close follow-up care *throughout* the pregnancy itself, can improve the outcome of these high-risk pregnancies. A strict diet low in phenylalanine and special formula of other amino acids is required.

Physiologic and Psychosocial Stress of Infant Growth

NORMAL GROWTH DEMANDS

Physical Growth Requirements

After the period of rapid fetal growth, the full-term neonate moves quickly at birth from a warm, protective and supportive uterine environment to the stress of the external world, literally cut off from its former umbilical nourishment. Survival demands immediate adaptation. Over the centuries, human milk has bountifully provided for the nutritional needs of the rapidly growing neonate and young infant, with 56% of its total kilocalories as well-absorbed fat and 38% as the sugar lactose producing major energy sources and the remaining 6% as highly digestible protein to promote continued growth. This ratio of basic energy and growth nutrients is well suited to meet appropriate growth demands over the first 4 to 6 months of the infant's life. By 6 months the infant will weigh twice what it weighed at birth, then three times what it weighed at birth by the end of the first year. During the first half-year of life, the infant's rapid growth and sharp increase in body fat to meet both fuel and body temperature needs demands a relatively high energy intake per kilogram body weight. The gradual decline in normal growth rate during the latter half of the first year is met by a continuing appropriate milk source with added solid foods. Any interference, through inadequate diet or disease, with this necessary nutritional support for the heightened metabolic demands of normal growth will add still more risk to life and health.

Psychosocial Development Needs

The core psychosocial stress during infancy is the development of *trust versus distrust* (p. 451). Feeding is the infant's main means of establishing human relationships vital to survival. The initial close mother-infant bonding in the feeding process fills this basic need to build the positive resource of trust. The need for sucking and the development of the lips and mouth as sensory organs represent adaptations that ensure an adequate early food intake. As a result, food becomes the infant's general means of exploring the environment. As described in Chapter 6, when neuromuscular coordination involving the central nervous system, the tongue, and the swallowing reflex develops,[19] infants gradually learn to eat a variety of semisolid foods, starting at about 6 months of age. Then as they continue to grow and develop, they will begin to evidence a desire for self-feeding. If their needs for food and love are fulfilled in these early relationships with mother, father, or other feeding adults, as well as broadening relationships with other family members, the anchor of trust is developed. Infants evidence this positively growing trust by their increasing capacity to wait for feedings until they are prepared.

HIGH-RISK INFANTS

Not all infants, however, are so fortunate in their development and growth experience during the stress of these early critical fetal-neonatal periods of life. Tiny babies born prematurely or small for their gestational age, having low birth weights and suffering some form of intrauterine growth retardation, those having birth defects, and those generally failing to thrive carry greatly increased risks and require special care.

Low Birth Weight

A low birth weight (LBW) of 2500 g (5 lb) or lower is a serious risk factor of great importance in neonatology and nutrition, given the incidence of the problem as well as its prognosis. The World Health Organization[20] reports that at least 15 million LBW babies are born every year worldwide, representing 17% of all newborns. Even in developed countries the incidence is highly significant—an estimated 1.3 million or 7% of all births. Villar and Cossio[21] identify a number of risk factors for LBW and its subgroups, intrauterine growth retardation (IUGR) and prematurity. Maternal characteristics associated with LBW include: (1) low prepregnancy weight, (2) short stature, (3) low gestational weight gain, and (4) low caloric intake during pregnancy. Additional maternal behavioral factors associated with increased incidence of IUGR include smoking and alcohol abuse. The subgroup IUGR refers to term babies born at 37 or more weeks of gestation, having both weight and length problems. The premature subgroup refers to preterm LBW babies born before week 37 of gestation. Additional maternal risk factors of caffeine consumption and physical activity are less clear and depend upon their extent. A moderate intake of caffeine-containing beverage, about one or two cups a day, does not appear to increase risk although this response is individual. The association of maternal physical activity appears to be selective, depending on the mother's social class, the family economic impact of her activities, and the type of work she does.[21] When work or physical exercise is strenuous, even in well-nourished women, it is associated with a 2% to 11% increase in the incidence of prematurity.[22,23] In general, the morbidity rates are significant in these high-risk LBW babies. From their studies, Villar and Belizan[24] report that all IUGR infants suffer a high degree of asphyxia, hypoglycemia, hypothermia, and hyperviscosity in the neonatal period, fail to reach the weight or length of normal–birth-weight newborns during the first year of life, and display long-term consequences in both physical growth and mental development. Although the risk of neonatal death is higher for premature than for IUGR infants, high LBW rates from either cause and high neonatal mortality coexist in adverse socioeconomic circumstances, another human toll of poverty.

Current Care of Low-Birth-Weight Infants

Over the past few years, tremendous strides have been made in the care of LBW infants and survival rates have improved. Better nutritional management and feeding methods, together with other aspects of care such as respiratory and environmental conditions, have produced a jump in survival rate from 10% or less in 1970 to about 90% in 1980.[25] Some of these tiny babies may do well on breast milk, while other infants will require and thrive on special newly developed commercial formulas (Table 11-3). Nutritional management also includes such changes as earlier feedings and use of continuous intragastric and transpyloric tube feeding techniques. Some LBW infants are started on regular strength formulas (67 kcal/dl), building to early follow-up use of special higher energy premature infant formulas (80 kcal/dl). Critical cases of special need may require parenteral nutritional support through vein feeding of specially formulated solutions.

Failure to Thrive

The general term *failure to thrive* has been used in pediatrics to describe any child who does not measure up to usual growth and development standards. Fomon's[26] early definition identified failure to thrive in precise physical growth terms: a rate of gain in weight or length less than the value corresponding to 2 standard deviations below the mean during an interval of at least 56 days for infants less than 5 months of age and during an interval of at least 3 months for older infants. In general, an infant is described as failing to thrive when there is poor weight gain without an immediate

TABLE 11-3 Nutritional Value of Special Formulas and Human Milk for the Preterm Infant

	Advisable Intake		Human Milk Content		Standard Formulas	Special Premature Formulas		
	Birth Weight							
Nutritional Component	1.0 kg (2.2 lb)	1.5 kg (3.3 lb)	Preterm	Mature	Enfamil* Similac† SMA‡	Enfamil Premature with Whey*	Similac Special Care†	"Preemie" SMA‡
Kilocalories/deciliter			73	73	67	81	81	81
Protein (g/100 kcal)	3.1	2.7	2.3§	1.5	2.2	3.0	2.7	2.5
Vitamins, fat-soluble								
D (IU/120 kcal/kg/day)	600	600	—	4.0	70-75	75	180	76
E (IU/120 kcal/kg/day)	30	30	—	0.3	2-3	2	4	2
Vitamins, water-soluble								
Folic acid (μg/120 kcal/kg/day)	60	60	—	8.0	9-19	36	45	14
Vitamin C (mg/120 kcal/kg/day)	60	60	—	7.0	10	10	45	10
Minerals								
Calcium (mg/100 kcal)	160	140	40.0	43.0	66-78	117	178	92
Phosphorus (mg/100 kcal)	108	95	18.0	20.0	49-66	58	89	49
Sodium (mEq/100 kcal)	2.7	2.3	1.5‖	0.8	1.0-1.8	1.7	1.9	1.7

*Mead Johnson Nutritional Division, Evansville, Ind.
†Ross Laboratories, Columbus, Ohio.
‡Wyeth Laboratories, Philadelphia.
§Range: 1.9-2.8 g/100 kcal.
‖Range: 0.9-2.3 mEq/100 kcal.

explanation. Powell[27] recommends an integrated view of the disorder and its care, combining both organic or intrinsic defect possibilities and nonorganic or extrinsic factors contributing to defective mother-infant interaction. The decreased energy (kilocalories) intake causes the lack of weight gain. Defective mother-infant interaction can cause the decreased energy intake, developmental delay, and abnormal behaviors. Careful nutrition and social assessment is required to identify underlying causes of feeding problems so that appropriate care can be planned. Numerous factors may be involved:

1. **Clinical disease.** There may be central nervous system disorders, endocrine disease, congenital defects, or partial obstruction. Neuromotor problems may be associated with poor suck, abnormal postural tone during feeding, and the retention of primitive reflexes that should have faded at an earlier age. Eating, chewing, and swallowing problems may be so severe in some children as to compromise their nutrient intake.
2. **Dietary practices.** Some infants may have suffered from inappropriate formula feeding, use of improper dilutions in mixing formulas, or other poor practices that result in an inadequate energy intake.
3. **Unusual nutrient needs or losses.** Other infants may receive an adequate diet to promote growth but suffer from inadequate nutrient absorption and therefore excessive fecal loss. In other cases a hypermetabolic state may require increased energy intake that is not being met.
4. **Psychosocial problems.** Early feeding problems during infancy may have psychosocial cause within the family. Such situations may turn into severe parent-child conflicts.

Often failure to thrive results from a complex of factors and there are no easy solutions. Careful history taking, supportive nutritional guidance, and much warm care are required to influence growth patterns. The full rehabilitation of these infants and young children demands not only full nutritional support but also careful and sensitive correction of social and environmental issues surrounding each individual problem. For example, failure to thrive in a vegan (strict vegetarian) infant or child may stem from deficiencies in energy, protein, calcium, iron, zinc, riboflavin, and vitamins B_{12} and D, which reflect vegan practices, such as limited food choices and use of low–caloric-density foods with restriction of number of meals and snacks, as well as the limited stomach capacity of all infants and young children.[28] Nutrition counseling would have to be based on the structure and food ways of the family. The practitioner must work within that belief system to explore with the family acceptable ways of increasing energy and nutrient intake.

Physiologic and Psychosocial Stress of Childhood Growth

PHYSICAL GROWTH

As indicated in the Chapter 2 discussion of comparative body composition, during the period of latent childhood growth between infancy and adolescence the growth of the child slows and is more erratic. However, continued growth places metabolic demands on the young body that gradually increase the energy and nutrient needs. In the preschool years especially, growth rates vary widely as resources are being laid down for the rapid adolescent growth ahead.

HIGH-RISK CHILDREN

Growth Failure

The growth potential of an individual is genetically determined. If conditions are favorable, each child will grow according to his own predetermined growth curve, as described in Chapter 7. This process is called "canalization" of growth along that individual's own growth channel.[29] Unfavorable conditions deflect a child away from the predetermined growth curve. The extent of the growth failure will depend upon the severity of the unfavorable conditions and how long the child is exposed to them without adequate relief, leaving them stunted and wasted. Depending upon the extent of damage and the quality of rehabilitation, "catch-up" growth may restore a child to his own growth channel in response to a high-energy diet with appropriate amounts of protein and trace elements. For example, a weight gain of 20 g/kg/day requires 174 kcal/kg/day and 4.8 g protein/kg/day, in order to achieve a self-correcting growth response.[29]

Developmental Disability

The developmentally disabled population is at high risk of nutritional deficiency and multiple health problems. These persons have sustained chronic physical or mental impairments during the growth years from numerous causes, including conditions such as cerebral palsy, spina bifida, and Down's syndrome. A myriad of psychosocial, economic, and physical stress factors face these persons and their families. These stresses must be considered in planning nutritional care in conjunction with other aspects of the total care plan. Wodarski[30] provides a comprehensive interdisciplinary model for achieving optimal nutritional health with a team of specialists such as a physician, nutritionist, nurse, social worker, speech therapist, psychologist, dentist, dental hygienist, occupational and physical therapists, pharmacist, and recreational therapist. Where such teamwork is not routine, it is the nutritionist's responsibility to recognize nutritional needs and initiate appropriate consultation and referral activities with available resource persons and agencies. In the care of any of these high-risk children, their development to the fullest extent possible of individual physical, mental, and emotional potential is based on adequate nutrition.

Chronic Disease Heritage

A number of the lipid disorders, as well as essential hypertension, which underlie potential development of cardiovascular disease, are familial. Children in such genetically high-risk families carry a strong predisposition risk for developing these chronic diseases. Thus both pediatricians and nutritionists have advised the adoption of prudent eating patterns in such families, giving appropriate attention to the total amount and kind of fat, as well as sodium, in the general family diet. Childhood obesity, a growing risk problem, is also receiving more current attention. Kolata[31] reports evidence of increased incidence accumulated by physicians studying data from the

National Health and Nutrition Examination Surveys (NHANES). These data indicate that over the past two decades the prevalence of obesity among 6- to 11-year-old American children increased by 54%; among 12- to 17-year-olds, by 39%. The picture is even worse for black children, the prevalence of obesity having increased almost twice as much in preadolescent black children as it has in preadolescent whites. The evidence is that a tendency to be obese is inherited and that fat children tend to remain fat.[31] Forty percent of children who are obese at age 7 become obese adults. Seventy percent of obese adolescents become obese adults. Thus in families carrying this risk factor, prudent attention to appropriate energy balance between food and exercise habits is indicated. Epstein and associates[32] have developed such a family-based behavioral weight control program in which they studied obese children aged 1 to 6 years, with improvements shown in nutrient density for all nutrients. Their results suggest that obesity can be managed successfully in young children without detrimental effect on growth or nutrient intake.

Physiologic and Psychosocial Stress of Adolescent Growth

PHYSICAL GROWTH

With the onset of puberty and the increased output of hormones flooding the body and regulating physical and sexual maturation, rapid growth creates physiologic stress. Body changes and development of sexual characteristics produce personal concerns about body size and shape. Figure-conscious young girls worry about increased fat deposits. Strength-minded young boys think about adequate muscle development. The growth spurt of the boy is generally later than that of the girl, but he soon passes her in weight and height. The magnitude of this adolescent growth and its related body composition changes in both sexes is described in Chapter 2.

PSYCHOSOCIAL DEVELOPMENT

Core Psychosocial Development Problem

Adolescence is an ambivalent period full of stresses and strains. On the one hand teenagers look back to the securities of earlier childhood; on the other, they reach for the maturity of adulthood. The core psychosocial problem adolescents struggle with is that of *identity versus role diffusion* (p. 451) with its eternal questions of "Who am I?" and "Where am I going?" The search for self begun in early childhood reaches a climax in the identity crisis of the teen years. The profound body changes associated with sexual development cause changes in body image and resulting tensions. Individual variance is great in response to these stressful tensions, depending on the resources that have been provided for them in earlier developmental years.

The Identity Crisis in a Complex Society

During the adolescent years, the identity crisis of "growing up" largely revolves around the process of sexual maturing and preparing for an adult role in a complex society. There is little wonder that this period is fraught with stress and its problems, many of which are carried into adulthood unresolved. This whole maturation process has never been easy, but in today's rapidly changing world it seems even more profound and produces many psychologic, emotional, and social tensions. The period of rapid physical growth is comparatively short, only 2 or 3 years. However, the attendant psychosocial development continues over a much longer period. In a technically developed society such as the United States, where values are placed on education and achievement, prolonged preparation for careers often delays marriage and establishment of a new family far beyond the beginning of the reproductive years. Social tensions and family conflicts are created. These conflicts may have nutritional consequences as teenagers eat away from home more often and develop snacking patterns of personal and peer group food choices. The pressure for peer group acceptance is strong and food fads are common.

HIGH-RISK ADOLESCENTS

Despite the increased physiologic demands of accelerated adolescent growth, nutritional status is compromised as some stressed teenagers carry additional risks from eating disorders, excessive athletic training, alcohol, or drugs.

Eating Disorders

In a modern society obsessed with thinness, especially for women, adolescent girls feel great pressure concerning body weight. Two factors combine to increase this stress, creating various degrees of eating disorders in some and increasing health risks: (1) Because of her normal physiologic sex differences associated with fat deposits during puberty, and her comparative lack of physical activity, she may gain weight easily; and (2) Social pressures and personal tensions concerning figure control may cause some girls to follow unwise self-imposed "crash" diets for weight loss. In such cases self-starvation regimens may develop into complex and far-reaching eating disorders such as *anorexia nervosa* and *bulimia,* which are discussed in detail in Chapter 8. In one high school survey of 1268 adolescent girls aged 13 to 19,[33] 36% said that they were currently "dieting" to lose weight, 69% had been dieting at some time before the survey, 52% had begun dieting before age 14, and 14% were "chronic dieters." Despite their average weight being below age norms, all of the subjects perceived themselves as overweight. As a result of such malnourishment of varying degrees at the very time when nutritional reserves for approaching reproduction are being stored, many teenage girls increase their risks of malnutrition and disease.

Athletics

The challenge and excitement of team sports sometimes push young preadolescents and adolescents to place added health risks on their bodies, already stressed by the normal physiologic surge of pubertal growth. Pressure to be admired by peers, to achieve approval of coach or parents, or to follow in the footsteps of a favored older brother or sister may lead some young boys and girls to exceed their physical capacity or sustain serious injury. The constant search for the "competitive edge" may lead to dietary misinformation and exploitation leading to nutritional problems. Scarcely any group of persons is more susceptible to myths and magic claims about foods and dietary supplements than are athletes and their coaches. Also, strenuous training and competition may bring health risks such as anemia or dehydration. So-called sports anemia is characterized by reduced hemoglobin and oxygen carrying capacity, thus having obvious implications for aerobic capacity and ability to sustain a heavy training schedule or excessive work load. With continued stress a transient anemia may become chronic and deplete iron stores in the young, growing athlete, which could pose long-term problems. The added problem of dehydration is a serious threat to health. Its extent depends on the intensity and duration of the exercise, the surrounding temperature, the level of fitness, and the preceding state of hydration. To prevent dehydration, athletes should drink more water than they think is needed, not depending on the normal thirst mechanism. Cold water is best, about the temperature inside a refrigerator, as it is absorbed more quickly from the stomach. Plain water is the rehydration fluid of choice; electrolytes will be replaced in the next meal.

Alcohol and Drug Abuse

As adolescents approach the drinking age in their community, alcohol begins to provide a more significant portion of their total energy intake. Pressured by peer groups, some begin to drink at younger and younger ages. Even mild alcohol abuse coupled with the increased nutritional requirements of adolescence can compromise nutritional status, especially in terms of such nutrients as folic acid, for example, which is destroyed by excessive amounts of alcohol. The extent of excessive social drinking among adolescents, as well as teenage alcoholism in susceptible persons, coupled with the increased risks of highway accidents involving death or serious injury, has led to the growth of a national organization—Students Against Drunk Driving (SADD). The high-risk population of young drug users has also brought devastating results to many young lives. Many have become addicted as early as elementary school, bringing physical and mental illness, malnutrition, disease, and death. A large part of any rehabilitation program must be optimal nutritional support.

Physiologic and Psychosocial Stress of Adulthood and Aging

PHYSIOLOGIC CHANGES

The changing body composition in adulthood and the aging process are described in Chapter 2 and the broader health and nutrition risks and problems in Chapter 10. This detailed background can be reviewed there. An important fact to remember is the *individuality* of the aging process. The biologic changes are general and persons in the advancing years of life experience the physiologic stress of aging in different ways, depending in large measure on their health status. They display a wide variety of individual reactions to normal body stress. They simply get old at different rates and in different ways. Upon individual genetic heritage, each person bears the imprint of unique health and disease experience. This combination has a direct effect on individual aging as the body's physical resources gradually decline and risk of disease and dependency increases.

PSYCHOSOCIAL PROBLEMS

In young and middle adulthood, personal stress relates mainly to striving to find one's way in the world with family and career. Greater stress and risks develop if disease, disability, or poverty is present, as described below. In older adulthood, as biologic changes occur, there often comes an increased concern about body functions, increasing social stress, personal losses, and diminished social opportunities to maintain self-esteem. Financial pressures and a decreasing sense of acceptance and accomplishment cause many elderly persons mental stress and loss of personal values. Many may feel inadequate. Often they are lonely, restless, unhappy, and uncertain. Primarily the greater part of the aging process in any area is culturally determined. Unfortunately in many instances Western culture imposes a set of negative roles on persons as they reach older age. All of these factors, both physical and psychosocial, increase health risks and vulnerability to disease and malnutrition in the aging population.

Physical Trauma and Disease

Throughout the life cycle, the presence of injury, disease, and disability adds more stress with increased health and nutrition risks to the general strains of human growth and development. These high-risk populations are found in hospitals and clinics, medical and rehabilitation centers, community agencies, and homes. In each case special nutritional care and support are needed to help reduce risks. Details of needed nutrition assessment to identify high-risk patients and plan their care have been provided in Chapter 3 and can be reviewed there.

CHILDHOOD DISEASE

Growing children are vulnerable to various forms of *protein-energy malnutrition,* especially children from poor homes and stressed families. The problem of child abuse in such stressed families is a serious one and adds more risk to their health and their lives. An underlying malnutrition is easily compounded by the stress of hospitalization and disease. Children with gastrointestinal problems that hinder food intake and utilization are at special risk of malnutrition and growth retardation. For example, malabsorption diseases, which often become chronic over time, such as inflammatory bowel disease—Crohn's disease and ulcerative colitis (p. 396), cystic fibrosis, celiac disease, short bowel syndrome, and infantile diarrhea, prevent absorption of needed nutrients and often stunt growth. Metabolic diseases such as IDDM and other genetic disorders carry risks of complications involving various organ systems and require specific individual management. Hypermetabolic diseases such as cancer may threaten life and require vigorous nutritional support.

TRAUMATIC INJURY AND DISABILITY

Persons of any age sustaining critical trauma such as extensive burns, spinal cord injury, or other serious injuries or disabilities, are at special risk. They require both immediate care and long-term rehabilitation by a nutrition support team of specialists. Three important factors guide this vital nutrition support: (1) need to replenish large catabolic losses, (2) essential anabolic healing demands, and (3) deep personal support needs. The plan of care for these high-risk patients and its outcome depend on several factors: (1) age—elderly persons and young children are more vulnerable; (2) health condition—any pre-existing condition, malnutrition or disease such as diabetes, cardiovascular or renal disease, complicates care; and (3) wound severity—location, extent, and time elapsed before treatment influence risk and outcome of care.

CHRONIC DISEASES OF AGING

High-risk populations among adults include persons with chronic diseases of aging and those carrying multiple risk factors for these diseases. For example, coronary heart disease, the major cause of death in the United States and most other Western societies, is a multifaceted disease with numerous risk factors, as summarized in Table 11-4. Some of these risk factors are personal ones that cannot be controlled. Others are background conditions for which screening and treatment are possible. Still others are learned behaviors, including the ability to cope with stress, which one can try to develop, or other harmful habits one can seek to change. Most of these interventions to reduce risk involve food patterns and nutrition. Another chronic disease, diabetes, carries risks of complications such as blindness, vascular disease, and renal failure. Continuing gastrointestinal disease and surgery carry added risks of malnutrition and debilitation. Chronic obstructive pulmonary disease (COPD), such as emphysema, brings added risk of respiratory failure. Alcoholism adds risk of liver disease and failure. All of these high-risk persons require special nutritional care and support.

Stress Related to Work, Increased Exercise, and Environment

Many persons are at increased risk due to the nature of their jobs, intensive exercise, and environmental factors. Increasing awareness of these problems, preventive measures to reduce risks, and health care for exposed population groups have begun

TABLE 11-4 Multiple Risk Factors in Cardiovascular Disease

Personal Characteristics (no control)	Learned Behaviors (intervene and change)	Background Conditions (screen-treat)
Sex	Stress/coping	Hypertension
Age	Smoking cigarettes	Diabetes mellitus
Family history	Sedentary life	Hyperlipidemia (especially hypercholesterolemia)
	Obesity	
	Food habits	
	Excess fat	
	Excess sugar	
	Excess salt	

to develop through work-site programs, sports medicine practice, and community health programs.

STRESS OF THE WORKPLACE

Increased physical risks occur in labor-intensive jobs and those with occupational safety and health hazards, such as those requiring use of heavy machinery or hazardous tools and heights. Poor lighting and ventilation, as well as smoking, present health risks in offices and industrial plants. Two special high-risk groups are: (1) migrant workers, whose lives involve multiple physical and psychosocial stress factors; and (2) workers in electronics, chemical industries, and those handling radioactive materials. Such groups of workers may be exposed to hazardous or carcinogenic substances. Also, in positions of management, the well known "executive syndrome" of stress-related ills—peptic ulcer, heart disease, hypertension, diabetes, alcohol and drug abuse—can result from the pressures of managing a business and meeting competition. These ills also affect workers suffering tensions of economic hardships and unemployment.

STRESS OF HEAVY EXERCISE

Aside from heavy labor on the job, many persons in athletics and intensive physical fitness programs also experience physical stress and risk injury. As indicated, heavy athletic exercise places great stress on the body. Heavy body-contact team sports, especially on professional teams where high stakes in money and competition are involved, carry tremendous risks of disabling injury. For every "star" there are hundreds of battered bodies who never made top billing or income, and every team member's playing life is short. Also, compulsive persons in individual athletic activities such as running, or in strenuous physical fitness programs, can experience severe injury. Compulsive runners share traits with compulsive dieters. Whereas the cadaverous anorexic victim always sees herself as fat, the compulsive runner always sees himself as out of shape. No goal, once attained, is sufficiently satisfying. If 5% body fat is achieved, the person strives for 4%. Such striving, often despite physical indications against it, has resulted in permanent disabilities and even death, sometimes from cardiac arrest caused by a linoleic acid deficiency.[34]

ENVIRONMENTAL STRESS FACTORS

Populations exposed to a variety of environmental stress factors carry additional risk factors to health. Air and water pollution is the price paid for an advanced technological society. Health problems accrue over time, for example, when buried radioactive chemical wastes leach out into ground water and contaminate public water sources, or when automobile and factory emissions contaminate air and increase respiratory problems. The ever increasing use of pesticides in agriculture, as target organisms develop tolerance levels, has accumulated and increased exposure of farm workers and consumers to a variety of potentially dangerous chemicals. Only recently, after a 14-year stalemate, have chemical companies and public-interest groups finally agreed on pesticide law reform, a significant part of which will speed up the safety review of old pesticides in long use.[35]

Poverty, Psychosocial Stress, and Mental Health

THE HIGH-RISK PROBLEM OF POVERTY

Poverty and Hunger

One is made increasingly aware through the daily news, or personal contact and experience in one's own community, that poverty and its consequences are hard realities for many persons. Extreme poverty and its ever present companion hunger, even to famine and death, exist in countries such as India, parts of Africa, and Middle Eastern nations. Closer to home, peoples of Central and South America are hard-pressed by social conditions such as inequity, revolution, and desperate poverty with multiple malnutrition problems (Fig. 11-3). But hunger does not stop at these nations'

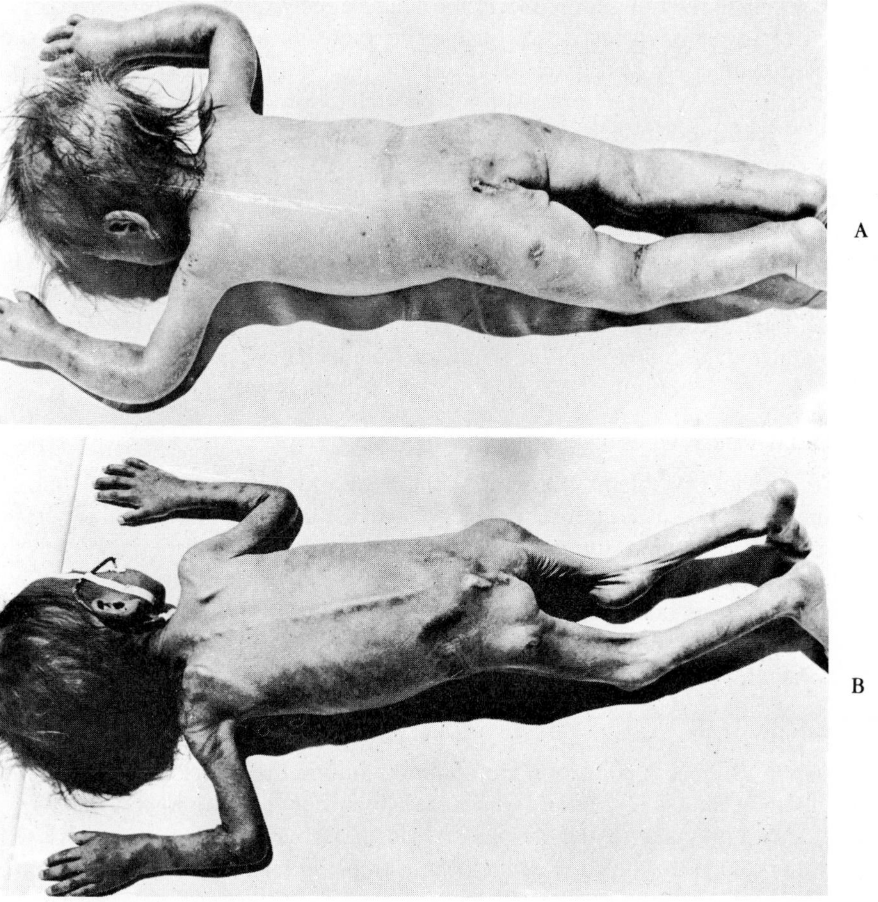

FIG. 11-3 **A**, Two-year-old child being treated for kwashiorkor. **B**, Two weeks after beginning treatment, edema has disappeared and skin lesions have improved. Note the muscular wasting that had been concealed by the edema.
(Courtesy Pan American Sanitary Bureau, Regional Office of The World Health Organization.)

borders. In the United States, one of the wealthiest countries on Earth, many studies document widespread hunger and its "growing epidemic" of malnutrition among the poor.[36] The 1985 Physician Task Force on Hunger in America found that in the United States alone, at least 20 million persons suffer from hunger some days each month. Worldwide about 40,000 to 50,000 people die *each day* from malnutrition, while an estimated 450 million to 1.3 billion people do not have enough to eat.[37] Hunger has been viewed mainly as a problem of overpopulation—world population has just passed the 5 billion mark, with exponential increases daily. Now, however, hunger is recognized as more than just a problem of numbers of people but as a major problem of the increasing gap between the rich and the poor, within and between countries.

Poverty and Politics

In recent times, hunger in America became extensive and was recognized by official sources. Government responses during the 1960s and 1970s almost eliminated the problem with special programs to reach and feed poor, high-risk population groups such as isolated elderly persons, poor pregnant women, mothers, infants, and children. Government policy changes in the early 1980s, however, effectively reduced help to the poor and caused more families to slip below the officially declared poverty line—$9287 or less annual income for a family of four. Together with economically depressed areas of unemployment and "new poor," some 12 million children and 8 million adults now suffer from hunger and varying levels of malnutrition.[38,39] Poverty and health problems among minority population groups in the United States bring special high risks (Fig. 11-4). For example, black infants have nearly twice the risk of dying during the first year of life that white infants have. The national infant mortality rate for blacks is about 22/1000 live births; for whites, it is 11.5/1000.

PSYCHOSOCIAL STRESS OF POVERTY

Tremendous problems exist among the poor and at times they seem almost insurmountable. Often a "culture of poverty" develops and is reinforced and perpetuated by society's values and attitudes, which wall off such persons more completely than do physical barriers. As a result of extreme pressures caused by living conditions, poverty-stricken persons become victims of negative attitudes and behaviors that influence their use of community health services. These psychosocial stresses further increase their health risks as they develop feelings of isolation, powerlessness, and insecurity.

Isolation

Strong feelings of alienation are common among the poor. In many communities few if any channels of communication are open between the lowest income groups and the rest of society, and this isolation leads to further withdrawal. Hazards to health are inherent in poor housing and poor nutrition, often compounded by distance from the sources of health care.

Powerlessness

It is ironic that often those persons most exposed to risks and emergencies have the fewest coping resources. Extreme frustration is inevitable and persons become over-

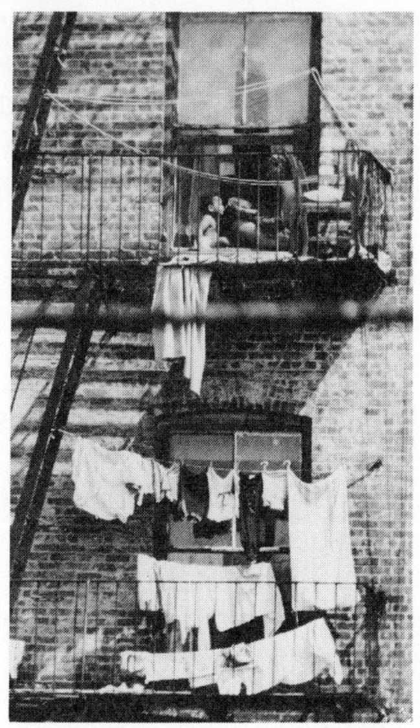

FIG. 11-4 Marasmus is most common in infants living in slum conditions.

whelmed. Why try, they conclude, if they have no control over the situation? Why plan, if there is no future different from today? In such a day-to-day struggle to exist, the poor person often sees little value in long-range preventive health measures.

Insecurity

Subjected to forces outside their control, poor individuals and families have little or no security. Insecurity, anxiety, and chronic stress often incapacitate them. In such a setting, where hunger may be a constant companion, food—which for poor people has the same deep psychologic and emotional meaning that it has for all people—assumes even greater meaning than it has for persons who rarely know hunger.

ROLE OF THE HEALTH WORKER

How can a concerned health worker help individuals and families conditioned by years of grinding poverty or those crushed by new poverty? In the face of such overpowering feelings of isolation, helplessness, and insecurity, what attitudes are necessary to help them? What methods and approaches are most likely to reach clients and patients and help supply their needs? Some basic principles can be helpful:

Self-Awareness

First, we must explore our own feelings about poor persons. We must be aware of our own class values and attitudes. If we are to be agents of constructive change, true "helping vehicles," we must first have some understanding of the person's situation and its broad social setting. We must understand ourselves better and our own cultural conditioning and biases.

Rapport

Genuine warmth, interest, friendliness, and kindness grow from within. *Rapport* is that feeling of relationship between persons that is born of mutual respect, regard, and trust. This sense of relationship gives both helper and helped a deep feeling of working *together*. Its most basic ingredient is a concern for people and for persons—a positive orientation toward human beings in general and a love and concern for individuals in particular.

Acceptance

This term is another way of stating the principle that one must begin where the client or patient is. Each person's own concerns should be the primary consideration. Often we work with other team specialists to cut through the maze of risk factors involved in a given situation before the client is ready to accept or even consider the health practice or nutrition counseling that is needed or desired. Much time may have to be spent, for example, in coming to understand the meaning of food to this person, before practical dietary matters can begin to be explored.

Listening

Here, more than elsewhere, the art of listening—positive, active, creative *listening*—is vital. Clients must tell their story in their own way, with no interruption by distracting statements or questions and no deflecting of the conversation to another's problems. This listening must also be observant. Sequence of statements, subjects introduced, areas of intense feelings and areas ignored give clues to real needs. Throughout we must proceed with sensitivity and create a relaxed, nonthreatening atmosphere in which persons feel free to talk—*and we must listen*. The reason that some frustrated persons finally take their problems to the streets may well be that *no one listens to them unless they do.*

MENTAL HEALTH NEEDS AND PROBLEMS

Human Needs and Strivings

In Erikson's frame of reference (p. 451), following the turbulent teen years, young adults, ages 18 to 40, must deal with the core psychosocial problem of *intimacy versus isolation.* In middle adulthood, ages 40 to 60, with a coming-to-terms with what life has offered, persons struggle with the core problem of *generativity versus self-absorption,* learning positive nurturing capacities to transmit culture from one generation to the next, or failing this, increasingly withdrawing from life. In the last stage of life, older adults, ages 60 to 80+, must resolve the final core problem of *integrity versus despair,* achieving a positive sense of wholeness and completeness, or failing this, developing negative attitudes of bitterness and distaste, poorly equipped to deal with adjustments and health problems that face them. These maturing processes blend with the human needs and strivings described by Maslow (p. 451) that characterize all persons' struggles to meet needs from basic survival necessities of food to appease hunger, to higher levels of safety, love, self-esteem, and self-fulfillment.

Mental Health Problems

For many persons, depending on their coping resources developed through the maturing process, life stresses produce increased risk of mental health problems, many of which clinicians see in primary health care daily. A recent National Institute of Mental Health study confirms relatively high rates of mental disorders among medical outpatient services in primary care settings, ranging between 19% and 27%.[40] An increasing number of these disorders were found to be in the substance abuse-dependency category centering on alcohol and drugs, the most prevalent disorder among male patients. Other categories included phobias and affective disorders such as depression, the two most prevalent disorders among female patients. Other depressive episodes recently studied include seasonal affective disorder (SAD), a disturbance in mood and behavior related to short winter days of decreased sunlight.[41] It has been successfully treated with extended hours of exposure to bright artificial light of higher intensity than is usually present in the home or workplace. This work provides a basis for re-evaluation of environmental lighting standards in home and workplace as a means of reducing mental health risks. All of these mental health problems involve a large high-risk population and have implications for public health, food behaviors, and nutritional status.

Long-Term Institutional Care

At special risk are populations in long-term institutional care facilities for both physical and mental disorders. Often increased numbers of patients and inadequate staff personnel result in limited individual attention with increased risk of nutrition and health problems.

Prison Populations

Increased crime rates, much of them drug-related, have increased prison populations to highly crowded situations in many instances. Such high-stress settings multiply both physical and mental health risks, and individual nutritional needs often suffer.

High-Risk Stress Management

As we have seen here, a key factor in the development of disease and risk of poor nutrition is stress, both physiologic and psychosocial. This basic risk factor permeates human life, with both positive and negative effects. The goal of health promotion, therefore, often centers upon managing stress in positive ways by identifying high-risk populations, recognizing key elements in daily stress management, and planning appropriate methods of reducing stress and its health risks, in the lives of our clients and in our own (p. 383).

KEY ELEMENTS IN DAILY STRESS MANAGEMENT

Personal Approaches

Building positive resources on a personal level for managing daily stress includes attention to key coping factors, such as having a sense of being in control of one's life, developing positive personality characteristics, and being able to do some self-assessment.

1. **Control of one's life.** Epidemiologic studies with various population groups, as well as laboratory research with animals, indicate that stress will be better tolerated and provoke fewer negative physiologic effects if the person has a measure of control over it.[19] Some stressors in life can be changed, many cannot. But the ultimate control lies within: one chooses how one will respond.
2. **Role of personality.** Such positive personality characteristics as hopefulness, a positive outlook or general life orientation, and ability to "go with the flow" have been found to correlate with a better ability to deal with life's stressors, and with a lowered risk of illness. On the other hand, a rigid "uptight" approach to life places that person at much greater risk. The familiar example of this high-risk person is one displaying "type A" behavior. This label was first applied by two San Francisco cardiologists, Friedman and Rosenman,[42] who gleaned a personality profile of the person most at risk for heart attack from their years of work with cardiac patients. This high-risk type A person, they found, is characterized by two basic behaviors: (1) **compulsion to work too hard**—tries to do too much in one space of time, expects a great deal from self and others beyond reasonable levels; and (2) **free-floating hostility**—loses temper easily, is impatient, struggles against time and other people. Type A behavior may not be easy to change. After all, it is basically the single-minded competitive productivity that American business and society rewards. But on the basis of healthier and happier living, some change on a personal level is worth the effort. Perhaps society needs to make some profound changes in its approach toward work and management style, human fulfillment, dignity, and reward.
3. **Self-assessment.** There are some important questions to ask oneself. "Do you know how you typically react, or what level of stress you are operating under, or what direction you seem to be taking?" One can then seek alternate ways of altering one's stress pattern: (1) Set priorities and values in life and avoid those stresses that can be avoided; and (2) displace stressors that cannot be eliminated with other positive activities to strengthen coping ability and more constructive type B behavior.[42] These activities include a focus on key elements that help displace and reduce stress: diet, exercise, relaxation, and personal interest areas, as described below.

Social Approaches

Human beings are by nature social beings and need other people in their lives to sustain positive health. Though some may at times cherish quiet times alone more than others, there are no true hermits. Everyone needs some kind of a social support system, a network of friends or family one can count on when help is needed. Everyone needs some kind of meaningful group support—church, school or special courses, community groups such as sports teams, personal interest or hobby group, music group or chorus, computer club, political group, volunteer work, or social club. There are many ways to develop a sense of belonging. This feeling, one of having something to contribute and having someone to turn to, is critical as a buffer from unavoidable life stresses.

METHODS OF REDUCING STRESS AND HEALTH RISKS

Positive Health Promotion

The preventive approach of developing positive health means changes wherever necessary to build positive attitudes and habits. This approach includes actions in three main areas—exercise, relaxation, and diet—to reduce stress-related risk factors and promote health.

Physical Activities

There are many beneficial effects of physical exercise. It improves both mental and physical health in many ways: (1) it drains off accumulated excess chemical messengers, catecholamines and hormones, triggered by the primitive "fight or flight" response to stress; (2) it increases rate and efficiency of metabolism; (3) it decreases individual "set point" for body fat deposits, thus helps maintain a healthy weight; (4) it increases blood levels of high-density lipoproteins, which help control cholesterol and decrease risk of coronary heart disease; (5) it dissipates anger and hostility; (6) it improves overall health and well-being and decreases risk of illness, which is itself a stressor; (7) it induces a meditation-like mental state, which brings a sense of detachment and mental relaxation; and (8) it brightens the mood, which helps to maintain a positive outlook.

Aerobic exercise best achieves the benefits described above. Exercise is considered aerobic if it raises the heart rate to a "submaximal" level and maintains it for at least 20 minutes. "Submaximal" level is estimated by subtracting the individual's age from 220 and multiplying the difference by 75%. Effective types of exercise include swimming, running, jogging, bicycle riding, team or individual sports, "aerobics" class—"jazzercise" or similar group—and walking. One of the most overlooked forms of exercise is walking—simple, regular, sustained walking. It can benefit heart, lungs, weight, state of mind, and peace with the earth. Take time along the way to notice where you are as you walk, be it wonders of nature along country trails or interests in human activity on city streets.

Relaxation Exercises

Relaxation is needed to balance with physical activity as a means of reducing stress and its high-risk effects. It helps to dissipate and diminish the harmful internal physiologic effects that stress creates in the body (p. 453). The ways that people unwind are as varied as people themselves. But what matters is that everyone must have some appropriate way to relax in a way that is satisfying to personal needs. For many persons, relaxation does not come easily or naturally. The Puritan work ethic heritage, a fast-paced demanding life style, and the too often over-riding cultural values on money and material goods as a measure of success, can lock one into mind sets, habits, and patterns of thinking and behaving that can be self-destructive. Moreover, a rigid and rapid lifestyle can cultivate some negative ways people physically reinforce stress in their lives, ways they "take it out" on others around them and on their own bodies. Muscle tension is a common example, as are headaches, backaches, and leg cramps, all classic symptoms of stress overload.

A number of useful techniques are available that focus on ways one can *learn* to relax. With *practice,* a necessity for any learning, one can not only feel relaxed but also help control such autonomic functions as breathing, pulse rate, electrical brain impulses, blood pressure, and peripheral blood circulation, as well as relax muscle tensions. These relaxation techniques include biofeedback, progressive muscle relaxation, clinical hypnosis, and meditation with visual imagery. Today a number of medical centers are studying the induced relaxation response, used with meditation and guided visual imagery together with other techniques, to help treat numerous health problems.[43] These researchers have found strong evidence that the calming effects of these relaxation techniques can relieve the body's stress and perhaps even boost the immune system (p. 458). Although individual methods of relaxation will vary, some assisted by background tapes, a significant personal pattern can meet one's own particular needs. In essence, to some degree people must change their lives and rethink their values if they want to avoid risks such as an early and possibly fatal heart attack.

Diet

First, a word of warning. Despite the great amount of food misinformation to the contrary, abroad today from many sources, there is no "wonder cure" for stress. Beware of the touted panacea, the wonder-food or claim, the so-called magic properties of any specific nutrient or food. Rather we seek a sound overall dietary pattern that meets both nutritional requirements and personal and health needs.

1. **Nutritional balance.** In general human beings need to eat a balanced diet that provides sufficient energy to maintain a healthy weight and all the necessary macro- and micro-nutrients. There is no scientific evidence that emotional stress increases the body's requirement for any specific nutrient above that which is already recommended for maintaining health. It is true, of course, that in instances of debilitation and malnourished states, more nutrient density would be needed to replenish stores. But in most instances of usual stress patterns of daily living, a reasonable and regular diet of sound nutrition in satisfying food choices is the need. A complex web of many different factors influences food choices, as shown in Table 11-5, and being aware of these influences may help in making more positive choices. Whatever the choices may be, the well-nourished person has a much better means of displacing stress, be it high-risk illness, disappointment, or job demands. Nonetheless, as easy as it sounds, surveys indicate that the American population as a whole eats a diet often deficient in basic nutrients such as iron, calcium, magnesium, zinc, vitamin A, vitamin C, and folic acid.[44] So the simple admonition to "eat right," which can have many variations in food choices yet follow wise health promotion guidelines, is in fact a prescription that society would do well to incorporate into a new lifestyle, along with relaxation and some form of daily exercise.

TABLE 11-5 Factors Determining Food Choices

Physical Factors	Social Factors	Physiologic Factors
Food supply available	Advertising	Allergy
Food technology	Culture	Disability
Geography, agriculture, distribution	Education, nutrition and general	Health-disease status
Personal economics, income	Political and economic policies	Heredity
Sanitation, housing	Religion and social custom	Personal food acceptance
Season, climate	Social class, role	Needs, energy or nutrients
Storage and cooking facilities	Social problems, poverty or alcoholism	Therapeutic diets

2. **Food and mood.** We all know from our own experience, as well as those of our clients and patients, that mood influences the food that one eats. Sometimes overeating or loss of appetite is associated with periods of depression. There is a place for "comfort foods" in dealing with stress. Plan for them at times of need.
3. **Food pattern and pace.** Food habits are hard to change. They're always tied to lifestyle. Many persons eat rapidly and irregularly, and suffer both physical and emotional consequences. One is better able to deal with stress if one simply slows the mode of eating, eats smaller "mini-meals" more frequently, and avoids the rich, heavy meals that too often make up the food pattern. Moderation and variety are key concepts. One should begin with breakfast, needed by the body after the overnight fast, continuing through the day with small amounts of food to refuel the body in a regular pattern. Avoid the excesses Americans tend to consume in fat, salt, and sugar, and in some cases caffeine, mostly in the form of coffee. Over 80% of American adults drink coffee; 75% of these coffee drinkers have two or more cups a day, and 16% drink over six cups a day.[45] Individual sensitivity to caffeine is highly variable, but it is a stimulant drug that many consider to be abused. In larger intakes, it depletes the body's vitamin C and thiamin stores, and even a mild deficiency of thiamin may create nervousness, irritability, loss of memory, or inability to concentrate.

Socioeconomic Needs

In cases of economic needs, various food assistance programs can be used to help supply needed foods. Details of these programs are described in the various age group chapters and in Chapter 12.

Hypermetabolic Needs

Additional energy and nutritive demands are posed by the physical and psychosocial stress of hypermetabolic conditions such as traumatic injury, surgery, infection, or cancer (p. 398). The magnitude of the metabolic response varies, but in any case it underscores the importance of good pre-stress nutritional status on a regular basis.

National Goals to Reduce Health Risks

BASIS OF HEALTH OBJECTIVES FOR THE NATION

Through previous chapters we have referred to national health goals based on health promotion and disease prevention by a concerted effort to reduce related risk factors. This current effort marks a significant redirection in public health care. Through the early 1970s, a growing concern among local and community groups about increasing health problems and costs led public health officials and government agencies to recognize the value of health promotion and risk-reduction principles, sowing the seeds for the far-reaching "revolution" in America's health care that is now under way.[46] In 1979, the United States Surgeon General issued an initial report identifying areas of potential disease prevention and controllable risk factors. This report set the course for specific objectives issued in 1980 for a national program aimed at health promotion and disease prevention, with target goals set for 1990.

PROGRESS TOWARD REDUCING RISKS AND IMPROVING HEALTH

At the halfway mark, in 1985, a mid-course progress review of the U.S. health goals and objectives was conducted, with findings published in 1986 by the Department of Health and Human Services. A summary of this progress review is given here in Table 11-6. It indicates important areas in which nutrition-related risk factors have been addressed. In a current evaluation of the program's overall progress, Sorenson[47] describes significant initial steps in a number of areas with several of the basic objectives "on track" for 1990 if present trends continue. Although we still have much work to do, an essential foundation is being laid upon which we need to build for the future.

Summary

The modern world is demanding and complex and exposes human beings to many risk factors affecting nutritional status and health. Among these risk factors, emotional stress plays a major role, triggering a cascade of primitive automatic physiologic events, designed as a "fight or flight" mechanism to protect the body through its general alarm and adaptive responses, but in a modern stress-filled world only compounding the problem and contributing to illness. Throughout the life cycle, physiologic and psychosocial stress attends growth and development, with special high-risk populations among pregnant women, infants, young children, adolescents, and elderly persons.

At any age additional stress factors may increase health risks for vulnerable population groups. These stress factors include physical trauma and disease, disability, environmental problems, the multiple problems of poverty and general economic stress with greater repercussions in minority populations, and mental health problems. High-stress management involves both personal and social approaches, based on identified individual and family needs, goals, and expectations. Methods of reducing stress and health risks focus on positive health and nutrition promotion helping to build greater coping capacity through sound diet, relaxation, and physical activity, with a strengthened personal support system.

TABLE 11-6 Progress Toward Meeting the 1990 Nutrition Objectives for the United States*

Objective	Baseline	Status
1. By 1990, the proportion of pregnant women with iron-deficiency anemia (as estimated by hemoglobin concentrations early in pregnancy) should be reduced to 3.5%.	In 1978, the proportion of pregnant women with iron deficiency anemia was 7.7%.	National data representative of the iron nutritional status of the population and its subsets during 1980–1985 are not available. In 1983, low hemoglobin values were reported as 17.3% and low hematocrits were observed as 25.8% in a limited sampling of low-income pregnant women.
2. By 1990, growth retardation of infants and children caused by inadequate diets should have been eliminated in the United States as a public health problem.	In 1972–1973, it was estimated that 10 to 15% of infants and children among migratory workers and certain poor rural populations suffered growth retardation due to diet inadequacies.	In 1983, data show that linear growth retardation remains at levels ranging from 10.9 to 23.6% in a selective group of low income children, ages 3 to 23 months, of all ethnic groups screened. In addition to these groups, linear growth retardation was 12.1% for Hispanic two- to five-year-olds; 22.4% for Asian two- to five-year-olds; and 16.6% for Hispanic six- to nine-year-old children. (The high prevalence among Asian children is because of the inclusion of the special population of Southeast Asian refugees.) Data are not available for the period 1983–1985.
3. By 1990, the prevalence of significant overweight (120% of "desired" weight) among the U.S. adult population should be decreased to 10% of men and 17% of women, without nutritional impairment.	In 1971–74, 14% of adult men and 24% of women were more than 120% of desired weight.	National data on the prevalence of overweight individuals, based on actual measurement, are not available for the period from 1980 to 1985. In 1976–80, 26.3% of adult men and 29.6% of adult women were overweight. NOTE: The NHANES II, conducted between 1976 and 1980, used the body mass index (BMI) measurement, where body weight is adjusted for height (BMI = Body Weight in Kilograms/ Height in Meters) to assess

*Data accumulated and published by the U.S. Department of Health and Human Services, 1986.

TABLE 11-6 Progress Toward Meeting the 1990 Nutrition Objectives for the United States—cont'd

Objective	Baseline	Status
		overweight conditions. Overweight was defined as BMI greater than or equal to 27.8 for males and 27.3 for females. Severe overweight was defined as BMI greater than or equal to 31.1 for males and 32.3 for females, these values being equal to the 95th percentile for males and females in the 20–29 year old age range. The appropriate language for this objective in terms of BMI would be: "By 1990, the prevalence of overweight (BMI or 27.8 or higher for men and 27.3 or higher for women) among the U.S. adult population should be reduced, without impairment of nutritional status, to approximately 18% of men and 21% of women.
4. By 1990, 50% of the overweight population should have adopted weight loss regimens, combining an appropriate balance of diet and physical activity.	Baseline data were not available.	Data from the Health Promotion/Disease Prevention Supplement to the 1985 National Health Interview Survey (NHIS) indicate that 27% of males and 46% of females say that they are trying to lose weight. About 30% of overweight females and 25% of overweight males reported adopting weight loss regimens that combine both exercise and diet restriction.
5. By 1990, the mean serum cholesterol level in the adult population 18 to 74 years of age should be at or below 200 milligrams per deciliter.	In 1971–74, for male and female adults aged 18 to 74, the mean serum cholesterol value was 223 milligrams per deciliter. NOTE: Because it is not adjusted to a standard reference (the Abell-Kendall method), 223 milligrams is 4.5 percent higher than the actual value.	In 1976–80, the mean serum cholesterol value for men and women ages 18 to 74 was, respectively, 211 and 215 milligrams per deciliter.

TABLE 11-6 Progress Toward Meeting the 1990 Nutrition Objectives for the United States—cont'd

Objective	Baseline	Status
6. By 1990, the mean serum cholesterol level in children aged one to 14 should be at or below 150 milligrams per deciliter (mg/dl).	In 1971-74, for children one to 17 years of age the mean serum cholesterol level was 176 mg/dl.	Recent national population data on mean serum cholesterol levels in children are not available.
7. By 1990, the average daily sodium ingestion (as measured by excretion) for adults should be reduced to at least the 3 to 6 g range.	In 1979, estimates ranged between averages of 4–10 g of sodium.	Recent population surveys to calculate sodium ingestion by measuring excretion are not available. However, recent estimates of adult intake have been made from dietary intakes. Data from the first two years of the revised FDA Total Diet Study (FY 82–84) indicate that average sodium intakes for adults, excluding salt added at the table, were within the Estimated Safe and Adequate Daily Dietary Intake (ESADDI) range of 1100 to 3300 mg established by the National Academy of Sciences in 1980. Very preliminary one-day data from the USDA indicate average sodium intakes for women ages 19 to 40 of about 2600 mg, also not including salt added at the table. However, data from both surveys indicate sodium intakes for children above the ESADDI for that age.
8. By 1990, the proportion of women who breast-feed their babies should be increased to 75% at hospital discharge and to 35% at six months of age.	In 1978, the proportion was 45% at hospital discharge and 21% at 6 months of age.	In 1983, the reported prevalences of breast-feeding among low-income women at 6 to 10 weeks post-parturition were as follows: 27.4% for white mothers, 44.3% for Native Americans, 28% for Hispanics and 13.6% for blacks. These CDC data are primarily from low-income women enrolled in the WIC program.

TABLE 11-6 Progress Toward Meeting the 1990 Nutrition Objectives for the United States—cont'd

Objective	Baseline	Status
		In 1984, a private survey conducted by Ross Laboratories (National Mothers' Survey) indicated that 61% of infants were breast-fed at 1 week of age and 27.5% at 6 months of age. (These data include infants receiving formula in addition to breastfeeding, and the survey excludes births to unwed mothers.)
9. By 1990, the proportion of the population that is able to correctly associate the principal dietary factors known or strongly suspected to be related to disease should exceed 75% for each of the following diseases: heart disease, high blood pressure, dental caries, and cancer.	Baseline data are largely unavailable. In 1978, 12 percent of adults were aware of the relationship between high blood pressure and sodium intake.	Data on the total population are not available; surveys of public knowledge primarily are on the adult population. It may be that progress toward this objective in the nonadult population could be assessed under the objective that addressed nutrition education in the school health curriculum at the elementary and secondary levels. FDA surveys in 1982 and 1984 indicate that about 50% of the adult population is aware of a suspected link between hypertension and sodium or salt consumption. The 1982 survey indicated that about 45% of adults were aware of a link between cardiovascular disease and saturated fats or cholesterol. The 1984 survey indicated about 78 percent were aware that there are health problems related to the consumption of fats. About 24 percent of adults related fat consumption to overweight or obesity, and of that percent, only 3% linked fat consumption to cancer, while about two-thirds linked fat to coronary heart disease. Another source indicates that 59% of the adult population

TABLE 11-6 Progress Toward Meeting the 1990 Nutrition Objectives for the United States—cont'd

Objective	Baseline	Status
		believe sodium is the substance most associated with high blood pressure. Of the adult population 86% indicate that high blood cholesterol increases the risk of having heart disease, and 80% are aware that eating a diet high in animal fat also increases a person's chances of getting heart disease. About 90% of the adult population indicates that avoiding between-meal sweets is important in reducing tooth decay.
10. By 1990, 70% of adults should be able to identify the major foods that are: low in fat content, low in sodium content, high in calories, high in sugars, good sources of fiber.	Baseline data were not available.	Data from both government and private surveys indicate that many U.S. adults know about nutrition and presumably have knowledge about the nutrient content of foods to some degree. One national survey has reported changes in eating habits, with six out of ten adults stating that they have changed their eating habits at home and four out of ten stating changes in eating away from home by either increasing consumption of fruits, vegetables or whole grains, or by decreasing consumption of refined sugar, animal fats or salt. Preliminary one-day data from USDA on dietary intakes of women 19 to 50 years of age and their children 1 to 5 years of age indicate that the intakes of both groups were lower in fat and higher in carbohydrates in 1985 than in 1977. Also, nutrition labeling on food labels has increased, with about 54% of sales of processed packaged foods carrying this information in 1984.

TABLE 11-6 Progress Toward Meeting the 1990 Nutrition Objectives for the United States—cont'd

Objective	Baseline	Status
11. By 1990, 90% of adults should understand that to lose weight people must either consume foods that contain fewer calories or increase physical activity or both.	Baseline data were not available.	In 1985, 74% of the population over 18 years of age believed that eating fewer calories is one of the two best ways to lose weight; 73% believed that increase in physical activity is one of the two best ways.
12. By 1990, the labels of all packaged foods should contain useful calorie and nutrient information to enable consumers to select diets that promote and protect good health. Similar information should be displayed where nonpackaged foods are obtained or purchased.	In 1978, about 42% of the sales of processed packaged foods had nutrition labeling.	In 1984, about 54% of the sales of packaged processed foods had nutrition labeling.
13. By 1990, sodium levels in processed food should be reduced by 20 percent from present levels.	No baseline data were available.	There is no available database designed to sample and measure the sodium content of the total processed food supply. As a surrogate measure, FDA's food label surveys of packaged processed foods show a decline in the average sodium content per serving between 1982 and 1983. However, this comparison is difficult to make because of the increasing number of sodium-labeled products in the marketplace and only a short period of time is included. Also, many lower sodium products have become available; between January 1981 and July 1985, 173 new lowered sodium brands were introduced into the marketplace.
14. By 1985, the proportion of employee and school cafeteria managers who are aware of and actively promoting USDA/DHHS dietary guidelines should be greater than 50%.	Data were not available.	No national statistics are available on the activities promoting the Dietary Guidelines for Americans in worksite feeding facilities and in school cafeterias.

TABLE 11-6 Progress Toward Meeting the 1990 Nutrition Objectives for the United States—cont'd

Objective	Baseline	Status
15. By 1990, all states should include nutrition education as part of required comprehensive school health education at the elementary and secondary levels.	In 1979, only 10 states mandated nutrition as a core content area in school health education.	In 1985, 12 states mandated nutrition as a core content area in school health education.
16. By 1990, virtually all routine health contacts with health professionals should include some element of nutrition education and nutrition counseling.	Baseline data were not available.	Data on a representative nationwide sample of health professionals such as physicians and other primary care providers and health clinic personnel are not available.
17. Before 1990, a comprehensive national nutrition status monitoring system should have the capability for detecting nutritional problems in special population groups, as well as for obtaining baseline data for decisions on national nutrition policies.	The proposal for a National Nutrition Monitoring System (NNMS) was submitted to Congress in 1978 by DHHS (then DHEW) and USDA. At that time baseline data were available from the 1977-1978 Nationwide Food Consumption Survey (NFCS) and the first National Health and Nutrition Examination Survey (NHANES I) which was conducted in 1971-74. Auxiliary components of NNMS, including Mortality and Natality Surveys, Food Label and Package Surveys (FLAPS), Multipurpose Consumer Survey, Total Diet Study, and Pregnancy and Pediatric Nutrition Surveillance Systems (PPNSS), were in place.	Implementation plans for the NNMS were submitted to Congress in 1981. The NHANES II survey was conducted from 1976-80 and results have been reported. The report from the Joint Nutrition Monitoring Evaluation Committee (JNMEC) to Congress was published in 1986. Through an interdepartmental committee, plans are in place for compatibility and linkages between NFCS and NHANES in upcoming surveys, where feasible. Recommendations have been submitted by various DHHS areas for dietary, biochemical and other measures for NHANES III. The USDA began a Continuing Survey of Food Intakes by Individuals (CSFII) in 1985. The PPNSS now collects data from 29 states and the District of Columbia. The other components of NNMS regularly collect data in their individual areas.

Review Questions

1. Describe the general adaptive syndrome identified by Selye, which the body activates in response to stress, in terms of basic physiologic events in each of its three stages. Why does this response pattern create problems in today's modern society?
2. Describe the normal physiologic stress of pregnancy. What factors would contribute to a high-risk pregnancy? Why?
3. What physiologic and psychosocial stress factors are involved in infant growth and development? Describe characteristics of high-risk infants.
4. Identify high-risk problems in young children and adolescents. Select several of these problems, describe their nature, and outline general care.
5. What physiologic and psychosocial factors present health and nutrition risks in older adults? Give reasons why elderly persons comprise a special high-risk population.
6. Describe additional high-risk stress conditions throughout the life cycle, giving approaches to planning nutrition and health care. Give special attention to the problem of poverty.
7. Identify and describe key elements in daily stress management and methods of reducing stress and health risks.

REFERENCES

1. Selye, H.: The stress of life, New York, 1956, McGraw-Hill Book Co.
2. Selye, H.: Hunger and stress, Nutrition Today **5**(1):2, Spring, 1970.
3. Erikson, E.: Childhood and society, New York, 1963, W.W. Norton & Co., Inc.
4. Hall, E.: A conversation with Erik Erikson, Psychol. Today **17**(6):22, 1983.
5. Maslow, A.H.: Motivation and personality, New York, 1954, Harper & Row Publishers, Inc.
6. Wallis, C.: Stress—can we cope? Time **121**(23):48, June 6, 1983.
7. Miller, J.A.: Immunity and crises, large and small, Science News **129**(22):340, 1986.
8. Rose, N.R.: Autoimmune diseases, Sci. Am. **244**(2):80, 1981.
9. Miller, J.A.: Double-duty cells in human immune system, Science News **123**(20):308, 1983.
10. Task Force on Nutrition: American College of Obstetrics and Gynecology and American Dietetic Association. Chicago, 1978.
11. King, J.C.: Dietary risk patterns during pregnancy. In Weininger, J., and Briggs, G., eds., Nutrition Update **1**:206, 1983.
12. Botti, J.J., and James, R.L.: Aerobic conditioning, nutrition, and pregnancy, Clin. Nutr. **4**(1):14, February 1985.
13. Weiner, L., and Rosett, H.L.: Pregnancy and alcohol, Clin. Nutr. **4**(1):10, February 1985.
14. Luke, B., Hawkins, M.M., and Petrie, R.H.: Influence of smoking, weight gain, and pregravid weight-for-height in intrauterine growth, Am. J. Clin. Nutr. **34**:1410, 1981.
15. Belizan, J.M., and Villar, J.: The relationship between calcium intake and edema-, proteinuria-, and hypertension-gestosis: an hypothesis, Am. J. Clin. Nutr. **33**:2202, 1980.
16. Willis, S.E., and Sharp, E.S.: Hypertension in pregnancy. I. Pathology. II. Prenatal detection and management, Am. J. Nurs. **82**:792, May 1982.
17. Weiner, C.P., and Verner, M.W.: Nutritional considerations in diabetic pregnancy, Clin. Nutr. **4**(1):5, February 1985.

18. Acosta, P.B., Blaskovics, M., Cloud, H., and others: Nutrition in pregnancy of women with hyperphenylalaninemia, J. Am. Diet. Assoc. **80**(5):443, 1982.
19. Bosma, J.F.: Development of feeding, Clin. Nutr. **5**(5):210, September-October 1986.
20. World Health Organization, Division of Family Health: The incidence of low birth weight: a critical review of available information, World Health Stat. Q. **33**:197, 1980.
21. Villar, J., and Cossio, T.G.: Nutritional factors associated with low birth weight and short gestational age, Clin. Nutr. **5**(2):78, March-April 1986.
22. Mamelle, N., Launon, B., and Lazar, P.: Prematurity and occupational activity during pregnancy, Am. J. Epidemiol. **119**:309, 1984.
23. Murphy, J.F., Dauncey, M., Newcombe, R., and others: Employment in pregnancy: prevalence, maternal characteristics, prenatal outcome, Lancet **1**:1163, 1984.
24. Villar, J., Belizan, J.M.: Growth and development of intrauterine growth-retarded infants, Clin. Nutr. **3**(6):198, November-December, 1984.
25. Owen, G.M., and Paige, D.M.: Childhood disease. In Paige, D.M., ed., Manual of clinical nutrition, Pleasantville, N.J., 1983, Nutrition Publications, Inc.
26. Fomon, S.J.: Infant nutrition, Philadelphia, 1974, W.B. Saunders Co.
27. Powell, G.F.: Nutrition in nonorganic failure to thrive, Clin. Nutr. **4**(2):54, April 1985.
28. Trusdell, D.D., and Acosta, P.B.: Feeding the vegan infant and child, J. Am. Diet. Assoc. **85**(7):837, July 1985.
29. Ashworth, A., and Millward, D.J.: Catch-up growth in children, Nutr. Rev. **44**:157, May 1986.
30. Wodarski, L.A.: Nutrition intervention in developmental disabilities: an interdisciplinary approach, J. Am. Diet. Assoc. **85**(2):218, February 1985.
31. Kolata, G.: Obese children: a growing problem, Science **232**(4746):20, April 4, 1986.
32. Epstein, L.H., and others: Family-based behavioral weight control in obese young children, J. Am. Diet. Assoc. **86**(4):481, April 1986.
33. Johnson, C.L., Lewis, C., Love, S., and others: A descriptive survey of dieting and bulimic behavior in a female, high-school population. In Understanding anorexia nervosa and bulimia, Columbus, Ohio, 1983, Ross Laboratories, Inc.
34. Herbert, W.: Runners: an ascetic disorder? Science News **123**(7):102, 1983.
35. Sun, M.: Antagonists agree on pesticide law reform. Science **232**(4746):16, April 4, 1986.
36. Physician Task Force on Hunger in America, The growing epidemic, Cambridge, Mass., 1985, Harvard University Press.
37. American Dietetic Association, Hunger: a worldwide problem, J. Am. Diet. Assoc. **86**(10):1414, October 1986.
38. Physician Task Force on Hunger in America, Increasing hunger and declining help: barriers to participation in the food stamp program, Cambridge, Mass., 1986, Harvard University Press.
39. Brown, J.L.: Hunger in the U.S., Sci. Am. **256**(2):37, February 1987.
40. Kessler, L.G., Burns, B.J., Shapiro, S., and others: Psychiatric diagnoses of medical service users: evidence from the Epidemiologic Catchment Area Program, Am. J. Public Health **77**(1):18, January 1987.
41. Jacobson, F.M., Wehr, T.A., Sack, D.A., and others: Seasonal affective disorder: a review of the syndrome and its public health implications, Am. J. Public Health **77**(1):57, January 1987.
42. Ferguson, T.: Type A behavior and the type B solution, Med. Self-Care **12**:36, Spring 1983.
43. Squires, S.: The power of positive imagery: visions to boost immunity, Am. Health **6**(6):56, July 1987.
44. Pao, E.M., and Mickle, S.J.: Problem nutrients in the United States, Food Technology **35**:58, September 1981.

45. Gelmch, W.H.: A regimen for stress reduction, Supervisory Management **27**:16, December 1982.
46. Califano, J.A., Jr: America's health care revolution: health promotion and disease prevention, J. Am. Diet. Assoc. **87**(4):437, April 1987.
47. Sorenson, A.W., Kavet, J., and Stephenson, M.G.: Health objectives for the nation: moving toward the 1990s, J. Am. Diet. Assoc. **87**(7):920, July 1987.

FURTHER READING

Bassett, M.T., and Krieger, N.: Social class and black-white differences in breast cancer survival, Am. J. Public Health **76**(12):1400, December 1986

Berdanier, C.D.: The many faces of stress, Nutr. Today **22**(2):12, April 1987.

This article clarifies the many ways that stress may affect nutrient needs, using helpful illustrations and a table showing the effect of stress on the basal requirements for selected nutrients.

Brown, J.L.: Hunger in the U.S., Sci. Am. **256**(2):37, February 1987.

This sensitive article by the chairman of the Physician Task Force on Hunger in America provides background about the devastating effects of poverty and hunger in the lives of an increasing high-risk population of Americans.

Clark, M., and Gelman, D.: A user's guide to hormones, Newsweek **109**(2):50, January 12, 1987.

This popular article provides a clearly written and illustrated background for understanding the integrated functions of hormones in relation to stress, health, and disease. The journalistic style and illustrations make it a good resource for public education.

Cross, A.T.: Politics, poverty, and nutrition, J. Am. Diet. Assoc. **87**(8):1007, August 1987; Endres, J., and others: Older pregnant women and adolescents: Nutrition data after enrollment in WIC, J. Am. Diet. Assoc. **87**(8):1011, August 1987; Lopez, L.M., and Habicht, J.: Food stamps and the energy status of the U.S. elderly poor, J. Am. Diet. Assoc. **87**(8):1020, August 1987.

These three articles explore political problems affecting poverty and nutrition and their relation to two U.S. food assistance programs for high-risk populations, WIC and Food Stamps. Cross, a sensitive nutritionist and attorney, makes a strong case for viewing adequate food and freedom from hunger and malnutrition as basic human rights. Authors of the companion articles illustrate the use of food programs in low-income, high-risk families.

Deykin, E.Y., and others: Adolescent depression, alcohol and drug abuse, Am. J. Public Health **77**(2):178, February 1987.

This article reports survey results showing incidence of major depressive disorder and associated abuse of alcolol and drugs among a sample population of 18- and 19-year old college students.

Fuchs, V.R.: Sex differences in economic well-being, Science **232**:459, April 25, 1986.

This timely article presents documentation to underscore the increasing emergence of sex differences in economic well-being, with women sustaining high-risk stress factors from their declining access to goods, services, and leisure, with increasing family support responsibilities in comparison to men.

Garre, M.A., Boles, J.M., and Youinou, P.Y.: Current concepts in immune derangement due to undernutrition, J. Parenteral Enteral Nutr. **11**(3):309, May-June 1987.

In this key article, a group of French researchers reviews and updates our current knowledge of the vital relationships between nutrition and immune function, and shows how protein-calorie malnutrition adversely affects all immune competent cells, increasing disease in high-risk populations.

Jacobson, M.L., and others: Tuberculosis risk among migrant farm workers on the Delmarva peninsula, Am. J. Public Health **77**(1):29, January 1987.

These current articles vividly illustrate the wide differences in disease incidence and outcome in two high-risk populations.

Owen, A.L., ed.: Community nutrition issue, Clin. Nutr. **3**(3) May-June, 1984.

This entire journal issue is devoted to four important articles describing implementation of the U.S. Health Goals for the Nation in nutrition services for high-risk groups such as pregnant women, infants, children, adolescents, adults and the elderly, as well as applications in clinical practice.

Stein, R.A.: Personal strategies for living with less stress, New York, 1983, John Gallagher Communications, Ltd.

This little paperback book by an experienced and sensitive physician is packed with practical information and guidelines for living a less stressful and healthier life. A good resource for clients and practitioners alike.

Basic Concepts

1. People may have appropriate nutrition information but they won't change their food behavior unless that information and action meets their personal goals and lifestyles.
2. An effective nutrition education program must first identify audience communication goals, then select a message and medium that best meets them.
3. Nutrition education for all ages includes a variety of strategies according to need.
4. Programs providing a served meal present opportunities for immediate practical nutrition education.

Chapter Twelve

Nutrition Education

Eleanor D. Schlenker

Nutrition education can be defined as the process of helping individuals develop the knowledge, skills, and motivation needed to make appropriate food choices throughout life. Although simple in definition, this task is complex in application.

Consumers are confused by conflicting views on nutrition issues appearing in the popular press and on television. And changing skills are needed for good food selection as a person moves through the life cycle. The teenager eats "on the run." The older widow prepares all her meals at home and eats alone. Peer pressure on one hand and persuasive advertising on the other compete with personal concerns about health.

In this chapter we will explore personal and environmental factors that affect individual food choices. We will see that educational strategies can be developed to intervene in these choices as needed.

Nutrition Knowledge, Motivation, and Food Behavior

BASIS OF NUTRITION BEHAVIOR

Establishing Food Patterns

What, when, where, or with whom one eats is determined mainly by personal psychosocial and cultural needs rather than by physiologic ones. Ethnic background, religious teaching, or geographic region can be strong determinants of food preferences. Food habits are learned in childhood. Yet adults may continue to choose homemade pasta or greens with salt pork long after leaving the family home.

Not only the kinds of food eaten as a child but also the way parents handled food behavior make lasting impressions. Foods used as rewards or special treats may continue to serve as comfort foods throughout life. Noting the time or passing a favorite restaurant can trigger feelings of hunger. Boredom, loneliness, or guilt can lead to eating, often to excessive eating. This interaction of factors contributing to development of personal lifestyle and food behavior is described in Fig. 12-1.

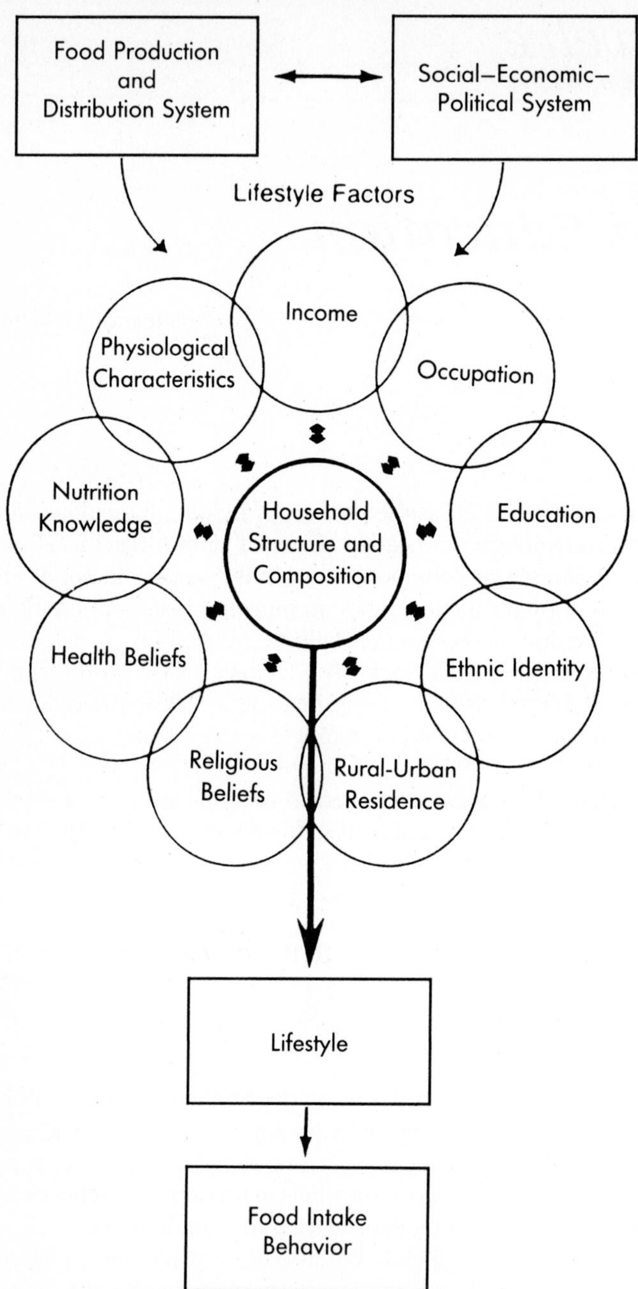

FIG. 12-1 Lifestyle model of dietary behavior.
(From Pelto, G.H.: Anthropological contributions to nutrition education research, J. Nutr. Educ. **13**[Suppl.]:2, 1981. © Society for Nutrition Education. Used by permission.)

Changing Food Patterns

Changing food behavior requires both direct and structural intervention.[1] *Direct intervention* includes such strategies as publications, public service announcements, or individual counseling to provide consumers and clients with knowledge that helps motivate them to make appropriate dietary changes. Ultimately personal motivation and decision must come from within, but sound knowledge at the right time can help provide a basic stimulus. *Structural intervention* includes such strategies as changing food production patterns or the economic environment to improve accessibility to nutritious food. Distributing food stamps to low-income families or developing convenience foods low in sodium or fat, as well as genetic production of leaner meat in response to market demands, are examples of structural interventions. Although nutrition educators traditionally have focused on direct intervention strategies, structural intervention will become increasingly important in solving contemporary nutrition problems.

Nutrition Knowledge and Behavior Change

A common belief is that acquiring nutrition knowledge will in itself lead to improved diet practices. This is rooted in the idea that it is lack of nutrition information that prevents people from making better food choices. Although practical knowledge is a necessary tool, it is of use only if and when a person makes a conscious decision to use it. Hochbaum[2] hypothesizes that a person must be emotionally "ready" to make a behavioral change for factual knowledge to be effective. Optimal health or prevention of disease has been considered an effective motivator and thus has been the foundation for many intervention programs for both children and adults. Some people do value health for its own sake and will deliberately select a lifestyle that will contribute to this end. But the majority of individuals select behaviors consistent with their personal goals regardless of their health-promoting qualities. Even people with a strong health orientation may experience conflicts relating to taste, cost, convenience, or peer acceptance of particular food items.

Food behavior is extremely complex. It frequently involves group as well as individual decisions. A child may not have the option of selecting a cereal lower in sugar if siblings favor a high-sugar brand. A working mother may choose prepared items although she considers fresh ingredients better nutritionally, because short-term goals at that moment take precedence over long-term advantages. Positive approaches that relate to practical concerns of daily living such as time, cost, and taste should be priority targets in nutrition education. Guidelines to assist in selecting essential food and nutrition information for all ages are provided here (see box, pp. 504–505).

NUTRITION KNOWLEDGE AND ATTITUDES

Children and Youth

Current findings[3,4] with both elementary and high school students indicate that although many have some understanding of the commonly used Basic Four Food Guide their knowledge of specific nutrients is limited. Number of years in school does not necessarily predict nutrition knowledge. For some items tested, grade school stu-

CONCEPTS FOR FOOD AND NUTRITION EDUCATION

Nutrition

Nutrition is the process by which food is selected and becomes part of the human body.

Food and Its Handling

A. Food contains nutrients that work together and interact with body chemicals to serve the needs of the body.
B. No one food, by itself, contains all the nutrients in the appropriate amounts and combinations needed for optimal growth and health.
C. Many different combinations of food can provide the needed nutrients in appropriate amounts.
D. Food contains important nonnutritive components, such as dietary fiber, which are needed for healthy functioning of the body.
E. Toxicants, additives, contaminants, and other nonnutritive factors in food affect its safety and quality.
F. The way food is grown, processed, stored, and prepared for eating influences the amount of nutrients in the food and its safety, appearance, taste, cost, and waste.
G. Varying amounts of energy and other resources are required to produce, process, package, and deliver it to the consumer.

Nutrients and Dietary Components

A. Nutrients in the food that we eat enable us to live, to grow, to keep healthy and well, and to be active.
B. Each nutrient—carbohydrates, protein, fats, vitamins, minerals, and water—has specific functions in the body.
C. Nutrients must be obtained from outside the body on a regular basis because the body cannot produce them in sufficient amounts.
D. Most healthy people can obtain all the nutrients, in the amounts needed, from a variety of foods.
E. Nutrients are distributed to and used by all parts of the body.
F. Nutrient interactions may affect the amounts of nutrients needed and their functioning.
G. The body stores some nutrients and withdraws them for use as needed.
H. Nutrients are found in varying amounts, proportions, and combinations in the plant and animal sources which serve as food.
I. Ongoing scientific research determines nutrients, their functions, and the amounts needed.
J. Both dietary excesses and nutrient deficiencies affect health.
K. Optimum intakes of nutrients and dietary components have both upper and lower limits.
L. All persons throughout life have need for the same nutrients, but the amounts of nutrients needed are influenced by age, sex, size, activity, specific activity, specific conditions of growth, state of health, pregnancy, lactation, and environmental stress.

CONCEPTS FOR FOOD AND NUTRITION EDUCATION—cont'd

Nutrition and Physical Activity

A. Balancing energy intake and energy expenditure is important for achieving and maintaining desirable body weight.
B. There is a synergistic relationship between nutrition and physical activity which affects health and well-being.

Food Selection

A. Food, that is, what people consider edible, is culturally defined.
B. Physiological, cultural, social, economic, psychological, and geographical factors influence food selection.
C. Knowledge, attitudes, and beliefs about food and nutrition affect food selection.
D. Food availability and merchandising influence food choices.

National and International Food Policy

A. Food plays an important role in the physical, psychological, and economic health of a society.
B. Food production, distribution, and merchandising systems have economic, social, political, and ecological consequences.
C. Effective utilization of individual and community resources is beneficial for the economic and nutritional well-being of the individual, family, and society.
D. The availability of food and maintenance of nutritional well-being is a matter of public policy.
E. Knowledge of food and nutrition combined with social consciousness enables citizens to understand and participate in the development and adoption of public policy affecting the nutritional well-being of societies.

Society for Nutrition Education: SNE concepts for food and nutrition education, J. Nutr. Educ. **14**:1, 1982. © Society for Nutrition Education. Concepts developed by the membership and approved by the Board of Directors. Used with permission.

dents knew more than those several years older. All age groups appeared to have some concept of the role of excess kilocalories in overweight, although none could select foods low in energy content. Younger children were better able to make practical choices of substitutes within the Basic Four Food Groups. They recognized items that might be used in place of meat or milk, or selected a balanced meal of less traditional foods such as a sandwich or pizza. The fact that younger children are better prepared to make alternative choices suggests a needed shift in recent years to a more liberal, less rigid approach to nutrition education.

Adults

Among adults nutrition knowledge is related to both age and level of education. Younger individuals and those with more years of formal education score higher on nutrition knowledge tests.[5] Men have high interest in nutrition information, particularly as related to health. Although nutrition materials and food classes have usually been directed toward women, the increasing number of single males, single-parent households headed by males, and two-parent households where food preparation activities are shared suggests a receptive audience for programs targeted toward men.

A problem among persons in all groups is the inability to evaluate the nutritional adequacy of their own individual diets. This may relate, in part, to the methods of evaluation currently available to consumers. In a recent survey,[5] individuals considered diets that met the criteria of the Basic Four Food Guide to be nutritionally adequate, although this is not always the case (p. 509). A diet can be planned by the Basic Four Food Guide and still be inadequate in specific nutrients. A priority in nutrition education must be the development of simple and appropriate tools for dietary evaluation.

CURRENT TRENDS IN CONSUMER ATTITUDES

Food quality, safety, and relation to health are growing concerns of the general public. Among supermarket shoppers surveyed by the Food Marketing Institute,[6] 63% were very concerned about the nutrient content of the food they eat and an additional 32% were somewhat concerned. Only 4% were not concerned. Over three-fourths of the shoppers reported selecting foods to achieve a balanced diet or serving nutritional snacks such as fruits and vegetables. Nearly half tried to select recipes on the basis of nutrient content and avoided buying foods with no nutritional value. Conversely, about one-fifth of the shoppers had no interest or concern about the nutritional value of the foods they purchased. Thirty-seven percent considered it the responsibility of the supermarket to provide nutrition and health information about the food being sold. Point-of-choice information can assist consumers in making food choices (p. 521).

The Learning Process

TEACHING VERSUS LEARNING

The terms *teaching* and *learning* are often confused. A teacher may assume that because information or materials have been provided the learner has acquired knowledge or skill. Moreover, the learner's interpretation of what has been said may differ from what the teacher intended. Emphasis on the importance of vitamins and minerals may motivate a mother to purchase a vitamin-mineral supplement for her child if it was not made clear that these nutrient requirements are best met by the selection of appropriate food items. To develop programs that not only provide useful information but also lead to appropriate behavior we need to understand how people learn.

STAGES IN THE LEARNING PROCESS

Personal Nature of Learning

Learning is a highly personal process. It relates directly to the personal needs and goals of the learner. Learning may take place to satisfy either a conscious or subconscious need, or to avoid a loss of privilege or a punishment. Current interests, ambitions, personal satisfactions from new activities, and past experiences all influence the learning process.

Learning Stages

For all of us, new ideas take time to grow. Actually, individuals adopt new ideas through several merging stages:[7]

- Becoming aware of a new idea or practice
- Developing an interest and seeking more information
- Evaluating advantages and disadvantages of the practice
- Trying it to test its usefulness
- Accepting or rejecting it for future use

Different types of information sources are more or less important depending on the stage in the adoption process.[7] Mass media—radio, television, or newspapers—are most important in the first two stages, making people more aware of new ideas and helping them obtain more information about them. Friends, neighbors, or professional sources, less important in early stages of the adoption process, exert the greatest influence in later stages as an individual evaluates, tests, and finally accepts or rejects the idea. Personal experience is the most important factor influencing the continued use of an idea or practice.

Implications for Nutrition Education

The relative importance of various information sources has implications for nutrition education at all ages. A child may be required to learn nutrition facts, but his choice of an after-school snack will likely depend on what his friend or sibling chooses to have. An overweight adult may be interested in a weight-loss program described in a newspaper article or leaflet from a local health agency, but long-term adherence to a weight-control program requires personal family support. Media impact in promoting initial recognition of an idea or problem points to the need of making more effective use of radio, television, and printed materials.

SOURCES OF NUTRITION INFORMATION

Types of Sources

The quality of the diet may be influenced by both the source of the nutrition information and the frequency of its use. Nutrition information is obtained from three main sources: (1) *casual sources:* articles or advertising read or seen and heard as a result of another activity such as watching television or reading; (2) *selective sources:* government pamphlets or special nutrition education programs; and (3) *significant persons:* persons in the immediate environment, such as family, friends, or neighbors.[8]

Sources Used by Children

For children and youth, casual sources are the most common. Television is usually the most frequent source. National surveys indicate that on the average children watch television 4 hours a day and see over 11,000 food commercials a year.[9] Children also receive food and nutrition information from their parents, but their peer group is an extremely important source of nutrition attitudes. Although nutrition education still receives only limited attention in the classroom, this setting has much potential for a graded, systematic treatment of essential information.

Sources Used by Adults

Information sources used by adults relate to age, sex, and stage in the family life cycle.[8] Young families in the process of developing appropriate food patterns are more likely to seek information from classes, government sources, parents, and relatives, and less likely to use advertisements and university extension programs. Older persons with established food patterns are less likely, but women as compared to men are more likely to seek out nutrition information from all sources. The 867 adult participants in a health survey[10] mentioned physicians most frequently as sources of credible nutrition information, followed by books, newspapers, and magazines. Only 12% of these adults used nutrition labels.

Unfortunately, many consumers do not know where to find reliable nutrition information. Therefore they depend on media sources that may present a biased point of view. Voluntary health organizations and government agencies need to cooperate in making appropriate information available to the public.

Food Guidance and Nutrition Education

NEED FOR FOOD GUIDES

The ultimate goal of nutrition education is to provide consumers of all ages with the information they need to plan, purchase, prepare, and consume wholesome, economical diets. Reaching this goal requires a food-selection guidance system that they can use as a model for planning and evaluating daily food intake. Several diet guides have been developed, but all have limitations that raise questions about their usefulness.

BASIS FOR DEVELOPMENT

Historically, food guidance systems were developed to translate dietary standards into simple and reliable tools that would be useful in planning day-to-day food intake. Several criteria must be considered in their development and evaluation. Food guides must:

- be consistent with known nutrient needs and provide adequate levels of protein, vitamins, and minerals without exceeding energy requirements.
- address current diet-health issues.
- be easily used and understood.
- be adaptable to a wide variety of cultural, religious, and regional food preferences and economic situations.
- be consistent with general food availability and, to the extent possible, generally accepted food patterns.

Food guides based on common food items rather than on abstract nutrient calculations are more easily used. Similarly, the closer the guide to current food intake the more likely it is to be adopted by consumers. A food guide requiring radical dietary changes is of limited use, if it is used at all.

GUIDES FOR FOOD SELECTION

Basic Four Food Groups

The Four Food Group plan, titled, "The Essentials of an Adequate Diet," was introduced by the U.S. Department of Agriculture in 1956.[11] Current criticisms of the plan, described in Table 12-1, relate to nutrient adequacy, diet-health problems, and usability. Diets fulfilling the criteria for adequacy can still be lacking in recommended levels of particular nutrients, especially vitamin E, vitamin B_6, folacin, iron, magnesium, and zinc.[12] These nutrients, however, are those for which food composition data are generally incomplete. Thus greater amounts may be consumed than are evident in calculated totals. On the other hand, these nutrients are often lost in processing and, with the exception of iron, are not added in the enrichment of refined breads and grain products.

The 1979 revision of the Four Food Group plan to include a fifth group called "fats, sweets, and alcohol" was an attempt to draw attention to the health issues related to overconsumption of energy, sugars, and fats.[11] This revision, published by USDA as the "Hassle-Free Food Guide," also noted the importance of specific vitamins and minerals within particular food groups, addressed the need for fiber, and encouraged the use of whole grains.

TABLE 12-1 Comparison of the Basic Four and Modified Basic Four Food Guides

Food Group	Basic Four	Modified Basic Four
Milk Group	2 servings	2 servings
Meat-Protein Group	2 servings	4 servings 2-animal protein 2-legumes or nuts
Fruit-Vegetable Group	4 servings citrus fruit daily dark green leafy or deep orange vegetables or fruit frequently	4 servings 1 citrus 1 dark green leafy 2 other
Grain Group	4 servings whole-grain, fortified or enriched products recommended	4 servings must be whole grain
Other	Use fats, sweets and alcohol in limited amounts	1 serving of vegetable oil or fat

From U.S. Dept. of Agriculture: Food, Home and Garden Bulletin no. 228, Washington, D.C., U.S. Government Printing Office, and King, J.C. and others: Evaluation and modification of the Basic Four Food Guide, J. Nutr. Educ. **10**:27, 1978.

Modified Basic Four Food Guide

The Modified Basic Four represents an effort to correct the nutrient inadequacies associated with the traditional Basic Four Food Groups (Table 12-1).[12] The inclusion of nuts and legumes and requirement for whole grains promotes higher intakes of iron, magnesium, zinc, and vitamin B_6. The dark-green leafy vegetable to be consumed daily contributes to folic acid and iron levels. Finally, the vegetable oil will supply vitamin E and linoleic acid to the diet. Acceptance of the Modified Basic Four by the general population is questionable in light of current trends toward processed breads and cereals and relatively low use of legumes and nuts, with the exception of peanut butter. Nevertheless, this modified guide does provide an alternative for motivated individuals willing to adjust their eating patterns.

Dietary Guidelines for Americans

In 1980 the United States Departments of Health and Human Services and of Agriculture issued a joint publication outlining what healthy Americans should eat or avoid to reduce the risk of chronic disease (Fig. 12-2). A 1985 revised edition incorporated new information on osteoporosis, eating disorders, alcohol in pregnancy, and serum cholesterol and blood pressure levels. A disadvantage of the Dietary Guidelines, however, is the lack of specific targets for intakes of particular nutrients.

Nutrition Labeling

Nutrition labeling guidelines, established by the Food and Drug Administration (FDA) in 1973, were developed to provide consumers with information regarding the nutrient content of food products. At present a food product is not required to carry a nutrition label unless: (1) it makes a nutritional claim of some type, or (2) nutrients have been added to the product, as is the case with enriched or fortified items. Although the nutrition label is not required on most food products, many now carry one.

Mandatory components of the nutrition label include an indication of serving size and the number of servings in the container. Nutrients that must be defined include: (1) energy in kilocalories; (2) fat, carbohydrate, and protein in g; and (3) protein, vitamins A and C, thiamin, riboflavin, niacin, calcium, and iron as percentage of the U.S. RDA. An extension of the law, effective in 1985, defined categories for stating sodium content. Nutrition labeling provides a means of evaluating the nutrient content of processed foods or comparing the nutrient content of different brands or products.

Food Exchange Lists

Exchange lists group foods that are similar in nutrient content and can be substituted for each other within the daily meal plan. Such a tool allows individuals to plan meals containing a variety of foods and yet stay within suggested limits of energy or other nutrients. The most common list, "Exchange Lists for Meal Planning," developed jointly by the American Dietetic Association and the American Diabetes Association, is based on kilocalories, protein, carbohydrate, and fat. The new 1986 revised edition incorporates current diet-health recommendations regarding starch, fiber, fat, and sodium, as well as providing expanded instructional material in a colorful format.

Dietary Guidelines
for Americans
Eat a Variety
of Foods
Maintain Desirable
Weight
Avoid Too Much Fat,
Saturated Fat, and
Cholesterol
Eat Foods with
Adequate Starch
and Fiber
Avoid Too Much
Sugar
Avoid Too Much
Sodium
If You Drink
Alcoholic
Beverages, Do So
in Moderation

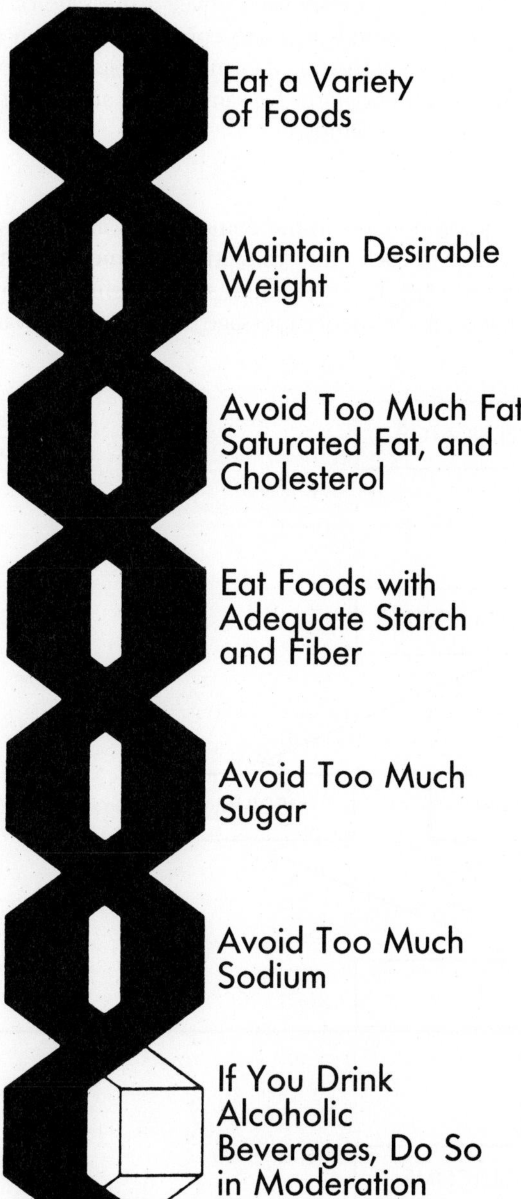

FIG. 12-2 Dietary Guidelines for Americans.

(From U.S. Dept. of Agriculture and U.S. Dept. of Health and Human Services: Nutrition and Your Health: Dietary Guidelines for Americans, 2nd ed., Home and Garden Bulletin No. 232, Washington, D.C., 1985, U.S. Government Printing Office.)

Developing Nutrition Education Programs

Communication is the transfer of ideas from one person to another. It can occur without speech or language. A smile, nod, or frown can convey a message of trust, understanding, or doubt. Although human beings learn to communicate at an early age, the effort to transfer ideas is not always successful. Many misunderstandings occur even when ethnic and educational backgrounds are the same. They are even more common between persons of different backgrounds.

A COMMUNICATION MODEL

A model that identifies important components in the communication process and describes how these components relate to each other can aid in planning and implementing nutrition education programs (Fig. 12-3). The first step is defining communication *goals* for the program, handout, or media message. What do you want to

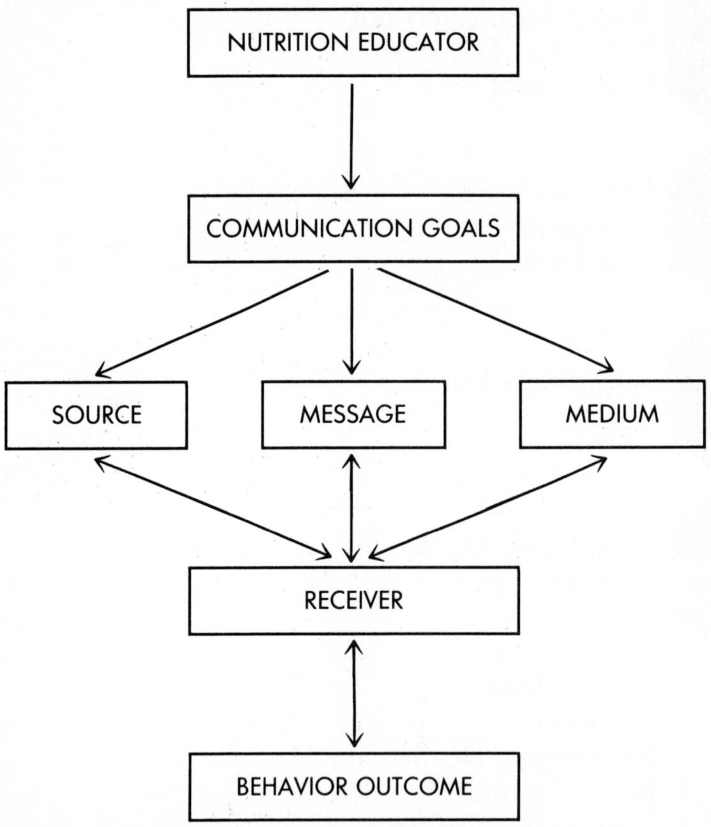

FIG. 12-3 A communication model for nutrition education.
(Developed with M.G. Ashman, Office of Information, College of Agriculture and Life Sciences, University of Vermont, Burlington.)

happen as a result of your nutrition message? You may have several goals in mind, both immediate and long term, as you plan.

One component in the communication model is the *source* of the nutrition message. If you are a community nutritionist you may be the source, working directly with individuals and families. Within a work-site fitness program you may be training and supervising workshop leaders who will be the source of nutrition information for their peers. The *message* component of the model is not only what you say but how you say it. The *medium* could be a face-to-face class or workshop, a handout to send by mail, or a radio message. Finally the *receiver* is the audience. What do you know about your audience? What are their needs? Before making any decisions, you must examine carefully each component in relation to your communication goals.

SELECTING COMMUNICATION GOALS

The general goal of nutrition education is to improve or enhance personal nutritional status, health, and well-being. When defining specific goals for a particular program or message, you must consider communication outcomes on three levels—cognitive, affective, and behavioral.[13]

Cognitive Goals

These goals relate to thinking skills and acquisition of knowledge. A cognitive goal for both children and adults could be learning to use nutrition labels to identify foods high in sodium and limit their use in the daily meal pattern.

Affective Goals

These goals relate to values and attitudes toward food, and whether proposed changes are good or desirable. A teenager may recognize that potato chips are high in fat but not desire to reduce intake.

Behavioral Goals

These goals relate to actual change in eating behavior. They are the most difficult to achieve. People are resistant to change, particularly in the short term. Repeated exposure to the same message over a long period of time is usually required for behavioral change unless motivation is extraordinary.[13] A woman who does not like milk may consume generous quantities during pregnancy but revert to her previous habits following the birth. Eppright and associates,[14] in their classic work on nutrition education, pointed out that changing the way people think about food may be less important than changing the way they feel about it.

SELECTING THE SOURCE

The source or apparent sender of the nutrition message influences the success of the message in several ways. First, the communication skills of the individual preparing the media presentation, written materials, or workshop will determine to a great extent the quality of the presentation. A second factor is the sender's depth of knowledge or familiarity with the subject area. A final issue is the credibility of the source with the population to be reached. An organization such as a hospital, government food program, or university extension service is usually recognized as a valid source of nutrition information.

SELECTING THE MESSAGE

For a message to be successful it must focus on the real-life situation of the audience. It must consider income, housing, accessibility to different types of food, and lifestyle. In a school or work-site program, the nutrition information should be consistent with the choices available in the school lunchroom or employee cafeteria. A message developed for low-income mothers must be based on food choices available to them. A message must also be reasonable in length and complexity. People soon lose interest in material that is difficult to understand. On the other hand, messages can be too simplistic and consequently misleading. For example, not all green vegetables are equally good sources of vitamin A.[13]

SELECTING THE MEDIUM

The medium for nutrition education depends on what you have to say and to whom. Interpersonal or face-to-face communication is ideal for small, well-defined groups. For reaching large numbers of persons, mass media (radio, television, telephone, newspapers) or printed materials are both efficient and cost-effective. A further consideration is the educational level of the audience. For persons with poor reading ability a face-to-face format with visual aids, or radio or television, is the logical choice. For teenagers radio messages scheduled after school on music stations would be appropriate. The Social Security office would be a location for reaching large numbers of older persons with a nutrition message.

Both children and adults learn more easily if several senses are stimulated simultaneously. A film followed by discussion, or a presentation describing the nutritional importance of dairy foods followed by tasting of milk-based recipe products, are examples of combinations that can lead to behavioral change. Table 12-2 describes some activity-oriented experiences that can be adapted for different age or educational levels.

ATTRACT THE AUDIENCE

People are being constantly bombarded with messages. They selectively choose those to which they will give attention. This selection process requires interaction between the audience, the message sender, and the message itself. This interactive process is described schematically on the model (Fig. 12-3) by the arrows going in both directions. If no interaction occurs, attention is lost.

Attention to the message depends on the extent to which it appears to meet an identified need. As Gillespie[13] points out, people who are not involved in meal-planning or food preparation may not realize that they can benefit from nutrition information. Attention-getting cues pointing to the importance or relevance of the message must precede or accompany it. Getting the most for your money or time, weight control, or pleasurable food experiences may be topics for such cues.

When developing communication goals, consider a measure by which you can

TABLE 12-2 Learning Activities for Nutrition Education

Type of Activity	Example
Demonstration	Prepare a "new" food or low-cost or low-kilocalorie food for tasting with directions or recipe handout for children or adults to try at home; lead the group in exercises that can be done at home
Skit; role playing	Have children write and perform skits of social situations relating to food such as selecting a fast food meal or snacks; volunteers in a work-site weight control support group may role play problems of people trying to lose weight.
Problem solving	Using newspapers with weekly food specials, select groceries for the week considering both nutritional adequacy and cost; keep diet diaries and evaluate using a food guide or computer program.
Field trip	Visit a grocery store, food cooperative or dairy (this may be a special treat for both children or adults who lack personal transportation).
Panel	Have several "experts" (group members or visitors) discuss or debate a topic, then continue discussion with the entire group. With adults topics might be food buying, use of food stamps or child-feeding problems; children might present a panel describing different types of exercise or the benefits of exercise; high school students might organize a debate on the benefits versus the risks of food additives.
Group activity	Develop and duplicate a "cookbook" applicable to the group (e.g., snack book or cooking for one or two); plant a vegetable garden outside or vegetables in containers under lights; prepare an exhibit for the school lunchroom, employee cafeteria, WIC center or senior center. (Such an activity provides a way for participants to get to know each other.)

evaluate the outcome of your program. Did it bring a change in nutrition knowledge (cognitive), nutrition attitudes (affective), or food selection (behavioral)? Examples of different types and methods of evaluation are given here in the following section.

Evaluating Nutrition Education Programs

Evaluation procedures must be developed as an integral component when the program is being planned. Accomplishments should be measured against specific objectives. Did a greater number of children select whole-grain than white bread following the classroom or lunchroom nutrition education program? Did participants in the weight-control support group maintain their weight loss over a six-month period? Such evaluation requires, however, that goals be stated in measurable terms.

TYPES OF EVALUATION

Evaluation is appropriate at many stages in a nutrition education program. *Continuous evaluation* provides ongoing information indicating whether or not changes are needed and if so what kinds. *Periodic evaluation* monitors progress and effectiveness. *Follow-up evaluation* conducted some time after completion of a project evaluates the extent to which desired outcomes were achieved or continued.

In addition to the desired or anticipated effects of an education program, there may be side effects or unanticipated results that are equally important. A nutrition education program in an elementary school may lead to increased consumption of milk with the school lunch. If, however, this is accompanied by reduced consumption of the bread and vegetable items, the behavior change, although intended, is not of benefit. Also, the characteristics of those who did not exhibit the behavior change are as important as those who did. The teaching method, communication medium, or message presented may not have been suitable for that audience.

METHODS OF EVALUATION

Nutrition Knowledge

The most common evaluation procedure in nutrition education is testing nutrition knowledge. Although children are accustomed to being tested, adults may resent the traditional pre-test, post-test approach. With adults a pre-test can serve as a teaching tool if class members keep their tests as a basis for the discussion to follow. If the knowledge tests are used, they must be pre-tested with individuals of similar age and background so that misunderstandings can be avoided.

Nutrition Attitudes

One alternative to testing nutrition knowledge is evaluating attitudes toward the information presented. Attitudes regarding the relative importance of nutrition and food choices have been strongly correlated with nutrition knowledge. An evaluation of workshops for adults might include such questions as, "Will the information presented today be of use to you (for example, in your food shopping, in controlling your weight)? If not, why not?" With children, true-false items could focus on food likes and dislikes or food behavior patterns, for example: "I like to try new foods."

Dietary Practices

The most desirable criterion for evaluating the effectiveness of a nutrition education program is food-related behavior. For example, observation of plate waste in the school lunchroom could measure any change resulting from nutrition activities in the classroom. Relative sales of broiled fish versus fried fish would indicate change resulting from a work-site fitness program.

Nutritional Status

If nutrition education is one component of a broad nutrition intervention program, an evaluation of nutritional status using dietary, clinical, and biochemical measurements may be possible. Because of the many uncontrollable factors influencing both the dietary intake and biochemical status of all age groups, it is often difficult to draw conclusions regarding the success of a nutrition intervention program. Moreover, a recent study[15] concluded that the personal attention received through diet counseling may result in nutritional improvement even if no additional foods are provided. The personal concern of the nutrition educator as perceived by the audience may be as important as the information provided in bringing about food behavior change.

Selecting Nutrition Education Materials

SOURCES OF MATERIALS

A nutrition educator may have neither the time nor the resources to prepare original materials. Instead existing materials must be adapted for the client group. Although a wide range of materials are available for school-age children and youth and for pregnant women, nutrition resources for other ages or target groups are limited. Professionals working with Spanish-speaking populations of all ages, preschoolers, the developmentally disabled, young adults, or the aged may have difficulty finding materials appropriate to the teaching level, income level, ethnic group, or topic of choice. Attractive, well-designed materials are often available free from companies or trade associations selling particular food products. But in some cases these materials are biased to promote the organization's products to best advantage.

CRITERIA FOR EVALUATING CONTENT

Materials from any source should be examined carefully as to content and presentation. The following criteria should be included in the evaluation:

Do They Present a Favorable Image of All Types of Individuals?

Persons of all nationalities, ethnic groups, ages, and physical status deserve to be described in a positive light. Stereotypic images (for example, an obese individual sitting before a plate heaped with food) or illustrations that are unrealistic in light of population trends (for example, presenting all food budgets based on two-parent households) can alienate the group being taught.

Are They Appropriate for the Particular Group?

Both subject matter and visual content enter into the evaluation of nutrition materials. Cartoons or stick figures, acceptable for a school-age group, can be insulting to an adult audience. Nutritional needs and problems also differ among age and sex groups. Posters encouraging children to "make your own milkshake" adding ice cream, juice or fruit, although encouraging the use of milk and dairy products, will not benefit weight-conscious young women who should increase their calcium intake.

Is the Information Presented with a Positive Approach?

Individuals of all ages are more receptive to learning principles that are positive in tone. Negative or unpleasant associations are shut out and are more likely to be forgotten. Food choices should be presented as options within the individual's control, not in the form of edicts.

Is the Information Accurate?

Extravagant claims regarding the nutrient contribution of any one food or food group can be misleading. Generalizations that present only part of the picture lead to inaccurate conclusions. For example, the comment that "high caloric foods must be eliminated from a weight reduction diet" does not deal with the issue of portion size.

Is the Information Practical?

Nutritional advice is of no value unless it can be put into practice. Thus aspects of cost, time, cooking skills, and available cooking facilities must be considered when selecting both lesson content and materials. Emphasis on the nutritional quality of fresh green leafy vegetables has little value for the low-income homemaker dependent on an inner-city convenience store that sells no fresh produce. Providing information to solve immediate problems should have priority in any nutrition education program.

CRITERIA FOR EVALUATING FORMAT

Materials that are dull, drab, or difficult to read will neither attract nor hold attention. A common mistake in preparing materials is including too many details and too many pictures. As a result, posters or handouts look crowded and confused. Keep wording as brief as possible and illustrations simple. Use real objects whenever practical.

NEED FOR PREVIEW

Regardless of source, no materials should be distributed or audiovisuals shown that have not been previewed carefully. Your use of a material implies that you endorse the facts or ideas presented. Although you might point out a specific inaccuracy, your clarification may be easily forgotten when your handout is read later at home. Your standards as a professional are reflected in the general appearance and quality of the materials. A copy that is so light or dark that it is barely legible or text that abounds in spelling or typographical errors suggests that you don't really care about the audience or the accuracy of the material being presented.

Current Strategies in Nutrition Education

Increasing emphasis on preventive health has led to the development and implementation of different educational strategies that meet the particular needs of individuals and programs. Efforts to reach greater numbers of people have led to the use of mass media as a means for communication. Nutrition intervention programs with individuals at risk because of body weight, serum lipid, or blood-pressure measurements have expanded the role of the nutrition counselor as a nutrition education provider.

GUIDELINES FOR NUTRITION COUNSELING

Nutrition counseling provides individualized instruction to assist a person in adjusting daily food intake to meet health or personal needs. Although diet counseling has been most commonly applied to patients assigned to a therapeutic regimen for treatment of a chronic disease, this mode of nutrition education is now being used in preventive care and health-fitness programs. Health or exercise clubs may provide nutrition counseling as one of their services to members.

Goal

The goal of nutrition counseling is development of a diet strategy that while meeting health and nutrition objectives will also be consistent with the client's lifestyle, ethnic food pattern, food preferences, and socioeconomic realities.

Process

The process of nutrition counseling involves several steps:

- Establish a positive, pleasant atmosphere for interaction.
- Define the client's objectives, purpose, or expectations regarding the outcomes of nutrition counseling.
- Gather information relating to current eating pattern, health status, and lifestyle.
- Assess the current food pattern.
- Develop an individualized nutritional care plan that addresses both long-term and short-term goals.
- Provide appropriate materials that support recommended changes.
- Provide continued follow-up and support.

Social Support

A critical component in achieving success with a diet plan is the support the client receives from family and friends. Involving the person who does the shopping and cooking in the counseling format may help avoid future problems. Also, for the recommended diet to be implemented, appropriate food must be available. Nutrition educators should be familiar with local food distribution programs that can provide assistance.

GROUP VERSUS INDIVIDUAL COUNSELING

The type of counseling to be provided is a decision related in part to the professional setting. In a clinic or hospital, when nutrition counseling focuses on a therapeutic regimen mandated by medical considerations, individual counseling is usually employed. In a work-site program or voluntary weight-control program, group counseling is more common. Group counseling has been considered an advantage in weight-control programs as it provides social support to the clients and reduces costs. On the other hand, the group process can be less effective if a member who is experiencing less success is negative in attitude or extremely vocal. The importance of social support should not be underestimated, as those who continue in a support group for one year are more likely to *sustain* their weight loss than those who discontinue attendance after the initial instruction period.[16]

NUTRITION EDUCATION AT THE WORK SITE

Escalating health care costs plus the expense of lost work time have led to the development of work-site health-promotion programs. Work-site programs offer particular advantages for nutrition educators. In the first place, workers are at the program location so attending class or obtaining materials is convenient. Secondly, since most work sites have lunch facilities, principles can be reinforced through visuals and the food options available.

Approaches to Work-Site Programs

Work-site health promotion programs include a wide range of topics. Although nutrition is not always included it is becoming more popular. Furthermore, the most common topics such as substance abuse, hypertension control, physical fitness, stress management, and smoking cessation all involve a nutrition component. Corporate wellness programs promote nutrition through direct and environmental approaches.[17] Direct approaches include nutrition classes or discussion groups, individual counseling, or distribution of printed materials. Environmental approaches that facilitate participation or awareness include released time for attending classes, appropriate food choices in cafeterias or vending machines, and nutrition information where food is served or consumed.

Nutrition Topics for Work-Site Programs

Programs may focus on individuals identified as at high risk based on cholesterol level, elevated blood pressure, or degree of overweight. Or the emphasis may be on general nutrition principles with all employees invited to participate. Usually programs have been developed around weight control or cardiovascular risk, although the Dietary Guidelines (p. 510), nutrition fallacies, and nutrient needs in pregnancy are sometimes included. As more women continue to work throughout pregnancy, the work site will become increasingly important as a site for prenatal care.

Evaluation

Evaluation of work-site programs has been limited. Over the short term, programs appear to be successful for weight control and for blood pressure and lipid management. Moreover, employers believe that work-site programs are cost effective in promoting health and employee morale. Long-term evaluation, however, is still necessary.

TELEVISION AND MASS MEDIA

Consumer surveys suggest that the average American spends more time watching television than doing anything else except sleeping.[9] Much has been written about the negative impact on children of television commercials for high-sugar cereals and snacks. On the other hand, Manoff[18] has pointed to the mass media as an untapped resource for spreading positive nutrition information. One effective use of television could be the short sequence, one minute or less, inserted as a public service announcement. Such a message demands neither interest nor motivation. It reaches its objective through repetition over days and weeks. Public service announcements may be most useful for simple messages such as announcing a congregate meal program, promoting the school lunch program, or giving a number to call for information about food stamps.

Television cooking shows attract many viewers and can provide important nutrition information in an entertaining format. Although nutritionists may wish to de-emphasize "cooking," the fact remains that persons not interested in nutrition may be attracted to such a program. Recipes low in fat, sugar, and sodium, and rich in vitamins and minerals could bring significant change in nutrient intake if incorporated in the diet as replacements for less nutrient-dense food items.

Most local television stations are required to provide time for nonprofit programming. Public television stations are also seeking educational programming. Pooling of resources by health agencies and community groups can make possible development of informative programming.

POINT-OF-CHOICE NUTRITION INFORMATION

A growing concept in nutrition education is providing food product information at the point of purchase. One application of the point-of-choice technique is a cafeteria serving either children or adults where visual aids highlight the nutrient content of one food choice as compared to another. Nutrient content information in a cafeteria appears to be more effective if presented with materials that point to the health benefit of a food lower in fat or sodium.[19] Point-of-choice information has also been used in supermarkets and does lead to demonstrable changes in items sold. In general, consumers appear willing to pay somewhat more for the item or brand higher in nutrient content.[20]

COMPUTERS IN NUTRITION EDUCATION

The rapid proliferation of microcomputers and nutrient-related software has made computer-assisted nutrition instruction a valuable tool in elementary and secondary classrooms and with adults. Computer programs for younger children evaluate diets according to servings from the different food groups. Older students and adults can calculate the nutrient content of their diets and compare the totals with recommended levels for their age, sex, and level of physical activity.

Interpretation of the findings, however, requires professional input. Individuals must be reminded that the nutrient intakes calculated are estimates, not absolute values. It must be made clear that individuals consuming less than recommended levels are not necessarily deficient. It is critical that individuals not be led to assume that intakes below the RDA require the use of vitamin and mineral supplements for improvement.

NUTRITION EDUCATION BY MAIL

With the increasing costs associated with face-to-face nutrition education programs, sending materials by mail can be an effective alternative. A series of three nutrition lessons directed to young families resulted in both cognitive and affective changes.[21] The families reported increased intakes of fruits and vegetables and other high-fiber items and decreased intakes of fat. It may be possible to further contain costs by including materials with other mailings such as pension checks or utility bills.

Food-Related Programs and Nutrition Education

Food programs developed and funded by the U.S. Departments of Agriculture and Health and Human Services reach pregnant and lactating mothers, children of all ages, low-income adults, and older adults. These existing programs provide a framework for nutrition education in population groups who can benefit from practical information on food selection and meal management.

NATIONAL SCHOOL LUNCH PROGRAM

The National School Lunch Program, begun in 1946, was developed to: (1) safeguard the health and well-being of the nation's children by providing them with nutritious food; and (2) support farm income by encouraging the use of agricultural commodities. About half of the cost of the lunch is met by cash reimbursements and donated commodity foods from the federal government. The remaining cost comes from local sources including the price paid by the students. Children falling under poverty guidelines are eligible for free or reduced-cost lunches. In recent years a school breakfast program was added to serve children in need of this meal.

Nutritional Impact

Under federal guidelines the school lunch is expected to provide one-third of the required nutrients for the day. Portion sizes vary according to the age of the child with the exception of milk, with all receiving 1 cup. The food items to be included in a Type A school lunch are listed below.

- Protein-rich food (one of the following or a combination thereof): meat, fish, poultry, egg, peanut butter, or cooked dry beans or peas
- Two or more vegetables or fruits
- Whole-grain or enriched bread or alternate (for example, rice, corn, waffle, or tortilla)
- Milk (whole, low-fat, skim, or buttermilk)

Children who participate in the school lunch program meet a higher percentage of their RDA for energy, protein, vitamin A, the vitamin B complex, and magnesium than nonparticipants similar in age and socioeconomic status.[22] Milk is an important contributor of nutrients, and students who consume a school lunch are more likely to meet the RDA for calcium.

Potential in Nutrition Education

The school lunch is a valuable tool in nutrition education, although this was not a major objective when it began. It provides an example of a basic meal pattern that includes foods from all the major food groups. Children can also be introduced to new foods. Nearly 70% of about 3000 students from grades 3 through 12 reported tasting foods in the school lunch that they had not eaten at home.[23] Nutrition education activities promoting good food choices, when integrated with the school lunch program, can increase not only participation in the program but also the amount of food in the lunch actually consumed.

NUTRITION EDUCATION AND TRAINING PROGRAM (NET)

A 1977 amendment to the Child Nutrition Act established the Nutrition Education and Training Program (NET). It was designed to encourage effective spread of scientifically valid food and nutrition information to children participating or eligible to participate in the school lunch program. Funds were made available to states to develop and implement nutrition education programs that would: (1) incorporate the school lunch program as a learning activity, and (2) integrate food and nutrition information with other subject matter such as health and physical education, science, social studies, or home economics. Schools with NET programs have reported increases in students' nutrition knowledge, improvement in attitudes toward nutrition, and selection of more appropriate snack foods both at home and at school.[24] Changes in food behavior are most likely to occur in programs with strong teacher, student, and school food-service involvement.

EXPANDED FOOD AND NUTRITION EDUCATION PROGRAM (EFNEP)

The Expanded Food and Nutrition Education Program (EFNEP) helps low-income individuals acquire the knowledge, skills, and attitudes necessary to select nutritionally sound diets. The primary audiences are low-income households, particularly those with young children, and 4–H youth in both urban and rural areas.

In EFNEP a priority concept has been the use of paraprofessionals working one-to-one with the individual in the household who is responsible for planning and preparing the family's food. These paraprofessionals, called nutrition or program aides, are selected from the target audience. They are given instruction in planning an adequate diet; food preparation, safety, and presentation; and family budgeting and financial management. Emphasis is placed on practical applications that can be carried out by a person with limited income, equipment, and skills. Although the one-on-one teaching method has proved to be highly successful with multi-problem families, it is extremely expensive. This cost factor limits the number of families who can be helped.

SPECIAL SUPPLEMENTAL FOOD PROGRAM FOR WOMEN, INFANTS, AND CHILDREN (WIC)

The Special Supplemental Food Program for Women, Infants, and Children (WIC) was established in 1972 to improve the diets of low-income pregnant and lactating mothers, and infants and children to age 5 who, because of poor nutritional patterns or inadequate health care, are at high risk. Foods provided to WIC recipients represent all four major food groups:

- Milk (skim, low-fat, whole, or buttermilk), infant formula, cheese
- Eggs and peanut butter
- Juice (orange, grapefruit, pineapple, tomato, or apple with vitamin C)
- Cereal (iron-fortified infant cereal; others for children, mothers)

The amounts of food provided are designed to include 3½ servings from the milk group, 1 serving from the meat group, 2 servings of fruit, and 1-2 servings of cereal for each participant per day. Although all WIC programs must provide foods from each major food group, there is some flexibility at the local level. For example, a program may choose to exclude sugar-coated cereals.

Although nutrition education is required, the level provided depends on the local program. In many situations nutrition education occurs only at the clinic visit required once every 6 months for recertification. A recent national study indicates that WIC families make better food choices with the money available for food than do nonWIC families of similar income.[25] This could reflect nutrition education focusing on wise buying practices.

CONGREGATE AND HOME-DELIVERED MEALS FOR THE AGED (TITLE III-C)

Congregate meal programs (see Chapter 10) and community senior centers provide excellent opportunities for nutrition education in a group setting. Some form of nutrition education is available at most meal sites, but the actual time spent and the type of instruction presented are quite varied. Distribution of printed materials or posting of visual materials is most common. Group discussion, tasting of recipe products, or market trips provide informal opportunities for older people to talk and learn about nutrition. Such activities can be more successful than a "lecture" session in teaching older adults. For those receiving home-delivered meals, including printed materials that suggest healthy snacks, or easy-to-prepare meals for use when no meals are delivered, would be of value. With older age groups, materials with large print that can be read easily are most appropriate.

Summary

Food habits are learned behaviors based on psychosocial and cultural rather than physiologic needs and tend to resist change. Nutrition knowledge will not result in improved food patterns unless the individual is motivated by personal goals or health concerns to initiate such a change. Nutrition educators seeking to help individuals make appropriate food choices must recognize the need to define such choices within the chosen lifestyle of the individual.

Whether or not an individual implements nutrition information may depend on the source or sender of the information, the media through which it is presented, and the ability of the message to meet identified personal needs. Mass media including radio, television, or newspapers are effective in making people aware of new ideas. But individuals are more likely to implement information received from a professional or reinforced by a friend or relative. Tests of nutrition knowledge are sometimes used to evaluate the effectiveness of nutrition education. Observed change in food behavior, although more difficult to measure, is the desired goal.

Increasing emphasis on preventive health has led to the development of innovative strategies to reach consumers at various locations, including the point of purchase (cafeteria or supermarket), the work site, or at home through television. Nutrition counseling on an individual or group basis has been used effectively in helping individuals adjust to therapeutic regimens, manage weight loss, or improve general dietary patterns. The school lunch or meals for the aged provide excellent opportunities to present practical nutrition information.

Review Questions

1. What is the basis for the food behavior of most individuals? Does nutrition information lead to changed food behavior? Explain.
2. What are the stages in the adoption of new ideas? How does the type of media interact at each stage?

3. Describe several food guides now used to evaluate dietary quality. What are the advantages and disadvantages of each?
4. Develop a nutrition education program for a group of your choice following the communication model given in this chapter. Briefly describe your: (1) communication goals, (2) message, (3) medium, (4) audience, and (5) method of evaluation.
5. Describe three government-sponsored programs that provide meals or supplemental foods to target populations. How can nutrition education be incorporated in each?

REFERENCES

1. Glanz, K.: Social psychological perspectives and applications to nutrition education, J. Nutr. Educ. **13**(Suppl.):66, 1981.
2. Hochbaum, G.M.: Strategies and their rationale for changing people's eating habits, J. Nutr. Educ. **13**(Suppl.):59, 1981.
3. Foley, C.S., Vaden, A.G., Newell, G.K., and Dayton, A.D.: Establishing the need for nutrition education. III. Elementary students' nutrition knowledge, attitudes, and practices, J. Am. Diet. Assoc. **83**(5):564, 1983.
4. Skinner, S.D., and Woodburn, M.J.: Nutrition knowledge of teenagers, J. Sch. Health **54**:71, 1984.
5. Spitze, H.T.: Nutrition knowledge of a sample of university-employed men, J. Nutr. Educ. **15**:54, 1983.
6. Food Marketing Institute: Trends, consumer attitudes and the supermarket update, Washington, D.C., 1984, Research Division, Food Marketing Institute.
7. Yarbrough, P.: Communication theory and nutrition education research, J. Nutr. Educ. **13**(Suppl.):16, 1981.
8. Schafer, R.B., and Keith, P.M.: Influences on food decisions across the family life cycle, J. Am. Diet. Assoc. **78**:144, 1981.
9. Jeffrey, D.B., McLellarn, R.W., and Fox, D.T.: The development of children's eating habits: the role of television commercials, Health Educ. Q. **9**:174, 1982.
10. Kunkel, M.E., Cody, M.M., Davis, R.J., and Wheeler, F.C.: Nutrition information sources used by South Carolina adults, J. Am. Diet. Assoc. **86**(3):371, 1986.
11. Light, L., and Cronin, F.J.: Food guidance revisited, J. Nutr. Educ. **13**:57, 1981.
12. King, J.C., and others: Evaluation and modification of the Basic Four Food Guide, J. Nutr. Educ. **10**:27, 1978.
13. Gillespie, A.H.: Planning and evaluating nutrition education programs: a communications approach. In Professional Perspectives, Division of Nutritional Sciences, Cornell University, January-February 1983.
14. Eppright, E., Pattison, M., Barbour, H.: Teaching nutrition, ed. 2, Ames, 1963, Iowa State University Press.
15. Gershoff, S.N., and others: Studies of the elderly in Boston. I. The effects of iron fortification on moderately anemic people, Am. J. Clin. Nutr. **30**:226, 1977.
16. Visocan, B.J., Dworkin, M.F., and Klein, L.W.: Effect of long-term group support on weight-loss maintenance, J. Nutr. Educ. **17**:3, 1985.
17. Glanz, K., and Seewald-Klein, T.: Nutrition at the worksite: an overview, J. Nutr. Educ. **18**(Suppl.):1, 1986.
18. Manoff, R.K.: Potential uses of mass media in nutrition programs, J. Nutr. Educ. **5**:125, 1973.

19. Davis-Chervin, D., Rogers, T., and Clark, M.: Influencing food selection with point-of-choice nutrition information, J. Nutr. Educ. **17**:18, 1985.
20. Muller, T.E.: The use of nutritive composition data at the point of purchase, J. Nutr. Educ. **16**:137, 1984.
21. Gillespie, A.H., Yarbrough, J.P., and Roderuch, C.E.: Nutrition communication program: a direct mail approach, J. Am. Diet. Assoc. **82**:254, 1983.
22. Hanes, S., Vermeersch, J., and Gale, S.: The national evaluation of school nutrition programs: program impact on dietary intake, Am. J. Clin. Nutr. **40**(Suppl.):390, 1984.
23. Singleton, N., and Rhoads, D.S.: Meal and snacking patterns of students, J. Sch. Health **52**:529, 1982.
24. Shannon, B., Graves, K., and Hart, M.: Food behavior of elementary school students after receiving nutrition education, J. Am. Diet. Assoc. **81**:428, 1982.
25. Rush, D.: National WIC evaluation, Public Health Currents **26**(4):1, 1986.

FURTHER READING

Engen, H.B., Iasiello-Vailas, L., and Smith, K.C.: Confrontation: a new dimension in nutrition counseling, J. Am. Diet. Assoc. **83**:34, 1983.

Confrontation is an important skill that when used constructively can help clients recognize and address specific attributes of their behavior that can be changed.

Hertzler, A.A.: Recipes and nutrition education, J. Am. Diet. Assoc. **83**:466, 1983.

Although nutrition educators have raised concerns about the use of recipes in nutrition education programs, this author points to their positive aspects in bringing about changes in food behavior. Client characteristics to be considered in the selection of recipes are presented.

Ip, S.-W., and Betts, N.M.: Food demonstrations as a means of nutrition education for Cambodian refugees, J. Nutr. Educ. **18**:104, 1986

This article describes a nutrition program to assist refugee families to learn to incorporate available and nutritious food items into their cultural food patterns. The methods used could be adapted to any ethnic or regional group.

Smicilklas-Wright, H., and others: Clients' comprehension of a computer-analyzed dietary intake printout, J. Nutr. Educ. **16**:67, 1984.

This article describes both problems and possible solutions in helping clients interpret computer generated dietary intake values.

Sunseri, A.J., and others: Ingredients in nutrition education: family involvement, reading, and race, J. Sch. Health **54**:193, 1984.

This article describes factors relating to both students and their families that were critical to the success of a school nutrition education program.

Appendix A

Physical Growth NCHS Percentiles

GIRLS: BIRTH TO 36 MONTHS
PHYSICAL GROWTH
NCHS PERCENTILES*

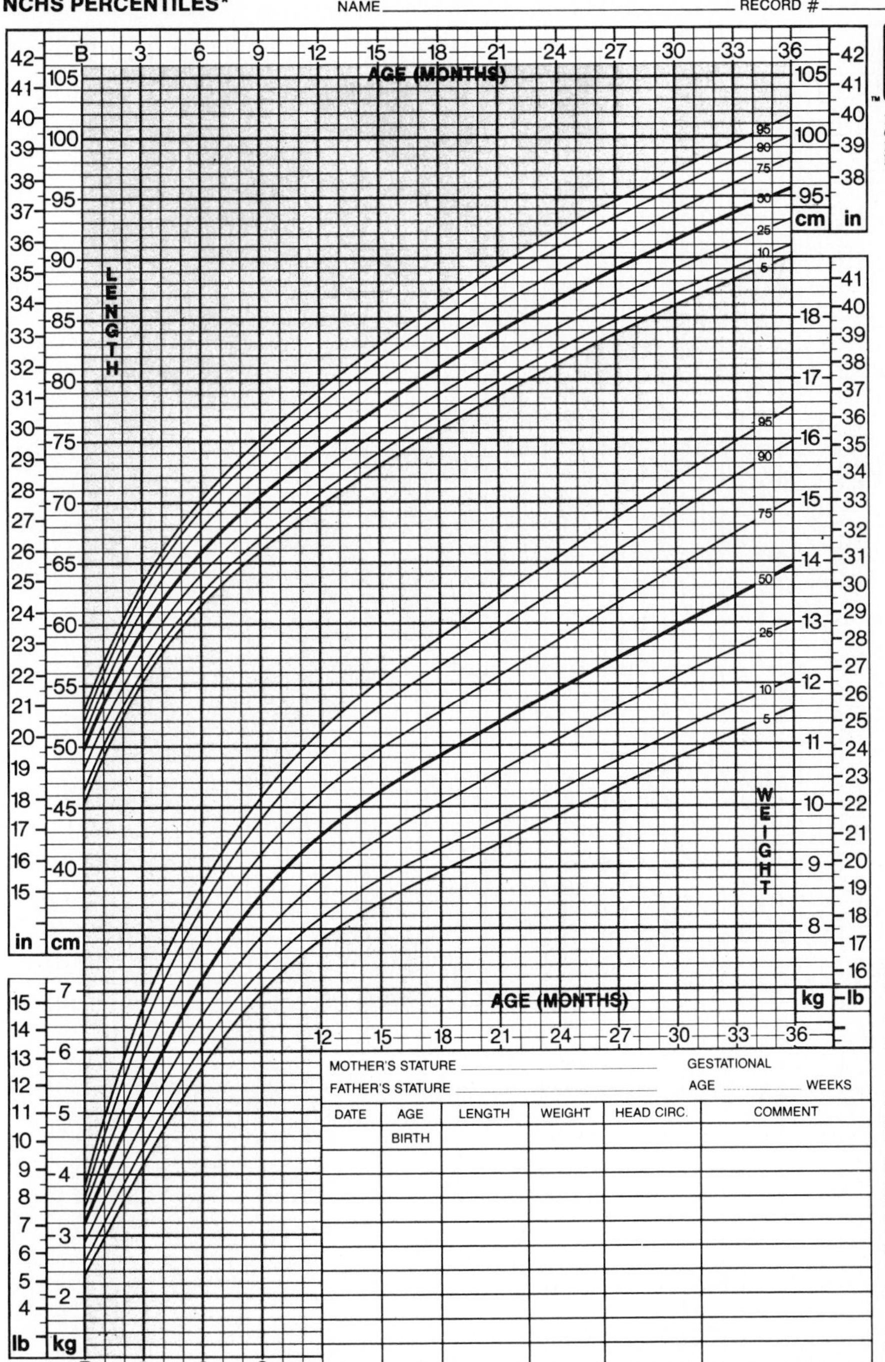

Ross Growth & Development Program

*Adapted from: Hamill PVV, Drizd TA, Johnson CL, Reed RB, Roche AF, Moore WM: Physical growth: National Center for Health Statistics percentiles. AM J CLIN NUTR 32:607-629, 1979. Data from the Fels Research Institute, Wright State University School of Medicine, Yellow Springs, Ohio.

BOYS: BIRTH TO 36 MONTHS PHYSICAL GROWTH NCHS PERCENTILES*

NAME ______________________ RECORD # ______________

Ross Growth & Development Program

AGE (MONTHS): B, 3, 6, 9, 12, 15, 18, 21, 24, 27, 30, 33, 36

LENGTH (in): 15–42; (cm): 40–105

Percentiles: 95, 90, 75, 50, 25, 10, 5

WEIGHT (kg): 2–18; (lb): 4–41

MOTHER'S STATURE ______________ GESTATIONAL

FATHER'S STATURE ______________ AGE ________ WEEKS

DATE	AGE	LENGTH	WEIGHT	HEAD CIRC.	COMMENT
	BIRTH				

*Adapted from: Hamill PVV, Drizd TA, Johnson CL, Reed RB, Roche AF, Moore WM: Physical growth: National Center for Health Statistics percentiles. AM J CLIN NUTR 32:607-629, 1979. Data from the Fels Research Institute, Wright State University School of Medicine, Yellow Springs, Ohio.

GIRLS: BIRTH TO 36 MONTHS PHYSICAL GROWTH NCHS PERCENTILES*

NAME______________________ RECORD #__________

AGE (MONTHS): B 3 6 9 12 15 18 21 24 27 30 33 36

HEAD CIRCUMFERENCE (cm): 31 32 33 34 35 36 37 38 39 40 41 42 43 44 45 46 47 48 49 50 51 52 53 54

HEAD CIRCUMFERENCE (in): 12 13 14 15 16 17 18 19 20 21

Percentiles: 95 90 75 50 25 10 5

WEIGHT (kg): 2 3 4 5 6 7 8 9 10 11 12 13 14 15 16 17 18 19 20 21

WEIGHT (lb): 4 6 8 10 12 14 16 18 20 22 24 26 28 30 32 34 36 38 40 42 44 46

LENGTH (cm): 50 55 60 65 70 75 80 85 90 95 100

LENGTH (in): 19 20 21 22 23 24 25 26 27 28 29 30 31 32 33 34 35 36 37 38 39 40

DATE	AGE	LENGTH	WEIGHT	HEAD CIRC.	COMMENT

*Adapted from: Hamill PVV, Drizd TA, Johnson CL, Reed RB, Roche AF, Moore WM: Physical growth: National Center for Health Statistics percentiles. AM J CLIN NUTR 32:607-629, 1979. Data from the Fels Research Institute, Wright State University School of Medicine, Yellow Springs, Ohio.

G106/JUNE 1983 LITHO IN USA

BOYS: BIRTH TO 36 MONTHS
PHYSICAL GROWTH
NCHS PERCENTILES*

NAME ______ RECORD # ______

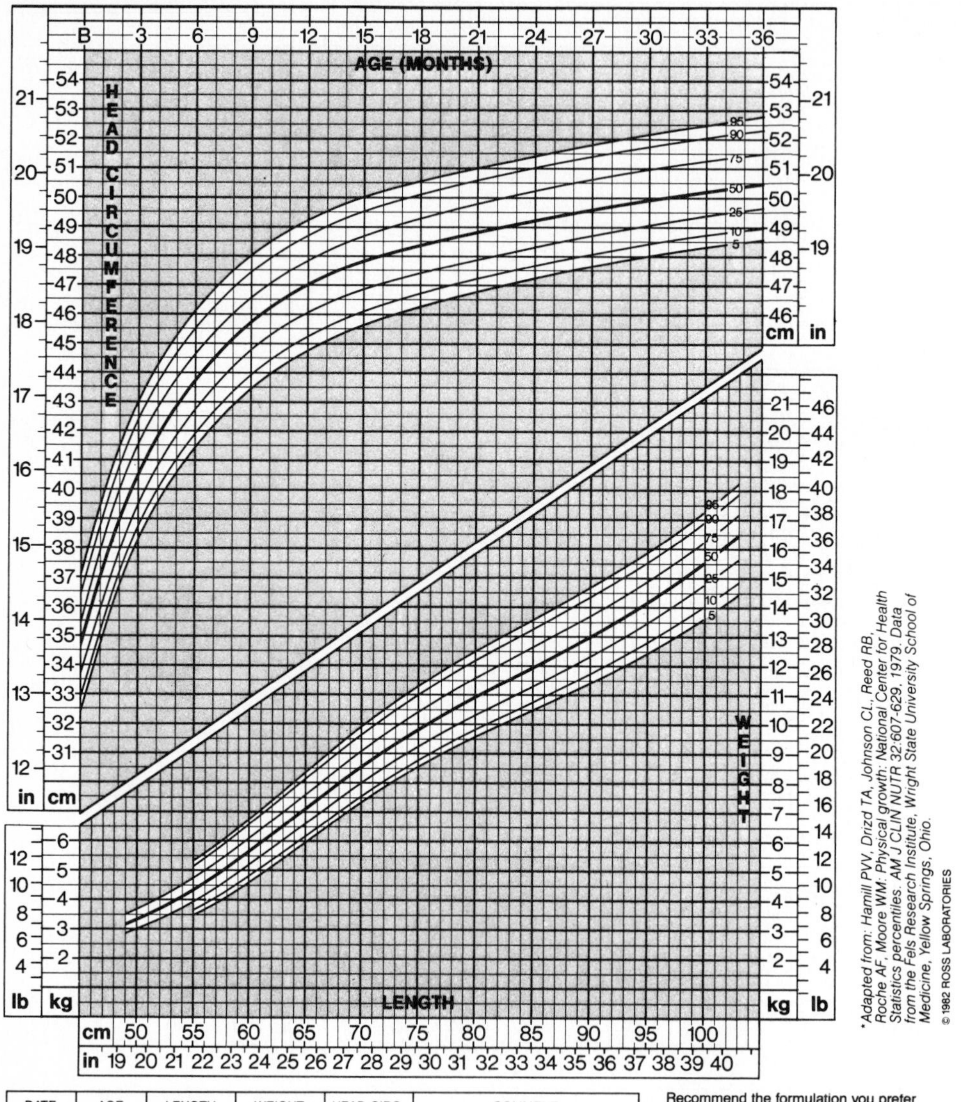

*Adapted from: Hamill PVV, Drizd TA, Johnson CL, Reed RB, Roche AF, Moore WM: Physical growth: National Center for Health Statistics percentiles. AM J CLIN NUTR 32:607-629, 1979. Data from the Fels Research Institute, Wright State University School of Medicine, Yellow Springs, Ohio.

DATE	AGE	LENGTH	WEIGHT	HEAD CIRC.	COMMENT

GIRLS: 2 TO 18 YEARS PHYSICAL GROWTH NCHS PERCENTILES*

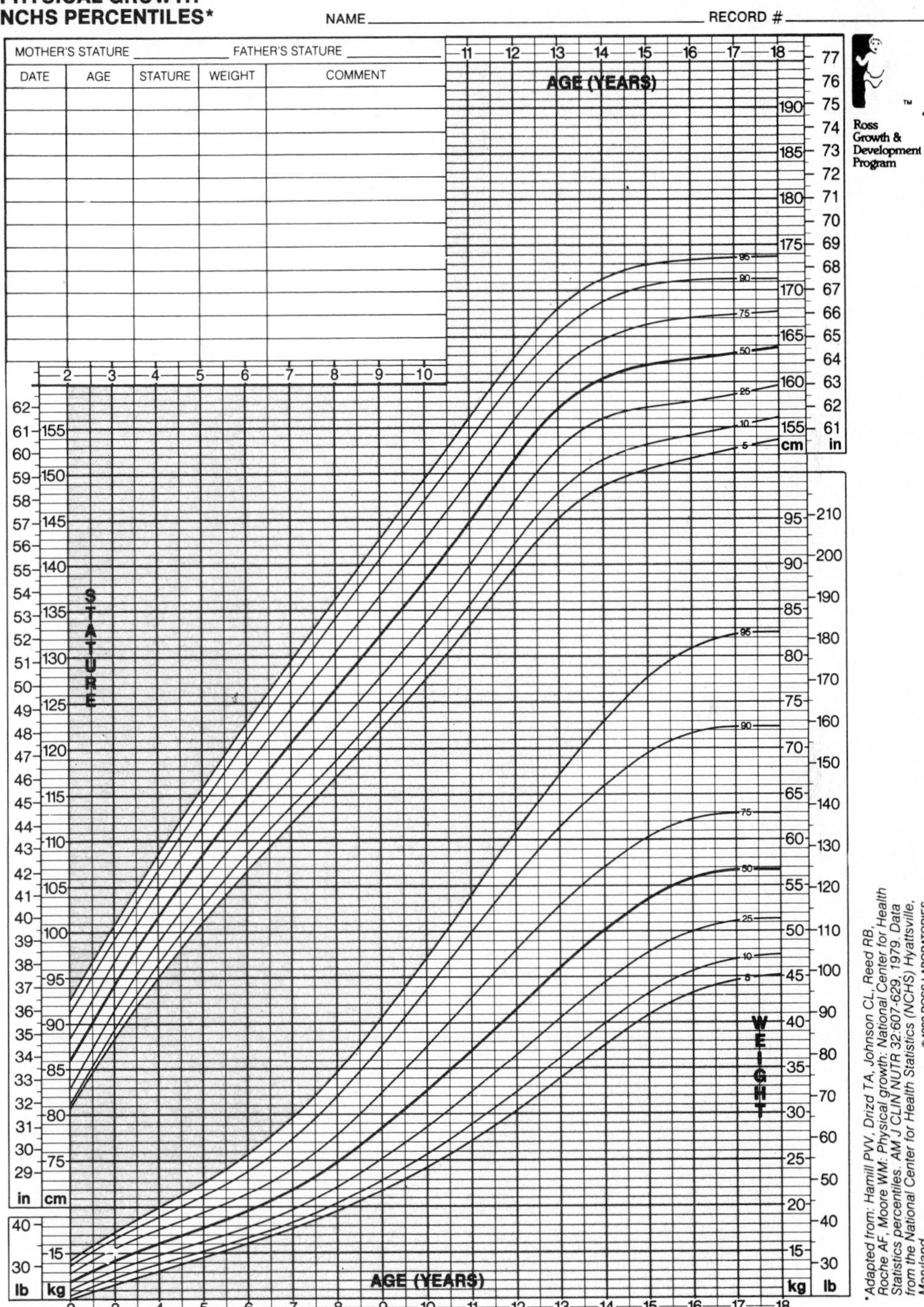

BOYS: 2 TO 18 YEARS
PHYSICAL GROWTH
NCHS PERCENTILES*

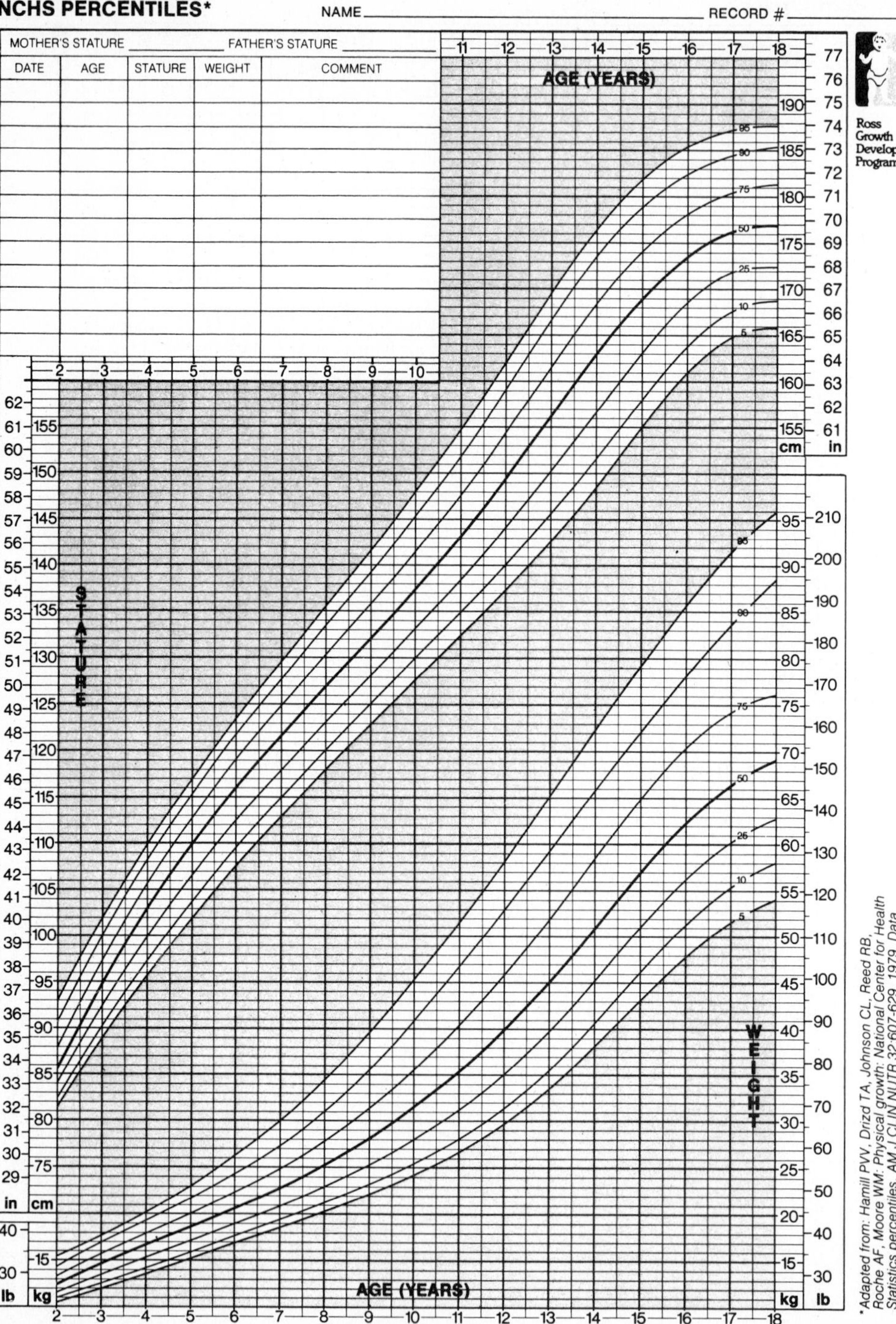

*Adapted from: Hamill PVV, Drizd TA, Johnson CL, Reed RB, Roche AF, Moore WM: Physical growth: National Center for Health Statistics percentiles. AM J CLIN NUTR 32:607-629, 1979. Data from the National Center for Health Statistics (NCHS), Hyattsville, Maryland.

GIRLS: PREPUBESCENT PHYSICAL GROWTH NCHS PERCENTILES*

NAME ______ RECORD # ______

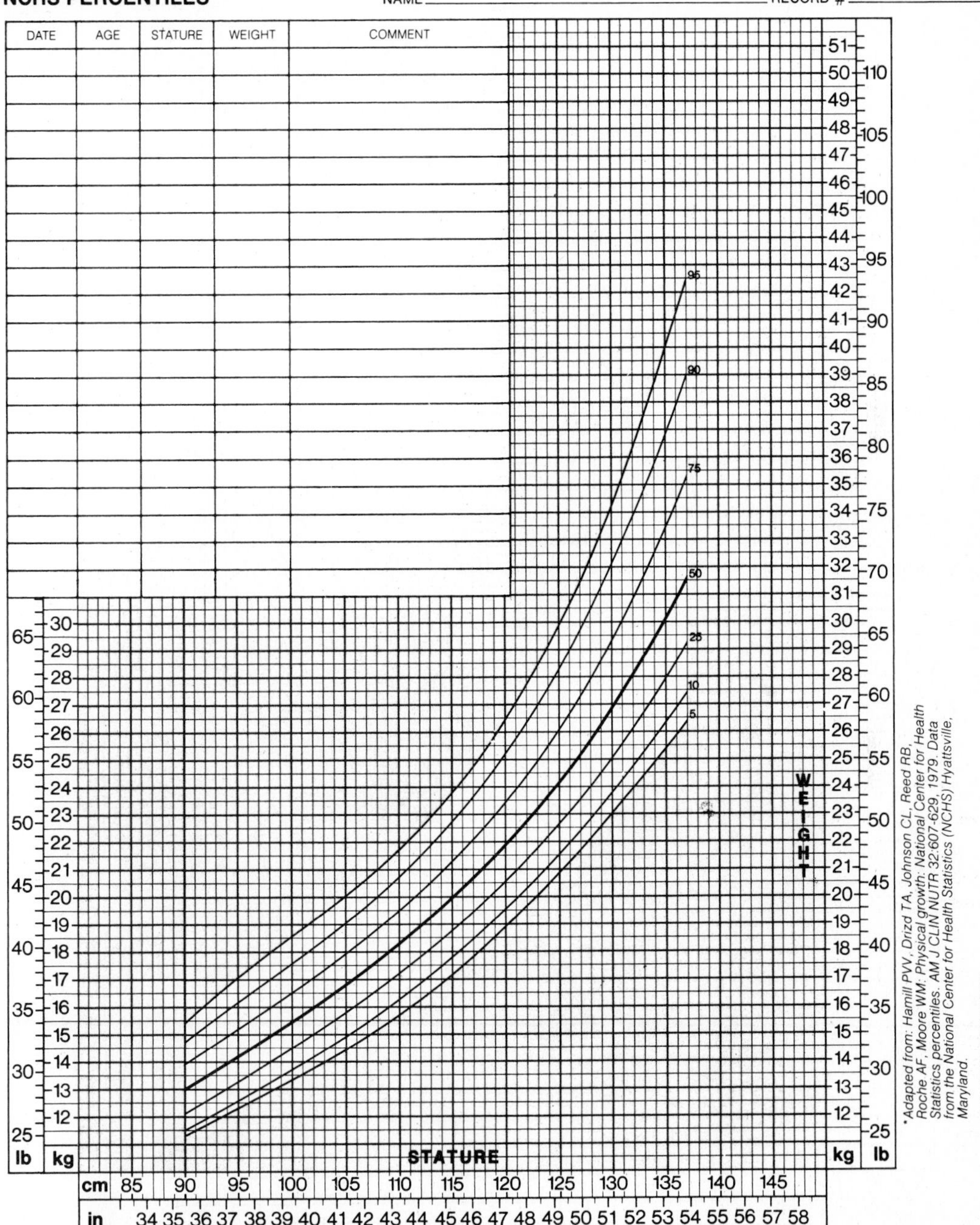

*Adapted from: Hamill PVV, Drizd TA, Johnson CL, Reed RB, Roche AF, Moore WM: Physical growth: National Center for Health Statistics percentiles. AM J CLIN NUTR 32:607-629, 1979. Data from the National Center for Health Statistics (NCHS) Hyattsville, Maryland.

BOYS: PREPUBESCENT PHYSICAL GROWTH NCHS PERCENTILES*

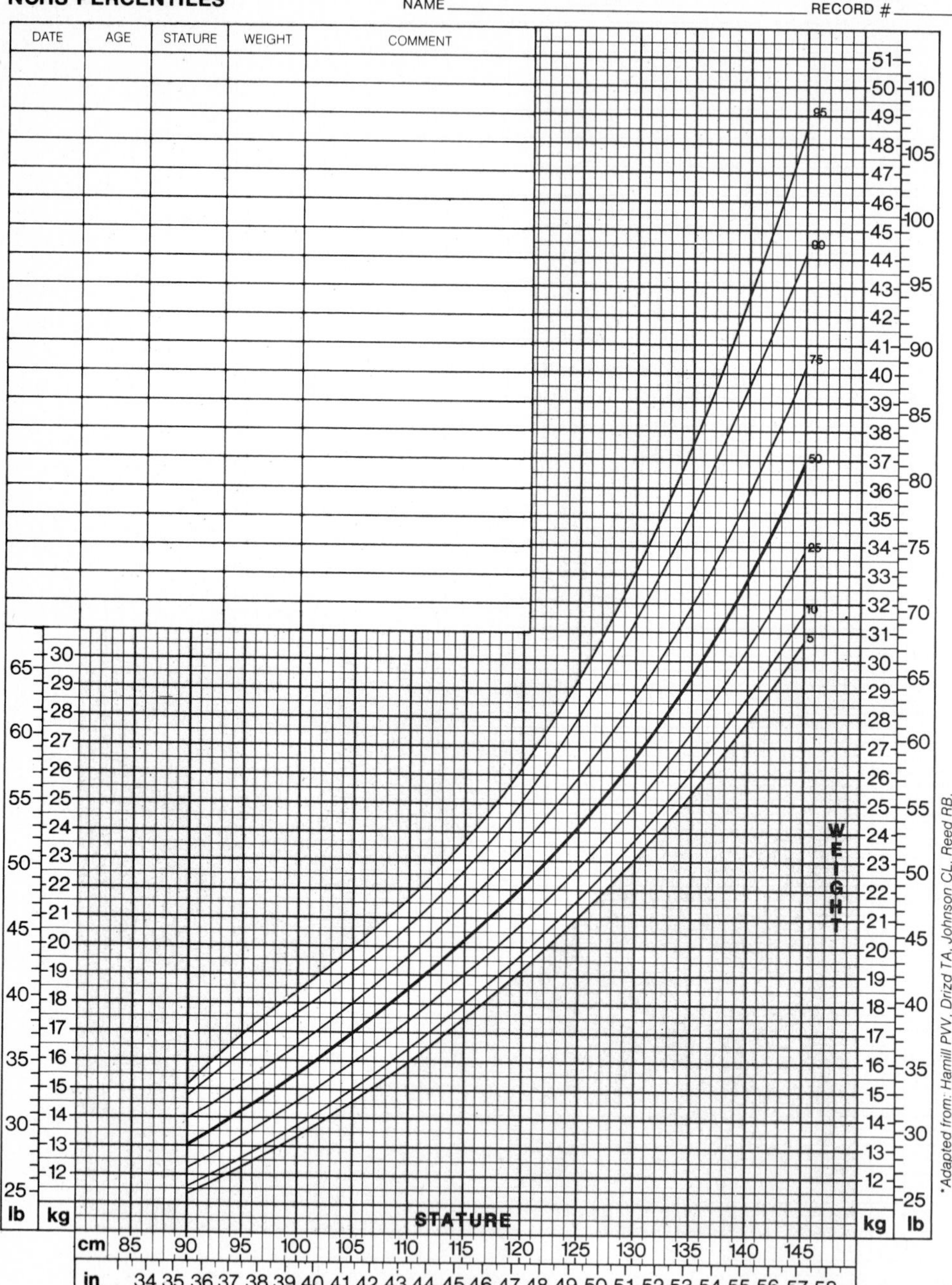

*Adapted from: Hamill PVV, Drizd TA, Johnson CL, Reed RB, Roche AF, Moore WM: Physical growth: National Center for Health Statistics percentiles. AM J CLIN NUTR 32:607-629, 1979. Data from the National Center for Health Statistics (NCHS) Hyattsville, Maryland.

Appendix B

Mid-Upper-Arm Circumference Percentiles (cm)

	Female Percentiles					Male Percentiles				
Age (yr)	5th	25th	50th	75th	95th	5th	25th	50th	75th	95th
1	13.8	14.8	15.6	16.4	17.7	14.2	15.0	15.9	17.0	18.3
2	14.2	15.2	16.0	16.7	18.4	14.1	15.3	16.2	17.0	18.5
3	14.3	15.8	16.7	17.5	18.9	15.0	16.0	16.7	17.5	19.0
4	14.9	16.0	16.9	17.7	19.1	14.9	16.2	17.1	18.0	19.2
5	15.3	16.5	17.5	18.5	21.1	15.3	16.7	17.5	18.5	20.4
6	15.6	17.0	17.6	18.7	21.1	15.5	16.7	17.9	18.8	22.8
7	16.4	17.4	18.3	19.9	23.1	16.2	17.7	18.7	20.1	23.0
8	16.8	18.3	19.5	21.4	26.1	16.2	17.7	19.0	20.2	24.5
9	17.8	19.4	21.1	22.4	26.0	17.5	18.7	20.0	21.7	25.7
10	17.4	19.3	21.0	22.8	26.5	18.1	19.6	21.0	23.1	27.4
11	18.5	20.8	22.4	24.8	30.3	18.6	20.2	22.3	24.4	28.0
12	19.4	21.6	23.7	25.6	29.4	19.3	21.4	23.2	25.4	30.3
13	20.2	22.3	24.3	27.1	33.8	19.4	22.8	24.7	26.3	30.1
14	21.4	23.7	25.2	27.2	32.2	22.0	23.7	25.3	28.3	32.3
15	20.8	23.9	25.4	27.9	32.2	22.2	24.4	26.4	28.4	32.0
16	21.8	24.1	25.8	28.3	33.4	24.4	26.2	27.8	30.3	34.3
17	22.0	24.1	26.4	29.5	35.0	24.6	26.7	28.5	30.8	34.7
18	22.2	24.1	25.8	28.1	32.5	24.5	27.6	29.7	32.1	37.9
19-25	21.1	24.7	26.5	29.0	34.5	26.2	28.8	30.8	33.1	37.2
25-35	23.3	25.6	27.7	30.4	36.8	27.1	30.0	31.9	34.2	37.5
35-45	24.1	26.7	29.0	31.7	37.8	27.8	30.5	32.6	34.5	37.4
45-55	24.2	27.4	29.9	32.8	38.4	26.7	30.1	32.2	34.2	37.6
55-65	24.3	28.0	30.3	33.5	38.5	25.8	29.6	31.7	33.6	36.9
65-75	24.0	27.4	29.9	32.6	37.3	24.8	28.5	30.7	32.5	35.5

Data derived from the Health and Nutrition Examination Survey data of 1971-1974, using same population samples as those of the National Center for Health Statistics (NCHS) growth percentiles for children. Adapted from Frisancho, A.R.: New norms of upper limb fat and muscle areas for assessment of nutritional status, Am. J. Clin. Nutr. 34:2540, 1981.

Appendix C

Triceps Skinfold Percentiles (mm)

	Female Percentiles					Male Percentiles				
Age (yr)	5th	25th	50th	75th	95th	5th	25th	50th	75th	95th
1	6	8	10	12	16	6	8	10	12	16
2	6	9	10	12	16	6	8	10	12	15
3	7	9	11	12	15	6	8	10	11	15
4	7	8	10	12	16	6	8	9	11	14
5	6	8	10	12	18	6	8	9	11	15
6	6	8	10	12	16	5	7	8	10	16
7	6	9	11	13	18	5	7	9	12	17
8	6	9	12	15	24	5	7	8	10	16
9	8	10	13	16	22	6	7	10	13	18
10	7	10	12	17	27	6	8	10	14	21
11	7	10	13	18	28	6	8	11	16	24
12	8	11	14	18	27	6	8	11	14	28
13	8	12	15	21	30	5	7	10	14	26
14	9	13	16	21	28	4	7	9	14	24
15	8	12	17	21	32	4	6	8	11	24
16	10	15	18	22	31	4	6	8	12	22
17	10	13	19	24	37	5	6	8	12	19
18	10	15	18	22	30	4	6	9	13	24
19-25	10	14	18	24	34	4	7	10	15	22
25-35	10	16	21	27	37	5	8	12	16	24
35-45	12	18	23	29	38	5	8	12	16	23
45-55	12	20	25	30	40	6	8	12	15	25
55-65	12	20	25	31	38	5	8	11	14	22
65-75	12	18	24	29	36	4	8	11	15	22

Data derived from the Health and Nutrition Examination Survey data of 1971-1974, using same population samples as those of the National Center for Health Statistics (NCHS) growth percentiles for children. Adapted from Frisancho, A.R.: New norms of upper limb fat and muscle areas for assessment of nutritional status, Am. J. Clin. Nutr. 34:2540, 1981.

Appendix D

Mid-Upper-Arm Muscle Circumference Percentiles (cm)

	Female Percentiles					Male Percentiles				
Age (yr)	5th	25th	50th	75th	95th	5th	25th	50th	75th	95th
1	10.5	11.7	12.4	13.9	14.3	11.0	11.9	12.7	13.5	14.7
2	11.1	11.9	12.6	13.3	14.7	11.1	12.2	13.0	14.0	15.0
3	11.3	12.4	13.2	14.0	15.2	11.7	13.1	13.7	14.3	15.3
4	11.5	12.8	13.8	14.4	15.7	12.3	13.3	14.1	14.8	15.9
5	12.5	13.4	14.2	15.1	16.5	12.8	14.0	14.7	15.4	16.9
6	13.0	13.8	14.5	15.4	17.1	13.1	14.2	15.1	16.1	17.7
7	12.9	14.2	15.1	16.0	17.6	13.7	15.1	16.0	16.8	19.0
8	13.8	15.1	16.0	17.1	19.4	14.0	15.4	16.2	17.0	18.7
9	14.7	15.8	16.7	18.0	19.8	15.1	16.1	17.0	18.3	20.2
10	14.8	15.9	17.0	18.0	19.7	15.6	16.6	18.0	19.1	22.1
11	15.0	17.1	18.1	19.6	22.3	15.9	17.3	18.3	19.5	23.0
12	16.2	18.0	19.1	20.1	22.0	16.7	18.2	19.5	21.0	24.1
13	16.9	18.3	19.8	21.1	24.0	17.2	19.6	21.1	22.6	24.5
14	17.4	19.0	20.1	21.6	24.7	18.9	21.2	22.3	24.0	26.4
15	17.5	18.9	20.2	21.5	24.4	19.9	21.8	23.7	25.4	27.2
16	17.0	19.0	20.2	21.6	24.9	21.3	23.4	24.9	26.9	29.6
17	17.5	19.4	20.5	22.1	25.7	22.4	24.5	25.8	27.3	31.2
18	17.4	19.1	20.2	21.5	24.5	22.6	25.2	26.4	28.3	32.4
19-25	17.9	19.5	20.7	22.1	24.9	23.8	25.7	27.3	28.9	32.1
25-35	18.3	19.9	21.2	22.8	26.4	24.3	26.4	27.9	29.8	32.6
35-45	18.6	20.5	21.8	23.6	27.2	24.7	26.9	28.6	30.2	32.7
45-55	18.7	20.6	22.0	23.8	27.4	23.9	26.5	28.1	30.0	32.6
55-65	18.7	20.9	22.5	24.4	28.0	23.6	26.0	27.8	29.5	32.0
65-75	18.5	20.8	22.5	24.4	27.9	22.3	25.1	26.8	28.4	30.6

Values derived by formula calculation. Data derived from the Health and Nutrition Examination Survey data of 1971-1974, using same population samples as those of the National Center for Health Statistics (NCHS) growth percentiles for children. Adapted from Frisancho, A.R.: New norms of upper limb fat and muscle areas for assessment of nutritional status, Am. J. Clin. Nutr. 34:2540, 1981.

Appendix E

*Weight-Height of Youths Aged 12-17 Years**

Weight-Height of Youths Aged 12 Years (kg/cm)

Sex and Height	n	N	$\overline{X}$	s	$s_{\overline{x}}$	Percentile						
						5th	10th	25th	50th	75th	90th	95th
MALE			IN KILOGRAMS									
Under 130 cm	5	15	*	*	*	*	*	*	*	*	*	*
130.0-134.9 cm	4	8	*	*	*	*	*	*	*	*	*	*
135.0-139.9 cm	34	111	32.50	3.741	0.727	26.6	27.6	30.2	31.6	34.7	37.7	39.4
140.0-144.9 cm	80	241	34.28	3.635	0.601	28.1	30.0	31.8	34.1	36.5	38.6	40.7
145.0-149.9 cm	123	386	39.27	6.243	0.615	32.1	33.2	35.7	38.2	40.9	46.1	52.5
150.0-154.9 cm	156	513	42.90	6.314	0.480	34.9	36.1	38.2	42.1	46.0	51.6	56.3
155.0-159.9 cm	135	432	47.35	7.551	0.769	38.3	39.4	41.9	46.2	50.5	57.4	61.9
160.0-164.9 cm	65	201	50.82	8.735	1.388	42.1	42.7	44.9	48.4	56.0	61.1	67.1
165.0-169.9 cm	29	88	55.75	8.811	2.031	43.3	46.4	49.0	54.4	59.9	68.3	76.6
170.0-174.9 cm	8	21	62.37	4.503	1.993	54.0	58.1	60.1	61.0	66.0	69.1	69.5
175.0-179.9 cm	3	10	*	*	*	*	*	*	*	*	*	*
180.0-184.9 cm	1	2	*	*	*	*	*	*	*	*	*	*
185.0-189.9 cm	—	—	—	—	—	—	—	—	—	—	—	—
190.0-194.9 cm	—	—	—	—	—	—	—	—	—	—	—	—
195.0 cm and over	—	—	—	—	—	—	—	—	—	—	—	—

NOTE: n = sample size; N = estimated number of youths in population in thousands; $\overline{X}$ = mean; s = standard deviation; $s_{\overline{x}}$ = standard error of the mean.

*From National Center for Health Statistics: Height and weight of youths 12-17 years, United States. In Vital and health statistics, series 11, no. 124, Health Services and Mental Health Administration, Washington, D.C., 1973, U.S. Government Printing Office.

Weight-Height of Youths Aged 12 Years (kg/cm) —cont'd

Sex and Height	n	N	$\overline{X}$	s	$s_{\overline{x}}$	Percentile						
						5th	10th	25th	50th	75th	90th	95th
FEMALE			IN KILOGRAMS									
Under 130 cm	—	—	—	—	—	—	—	—	—	—	—	—
130.0-134.9 cm	3	10	*	*	*	*	*	*	*	*	*	*
135.0-139.9 cm	12	44	29.41	3.372	0.914	25.0	25.0	26.4	28.9	32.1	34.1	34.2
140.0-144.9 cm	32	116	38.30	7.314	1.194	28.8	30.6	33.3	36.8	41.4	49.2	55.1
145.0-149.9 cm	72	258	39.78	6.205	0.975	31.8	32.8	35.5	38.5	42.8	48.3	50.6
150.0-154.9 cm	147	517	44.00	7.421	0.677	34.4	35.8	38.9	42.8	47.4	52.9	57.4
155.0-159.9 cm	144	525	48.74	8.369	0.714	37.9	39.2	43.0	46.8	53.8	60.7	63.5
160.0-164.9 cm	95	336	53.06	8.010	0.658	42.5	43.9	47.2	51.1	57.2	65.6	69.6
165.0-169.9 cm	31	117	54.89	7.022	1.384	43.9	47.1	50.4	53.1	59.7	64.5	71.3
170.0-174.9 cm	11	42	63.66	14.501	6.214	48.7	50.1	50.8	56.7	82.2	86.0	86.1
175.0-179.9 cm	—	—	—	—	—	—	—	—	—	—	—	—
180.0-184.9 cm	—	—	—	—	—	—	—	—	—	—	—	—
185.0-189.9 cm	—	—	—	—	—	—	—	—	—	—	—	—
190.0-194.9 cm	—	—	—	—	—	—	—	—	—	—	—	—
195.0 cm. and over	—	—	—	—	—	—	—	—	—	—	—	—

NOTE: n = sample size; N = estimated number of youths in population in thousands; $\overline{X}$ = mean; s = standard deviation; $s_{\overline{x}}$ = standard error of the mean.

Weight-Height of Youths Aged 13 Years (kg/cm)

Sex and Height	n	N	$\overline{X}$	s	$s_{\overline{x}}$	Percentile						
						5th	10th	25th	50th	75th	90th	95th
			IN KILOGRAMS									
MALE												
Under 130 cm	—	—	—	—	—	—	—	—	—	—	—	—
130.0-134.9 cm	2	5	*	*	*	*	*	*	*	*	*	*
135.0-139.9 cm	6	25	32.62	5.624	7.716	27.2	27.6	28.9	31.0	34.9	43.1	43.2
140.0-144.9 cm	18	56	36.54	5.852	1.607	30.0	30.5	32.1	36.1	39.2	41.7	53.2
145.0-149.9 cm	65	204	39.03	5.270	0.662	32.4	33.9	36.1	37.9	41.2	44.5	46.4
150.0-154.9 cm	99	312	42.58	6.724	0.865	34.8	36.2	37.9	41.0	45.5	49.4	61.0
155.0-159.9 cm	131	421	47.27	7.482	0.717	37.8	39.2	41.7	45.8	51.1	58.7	61.7
160.0-164.9 cm	125	393	53.01	9.324	0.916	41.5	43.7	46.9	50.4	58.2	64.4	72.5
165.0-169.9 cm	91	285	55.92	8.560	0.833	46.3	47.5	49.3	53.6	59.4	69.0	75.0
170.0-174.9 cm	63	215	62.01	10.362	1.033	51.2	51.6	53.7	60.1	67.0	76.0	85.0
175.0-179.9 cm	19	68	67.92	12.085	3.428	56.3	57.9	60.1	63.3	70.3	88.3	89.0
180.0-184.9 cm	5	15	*	*	*	*	*	*	*	*	*	*
185.0-189.9 cm	—	—	—	—	—	—	—	—	—	—	—	—
190.0-194.9 cm	—	—	—	—	—	—	—	—	—	—	—	—
195.0 cm. and over	—	—	—	—	—	—	—	—	—	—	—	—
FEMALE												
Under 130 cm	—	—	—	—	—	—	—	—	—	—	—	—
130.0-134.9 cm	1	3	*	*	*	*	*	*	*	*	*	*
135.0-139.9 cm	—	—	—	—	—	—	—	—	—	—	—	—
140.0-144.9 cm	15	51	37.13	7.317	2.259	26.6	27.5	30.5	36.7	40.1	44.5	56.1
145.0-149.9 cm	47	165	42.23	6.880	0.888	34.7	35.6	38.2	40.5	44.2	53.6	57.6
150.0-154.9 cm	98	329	44.32	7.029	0.787	35.6	36.5	39.2	42.9	47.3	53.7	57.9
155.0-159.9 cm	152	499	49.75	8.757	0.699	39.1	39.9	43.8	48.4	53.8	61.0	65.9
160.0-164.9 cm	156	515	53.16	8.399	0.522	41.2	43.9	47.7	52.2	57.0	63.8	68.5
165.0-169.9 cm	86	284	58.17	9.125	0.921	46.2	47.4	52.2	58.1	61.5	69.3	76.2
170.0-174.9 cm	24	87	58.11	13.209	2.343	46.2	47.1	48.4	52.9	65.3	68.6	96.8
175.0-179.9 cm	3	10	*	*	*	*	*	*	*	*	*	*
180.0-184.9 cm	—	—	—	—	—	—	—	—	—	—	—	—
185.0-189.9 cm	—	—	—	—	—	—	—	—	—	—	—	—
190.0-194.9 cm	—	—	—	—	—	—	—	—	—	—	—	—
195.0 cm. and over	—	—	—	—	—	—	—	—	—	—	—	—

NOTE: n = sample size; N = estimated number of youths in population in thousands; $\overline{X}$ = mean; s = standard deviation; $s_{\overline{x}}$ = standard error of the mean.

Weight-Height of Youths Aged 14 Years (kg/cm)

Sex and Height	n	N	$\overline{X}$	s	$s_{\overline{x}}$	Percentile 5th	10th	25th	50th	75th	90th	95th
			IN KILOGRAMS									
MALE												
Under 130 cm	—	—	—	—	—	—	—	—	—	—	—	—
130.0-134.9 cm	—	—	—	—	—	—	—	—	—	—	—	—
135.0-139.9 cm	2	7	*	*	*	*	*	*	*	*	*	*
140.0-144.9 cm	3	13	*	*	*	*	*	*	*	*	*	*
145.0-149.9 cm	11	42	40.51	1.829	0.644	36.9	38.6	39.6	40.6	42.0	42.5	42.7
150.0-154.9 cm	45	135	43.63	6.277	1.182	36.2	37.0	39.0	41.4	48.0	51.7	55.3
155.0-159.9 cm	83	261	47.42	7.822	0.872	37.7	38.7	41.8	46.1	51.2	58.0	62.7
160.0-164.9 cm	96	299	52.28	6.785	0.584	42.5	44.0	47.5	52.1	56.3	61.5	65.1
165.0-169.9 cm	134	432	58.07	9.416	1.054	47.7	49.3	51.6	55.4	62.3	70.6	75.7
170.0-174.9 cm	144	435	62.37	11.516	1.095	49.7	51.0	55.0	59.4	65.6	79.2	86.3
175.0-179.9 cm	71	228	65.54	9.704	1.306	50.9	55.1	58.5	64.7	69.9	74.5	84.0
180.0-184.9 cm	25	81	72.44	13.014	2.298	59.6	60.0	65.1	69.4	77.0	83.0	94.3
185.0-189.9 cm	3	9	*	*	*	*	*	*	*	*	*	*
190.0-194.9 cm	1	3	*	*	*	*	*	*	*	*	*	*
195.0 cm. and over	—	—	—	—	—	—	—	—	—	—	—	—
FEMALE												
Under 130 cm	—	—	—	—	—	—	—	—	—	—	—	—
130.0-134.9 cm	—	—	—	—	—	—	—	—	—	—	—	—
135.0-139.9 cm	1	2	*	*	*	*	*	*	*	*	*	*
140.0-144.9 cm	2	6	*	*	*	*	*	*	*	*	*	*
145.0-149.9 cm	17	52	42.00	5.879	1.683	32.0	35.3	36.3	42.3	47.5	49.5	51.1
150.0-154.9 cm	64	196	48.26	6.797	0.926	37.7	39.2	42.5	47.9	53.3	55.9	58.8
155.0-159.9 cm	157	508	51.35	7.705	0.520	42.1	43.4	46.3	49.6	55.6	62.2	64.3
160.0-164.9 cm	186	603	54.59	8.810	0.707	43.0	45.0	48.4	53.0	59.7	66.7	70.7
165.0-169.9 cm	114	372	58.46	10.185	0.955	45.9	47.5	52.1	56.8	61.8	70.5	76.4
170.0-174.9 cm	36	121	64.37	15.821	2.814	49.2	52.1	56.2	59.8	70.5	72.9	99.4
175.0-179.9 cm	7	28	61.33	5.496	2.620	51.7	52.0	57.7	59.8	64.6	70.2	70.6
180.0-184.9 cm	2	7	*	*	*	*	*	*	*	*	*	*
185.0-189.9 cm	—	—	—	—	—	—	—	—	—	—	—	—
190.0-194.9 cm	—	—	—	—	—	—	—	—	—	—	—	—
195.0 cm. and over	—	—	—	—	—	—	—	—	—	—	—	—

NOTE: n = sample size; N = estimated number of youths in population in thousands; $\overline{X}$ = mean; s = standard deviation; $s_{\overline{x}}$ = standard error of the mean.

Weight-Height of Youths Aged 15 Years (kg/cm)

Sex and Height	n	N	$\overline{X}$	s	$s_{\overline{x}}$	Percentile						
						5th	10th	25th	50th	75th	90th	95th
MALE			IN KILOGRAMS									
Under 130 cm	—	—	—	—	—	—	—	—	—	—	—	—
130.0-134.9 cm	—	—	—	—	—	—	—	—	—	—	—	—
135.0-139.9 cm	—	—	—	—	—	—	—	—	—	—	—	—
140.0-144.9 cm	—	—	—	—	—	—	—	—	—	—	—	—
145.0-149.9 cm	1	2	*	*	*	*	*	*	*	*	*	*
150.0-154.9 cm	10	30	45.72	8.582	3.550	35.7	39.2	42.6	44.7	46.0	48.7	76.1
155.0-159.9 cm	34	99	52.81	10.552	1.695	40.3	43.1	46.7	49.2	56.7	69.6	76.3
160.0-164.9 cm	71	206	53.01	8.417	0.986	42.7	44.1	46.9	51.5	56.3	65.3	68.8
165.0-169.9 cm	132	404	57.72	8.503	0.819	48.0	48.8	53.1	56.4	61.3	67.1	73.3
170.0-174.9 cm	176	574	62.88	8.464	0.633	51.6	53.4	56.7	61.9	67.2	72.9	78.1
175.0-179.9 cm	118	374	65.80	9.457	1.045	53.1	55.6	59.7	64.3	69.5	80.2	89.2
180.0-184.9 cm	51	144	72.00	11.928	1.724	54.6	60.3	64.4	70.2	68.4	84.4	96.6
185.0-189.9 cm	14	48	74.21	15.035	5.200	58.3	58.5	62.9	70.7	84.6	92.4	110.8
190.0-194.9 cm	6	15	83.39	16.431	10.332	66.4	66.7	69.6	73.8	103.0	105.7	106.2
195.0 cm. and over	—	—	—	—	—	—	—	—	—	—	—	—
FEMALE												
Under 130 cm	—	—	—	—	—	—	—	—	—	—	—	—
130.0-134.9 cm	—	—	—	—	—	—	—	—	—	—	—	—
135.0-139.9 cm	—	—	—	—	—	—	—	—	—	—	—	—
140.0-144.9 cm	2	5	*	*	*	*	*	*	*	*	*	*
145.0-149.9 cm	15	51	47.91	7.875	3.623	36.0	39.4	42.1	45.4	52.7	55.7	66.3
150.0-154.9 cm	69	242	49.69	8.895	1.190	39.1	40.6	44.3	48.1	52.8	60.5	68.3
155.0-159.9 cm	111	400	51.52	8.473	0.934	41.4	43.5	46.3	50.8	55.1	59.8	65.2
160.0-164.9 cm	137	509	57.03	10.828	0.875	45.1	47.3	50.2	55.0	60.2	71.7	77.7
165.0-169.9 cm	109	398	60.71	10.357	1.053	47.5	49.3	55.1	58.4	65.7	74.1	81.0
170.0-174.9 cm	49	188	65.27	10.730	1.880	49.7	53.6	57.2	61.2	71.6	85.3	86.4
175.0-179.9 cm	7	23	63.30	8.872	4.807	49.7	49.9	53.8	62.4	71.1	71.9	79.2
180.0-184.9 cm	3	26	*	*	*	*	*	*	*	*	*	*
185.0-189.9 cm	1	3	*	*	*	*	*	*	*	*	*	*
190.0-194.9 cm	—	—	—	—	—	—	—	—	—	—	—	—
195.0 cm. and over	—	—	—	—	—	—	—	—	—	—	—	—

NOTE: n = sample size; N = estimated number of youths in population in thousands; $\overline{X}$ = mean; s = standard deviation: $s_{\overline{x}}$ = standard error of the mean.

Weight-Height of Youths Aged 16 Years (kg/cm)

Sex and Height	n	N	$\overline{X}$	s	$s_{\overline{x}}$	Percentile 5th	10th	25th	50th	75th	90th	95th
MALE						IN KILOGRAMS						
Under 130 cm	—	—	—	—	—	—	—	—	—	—	—	—
130.0-134.9 cm	—	—	—	—	—	—	—	—	—	—	—	—
135.0-139.9 cm	—	—	—	—	—	—	—	—	—	—	—	—
140.0-144.9 cm	—	—	—	—	—	—	—	—	—	—	—	—
145.0-149.9 cm	1	1	*	*	*	*	*	*	*	*	*	*
150.0-154.9 cm	4	12	*	*	*	*	*	*	*	*	*	*
155.0-159.9 cm	11	33	49.89	7.323	3.572	42.0	42.2	44.7	46.8	54.4	59.8	67.2
160.0-164.9 cm	32	108	53.09	6.459	1.273	44.2	44.9	48.2	51.4	58.0	60.9	66.1
165.0-169.9 cm	87	275	59.39	9.178	0.981	48.5	49.8	52.7	58.0	63.9	69.3	75.9
170.0-174.9 cm	166	552	62.66	7.556	0.629	51.6	53.8	57.5	61.6	67.1	73.1	78.0
175.0-179.9 cm	149	511	67.33	9.018	0.856	56.3	58.2	61.0	65.4	72.5	80.1	83.8
180.0-184.9 cm	72	227	72.38	12.485	1.993	58.3	59.3	64.4	68.9	76.5	90.2	96.9
185.0-189.9 cm	29	95	81.06	14.268	3.265	63.7	66.6	69.7	78.4	90.3	97.0	111.4
190.0-194.9 cm	3	10	*	*	*	*	*	*	*	*	*	*
195.0 cm. and over	2	7	*	*	*	*	*	*	*	*	*	*
FEMALE												
Under 130 cm	—	—	—	—	—	—	—	—	—	—	—	—
130.0-134.9 cm	—	—	—	—	—	—	—	—	—	—	—	—
135.0-139.9 cm	—	—	—	—	—	—	—	—	—	—	—	—
140.0-144.9 cm	2	5	*	*	*	*	*	*	*	*	*	*
145.0-149.9 cm	10	33	52.58	8.198	3.191	43.9	44.1	44.9	51.0	54.5	72.0	72.1
150.0-154.9 cm	57	178	51.79	10.457	1.053	41.4	42.0	45.8	48.9	54.1	61.5	83.3
155.0-159.9 cm	117	354	53.20	7.766	0.734	44.0	45.6	48.4	51.6	56.4	61.9	69.0
160.0-164.9 cm	160	547	57.71	11.129	1.246	46.1	47.3	51.5	55.5	61.2	69.5	75.1
165.0-169.9 cm	122	450	61.72	11.998	0.802	47.1	48.8	53.3	59.1	67.3	78.7	86.7
170.0-174.9 cm	53	170	63.61	8.734	1.126	52.9	53.8	58.1	62.1	66.8	73.8	84.2
175.0-179.9 cm	14	45	72.55	15.012	5.224	58.6	58.8	61.7	65.9	80.6	99.1	105.5
180.0-184.9 cm	1	2	*	*	*	*	*	*	*	*	*	*
185.0-189.9 cm	—	—	—	—	—	—	—	—	—	—	—	—
190.0-194.9 cm	—	—	—	—	—	—	—	—	—	—	—	—
195.0 cm. and over	—	—	—	—	—	—	—	—	—	—	—	—

NOTE: n = sample size; N = estimated number of youths in population in thousands; $\overline{X}$ = mean; s = standard deviation: $s_{\overline{x}}$ = standard error of the mean.

Weight-Height of Youths Aged 17 Years (kg/cm)

Sex and Height	n	N	$\overline{X}$	s	$s_{\overline{x}}$	Percentile 5th	10th	25th	50th	75th	90th	95th
MALE						IN KILOGRAMS						
Under 130 cm	—	—	—	—	—	—	—	—	—	—	—	—
130.0-134.9 cm	—	—	—	—	—	—	—	—	—	—	—	—
135.0-139.9 cm	—	—	—	—	—	—	—	—	—	—	—	—
140.0-144.9 cm	—	—	—	—	—	—	—	—	—	—	—	—
145.0-149.9 cm	—	—	—	—	—	—	—	—	—	—	—	—
150.0-154.9 cm	1	3	*	*	*	*	*	*	*	*	*	*
155.0-159.9 cm	11	39	54.63	9.397	3.414	43.8	46.4	48.2	49.7	57.8	69.9	73.2
160.0-164.9 cm	25	81	57.75	6.503	1.355	49.7	51.1	52.5	56.9	61.6	70.1	70.8
165.0-169.9 cm	63	248	62.57	8.344	1.224	50.2	53.2	56.4	61.5	66.9	72.7	77.3
170.0-174.9 cm	115	396	67.06	11.163	0.704	53.3	55.5	59.5	64.6	71.9	80.9	91.6
175.0-179.9 cm	151	537	68.37	9.907	0.831	56.9	58.9	61.5	66.5	73.6	79.4	88.4
180.0-184.9 cm	80	297	73.31	12.454	1.335	59.6	61.0	65.1	71.2	78.4	91.8	102.7
185.0-189.9 cm	36	133	76.03	9.171	1.301	62.4	66.3	70.5	75.3	80.8	90.3	92.9
190.0-194.9 cm	7	25	81.40	10.985	7.588	62.9	62.9	67.8	87.3	90.3	90.6	90.6
195.0 cm. and over	—	—	—	—	—	—	—	—	—	—	—	—
FEMALE												
Under 130 cm	—	—	—	—	—	—	—	—	—	—	—	—
130.0-134.9 cm	—	—	—	—	—	—	—	—	—	—	—	—
135.0-139.9 cm	—	—	—	—	—	—	—	—	—	—	—	—
140.0-144.9 cm	2	5	*	*	*	*	*	*	*	*	*	*
145.0-149.9 cm	8	26	43.49	3.939	1.604	38.6	38.8	40.1	45.1	45.7	51.1	51.2
150.0-154.9 cm	43	151	49.96	6.508	0.827	41.6	42.3	44.6	48.9	53.5	59.2	64.1
155.0-159.9 cm	103	385	54.71	9.903	0.775	44.4	45.5	48.7	53.2	57.7	61.6	76.2
160.0-164.9 cm	133	506	57.79	10.620	1.028	46.8	48.0	50.2	55.4	61.5	72.3	82.3
165.0-169.9 cm	116	433	60.63	10.117	1.182	47.9	50.3	55.1	59.3	65.1	69.4	71.6
170.0-174.9 cm	51	186	62.18	9.132	1.407	50.6	52.9	55.5	60.2	65.7	76.1	82.7
175.0-179.9 cm	12	47	65.76	8.405	2.229	54.9	56.7	60.1	61.7	75.2	75.9	83.0
180.0-184.9 cm	1	2	*	*	*	*	*	*	*	*	*	*
185.0-189.9 cm	—	—	—	—	—	—	—	—	—	—	—	—
190.0-194.9 cm	—	—	—	—	—	—	—	—	—	—	—	—
195.0 cm. and over	—	—	—	—	—	—	—	—	—	—	—	—

NOTE: n = sample size; N = estimated number of youths in population in thousands; $\overline{X}$ = mean; s = standard deviation; $s_{\overline{x}}$ = standard error of the mean.

Weight-Height of Youths Aged 12 Years (lb/in)

Sex and Height	n	N	$\overline{X}$	s	$s_{\overline{x}}$	Percentile						
						5th	10th	25th	50th	75th	90th	95th
MALE			IN POUNDS									
Under 51.18 in	5	15	*	*	*	*	*	*	*	*	*	*
51.18-53.15 in	4	8	*	*	*	*	*	*	*	*	*	*
53.15-55.12 in	34	111	71.65	8.248	1.603	54.6	60.8	66.6	69.7	76.5	83.1	86.9
55.12-57.09 in	80	241	75.57	8.014	1.325	61.9	66.1	70.1	75.2	80.5	85.1	89.7
57.09-59.06 in	123	386	86.58	13.764	1.356	70.8	73.2	78.7	84.2	90.2	101.6	115.7
59.06-61.02 in	156	513	94.58	13.920	1.058	76.9	79.6	84.2	92.8	101.4	113.8	124.1
61.02-62.99 in	135	433	104.39	16.647	1.695	84.4	86.9	92.4	101.9	111.3	126.5	136.5
62.99-64.96 in	65	201	112.04	19.257	3.060	92.8	94.1	99.0	106.7	123.5	134.7	147.9
64.96-66.93 in	29	88	122.91	19.425	4.478	95.5	102.3	108.0	119.9	132.1	150.6	168.9
66.93-68.90 in	8	21	137.50	9.927	4.394	119.0	128.1	132.5	134.5	145.5	152.3	153.2
68.90-70.87 in	3	10	*	*	*	*	*	*	*	*	*	*
70.87-72.83 in	1	2	*	*	*	*	*	*	*	*	*	*
72.83-74.80 in	—	—	—	—	—	—	—	—	—	—	—	—
74.80-76.77 in	—	—	—	—	—	—	—	—	—	—	—	—
76.77 and over	—	—	—	—	—	—	—	—	—	—	—	—
FEMALE												
Under 51.18 in	—	—	—	—	—	—	—	—	—	—	—	—
51.18-53.15 in	3	10	*	*	*	*	*	*	*	*	*	*
53.15-55.12 in	12	44	64.84	7.434	2.015	55.1	55.1	58.2	63.7	70.8	75.2	75.4
55.12-57.09 in	32	116	84.44	16.125	2.632	63.5	67.5	73.4	81.1	91.3	108.5	121.5
57.09-59.06 in	72	258	87.70	13.680	2.150	70.1	72.3	78.3	78.9	94.4	106.5	111.6
59.06-61.02 in	147	517	97.00	16.361	1.493	75.8	78.9	85.8	94.4	104.5	116.6	126.5
61.02-62.99 in	144	525	107.45	18.451	1.574	83.6	86.4	94.8	103.2	118.6	133.8	140.0
62.99-64.96 in	95	336	117.00	17.659	1.451	93.7	96.8	104.1	112.7	126.1	144.6	153.4
64.96-66.93 in	31	117	121.01	15.481	3.051	96.8	103.8	111.1	117.1	131.6	142.2	157.2
66.93-68.90 in	11	42	140.35	31.969	13.700	107.4	110.5	112.0	125.0	181.2	189.6	189.8
68.90-70.87 in	—	—	—	—	—	—	—	—	—	—	—	—
70.87-72.83 in	—	—	—	—	—	—	—	—	—	—	—	—
72.83-74.80 in	—	—	—	—	—	—	—	—	—	—	—	—
74.80-76.77 in	—	—	—	—	—	—	—	—	—	—	—	—
76.77 in. and over	—	—	—	—	—	—	—	—	—	—	—	—

NOTE: n = sample size; N = estimated number of youths in population in thousands; $\overline{X}$ = mean; s = standard deviation; $s_{\overline{x}}$ = standard error of the mean.

Weight-Height of Youths Aged 13 Years (lb/in)

Sex and Height	n	N	$\overline{X}$	s	$s_{\overline{x}}$	Percentile						
						5th	10th	25th	50th	75th	90th	95th
MALE			IN POUNDS									
Under 51.18 in	—	—	—	—	—	—	—	—	—	—	—	—
51.18-53.15 in	2	5	*	*	*	*	*	*	*	*		
53.15-55.12 in	8	25	71.91	12.399	17.011	60.0	60.8	63.7	68.3	76.9	95.0	95.2
55.12-57.09 in	18	56	80.56	12.902	3.543	66.1	67.2	70.8	79.6	86.4	91.9	117.3
57.09-59.06 in	65	204	86.05	11.618	1.460	71.4	74.7	79.6	83.6	90.8	98.1	102.3
59.06-61.02 in	99	312	93.87	14.824	1.907	76.7	79.8	83.6	90.4	100.3	108.9	134.5
61.02-62.99 in	131	421	104.21	16.495	1.581	83.3	86.4	91.9	101.0	112.7	129.4	136.0
62.99-64.96 in	125	393	116.87	20.556	2.019	91.5	96.3	103.4	111.1	128.3	142.0	159.8
64.96-66.93 in	91	285	123.28	18.872	1.837	102.1	104.7	108.7	118.2	131.0	152.1	165.3
66.93-68.90 in	63	215	136.71	22.844	2.277	112.9	113.8	118.4	132.5	147.7	167.6	187.4
68.90-70.87 in	19	68	149.72	26.643	7.557	124.1	127.6	132.5	139.6	155.0	194.7	196.2
70.87-72.83 in	5	15	*	*	*	*	*	*	*	*	*	*
72.83-74.80 in	—	—	—	—	—	—	—	—	—	—	—	—
74.80-76.77 in	—	—	—	—	—	—	—	—	—	—	—	—
76.77 in. and over	—	—	—	—	—	—	—	—	—	—	—	—
Female												
Under 51.18 in	—	—	—	—	—	—	—	—	—	—	—	—
51.18-53.15 in	1	3	*	*	*	*	*	*	*	*	*	*
53.15-55.12 in	—	—	—	—	—	—	—	—	—	—	—	—
55.12-57.09 in	15	51	81.86	16.131	4.980	58.6	60.6	67.2	80.9	88.4	98.1	123.7
57.09-59.06 in	47	165	93.10	15.168	1.958	76.5	78.5	84.2	89.3	97.4	118.2	127.0
59.06-61.02 in	98	329	97.71	15.496	1.735	78.7	80.5	86.4	94.6	104.3	118.4	127.6
61.02-62.99 in	152	499	109.68	19.306	1.541	86.2	88.0	96.6	106.7	118.6	134.5	145.3
62.99-64.96 in	156	515	117.20	18.517	1.151	90.8	96.8	105.2	115.1	125.7	140.7	151.0
64.96-66.93 in	86	284	128.24	20.117	2.031	101.9	104.5	115.1	128.1	135.6	152.8	168.0
66.93-68.90 in	24	87	128.11	29.121	5.165	101.9	103.8	106.7	116.6	144.0	151.2	213.4
68.90-70.87 in	3	10	*	*	*	*	*	*	*	*	*	*
70.87-72.83 in	—	—	—	—	—	—	—	—	—	—	—	—
72.83-74.80 in	—	—	—	—	—	—	—	—	—	—	—	—
74.80-76.77 in	—	—	—	—	—	—	—	—	—	—	—	—
76.77 in. and over	—	—	—	—	—	—	—	—	—	—	—	—

NOTE: n = sample size; N = estimated number of youths in population in thousands; $\overline{X}$ = mean; s = standard deviation; $s_{\overline{x}}$ = standard error of the mean.

Weight-Height of Youths Aged 14 Years (lb/in)

Sex and Height	n	N	$\overline{X}$	s	$s_{\overline{x}}$	Percentile						
						5th	10th	25th	50th	75th	90th	95th
MALE			IN POUNDS									
Under 51.18 in	—	—	—	—	—	—	—	—	—	—	—	—
51.18-53.15 in	—	—	—	—	—	—	—	—	—	—	—	—
53.15-55.12 in	2	7	*	*	*	*	*	*	*	*	*	*
55.12-57.09 in	3	13	*	*	*	*	*	*	*	*	*	*
57.09-59.06 in	11	42	89.31	4.032	1.420	81.4	85.1	87.3	89.5	92.6	93.7	94.1
59.06-61.02 in	45	135	96.19	13.838	2.606	79.8	81.6	86.0	91.3	106.8	114.0	121.9
61.02-62.99 in	83	261	104.54	17.245	1.922	83.1	85.3	92.2	101.6	112.9	127.9	138.2
62.99-64.96 in	96	299	115.26	14.958	1.288	93.7	97.0	104.7	114.9	124.1	135.6	143.5
64.96-66.93 in	134	432	128.02	20.759	2.324	105.2	108.7	113.8	122.1	137.4	155.6	166.9
66.93-68.90 in	144	435	137.50	25.388	2.414	109.6	112.4	121.3	131.0	145.0	165.2	185.2
68.90-70.87 in	71	228	144.49	21.394	2.879	112.2	121.5	129.0	142.6	154.1	174.1	190.3
70.87-72.83 in	25	81	159.70	28.691	5.066	131.4	132.3	143.5	153.0	170.9	183.0	207.9
72.83-74.80 in	3	9	*	*	*	*	*	*	*	*	*	*
74.80-76.77 in	1	3	*	*	*	*	*	*	*	*	*	*
76.77 in. and over	—	—	—	—	—	—	—	—	—	—	—	—
FEMALE												
Under 51.18 in	—	—	—	—	—	—	—	—	—	—	—	—
51.18-53.15 in	—	—	—	—	—	—	—	—	—	—	—	—
53.15-55.12 in	1	2	*	*	*	*	*	*	*	*	*	*
55.12-57.09 in	2	6	*	*	*	*	*	*	*	*	*	*
57.09-59.06 in	17	52	92.59	12.961	3.710	70.5	77.8	80.0	93.3	104.7	109.1	112.7
59.06-61.02 in	64	196	106.40	14.985	2.042	83.1	86.4	93.7	105.6	117.5	123.2	129.6
61.02-62.99 in	157	508	113.21	16.987	1.146	90.8	95.7	102.1	109.3	122.6	137.1	141.8
62.99-64.96 in	186	603	120.35	19.423	1.559	94.8	99.2	106.7	116.8	131.6	147.0	155.0
64.96-66.93 in	114	372	128.88	22.454	2.105	101.2	104.7	114.9	125.2	136.2	155.4	168.4
66.93-68.90 in	36	121	141.91	34.879	6.204	108.5	114.9	123.9	131.8	155.4	160.7	219.1
68.90-70.87 in	7	28	135.21	12.117	5.776	114.0	114.6	127.2	131.8	142.4	154.8	155.6
70.87-72.83 in	2	7	*	*	*	*	*	*	*	*	*	*
72.83-74.80 in	—	—	—	—	—	—	—	—	—	—	—	—
74.80-76.77 in	—	—	—	—	—	—	—	—	—	—	—	—
76.77 in. and over	—	—	—	—	—	—	—	—	—	—	—	—

NOTE: n = sample size; N = estimated number of youths in population in thousands; $\overline{X}$ = mean; s = standard deviation; $s_{\overline{x}}$ = standard error of the mean.

Weight-Height of Youths Aged 15 Years (lb/in)

Sex and Height	n	N	$\overline{X}$	s	$s_{\overline{x}}$	Percentile						
						5th	10th	25th	50th	75th	90th	95th
MALE						IN POUNDS						
Under 51.18 in	—	—	—	—	—	—	—	—	—	—	—	—
51.18-53.15 in	—	—	—	—	—	—	—	—	—	—	—	—
53.15-55.12 in	—	—	—	—	—	—	—	—	—	—	—	—
55.12-57.09 in	—	—	—	—	—	—	—	—	—	—	—	—
57.09-59.06 in	1	2	*	*	*	*	*	*	*	*	*	*
59.06-61.02 in	10	30	100.80	18.920	7.826	78.7	86.4	93.9	98.5	101.4	107.4	167.8
61.02-62.99 in	34	99	116.43	23.263	3.737	88.8	95.0	103.0	108.5	125.0	153.4	168.2
62.99-64.96 in	71	206	116.87	18.556	2.174	94.1	97.2	103.4	113.5	124.1	144.0	151.7
64.96-66.93 in	132	404	127.25	18.746	1.806	105.8	107.6	117.1	124.3	135.1	147.9	161.6
66.93-68.90 in	176	574	138.63	18.660	1.396	113.8	117.7	125.0	136.5	148.2	160.7	172.2
68.90-70.87 in	118	374	146.06	20.849	2.304	117.1	122.6	131.6	141.8	153.2	176.8	196.7
70.87-72.83 in	51	144	158.73	26.297	3.801	120.4	132.9	142.0	154.8	172.8	186.1	213.0
72.83-74.80 in	14	48	163.61	33.147	11.464	128.5	129.0	138.7	155.9	186.5	203.7	244.3
74.80-76.77 in	6	15	183.84	36.224	22.778	146.4	147.0	153.4	162.7	227.1	233.0	234.1
76.77 in. and over	—	—	—	—	—	—	—	—	—	—	—	—
FEMALE												
Under 51.18 in	—	—	—	—	—	—	—	—	—	—	—	—
51.18-53.15 in	—	—	—	—	—	—	—	—	—	—	—	—
53.15-55.12 in	—	—	—	—	—	—	—	—	—	—	—	—
55.12-57.09 in	2	5	*	*	*	*	*	*	*	*	*	*
57.09-59.06 in	15	51	105.62	17.361	7.987	79.4	86.9	92.8	100.1	116.2	122.8	146.2
59.06-61.02 in	69	242	109.55	19.610	2.624	86.2	89.5	97.7	106.0	116.4	133.4	150.6
61.02-62.99 in	111	400	113.58	18.680	2.059	91.3	95.9	102.1	121.0	121.5	131.8	143.7
62.99-64.96 in	137	509	125.73	23.872	1.929	99.4	104.3	110.7	121.3	132.7	158.1	171.3
64.96-66.93 in	109	398	133.84	22.833	2.322	104.7	108.7	121.5	128.8	144.8	163.4	178.6
66.93-68.90 in	49	188	143.90	23.656	4.145	109.6	118.2	126.1	134.9	157.9	188.1	190.5
68.90-70.87 in	7	23	139.55	19.559	10.598	109.6	110.0	118.6	137.6	156.1	158.5	174.6
70.87-72.83 in	3	26	*	*	*	*	*	*	*	*	*	*
72.83-74.80 in	1	3	*	*	*	*	*	*	*	*	*	*
74.80-76.77 in	—	—	—	—	—	—	—	—	—	—	—	—
76.77 in. and over	—	—	—	—	—	—	—	—	—	—	—	—

NOTE: n = sample size; N = estimated number of youths in population in thousands; $\overline{X}$ = mean; s = standard deviation; $s_{\overline{x}}$ = standard error of the mean.

Weight-Height of Youths Aged 16 Years (lb/in)

Sex and Height	n	N	$\overline{X}$	s	$s_{\overline{x}}$	Percentile						
						5th	10th	25th	50th	75th	90th	95th
MALE			IN POUNDS									
Under 51.18 in	—	—	—	—	—	—	—	—	—	—	—	—
51.18-53.15 in	—	—	—	—	—	—	—	—	—	—	—	—
53.15-55.12 in	—	—	—	—	—	—	—	—	—	—	—	—
55.12-57.09 in	—	—	—	—	—	—	—	—	—	—	—	—
57.09-59.06 in	1	1	*	*	*	*	*	*	*	*	*	*
59.06-61.02 in	4	12	*	*	*	*	*	*	*	*	*	*
61.02-62.99 in	11	33	109.99	16.145	7.875	92.6	93.0	98.5	103.2	119.9	131.8	148.2
62.99-64.96 in	32	108	117.04	14.240	2.807	97.4	99.0	106.3	113.3	127.9	134.3	145.7
64.96-66.93 in	87	275	130.93	20.234	2.163	106.9	109.8	116.2	127.9	140.9	152.8	167.3
66.93-68.90 in	166	552	138.14	16.658	1.387	113.8	118.6	126.8	135.8	147.9	161.2	172.0
68.90-70.87 in	149	511	148.44	19.881	1.887	124.1	128.3	134.5	144.2	159.8	176.6	184.7
70.87-72.83 in	72	227	159.57	27.525	4.394	128.5	130.7	142.0	151.9	168.7	198.9	213.6
72.83-74.80 in	29	95	178.71	31.456	7.198	140.4	146.8	153.7	172.8	199.1	213.8	245.6
74.80-76.77 in	3	10	*	*	*	*	*	*	*	*	*	*
76.77 in. and over	2	7	*	*	*	*	*	*	*	*	*	*
FEMALE												
Under 51.18 in	—	—	—	—	—	—	—	—	—	—	—	—
51.18-53.15 in	—	—	—	—	—	—	—	—	—	—	—	—
53.15-55.12 in	—	—	—	—	—	—	—	—	—	—	—	—
55.12-57.09 in	2	5	*	*	*	*	*	*	*	*	*	*
57.09-59.06 in	10	33	115.92	18.074	7.035	96.8	97.2	99.0	112.4	120.2	158.7	158.9
59.06-61.02 in	57	178	114.18	23.054	2.322	91.3	92.6	101.0	107.8	119.3	135.6	183.6
61.02-62.99 in	117	354	117.29	17.121	1.618	97.0	100.5	106.7	113.8	124.3	136.5	152.1
62.99-64.96 in	160	547	127.23	24.535	2.747	101.6	104.3	113.5	122.4	134.9	153.2	165.6
64.96-66.93 in	122	450	136.07	26.451	1.768	103.8	107.6	117.5	130.3	148.4	173.5	191.1
66.92-68.90 in	53	170	140.24	19.255	2.482	116.6	118.6	128.1	136.9	147.3	173.7	185.6
68.90-70.87 in	14	45	159.95	33.096	11.517	129.2	129.6	136.0	145.3	177.7	218.5	232.6
70.87-72.83 in	1	2	*	*	*	*	*	*	*	*	*	*
72.83-74.80 in	—	—	—	—	—	—	—	—	—	—	—	—
74.80-76.77 in	—	—	—	—	—	—	—	—	—	—	—	—
76.77 in. and over	—	—	—	—	—	—	—	—	—	—	—	—

NOTE: n = sample size; N = estimated number of youths in population in thousands; $\overline{X}$ = mean; s = standard deviation; $s_{\overline{x}}$ = standard error of the mean.

Weight-Height of Youths Aged 17 Years (lb/in)

Sex and Height	n	N	$\overline{X}$	s	$s_{\overline{x}}$	Percentile						
						5th	10th	25th	50th	75th	90th	95th
MALE			IN POUNDS									
Under 51.18 in	—	—	—	—	—	—	—	—	—	—	—	—
51.18-53.15 in	—	—	—	—	—	—	—	—	—	—	—	—
53.15-55.12 in	—	—	—	—	—	—	—	—	—	—	—	—
55.12-57.09 in	—	—	—	—	—	—	—	—	—	—	—	—
57.09-59.06 in	—	—	—	—	—	—	—	—	—	—	—	—
59.06-61.02 in	1	3	*	*	*	*	*	*	*	*	*	*
61.02-62.99 in	11	39	120.44	20.717	7.527	96.6	102.3	106.3	109.6	127.4	154.1	161.4
62.99-64.96 in	25	81	127.32	14.337	2.987	109.6	112.7	115.7	125.4	135.8	154.5	156.1
64.96-66.93 in	63	248	137.94	18.395	2.699	110.7	117.3	124.3	135.6	147.5	160.3	170.4
66.93-68.90 in	115	396	147.84	24.610	1.552	117.5	122.4	131.2	142.4	158.5	178.4	202.2
68.90-70.87 in	151	537	150.73	21.841	1.832	125.4	129.9	135.6	146.6	162.3	175.0	194.9
70.87-72.83 in	80	297	161.62	27.456	2.943	131.4	134.5	143.5	157.0	172.8	202.4	226.4
72.83-74.80 in	36	133	167.62	20.219	2.868	137.6	146.2	155.4	166.0	178.1	199.1	204.8
74.80-76.77 in	7	25	179.46	24.218	16.729	138.7	138.7	149.5	192.5	199.1	199.7	199.7
76.77 in and over	—	—	—	—	—	—	—	—	—	—	—	—
FEMALE												
Under 51.18 in	—	—	—	—	—	—	—	—	—	—	—	—
51.18-53.15 in	—	—	—	—	—	—	—	—	—	—	—	—
53.15-55.12 in	—	—	—	—	—	—	—	—	—	—	—	—
55.12-57.09 in	2	5	*	*	*	*	*	*	*	*	*	*
57.09-59.06 in	8	26	95.88	8.684	3.536	85.1	85.5	88.4	99.4	100.8	112.7	112.9
59.06-61.02 in	43	151	110.14	14.348	1.823	91.7	93.3	98.3	107.8	117.9	130.5	141.3
61.02-62.99 in	103	385	120.61	21.832	1.709	97.9	100.3	107.4	117.3	127.2	135.8	168.0
62.99-64.96 in	133	506	127.41	23.413	2.266	103.2	105.8	110.7	122.1	127.2	159.4	181.4
64.96-66.93 in	116	433	133.67	22.304	2.606	105.6	110.9	121.5	130.7	143.5	153.0	157.9
66.93-68.90 in	51	186	137.08	20.133	3.102	111.6	116.6	122.4	132.7	144.8	167.8	182.3
68.90-70.87 in	12	47	144.98	18.530	4.914	121.0	125.0	132.5	136.0	165.8	167.3	183.0
70.87-72.83 in	1	2	*	*	*	*	*	*	*	*	*	*
72.83-74.80 in	—	—	—	—	—	—	—	—	—	—	—	—
74.80-76.77 in	—	—	—	—	—	—	—	—	—	—	—	—
76.77 in. and over	—	—	—	—	—	—	—	—	—	—	—	—

NOTE: n = sample size; N = estimated number of youths in population in thousands; $\overline{X}$ = mean; s = standard deviation; $s_{\overline{x}}$ = standard error of the mean.

Appendix F

Food Guide: Exchange Lists for Meal Planning (1986 Revision)

The *exchange system of dietary control,* developed by two professional organizations—the American Dietetic Association and the American Diabetes Association—is based on a simple grouping of common foods according to generally equivalent nutritional values. This system may be used for any situation requiring caloric and food value control.

The foods are divided into six basic groups (with subgroups), called the "exchange lists." Each food item within a group or subgroup contains about the same food value as other food items in that group, allowing for exchange within groups, thus providing for variety in food choices as well as food value control. Hence the term *food exchanges* is sometimes used to refer to food choices or servings. The total number of "exchanges" per day depends on individual nutritional needs, based on normal nutrition standards. Although there is some variation in the composition of foods within the exchange groups, for simplicity the following values for carbohydrate, protein, fat, and kilocalories are used.

Exchange Lists

Food Groups	Carbohydrate (g)	Protein (g)	Fat (g)	Kilocalories
Starch/Bread	15	3	trace	80
Meat				
lean	—	7	3	55
medium-fat	—	7	5	75
high-fat	—	7	8	100
Vegetable	5	2	—	25
Fruit	15	—	—	60
Milk				
skim	12	8	trace	90
low-fat	12	8	5	120
whole	12	8	8	150
Fat	—	—	5	45

List 1: Starch/Bread List

Whole grain foods have about 2 g fiber/serving. Foods containing 3 g fiber/serving or more are marked with the symbol *.

Food	Serving
Cereals/Grains/Pasta	
*Bran cereals, concentrated	⅓ cup
*Bran cereals, flaked (such as Bran Buds, All Bran)	½ cup
Bulgur (cooked)	½ cup
Cooked cereals	½ cup
Cornmeal (dry)	2½ tbsp
Grapenuts	3 tbsp.
Grits (cooked)	½ cup
Other ready-to-eat unsweetened cereals	¾ cup
Pasta (cooked)	½ cup
Puffed cereal	1½ cup
Rice, white or brown (cooked)	⅓ cup
Shredded Wheat	½ cup
*Wheat germ	3 tbsp
Dried Beans/Peas/Lentils	
*Beans and peas (cooked; such as kidney, white, split, black-eyed)	⅓ cup
*Lentils (cooked)	⅓ cup
*Baked beans	¼ cup
Starchy Vegetables	
*Corn	½ cup
*Corn on cob, 6 in. long	1
*Lima beans	½ cup
*Peas, green (fresh, frozen, or canned)	½ cup
*Plantain	½ cup
Potato, baked	1 small (3 oz)
Potato, mashed	½ cup
Squash, winter (acorn, butternut)	¾ cup
Yam, sweet potato, plain	⅓ cup
Bread	
Bagel	½ (1 oz)
Bread sticks, crisp (4 in long × ½ in)	2 (⅔ oz)
Croutons, low fat	1 cup
English muffin	½
Frankfurter bun or hamburger bun	½ (1 oz)
Pita (6 in. across)	½
Plain roll, small	1 (1 oz)
Raisin, unfrosted	1 slice (1 oz)
*Rye, pumpernickel	1 slice (1 oz)
Tortilla, 6 in. across	1
White (including French, Italian)	1 slice (1 oz)
Whole wheat	1 slice (1 oz)
Crackers/Snacks	
Animal crackers	8
Graham crackers (2½ in square)	3
Matzoth	¾ oz

Melba toast	5 slices
Oyster crackers	24
Popcorn (popped, no fat added)	3 cups
Pretzels	¾ oz
Rye crisp (2 in × 3½ in)	4
Saltine-type crackers	6
Whole wheat crackers, no fat added (crisp breads, such as Finn, Kavli, Wasa)	2-4 slices (¾ oz)

Starch Foods Prepared with Fat
(Count as 1 starch/bread serving + 1 fat.)

Biscuit (2½ in across)	1
Chow mein noodles	½ cup
Corn bread (2 in cube)	1 (2 oz)
Cracker, round butter type	6
French fried potatoes (2 in to 3½ in long)	10 (1½ oz)
Muffin, plain, small	1
Pancake (4 in across)	2
Stuffing, bread (prepared)	¼ cup
Taco shell (6 in across)	2
Waffle (4½ in square)	1
Whole wheat crackers, fat added (such as Triscuits)	4-6 (1 oz)

List 2: Meat and Meat Substitutes List

To reduce fat intake, choose items mainly from the lean and medium-fat groups, using more fish and poultry (remove skin) as meat choices, and trimming fat from all meats. Items having 400 mg sodium or more/exchange are marked with the symbol **. None of the items on this list contributes fiber to the diet. One exchange is equal to the amount listed for each item. In the case of meat, for example, a serving may be 2-3 exchanges (2-3 oz).

Lean Meat and Substitutes

Beef	USDA Good or Choice grades of lean beef, such as round, sirloin, and flank steak; tenderloin; and chipped beef**	1 oz
Pork	Lean pork, such as fresh ham; canned, cured, or boiled ham**; Canadian bacon**, tenderloin	1 oz
Veal	All cuts except for veal cutlets (ground or cubed)	1 oz
Poultry	Chicken, turkey, Cornish hen (without skin)	1 oz
Fish	All fresh and frozen fish	1 oz
	Crab, lobster, scallops, shrimp, clams (fresh or canned in water**)	2 oz
	Oysters	6 medium
	Tuna** (canned in water)	¼ cup
	Herring (uncreamed or smoked)	1 oz
	Sardines (canned)	2 medium
Wild Game	Venison, rabbit, squirrel	1 oz
	Pheasant, duck, goose (without skin)	1 oz
Cheese	Any cottage cheese	¼ cup
	Grated parmesan	2 tbsp
	Diet cheeses** (less than 55 kcal/oz)	1 oz

Other	95% fat-free luncheon meat	1 oz slice
	Egg whites	3 whites
	Egg substitutes (less than 55 kcal/¼ cup)	¼ cup
Medium-Fat Meat and Substitutes		
Beef	Ground beef, roast (rib, chuck, rump), steak (cubed, Porterhouse, T-bone), and meatloaf (Most beef products are in this category.)	1 oz
Pork	Chops, loin roast, Boston butt, cutlets (Most pork products fall into this category.)	1 oz
Lamb	Chops, leg, and roast (Most lamb products fall into this category)	1 oz
Veal	Cutlet (ground or cubes, unbreaded)	1 oz
Poultry	Chicken (with skin), domestic duck or goose (well-drained of fat), ground turkey	1 oz
Fish	Tuna** (canned in oil and drained)	¼ cup
	Salmon** (canned)	¼ cup
Cheese	Skim or part-skim cheeses, such as:	
	Ricotta	¼ cup
	Mozzarella	1 oz
	Diet cheeses** (56-80 kcal/oz)	1 oz
Other	86% fat-free luncheon meat**	1 oz
	Egg (high in cholesterol, limit to 3/week)	1
	Egg substitutes (56-80 kcal per ¼ cup)	¼ cup
	Tofu (2½ in × 2¾ in × 1 in)	4 oz
	Liver, heart, kidney, sweetbreads (high in cholesterol, limit use)	1 oz
High-Fat Meat and Substitutes (These items are high in saturated fat, cholesterol, and kilocalories; limit to 3 times/week.)		
Beef	USDA Prime cuts, ribs; corned beef**	1 oz
Pork	Spareribs, ground pork, pork sausage**	1 oz
Lamb	Ground lamb patties	1 oz
Fish	Any fried fish product	1 oz
Cheese	Regular cheeses**, such as American, Blue, Swiss	1 oz
Other	Luncheon meat**, such as bologna, salami, pimento loaf	1 oz slice
	Sausage**, such as Polish, Italian	1 oz
	Knockwurst, smoked	1 oz
	Bratwurst**	1 oz
	Frankfurter** (turkey or chicken)	1 frank (10/lb)
	Frankfurter** (beef, pork, or combination) (count as 1 high-fat meat + 1 fat)	1 frank (10/lb)
	Peanut butter	1 tbsp

List 3: Vegetable List

Unless otherwise noted, one vegetable exchange is 1 cup raw vegetable or ½ cup cooked vegetable or vegetable juice. Vegetables containing 400 mg sodium or more/serving are marked with the symbol **. Fresh and frozen vegetables have less added salt. Canned vegetables contain more salt, but rinsing will help remove much of it. In general, vegetables contain 2-3 g dietary fiber/serving. Starchy vegetables are found in the Starch/Bread List. Other free vegetables are in the Free Food List.

Artichoke (½ medium)
Asparagus
Beans (green, wax, Italian)
Bean sprouts
Beets
Broccoli
Brussels sprouts
Cabbage
Carrots
Cauliflower
Eggplant
Greens (collard, mustard, turnip)
Kohlrabi
Leeks
Mushrooms, cooked
Okra
Onions
Pea pods
Peppers (green)
Rutabaga
Sauerkraut**
Spinach
Summer squash (crookneck)
Tomato (1 large)
Tomato/vegetable juice
Turnips
Water chestnuts
Zucchini

List 4: Fruit List

Fruits containing 3 g dietary fiber or more/serving are marked with the symbol *. Portions are usual serving sizes of commonly eaten fruits.

Fresh, Unsweetened Frozen, and Unsweetened Canned Fruit

Apple (raw, 2 in across)	1 apple
Applesauce (unsweetened)	½ cup
Apricots (medium, raw)	4 apricots
Apricots (canned)	½ cup or 4 halves
Banana (9 in long)	½ banana
*Blackberries (raw)	¾ cup
*Blueberries (raw)	¾ cup
Canteloupe (5 in across)	⅓ melon
Canteloupe (cubes)	1 cup
Cherries (large, raw)	12 cherries
Cherries (canned)	½ cup
Figs (raw, 2 in across)	2 figs
Fruit cocktail (canned)	½ cup
Grapefruit (medium)	½ grapefruit
Grapefruit (segments)	¾ cup
Grapes (small)	15 grapes
Honeydew melon (medium)	⅛ melon
Honeydew melon (cubes)	1 cup
Kiwi fruit (large)	1 kiwi fruit
Mandarin oranges (segments)	¾ cup
Mango (small)	½ mango
*Nectarine (1½ in across)	1 nectarine
Orange (2½ in across)	1 orange
Papaya (small cubes or balls)	1 cup
Peach (2¾ in across)	1 peach
Peach (slices)	¾ cup
Peaches (canned)	½ cup or 2 halves

Pear	½ large pear or 1 small
Pears (canned)	½ cup or 2 halves
Persimmon (medium, native)	2 persimmons
Pineapple (raw, cubes)	¾ cup
Plum (raw, 2 in across)	2 plums
*Pomegranate	½ pomegranate
*Raspberries (raw)	1 cup
*Strawberries (raw, whole)	1¼ cups
Tangerine (2½ in across)	2 tangerines
Watermelon (cubes or balls)	1¼ cup
Dried Fruit	
*Apples	4 rings
*Apricots	7 halves
Dates	2½ medium
*Figs	1½
*Prunes	3 medium
Raisins	2 tbsp
Fruit Juice	
Apple juice or cider	½ cup
Cranberry juice cocktail	⅓ cup
Grapefruit juice	⅓ cup
Grape juice	⅓ cup
Orange juice	½ cup
Pineapple juice	½ cup
Prune juice	⅓ cup

List 5: Milk List

Milk may be used alone or in combination with other foods. See the Combination Foods List.

Skim and Very Lowfat Milk	
Skim or nonfat milk	1 cup
½% milk	1 cup
1% milk	1 cup
Lowfat buttermilk	1 cup
Evaporated skim milk	½ cup
Dry nonfat milk	⅓ cup
Plain nonfat yogurt	8 oz
Lowfat Milk	
2% milk	1 cup
Plain lowfat yogurt (with added nonfat milk solids)	8 oz
Whole Milk (more than 3¼% butterfat; limit use)	
Whole milk	1 cup
Evaporated whole milk	½ cup
Whole plain yogurt	8 oz

List 6: Fat List

Measure carefully; use mainly unsaturated fats. Sodium content varies widely, so check labels.

Unsaturated Fats	
Avocado	⅛ medium
Margarine	1 tsp
Margarine, diet	1 tbsp
Mayonnaise	1 tsp
Mayonnaise, reduced kcalories	1 tbsp
Nuts and seeds:	
Almonds, dry roasted	6 whole
Cashews, dry roasted	1 tbsp
Pecans	2 whole
Peanuts	20 small or 10 large
Walnuts	2 whole
Other nuts	1 tbsp
Seeds, pine nuts, sunflower (shelled)	1 tbsp
Pumpkin seeds	1 tsp
Oil (corn, cottonseed, safflower, soybean, sunflower, olive, peanut)	1 tsp
Olives	10 small or 5 large
Salad dressing, mayonnaise type	2 tsp
Salad dressing, mayonnaise type, low kcal	1 tbsp
Salad dressing (all varieties)	1 tbsp
*Salad dressing, low kcal	2 tbsp
(2 tbsp low-caloric salad dressing is a free food)	

Saturated Fats	
Butter	1 tsp
Bacon	1 slice
Chitterlings	½ oz
Coconut, shredded	2 tbsp
Coffee whitener, liquid	2 tbsp
Coffee whitener, powder	4 tsp
Cream (light, coffee, table)	2 tbsp
Cream, sour	2 tbsp
Cream (heavy, whipping)	1 tbsp
Cream cheese	1 tbsp
Salt pork	¼ oz

Free Foods

Any food or drink containing less than 20 kcal/serving is "free." If a serving size is given, 2-3 servings/day are sufficient. Higher fiber* and sodium** foods are indicated. Use *nonstick pan spray* for cooking as desired.

Drink
- Bouillon** or broth, fat-free
- Bouillon, low sodium
- Carbonated drinks, sugar-free

Fruits

Cranberries, unsweetened	½ cup
Rhubarb, unsweetened	½ cup

Vegetables

Carbonated water	
Club soda	
Cocoa powder, unsweetened	1 tbsp.
Coffee/Tea	
Drink mixes, sugar-free	
Tonic water, sugar-free	
Condiments	
Catsup	1 tbsp
Horseradish	
Mustard	
Pickles**, dill, unsweetened	
Salad dressing, low kcal	2 tbsp
Taco sauce	1 tbsp
Vinegar	
Seasonings	
Basil (fresh)	
Celery seeds	
Cinnamon	
Chili powder	
Chives	
Curry	
Dill	
Flavoring extracts (vanilla, almond, walnut, butter)	
Garlic, fresh and powder	
Herbs, spices	
Hot pepper sauce and flakes	
Lemon, juice and zest (outer skin)	
Lemon pepper	
Lime, juice and zest	
Mint, fresh leaves	
Onion powder	
Oregano	
Paprika	
Parsley	
Pepper	
Pimento	
Soy sauce**	
Soy sauce, low sodium—"lite"	
Wine, used in cooking	¼ cup
Worcestershire sauce	

Cabbage	
Celery	
Chinese cabbage*	
Cucumber	
Green onion	
Hot peppers	
Mushrooms	
Radishes	
Zucchini*	
Salad Greens	
Endive	
Escarole	
Lettuce	
Romaine	
Spinach	
Sweet Substitutes	
Candy, hard, sugar-free	
Gelatin dessert, sugar free	
Gum, sugar-free	
Jam/Jelly, sugar-free	2 tsp
Pancake syrup, sugar-free	1-2 tbsp
Sugar substitutes (saccharin, aspartame)	
Whipped topping	2 tbsp

Combination Foods

Check the *American Dietetic Association/American Diabetes Association Family Cookbooks* and the *American Diabetes Association Holiday Cookbook* for many recipes and much information, including combination foods.

Food	*Amount*	*Exchanges*
Casseroles, homemade	1 cup (8 oz)	2 starch, 2 medium-fat meat, 1 fat
Cheese pizza**, thin crust	¼ of 10 in	2 starch, 1 medium-fat meat, 1 fat
Chili beans* **	1 cup (8 oz)	2 starch, 2 medium-fat meat, 2 fat
Chow mein* ** (without noodles or rice)	2 cups	1 starch, 2 vegetables, 2 lean meat
Macaroni and cheese**	1 cup	2 starch, 1 medium-fat meat, 2 fat
Spaghetti and meatballs (canned)	1 cup	2 starch, 1 medium-fat meat, 1 fat
Sugar-free pudding (made with skim milk)	½ cup	1 starch
Soup		
Bean* **	1 cup	1 starch, 1 vegetable, 1 lean meat
Chunky, all varieties**	10¾ oz can	1 starch, 1 vegetable, 1 medium-fat meat
Cream** (made with water)	1 cup	1 starch, 1 fat
Vegetable** or broth**	1 cup	1 starch
Beans used as a meat substitute		
Dried beans*, peas*, lentils* (cooked)	1 cup	2 starch, 1 lean meat

Foods for Occasional Use

Food	*Amount*	*Exchanges*
Angel food cake	1/12 cake	2 starch
Plain cake, no icing	1/12 cake or 3 in square	2 starch, 2 fat
Cookies	2 small (¾ in across)	1 starch, 1 fat
Frozen fruit yogurt	⅓ cup	1 starch
Gingersnaps	3	1 starch
Granola	¼ cup	1 starch, 1 fat
Granola bars	1 small	1 starch, 1 fat
Ice cream, any flavor	½ cup	1 starch, 2 fat
Ice milk, any flavor	½ cup	1 starch, 1 fat
Sherbet, any flavor	¼ cup	1 starch
Snack chips**, all varieties	1 oz	1 starch, 2 fat
Vanilla wafers	6 small	1 starch, 1 fat

Glossary

Abruptio placentae (L. *abruptio,* a sudden breaking off; *plakoeis,* a flat cake) Premature separation of a normally situated placenta.

Achlorhydria (L. *a-,* negative; *chlorhydria,* hydrochloric acid) Absence or reduced amounts of hydrochloric acid in the gastric secretions.

Adipocyte (L. *adipis,* fat; *kytos,* hollow vessel, anything that contains or covers) A fat cell.

Alveoli (L. *alveolus,* hollow structure) Collections of glandular cells; milk-producing cells in the mammary glands.

Alzheimer's disease A type of senile dementia (Alois Alzheimer, German neurologist, 1864–1915); progressive irreversible degenerative changes in the brain resulting in loss of neuromuscular function and mental capability.

Amenorrhea (L. *a-,* negative; Gr. *men,* month; *rhoia,* flow) Abnormal absence or suppression of menstruation.

Amniotic fluid (Gr. *amnion,* bowl, membrane enveloping the fetus) The albuminous fluid in the amniotic sac in which the fetus floats during gestation.

Anemia (Gr. *an-,* negative prefix; *haima,* blood) Blood condition marked by decrease in number of circulating red blood cells, hemoglobin, or both.

Anorexia nervosa (Gr. *anorektos,* without appetite; *neuron,* nerve) An eating disorder, psychophysiologic condition characterized by distorted body image and severe and prolonged inability or refusal to eat, usually seen in girls and young women; a form of self-starvation sometimes accompanied by induced vomiting and resulting in extreme emaciation.

Anthropometry (Gr. *anthropos,* man; *metron,* measure) Science dealing with the measurement of the human body in size, weight, and proportions.

Antibodies Specific protein substances circulating in the blood designed to interact with and destroy their specific disease agents—*antigens.*

Antidiuretic hormone (ADH) Secreted by the posterior pituitary gland in response to body stress; acts on the distal tubules of the kidney's nephrons to cause water reabsorption and thus protect vital body water. It is also called *vasopressin.*

Antigens (*antibody* + Gr. *gennan,* to produce) Any disease agents, such as toxins, bacteria, viruses, or other foreign substances, that stimulate the production of specific *antibodies* to combat them.

Antioxidant (Gr. *anti-,* against; *oxys,* keen) A substance that inhibits oxidation of unsaturated fatty acids and formation of free radicals in the cell.

Apgar score A method of estimating an infant's condition at birth by scoring the heart rate, respiration effort, muscle tone, reflex irritability, and color. Developed by Virginia Apgar (1909–1974), American anesthesiologist.

Areola (L. *aerola,* area, space) The circular pigmented area around the nipple of the breast.

Atherosclerosis (Gr. *athere,* gruel; *sklerosis,* hardness) Condition in which yellowish fatty plaques *(athromas)* form within the medium and large arteries, eventually filling in the vessel at that point and blocking blood circulation.

Autonomy (Gr. *auto-,* self; *nomos,* law) State of being independent; self-governing.

Balance (L. *balanx,* balance) The harmonious adjustment of parts or performance of functions; a dynamic equilibrium maintained in the human body by numerous interrelated mechanisms.

Basal metabolism (Gr. *basis,* base; *metabole,* change) The amount of energy needed by the body for maintenance of life when the person is at digestive, physical, and emotional rest. Measured in terms of oxygen consumption, this basal metabolic rate (BMR) is reported as the percent of variation in the person above or below the normal number of kilocalories required for a person of like height, weight, and gender.

Biologic age The relative age of an individual based on physiologic capacity and measurements.

Blastocyst (Gr. *blastos,* germ; *kystis,* bladder) The stage in the development of the embryo in which cells are arranged in a single layer to form a hollow sphere.

Body image The thoughts, feelings, and perceptions a person has of his or her physical being.

Bulimia (L. *bous,* ox; *limos,* hunger) A form of abnormal eating behavior characterized by consumption of huge amounts of food to point of discomfort then induced vomiting to get rid of it; underlying psychophysiologic fear of fatness.

Cachexia (Gr. *kakos,* bad; *hexis,* habit) A specific profound effect caused by a disturbance in glucose metabolism usually seen in patients with advanced cancer; general poor health and malnutrition usually indicated by an emaciated appearance.

Calcitonin (L. *calx,* lime, calcium; *tonus,* tension, balance) A polypeptide hormone secreted by the thyroid gland in response to hypercalcemia, which lowers both calcium and phosphate in the plasma.

Candida (L. *candidus,* glowing white) A genus of fungi causing a variety of common infections; part of the normal flora of the skin and internal epithelial linings of the mouth, intestinal tract, and vagina.

Cardiac output Total amount of blood pumped by the heart per minute.

Carnitine A naturally occurring amino acid required for the metabolism of fatty acids.

Cathartic (Gr. *katharsis,* a cleansing) A drug that hastens and increases the emptying of the bowels; called also a *purgative.*

Cerebral hemorrhage Rupture of an artery in the brain; stroke.

Cholesterol (Gr. *chole,* bile; *steros,* solid) A fat-related compound, a sterol, found only in animal tissue; a normal constituent of bile and a principal constituent of gallstones. In the body, cholesterol is synthesized mainly by the liver. In the diet, it occurs only in foods of animal sources. In human body metabolism, cholesterol is important as a precursor of various steroid hormones such as sex hormones and adrenal cordicoids, as well as vitamin D hormone. However, in disorders of lipid metabolism, it is a major factor in *atherosclerosis,* the underlying pathology of heart disease.

Chronic (Gr. *chronos,* time) Of long duration.

Chronologic age Age of an individual based on the number of years lived.

Cineradiography (Br. *cinema,* motion pictures; L. *radius,* ray; Gr. *graphein,* to write) Process of making a motion picture record of the successive images appearing on a fluoroscopic screen.

Cognitive (L. *cognito,* to know) Related to the process of knowing and learning; mental processes of thinking and remembering.

Cohort (L. *cohors,* farmyard, armed force from a particular place) A group of persons falling within a specified age range.

Colostrum (L. *colostrum,* bee-stings) A thin, white, opalescent fluid, the first milk secreted at the termination of a pregnancy; foremilk. It contains more lactalbumin and lactoprotein than milk secreted later, as well as various immunoglobulins representing the antibodies found in maternal blood.

Compartment Physiologic term used in the collective sense to designate the total body amount of a substance actually occurring in different body tissues.

Congregate meals (L. *congregare,* to flock together) Group meals for older people served in a social setting and usually funded by Title III-C of the Older Americans Act.

Constipation (L. *constipatio,* a crowding together) Infrequent and difficult passage of dry stool.

Cyclamate An artificial sweetener popular in the 1960s but banned for use in the United States in 1969. Current efforts are being made to regain its use.

Dependency ratio The number of individuals age 65 and over divided by the number of individuals of working age (age 18 to 64).

Developmental Related to the process of changing from a less mature to a more mature state.

Dyspepsia (Gr. *dys-,* painful; *peptein,* to digest) Indigestion; upset stomach.

Dysphagia (Gr. *dys-* + *phagein,* to eat) Difficulty in swallowing.

Edentulous (L. *e-,* without; *dens,* tooth) Absence of natural teeth.

Endometrial lining (Gr. *endon,* within; *metra,* uterus) Inner mucous membrane of the uterine wall; is sloughed or shed each month if a pregnancy does not occur.

Enmeshment To be so entangled that escape is difficult.

Erythrocyte (Gr. *erythros,* red; *kytos,* hollow vessel) Mature red blood cell.

Erythropoiesis (Gr. *erythro-* + *poiesis,* making) The formation of red blood cells.

Essential hypertension High blood pressure of unknown cause; usually related to a strong family history of hypertension and beginning during the rapid growth period of adolescence or in young adulthood.

Etiology (Gr. *aitia,* cause + *-ology,* study) Theory or study of the causes of a disease or disorder.

Food guide A model for planning and evaluating a daily diet.

Frontal bossing (L. *frontalis,* forehead; M.E. *boce,* lump, growth) A condition in which the front portion of the skull protrudes.

Functional disability Disability that interferes with activities of daily living, such as bathing, dressing, shopping, preparing meals, eating.

Galactosemia A rare genetic disease in newborns; an inborn error in the metabolism of galactose, causing it to accumulate in unusually large amounts in the blood. Untreated it causes mental and physical retardation, galactose and amino acids in the urine, enlargement of liver and spleen, osteoporosis, and cataracts. Mandatory screening laws now identify these infants at birth; special galactose-free diet allows them to grow and develop normally.

Gastrectomy Surgical removal of all or part of the stomach.

Gastrocnemius muscle (Gr. *gastrokneme,* calf of the leg) The large muscle of the calf; it plantar flexes the foot (lifts the foot when standing on toes) and flexes the knee joint.

Genitalia (L. *genitalis,* belonging to a birth) The reproductive organs; especially the external sex organs.

Geriatrics (Gr. *geras,* old age) The medical specialty concerned with chronic disease and physical health in older adults.

Gerontology The study of aging including biologic, physiologic, psychologic, and sociologic aspects.

Gestation (L. *gestare,* to bear) The development of the new individual within the uterus from conception to birth.

Gingivitis (L. *gingiva,* gum of the mouth) Inflammation of the gums.

Glomerular filtration rate A measure of the amount of blood filtered by the kidneys' nephrons per unit of time (ml/min).

Guiac test A test for occult (unseen) blood in the stool.

HANES The Health and Nutrition Examination Survey conducted periodically to evaluate the nutritional status of the United States population.

Health maintenance organization (HMO) A prepaid health plan in which members receive all necessary medical and health services.

Home health agency A community organization providing nursing and personal care services and/or homemaking services to homebound aged persons under the supervision of a physician.

Homeostasis (Gr. *homoios,* like, unchanging; *stasis,* standing, steady) State of relative dynamic equilibrium within the body's internal environment; a biochemical and physiologic balance achieved through the constant operation of numerous interrelated homeostatic mechanisms.

Human chorionic gonadotropin A placental hormone, released in large amounts during early pregnancy, responsible for stimulating the corpus luteum in the maternal ovary. This stimulus promotes the continued production of estrogen and progesterone by the corpus luteum.

Human chorionic somatomammotropin A hormone secreted by the placenta during pregnancy; stimulates protein metabolism and alters carbohydrate metabolism by diminishing insulin action and increasing mobilization of free fatty acids from maternal peripheral fat depots; has a lactogenic effect on mammary glands.

Human chorionic thyrotropin A placental hormone that stimulates the maternal thyroid gland to increase its production of thyroid hormones.

Human placental lactogen See Human chorionic somatomammotropin.

Hydrocephalus (Gr. *hydro-,* water; *kephale,* head) A condition characterized by enlargement of the cranium caused by abnormal accumulation of fluid.

Hydroxyapatite Compound forming the main constituent of bones and teeth.

Hygroscopic (Gr. *hygros,* moist) Taking up and retaining moisture readily.

Hyperkinetic (Gr. *hyper-,* above; *kinesis,* motion) Abnormally increased motor function or activity.

Hyperlipoproteinemias A group of conditions in which serum lipids and lipoproteins are abnormally high; often associated with increased risk of cardiovascular disease.

Hypochromic (Gr. *hypo-,* under; *chroma,* color) Form of anemia characterized by low hemoglobin concentration in red blood cells.

Hypogeusia (Gr. *hypo-,* under; *geusis,* taste) Abnormally diminished acuteness of the sense of taste.

Hyponatremia Abnormally low levels of sodium in the blood.

Hypophysectomy (Gr. *hypo-,* under; *phyein,* to grow; *ektome,* excision) Surgical removal of the *hypophysis*—the pituitary gland.

Hypoplasia (Gr. *hypo-,* under; *plasis,* formation) Incomplete development of an organ or tissue.

Hypothalamus A region of the brain between the thalamus and the midbrain that functions as the main control center for the autonomic, or sympathetic, nervous system.

Ideal weight Optimal body weight for an individual of a given height, sex, or age.

Ketones Intermediate products of fat metabolism; acids such as acetone.

Ketoacidosis Abnormally high concentration of ketone bodies in the body tissues and fluids; a form of metabolic acidosis with markedly increased production of ketoacids; breath may have a fruity or acetone odor. Is also a complication of diabetes mellitus and starvation.

Ketonuria Appearance of ketone bodies in the urine.

Ketosis General synonymous term for ketoacidosis.

Kilocalorie (Fr. *chilioi,* thousand; L. *calor,* heat) The general term *calorie* refers to a unit of heat measure and is used alone to designate the *small calorie.* The calorie used in nutritional science and the study of metabolism is the *large calorie,* 1000 calories, or kilocalorie, to be more accurate and avoid the use of very large numbers in calculations.

Lacteals (L. *lacteus,* milky) A collection of lymphatic vessels in the mesentery conveying fatty chyle from the intestine.

La Leche League A long-standing breastfeeding support organization.

Lanugo (L. *lana,* wool) Soft downy hair growth covering the fetus and newborn.

Life expectancy The average remaining lifetime in years for a person of a given age.

Long-term care Medical, personal, or homemaking services provided within an institution or in the community for older adults who are no longer able to care for their own needs.

Lymphocytes (L. *lympha,* water; *kytos,* hollow vessel, anything that contains or covers) Special white blood cells that function as components of the body's immune system.

Lyophilization (Gr. *lyein,* to dissolve; *philein,* to love) Process for making stable biologic preparations such as blood plasma and serum by rapid freezing followed by drying under a vacuum.

Macrophages (Gr. *macro-,* large; *phagein,* to eat) Large reticuloendothelial cells that are components of the body's immune system; mononuclear phagocytes that interact with B and T lymphocytes to facilitate production of antibodies; found in various tissues and organs of the body, such as the spleen, lymph nodes, liver, lungs, bone marrow, brain, and spinal cord.

Mastitis (Gr. *mastos,* breast) Inflammation of the breast.

Maternal mortality The number of women who die of conditions related to pregnancy during the gestational period, labor and birth, and 90 days following birth in a given year over the number of infants born alive in that same year. Usually expressed as number of deaths per 100,000 live births.

Mean Mathematical term for the average numerical value of a group of numbers.

Mean corpuscular hemoglobin concentration Index to express the hemoglobin content of red blood cells. Expressed as hemoglobin grams per 100 dl red blood cells.

Meconium (Gr. *mekonion*) The first intestinal discharges of the newborn infant, greenish and consisting of epithelial cells, mucus, and bile.

Median (L. *medianus,* middle) The middle value in a distribution of numbers with half of the values falling above and half falling below.

Megaloblast (Gr. *megalo-,* great size; *blaston,* germ, immature cell) An abnormally large immature red blood cell, formed in *megaloblastic anemia* in relation to a deficiency of folic acid.

Menarche (Gr. *men,* month; *arche,* beginning) Initiation of the menstrual cycle.

Micelle (L. *micella,* small body) A microscopic colloid particle of fat and bile formed in the small intestine for initial stage of fat absorption.

Microcytic (Gr. *micro-,* small; *kystis,* sac, bladder) Small sized body; abnormally small red blood cells.

Microphthalmia (Gr. *micro-* small; *ophthalmos,* eye) The condition of abnormally small eyes.

Mortality ratio Total number of deaths in a specific category divided by the total number of deaths.

Morula (L. *morus,* mulberry) The initial ball of 12 to 16 cells created by the division of the fertilized ovum (egg cell).

Multigravida (L. *multus,* many, much; *gravida,* pregnancy) A woman with the condition of pregnancy for the second time or more; *primigravida* is a woman who is pregnant for the first time.

Neonatal mortality The number of infant deaths during the first 28 days of life per 1000 live births.

Nullipara (L. *nullus,* none; *parere,* to bring forth, produce) A woman who has never borne a viable child; written *para 0.*

Nutrient density The nutrient concentration of protein, vitamin, or mineral content of a food expressed in relation to its energy (kilocalories) content.

Nutrition (L. *nutritio,* nourishment) The sum of the processes involved in obtaining and taking in nutrients, assimilating and using them to maintain body tissues and provide energy; a foundation for life and health.

Nutrition education The process of helping individuals obtain the knowledge, skills, and motivation needed to make appropriate food choices for positive health throughout life.

Nutritional science The body of science, developed through controlled research, that relates to the processes involved in nutrition—physiologic, biochemical, and clinical, as well as psychologic, sociologic, cultural, economic, agricultural, technologic, environmental, and political.

Oligosaccharides (Gr. *oligo-,* few, little; L. *saccharide,* sugar) A carbohydrate compound composed of a small number (about 4 to 10) of simple sugar units; usually produced in intermediary stages of polysaccharide hydrolysis.

Osmolality (Gr. *osmos,* impulsion through a membrane) Property of a solution that depends on the concentration of the particles (solutes) in solution per unit of solvent base.

Osteomalacia (Gr. *osteon,* bone; *malakaia,* softness) Condition characterized by softening of the bones because of impaired mineralization, with symptoms of pain, tenderness, muscular weakness, and loss of appetite.

Osteoporosis (Gr. *osteo-* + *poros,* passageway) Abnormal loss of bone mineral, seen more in elderly persons, producing more porous fragile bone tissue prone to fracture or deformity.

Ovulation (L. *ovum,* egg) Production and discharge of ova by the ovary.

Oxytocin (Gr. *tokos,* birth) Hormone from the posterior pituitary gland with pronounced uterine-contracting and milk-releasing action.

Palmar grasp (L. *palma,* palm of the hand) A crude grasp of objects by infants with the palm and fingers.

Parietal cells (L. *parietes,* wall) Cells lining the stomach that secrete hydrochloric acid.

Parity (L. *parere,* to bring forth, produce) Condition of a woman in reference to the number and frequency of live offspring she has borne.

Perception (L. *perceptio,* a gathering together) A conscious mental taking in of sensory stimuli; an impression developed by the mind.

Perinatal mortality (Gr. *peri-,* around, surrounding; L. *natus,* birth) Number of deaths of offspring during the late fetal period and first 28 days of life per 1000 live births.

Peyer's patches Aggregates of lymphoid nodules in the submucosa of the lower small intestine (Johann Conrad Peyer, Swiss anatomist, 1653–1712).

Phagocytes (Gr. *phagein,* to eat; *kytos,* hollow vessel) Cells that defend the body by ingesting microorganisms, foreign particles, or other cells.

Pharmacologic Pertaining to drugs and drug dosages; use of a substance as a drug, in greater amounts than regular usage, e.g., megadoses of vitamins.

Phenylketonuria (PKU) Genetic disease, now screened at birth; results from inability to metabolize the essential amino acid phenylalanine because of a deficiency of phenylalanine hydroxylase, the cell enzyme controlling the conversion of phenylalanine to tyrosine. Immediate treatment with a low-phenylalanine diet allows affected infants and children to grow normally. Untreated they are subject to brain damage and severe mental retardation.

Pincer grasp (M.E. *pinceour,* to pinch) Maturing ability of young children pick up very small objects with a discrete grasp between the thumb and first or index finger.

Pinocytosis (Gr. *pinein,* to drink; *kytos,* cell) The uptake of fluid material by a living cell; engulfing of nutrient solutions by cells as a means of absorption; "cell drinking."

Poverty line The minimum income, as determined by the federal government, required to provide basic necessities of food, clothing, and shelter; the level of income or below that qualifies persons and families to receive aid from government-funded programs.

Preeclampsia (L. *prae,* before; *eklampsis,* sudden development) Complicating condition of pregnancy, characterized by hypertension, proteinuria, and edema, developing during the latter half of gestation, sometimes leading to the stage of convulsions (eclampsia); also called *pregnancy-induced hypertension (PIH).*

Preferred physician organization (PPO) A health care plan in which members contract for medical and health services to be provided at a set fee from designated physicians, usually in a group medical practice.

Primigravida (L. *primus,* first; *gravida,* heavy, loaded) The condition of pregnancy for the first time.

Proctocolitis (Gr. *proktos,* anus; *kolon,* colon) Inflammation of both colon and rectum.

Prolactin A hormone from the anterior lobe of the pituitary gland that stimulates the synthesis and secretion of milk.

Prostaglandins A group of substances (named for their initial identification in semen) with many effects in mammalian organisms, including strong contraction of smooth muscle and dilation of certain vascular beds.

Psychosocial The psychologic and social aspects of human growth and development compared with the physical and physiologic aspects of life.

Psychosomatic reflex (Gr. *psycho-,* mind; *soma,* body) An automatic reaction dictated by influences of the mind or higher functions of the brain, such as emotions, fears, and desires.

Pubescence (L. *pubertas,* puberty) Reaching and having reached the state of puberty, the period of developing secondary sex characteristics and physical capacity for sexual reproduction.

Residual volume Amount of air remaining in the lungs after the individual has exhaled.

Rooting reflex The reflex action, fully developed at birth, which causes the newborn, when touched on the cheek or lips, to turn the head toward the stimulus and seek to contact it with the mouth. Designed to assist initial attempts of the infant to find the nipple and secure breast milk.

Salicylate Any salt of salicylic acid; component of drugs such as aspirin.

Secular (L. *saeculum,* long period of time) Activities developing over a period of time; going on from age to age; occurring as a function of time.

Self-esteem Respect for and belief in oneself.

Spontaneous abortion Expulsion of the fetus before it is viable.

Stillbirth Birth of a dead child.

Tachycardia (Gr. *tachys,* swift; *kardia,* heart) Rapid heart beat.

Teratogenesis (Gr. *teratos,* monster; *genesis,* production) The process by which an agent or disease state causes congenital malformations or other serious deviations from normal fetal development.

Title III-C The statute of the Older Americans Act authorizing congregate and home-delivered meals and social services for people age 60 and over.

Transaminases Enzymes that catalyze the transfer of an amino group from one molecule to another.

Trophoblast (Gr. *trophe,* nutrition; *blastos,* germ) Extraembryonic ectodermal tissue on the surface of the cleaving fertilized ovum, which is responsible for contact with maternal circulation and supply of nutrients to the embryo.

Viscera (L. *viscus,* large body organ) Large internal organs of the body located in the chest and abdomen.

Vital capacity Volume of air moved in and out of the lungs with each breath.

Index

C

I

N

O

R

Metropolitan Life Insurance Company Height-Weight Data, Revised 1983

Women					Men				
Height		Frame*			Height		Frame*		
Ft	In	Small	Medium	Large	Ft	In	Small	Medium	Large
4	10	102-111	109-121	118-131	5	2	128-134	131-141	138-150
4	11	103-113	111-123	120-134	5	3	130-136	133-143	140-153
5	0	104-115	113-126	122-137	5	4	132-138	135-145	142-156
5	1	106-118	115-129	125-140	5	5	134-140	137-148	144-160
5	2	108-121	118-132	128-143	5	6	136-142	139-151	146-164
5	3	111-124	121-135	131-147	5	7	138-145	142-154	149-168
5	4	114-127	124-138	134-151	5	8	140-148	145-157	152-172
5	5	117-130	127-141	137-155	5	9	142-151	148-160	155-176
5	6	120-133	130-144	140-159	5	10	144-154	151-163	148-180
5	7	123-136	133-147	143-163	5	11	146-157	154-166	161-184
5	8	126-139	136-150	146-167	6	0	149-160	157-170	164-188
5	9	129-142	139-153	149-170	6	1	152-164	160-174	168-192
5	10	132-145	142-156	152-173	6	2	155-168	164-178	172-197
5	11	135-148	145-159	155-176	6	3	158-172	167-182	176-202
6	0	138-151	148-162	158-179	6	4	162-176	171-187	181-207

Based on a weight-height mortality study conducted by the Society of Actuaries and the Association of Life Insurance Medical Directors of America, Metropolitan Life Insurance Company, revised 1983.

*Weights at ages 25 to 59 based on lowest mortality. Height includes 1-in heel. Weight for women includes 3 lb for indoor clothing. Weight for men includes 5 lb for indoor clothing. (See p. 479 for controversy surrounding the use and abuse of these tables over the years.)